Breast Cancer and Gynecologic Cancer Rehabilitation

Breast Cancer and Gynecologic Cancer Rehabilitation

EDITED BY

ADRIAN CRISTIAN MD MHCM FAAPMR

Chief, Cancer Rehabilitation, Miami Cancer Institute, Miami, FL, United States
Professor, Florida International University, Herbert Wertheim College of Medicine, Miami, FL, United States

ELSEVIER

Elsevier
Radarweg 29, PO Box 211, 1000 AE Amsterdam, Netherlands
The Boulevard, Langford Lane, Kidlington, Oxford OX5 1GB, United Kingdom
50 Hampshire Street, 5th Floor, Cambridge, MA 02139, United States

Notices

Knowledge and best practice in this field are constantly changing. As new research and experience broaden our understanding, changes in research methods, professional practices, or medical treatment may become necessary.

Practitioners and researchers must always rely on their own experience and knowledge in evaluating and using any information, methods, compounds, or experiments described herein. In using such information or methods they should be mindful of their own safety and the safety of others, including parties for whom they have a professional responsibility.

To the fullest extent of the law, neither the Publisher nor the authors, contributors, or editors, assume any liability for any injury and/or damage to persons or property as a matter of products liability, negligence or otherwise, or from any use or operation of any methods, products, instructions, or ideas contained in the material herein.

British Library Cataloguing-in-Publication Data
A catalogue record for this book is available from the British Library

Library of Congress Cataloging-in-Publication Data
A catalog record for this book is available from the Library of Congress

ISBN: 978-0-323-72166-0

Publisher: Cathleen Sether
Acquisitions Editor: Humayra Rahman
Editorial Project Manager: Megan Ashdown
Production Project Manager: Kiruthika Govindaraju
Cover Designer: Alan Studholme

Typeset by MPS Limited, Chennai, India

To Eliane, my wife and best friend, for her unwavering love, support, encouragement, and belief that we have the power to make the world a better place,

To my children, Alec and Chloe for their love, support, and boundless optimism,

To my colleagues at the Miami Cancer Institute for their dedication to the compassionate care of our patients,

To my patients, for the privilege of allowing me to be part of their life and for teaching me about strength, resilience, and dignity in the face of adversity.

Contents

List of Contributors

Meryl J. Alappattu, PT, PhD

Department of Physical Therapy, University of Florida, Gainesville, FL, United States

Angel Amadeo, BS

Bachelor of Science (BS), University of Central Florida, Orlando, FL, United States

Carla Araya, MPH, RDN, LDN

Clinical Nutrition Specialist, Miami Cancer Institute, Miami, FL, United States

Mirza Baig, BS

Herbert Wertheim College of Medicine at Florida International University, Miami, FL, United States

Betty Chernack, MD

Department of Physical Medicine and Rehabilitation, University of Pennsylvania, Philadelphia, PA, United States

Adrian Cristian, MD, MHCM

Cancer Rehabilitation, Miami Cancer Institute, Miami, FL, United States; Professor, Department of Translational Medicine Herbert Wertheim School of Medicine, Florida International University, Miami, FL, United States

Mary Crosswell, PT DPT CLT

Supervisor of Rehabilitation Services, South Miami Hospital, Baptist Health South Florida, Miami, FL, United States

M. Beatriz Currier, MD

Miami Cancer Institute, Cancer Patient Support Center at Baptist Health South Florida, Miami, FL, United States

Christian M. Custodio, MD

Memorial Sloan Kettering Cancer Center, New York, NY, United States; Weill Cornell Medicine, New York, NY, United States

John P. Diaz, MD, FACOG

Director of Minimally Invasive Gynecologic Surgery, Lead Physician Research Gynecologic Oncology, Division of Gynecologic Oncology, Miami Cancer Institute, Baptist Health South Florida, Miami, FL, United States

Claudia Ferri, MS, RD, CSO, LDN

Baptist Health South Florida, Miami Cancer Institute, Miami, FL, United States

Kristen M. Galamaga, LMT

Miami Cancer Institute, Miami, FL, United States

Allie Garcia-Serra, MD

Radiation Oncologist, Innovative Cancer Institute, Miami, FL, United States

Monica Gibilisco, DO

NYIT College of Osteopathic Medicine

Louise V. Gleason, MSPT, PRPC

Pelvic Health & Continence Testing Department, Center for Women and Infants: South Miami Hospital, Miami, FL, United States

Alexandra I. Gundersen, MD

Harvard Medical School, Boston, MA, United States; Department of Physical Medicine and Rehabilitation, Spaulding Rehabilitation Hospital, Boston, MA, United States

Richard A. Hamilton, PhD

Miami Cancer Institute, Cancer Patient Support Center at Baptist Health South Florida, Miami, FL, United States

Shana E. Harrington, PT, PhD

Physical Therapy Program, University of South Carolina, Columbia, SC, United States

Sherry Hite, MOT, OTR/L

Department of Rehabilitation, City of Hope National Medical Center, Duarte, CA, United States

Ashish Khanna, MD

Cancer Rehabilitation Medicine, The Kessler Institute for Rehabilitation, West Orange, NJ, United States; Department of Physical Medicine & Rehabilitation, Rutgers New Jersey Medical School, West Orange, NJ, United States

Vinita Khanna, LCSW, MPH, ACHP-SW, OSW-C

Department of Clinical Social Work, USC Norris Comprehensive Cancer Center, Los Angeles, CA, United States

Mariana Khawand-Azoulai, MD

Medicine/Palliative Care; University of Miami/Jackson Hospice and Palliative Medicine; Medical Director - Palliative Medicine Services Uhealth

Lynn Kim, OTD, OTR/L

Department of Rehabilitation, City of Hope National Medical Center, Duarte, CA, United States

Sasha E. Knowlton, MD

Assistant Director of Cancer Rehabilitation, Instructor in Physical Medicine and Rehabilitation, Harvard Medical School, Boston, MA, United States

Franchesca König, MD

Memorial Sloan Kettering Cancer Center, New York, NY, United States; Weill Cornell Medicine, New York, NY, United States

Nicholas C. Lambrou, MD

Miami Cancer Institute, Miami, FL, United States; Baptist Health South Florida, South Miami, FL, United States

Susan Maltser, DO

Donald and Barbara Zucker School of Medicine at Hofstra/Northwell, Manhasset, NY, United States; Glen Cove Hospital, Glen Cove, NY, United States

Miguel A. Medina, III, MD

Plastic and Reconstructive Surgery; Director of Microsurgery Miami Cancer Institute at Baptist Health South Florida, Miami, FL, United States

Suleyki Medina, MD

Palliative Medicine Physician, Symptom Management and Palliative Medicine, Miami Cancer Institute, Baptist Health South Florida, Miami, FL, United States

Elina Melik-Levine, ARNP

Miami Cancer Institute, Baptist Health South Florida, Miami, FL, United States

Jane Mendez, MD

Chief Breast Surgery, Miami Cancer Institute, Baptist Health South Florida, FL, United States

Charles Mitchell, DO

Department of Physical Medicine and Rehabilitation, Atrium Health Carolinas Rehabilitation, Charlotte, NC, United States; Department of Supportive Care Oncology, Levine Cancer Institute, Charlotte, NC, United States; Atrium Health, Charlotte, NC, United States

Diana Molinares, MD

Cancer Rehabilitation Medicine Director for Sylvester Cancer Center, Department of Physical Medicine and Rehabilitationm, University of Miami-Miller School of Medicine, Miami, FL, United States

Aileen M. Moreno, LCSW

Miami Cancer Institute, Cancer Patient Support Center at Baptist Health South Florida, Miami, FL, United States

Karla Otero, MS, RDN, LDN, CSO, CDE

Supervisor of Clinical Nutrition Cancer Patient Support Center, Miami Cancer Institute, Miami, FL, United States

Theresa Pazionis, MD, MA, FRCSC

Assistant Professor, Orthopedic Surgery and Sports Medicine, Lewis Katz School of Medicine at Temple University, Philadelphia, PA, United States

Austin J. Pourmoussa

Medical Student Herbert Wertheim School of Medicine Florida International University, Miami, FL, United States

Terrence MacArthur Pugh, MD

Department of Physical Medicine and Rehabilitation, Atrium Health Carolinas Rehabilitation, Charlotte,

NC, United States; Department of Supportive Care Oncology, Levine Cancer Institute, Charlotte, NC, United States; Atrium Health, Charlotte, NC, United States; University of North Carolina School of Medicine, Chapel Hill, NC, United States

Vishwa S. Raj, MD

Vice-Chair for Clinical Operations, Department of Physical Medicine and Rehabilitation, Atrium Health Carolinas Rehabilitation, Charlotte, NC, United States; Chief, Section of Rehabilitation, Department of Supportive Care Oncology, Levine Cancer Institute, Charlotte, NC, United States; Atrium Health, Charlotte, NC, United States; Medical Director, Director of Oncology Rehabilitation, Carolinas Rehabilitation, Charlotte, NC, United States

Julia M. Reilly, MD

Attending Physiatrist, Memorial Sloan-Kettering Cancer Center, New York, NY, United States

Angelique Ellerbee Richardson, MD, Phd

University of California in San Diego, CA, United States

Maria-Amelia Rodrigues, MD

Department of Radiation Oncology, Miami Cancer Institute, Baptist Health South Florida, Florida, FL, United States

Carly Rothman, DO

Donald and Barbara Zucker School of Medicine at Hofstra/Northwell, Manhasset, NY, United States

Harry M. Salinas, MD

Plastic and Reconstructive Surgery, Miami Cancer Institute, Baptist Health South Florida, Miami, FL, United States

Ana Cristina Sandoval Leon, MD

Medical Oncologist, Miami Cancer Institute, Miami, FL, United States

Jonas M. Sokolof, DO

Clinical Associate Professor of Rehabilitation Medicine NYU Grossman School of Medicine Director of Oncological Rehabilitation at NYU-Langone Health

Nicole L. Stout, DPT, CLT-LANA, FAPTA

West Virginia University Cancer Institute, Morgantown, WV, United States

Rachel Thomas

Medical Student Lewis Katz School of Medicine at Temple University, Philadelphia, PA, United States

Erin M. Wolfe, BS

Miller School of Medicine, University of Miami, Miami, FL, United States

Vanessa Yanez, MOT, OTR/L

Department of Rehabilitation, City of Hope National Medical Center, Duarte, CA, United States

Jasmine Zheng, MD

Department of Physical Medicine and Rehabilitation, University of Pennsylvania, Philadelphia, PA, United States

Preface

Advances in earlier detection and improved treatment options have led to increased survival rates for persons diagnosed with breast and gynecologic cancer. Yet, in spite of these increased survival rates, people often develop various physical and psychological impairments that have an adverse impact on their level of function in performing self-care as well as engaging in work, school, or avocational activities.

Rehabilitation medicine has a vital role in minimizing impairments and maximizing the quality of life. To be successful, it often requires a collaborative effort among physiatrists, medical, surgical, orthopedic and radiation oncologists, palliative care physicians, nutritionists, physical therapists, occupational therapists, psychologists, psychiatrists, social workers, massage therapists, and advanced care providers.

This book is meant to provide the reader with a multidisciplinary and holistic approach to the care of the person with breast cancer and/or gynecologic cancer. It is separated into two broad sections that provide content for each of these types of cancer. This includes cancer treatment using medical, surgical, and radiation therapy interventions followed by content on commonly seen impairments and their treatment.

I am extremely grateful to the authors for their important contribution to this book and help in making it a reality. My hope is that health-care providers reading it will have a better appreciation of the complexities involved in the care of people affected by these types of cancers and subsequently provide compassionate and effective care to them.

Adrian Cristian
Cancer Rehabilitation, Miami Cancer Institute, Miami, FL, United States

SECTION I

CHAPTER 1

Cascade of Disability in Breast and Gynecologic Cancer

ADRIAN CRISTIAN, MD, MHCM

INTRODUCTION

According to the American Cancer Society, as of January 1, 2019, there were 3,861,520 women living with breast cancer; 807,860 women living with uterine cancer; 283,120 women living with cervical cancer; and 249,320 women living with ovarian cancer. The 5-year survival rates are 91% for breast cancer, 65.8% for cervical cancer, 81.2% for uterine cancer, and 47.6% for ovarian cancer.[1–3] As women are surviving breast and gynecologic cancers longer, it is perhaps not surprising that the projection for people living with breast and gynecologic cancers is to see these numbers increase. The projection is that by 2030 there will be 4,957,960 living with breast cancer; 1,023,290 living with uterine cancer; 297,580 living with ovarian cancer; and 288,710 living with uterine cervix cancer. Women are also living substantially longer post diagnosis as well. For example, 19% of women are living 20+ years since diagnosed with breast cancer, 29% since diagnosed with ovarian cancer, 49% since diagnosed with cervical cancer, and 22% with uterine cancer. The number of women living with metastatic breast cancer is greater than 150,000. Women are also diagnosed with breast or gynecologic cancer more often later in life. For example, age at prevalence for women diagnosed with breast cancer in the 65–84 age-group was 51% for breast cancer, 47% for ovarian cancer, 39% for uterine cancer, and 56% for uterine corpus.

These statistics illustrate that there are a significant number of women diagnosed with breast and gynecologic cancers, often later in life and living longer post treatments for their cancer. The most common treatments for these types of cancers include a combination of surgery, radiation therapy, chemotherapy, and antihormonal therapy. Whereas these treatments can be very successful in treating the cancer, they can also have an adverse impact on healthy tissues such as muscle, nerve, and connective. The adverse impact on healthy tissues can at times be very close to the onset of the treatment; however, these adverse effects often develop slowly over time leading to a gradual loss of function that can be imperceptible to both the individual and the treatment team. Often the loss of function cannot be directly linked to any one treatment, but rather to a combined effect of several treatments as well the patient's own precancer state of health, nutritional status, and preexisting diseases such as diabetes mellitus.

Rehabilitation medicine should be an integral part of the care of the person with breast or gynecologic cancer from time of diagnosis, through active treatment and in the survivorship period. Following diagnosis and precancer treatment, physiatrists can assess the patient for any preexisting physical impairments of key body structures that would be subjected to the effects of multimodality cancer treatment. For the person with newly diagnosed breast cancer, this can include shoulder dysfunction, assessment of preexisting peripheral neuropathy, preexisting painful joint conditions affecting the hands, knees, and lower back, and lymphedema. For the person with newly diagnosed gynecologic cancer, this can include assessment of preexisting peripheral neuropathy, preexisting lymphedema of leg, impaired balance, decreased fine motor skills and strength in hands, and history of pelvic floor dysfunction. In addition, an assessment of nutritional status, preexisting cognitive impairment, depression, and anxiety is also very important.

Breast Cancer and Gynecologic Cancer Rehabilitation DOI: https://doi.org/10.1016/B978-0-323-72166-0.00001-3

Physiatrists can also provide useful and timely information to medical, surgical, and radiation oncologists with respect to potential impact of cancer treatment on loss of function, which can then in turn be useful in the planning of the cancer treatment. This is based on their knowledge of functional anatomy of the musculoskeletal and nervous systems as well as assessment of functional loss. This information would ideally be discussed at multidisciplinary tumor boards. Another role that physiatrists can have in the planning of cancer treatment is to assess the patient for frailty since frailty can have an adverse impact on a person's ability to tolerate cancer treatments.

Once these preexisting impairments are identified, a coordinated effort of various team members such as physical therapy, occupational therapy, psychology, and nutrition to minimize them is critical. At times, it is not realistic to address all of these impairments prior to start of treatment since the patient's focus as well as that of the cancer treatment team is on initiating treatment as soon as possible, therefore prioritization is key. For example, a patient with a preexisting reduction in range of motion of the shoulder would need this limitation to be addressed to help her undergo radiation therapy. Rehabilitative interventions can be continued during active cancer treatment; however, this depends on the patient's ability to tolerate both cancer treatment and rehabilitative interventions concurrently. Periodic surveillance for subjective and objective evidence of loss of physical function becomes important at times during active treatment as well as during survivorship.

ASSESSMENT OF BREAST AND GYNECOLOGIC CANCER PATIENT WITH A FOCUS ON PHYSICAL IMPAIRMENTS AND LOSS OF FUNCTION

The physiatrist should approach the assessment of the person with breast or gynecologic cancer by having a good working knowledge of the common physical, cognitive, and psychologic impairments affecting the breast and gynecologic cancer patients and utilizing appropriate clinical assessment tools.

A review of pertinent past medical history and past surgical history can help identify the areas of potential loss of function. For example, preexisting peripheral neuropathy from diabetes may worsen once the patient is treated with chemotherapy, thereby adversely affecting hand function and balance. Another example is a patient with a history of limited shoulder function due to adhesive capsulitis that could potentially lead to a worsening of the condition following treatment of breast cancer with surgery and radiation therapy.

Review of prior imaging studies such as PET/CT scans, bone scans, MRIs, and plain X-rays can help identify the areas with metastatic disease. Results of echocardiograms and pulmonary function studies, if available, can provide information about heart and lung function, respectively. That knowledge can then be used in setting precautions during rehabilitation to minimize the risk of harm for the patient. Review of laboratory studies such as hemoglobin, platelet, and white blood cell counts can yield important information that can be used in generating additional hematological precautions in the rehabilitation prescription. This information as well as review of liver and renal function tests and medications for pertinent drug–drug and drug–disease interactions can be very useful when prescribing medications for the treatment of painful conditions.

The review of systems can serve as a useful "checklist" of areas of potential concern with respect to loss of function post breast and gynecologic cancer treatment. Table 1.1 provides an example of such a checklist as well as possible treatment interventions. In addition to those listed, other areas of interest include symptoms pertaining to the cardiovascular, pulmonary, and nervous systems as well as changes in weight and appetite.

It is also important to assess the patient's level of function in their home, community, and work settings. Pertinent questions about the person's ability to perform self-care activities such as bathing and dressing and limitations or need for additional assistance are important. Household and community mobility, need for assistive devices for walking, ability to drive, shop for food, and managing finances can all yield important information about functional loss.

If the patient is working, it is important to inquire about the specific tasks involved in their work and any current limitations in their ability to perform their work. For example, a person with breast cancer who works as a hairdresser may have difficulty raising her arm overhead following breast cancer surgery, which can adversely affect her ability to perform her job. Another example is a person with gynecologic cancer that develops lymphedema of the lower extremity as well as peripheral neuropathy, both of which can make it difficult for her to maintain her balance and walk. This in turn can have an adverse effect on her job as a flight attendant for example. It is also important to ask the person about any

TABLE 1.1
Breast and Gynecologic Cancer Impairment Checklist

Impairment	Sample Interventions
Fatigue	Medication review Treat underlying anemia and hypothyroidism if present Treat depression if present Exercise program
General weakness	Exercise program
Obesity	Nutrition referral, exercise
Shoulder dysfunction	Physical therapy Nonsteroidal antiinflammatory drugs
Aromatase inhibitor musculoskeletal symptoms	Physical and occupational therapy Nutrition referral if obesity is present Nonsteroidal antiinflammatory drugs Injections
Lymphedema	Lymphedema therapy, compression sleeve, compression pump, patient education Nutrition referral if obese Arm-strengthening exercises
Peripheral neuropathy	Physical therapy Occupational therapy Medications—duloxetine, pregabalin, gabapentin Topical medications
Cognitive impairment	Neuropsychological evaluation Occupational and speech therapy
Psychosocial distress	Psychiatry, psychology, social work referral
Adverse impact of impairments on work	Physical and occupational therapy Driver training Ergonomic evaluation, functional capacity evaluation

problems with concentration, memory loss, or difficulty performing activities that require the use of executive functioning skills for either work, school, hobbies, or family life.

Lastly, inquiring about the patient's ability to function in their various life roles such as spouse or partner, daughter, and/or parent can yield useful information about additional functional limitations. For example, are there difficulties with child rearing due to shoulder or other joint pains or impaired balance associated with neuropathy? Another example, is there sexual dysfunction associated with treatment for gynecologic cancer that included surgery and radiation therapy?

Since exercise is an important part of the lives of many patients with breast and gynecologic cancers, it is useful to inquire about any limitations in the person's ability to engage in different forms of exercise due to their cancer and cancer treatment. For example, a person may be reluctant to participate due to joint pains or concerns about safely exercising if they have metastatic bone disease.

The physical examination of the breast and gynecologic cancer patients should include a thorough assessment of the nervous and musculoskeletal system that includes inspection, palpation, range of motion, as well as special diagnostic tests of interest. Inspection and palpation of surgical scars can yield useful information about structures that can be a source of pain.

Muscle strength testing of key muscle groups of the upper and lower extremities, testing of muscle stretch reflexes of the upper and lower extremities, as well as sensory testing of the extremities utilizing tests for light touch, pinprick, vibration, proprioception, cold testing, and monofilament testing to name a few can be useful. Assessment for the presence of lymphedema should include obtaining circumferential measurements of the arms or legs as necessary to either establish a baseline level for the patient prior to start of breast or gynecologic cancer treatment, respectively, as well as posttreatment.

Functional examination in the clinic setting can provide useful information about strength, fall risk, as well as presence of frailty. Sample tests include (1) Timed Up and Go Test, (2) sit-to-stand test, (3) balance test, and (4) grip strength. Self-reported outcome measures can also provide useful information about general physical function and fatigue.

CASCADE OF DISABILITY

Treatments for breast and gynecologic cancers can have significant adverse effects on the individual affected by these cancers. One way to think about this is through a *layering of impairments*. There are several layers of potential issues affecting the person with breast or gynecologic cancer: (1) aging-related changes; (2) presence of comorbid conditions such as diabetes, cardiac disease, and connective tissue disorders; (3) cancer characteristics such as tumor size and location, lymph node involvement, and presence of metastatic disease; and (4) cancer treatment–related injury to healthy tissues from surgery, chemotherapy, radiation therapy, antihormonal therapies (Figs. 1.1 and 1.2).

The combination of factors such as a preexisting sedentary lifestyle, obesity, preexisting peripheral neuropathy associated with diabetes mellitus and joint pains from degenerative changes in knees can each lead to physical impairments and a gradual loss of function. The diagnosis and treatment of breast or gynecologic cancer can lead to additional impairments that when superimposed on existing impairments can lead to a significant functional decline, or a *cascade of disability*.

	Layers	Examples
First	Age-related changes	Shoulder tendinopathy, muscle and peripheral nerve changes
Second	Coexisting medical conditions	Diabetes mellitus, cardiac disease,
Third	Preexisting conditions	Rotator cuff injury, adhesive capsulitis of shoulder, peripheral neuropathy, carpal tunnel syndrome, osteoarthritis of knees, hands, obesity
Fourth	Cancer characteristics	Tumor size, lymph node involvement, metastatic disease
Fifth	Cancer treatment-related toxicities	Shoulder dysfunction, lymphedema of upper extremity, aromatase inhibitor musculoskeletal syndrome, cognitive impairment, peripheral neuropathy

FIGURE 1.1 Layers of impairments—breast cancer.

	Layers	Examples
First	Age-related changes	Muscle and peripheral nerve changes
Second	Coexisting medical conditions	Diabetes mellitus
Third	Preexisting conditions	Peripheral neuropathy, osteoarthritis of knees, obesity
Fourth	Cancer characteristics	Tumor size, lymph node involvement, metastatic disease
Fifth	Cancer treatment-related toxicities	Peripheral neuropathy, lymphedema of lower extremity, pelvic floor dysfunction, cognitive impairment

FIGURE 1.2 Layers of impairments—gynecologic cancer.

One example of this cascade of disability could be seen in loss of arm function in breast cancer. Surgery and radiation therapy for breast cancer can lead to shoulder dysfunction and lymphedema of the ipsilateral arm thereby limiting the use of the affected arm for self-care activities such as bathing and dressing. The use of aromatase inhibitor can also contribute to shoulder and hand pain leading to further reduction in use of arm. Chemotherapy treatment with carboplatin or cisplatin can lead to neuropathic pain in the hands as well as decreased hand strength and sensation, further limiting the use of the hands. This in turn can impact on the person's ability to use their hands for work. Chemotherapy-related peripheral neuropathy can also cause pain and altered sensation in the feet. The altered or diminished sensation can adversely affect balance, which can in turn contribute to falls. Pain in the joints of the feet, knees, and hips due to side effects associated with the use of aromatase inhibitors can also make it difficult for the person to walk making them more sedentary, which can in turn contribute to increased weight gain. Pain in the legs, coupled with impaired sensation and weakness as well as decreased use of hands, can also affect the person's ability to drive. Fatigue can also contribute to loss of function. This can be secondary to chemotherapy, radiation therapy, anemia, impaired sleep from pain in shoulders and other joints, and pain medications, all of which can affect daytime function at work, school, and in various life roles mentioned earlier. Cognitive impairment, anxiety, and depression can all also lead to a loss of function as well (Fig. 1.3).

The fatigue, diminished mobility in home and community, impaired balance, and decreased use of ipsilateral arm and hands can all adversely affect the person's ability to work. If the person cannot work, there is the potential for a drop in income, loss of or significant reduction of health insurance benefits, and subsequent worsening of health. The person's ability to function as a parent, spouse, and care giver to family members and engage in hobbies can also be diminished.

Another example of the cascade of disability as it applies to the person with gynecologic cancer is in the combination of chemotherapy-induced peripheral neuropathy associated with lymphedema of the leg. This can contribute to impaired balance and an increased risk of falls, which can also affect ability to work in jobs or engage in life roles that require an intact balance. Hand use can also be affected as described previously for breast cancer patients. Fatigue, cognitive impairment, and psychosocial distress can also be present and adversely affect quality of life. In addition, gynecologic surgery and radiation therapy can adversely affect pelvic floor function potentially contributing to bowel, bladder, and sexual dysfunction—all of which can have a profound effect on the individual's quality of life (Fig. 1.4).

Any of the abovementioned cancer-related impairments can have an adverse effect on an individual's level of function. What is striking is that the breast and gynecologic cancer patients face many of them at the same time during and after cancer treatment is completed. The loss of function can be very dramatic such as the person who cannot lift their arm after

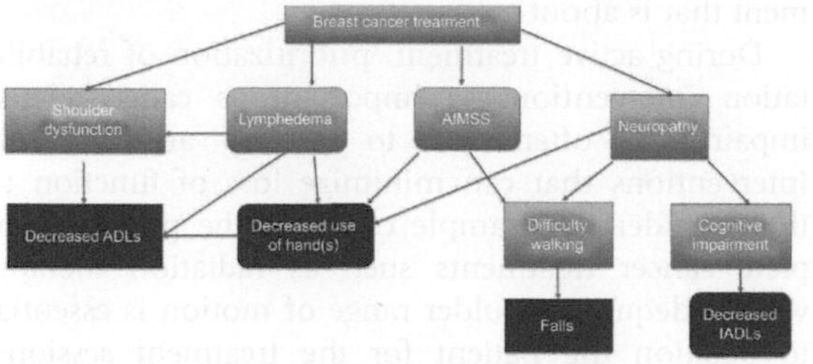

FIGURE 1.3 Cascade of disability in breast cancer. *ADLs*, Activities of daily living; *AIMSS*, aromatase inhibitor musculoskeletal syndrome; *IADLs*, instrumental activities of daily living. Each of the arrows also represents points where rehabilitative interventions can be used to either prevent impairment or minimize their functional impact on the individual if they should develop.

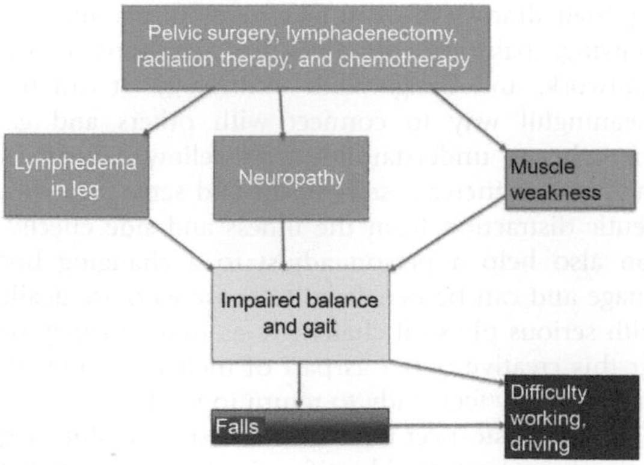

FIGURE 1.4 Cascade of disability in gynecologic cancer.

breast cancer surgery, or the development of lymphedema in the leg following gynecologic surgery and radiation therapy for gynecologic cancer; however, in many instances the loss of function is gradual so that the person needs to learn to compensate and accept a new normal that is less than their prior level of function.

RETURN TO WORK IN BREAST AND GYNECOLOGIC CANCERS

Work is an important part of life with substantial physical and mental health benefits. As mentioned before, persons with breast and gynecologic cancers face significant barriers in ability to return to work. In addition to physical impairments associated with the cancer and its treatment, there are the additional challenges associated with work interruption such as chemotherapy and radiation therapy treatment sessions, doctor visits, as well as treatment side effects (Fig. 1.5).

In the general cancer population, it has been reported that 63.5% of cancer survivors return to work and that mean duration of absence from work is 151 days. Around 26%–53% of cancer survivors lose their job or quit working over a 72-month period post diagnosis.[4] For survivors of breast cancer and cancer of female reproductive organs, unemployment rates are higher compared to healthy control participants.[5]

Noeres et al. reported on return to work following breast cancer in Germany. It was noted that 1 year after primary breast cancer surgery, patients were almost three times more likely to leave their job compared to a reference group. At 6 years the possibility of returning to work was only 50% that of a reference group. Factors associated with this included a lower level of education, part-time employment,

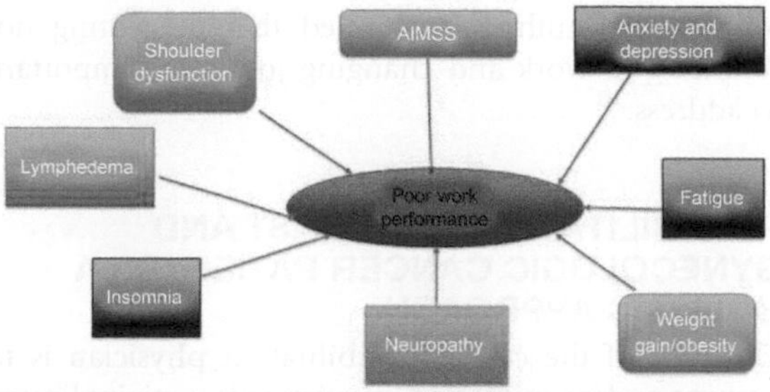

FIGURE 1.5 Factors adversely affecting work performance in persons with breast and gynecologic cancer. *AIMSS*, Aromatase inhibitor musculoskeletal syndrome.

work-related difficulties, age, tumor stage, and severity of side effects.[6] Schmidt et al. reported that 1 year following breast cancer surgery, 57% of survivors worked with the same working time and 22% worked with reduced working time compared to prediagnosis. Significant association with respect to return to work 1 year later included the presence of depressive symptoms, arm morbidity, cognitive impairment, lower education, younger age, and persistent fatigue. Cessation of work after breast cancer was associated with a worse quality of life.[7] A history of use of psychiatric medications prior to the diagnosis of breast cancer led to a small yet statistically significant reduction in return to work 1 year after breast cancer diagnosis. Factors such as high income and older age had a positive correlation with returning to work.[8]

Stergiou-Kita et al. reported that in assessing whether or not a cancer survivor can return to work, key areas that need to be focused on include (1) assessment of the person's functional abilities in relation to job demands, (2) identifying the cancer survivors individual strengths and barriers as they pertain to their work, and (3) identifying support systems in the workplace for the survivor. They concluded that clinicians should determine if the cancer survivor is "physically, cognitively, and emotionally" ready to return to work and if their workplace has the necessary support system in place to have them return to work.[9] For gynecologic cancer patients, less has been reported to date on return to work compared to breast cancer; however, in Japan, one study found that 71.3% of patients returned to work in the same workplace and 83.9% of persons who had worked prior to the gynecologic cancer diagnosis were able to return to work. Among those who could not return to work, 9.7% were self-employed, 5.9% were regularly employed, and 30.5% were nonregularly employed. Nonregular employment was the most common variable to have a negative effect on return to work and job change. Authors concluded that preventing not returning to work and changing jobs were important to address.[10]

REHABILITATION OF BREAST AND GYNECOLOGIC CANCER PATIENTS—A HOLISTIC APPROACH

The goal of the cancer rehabilitation physician is to prevent and/or minimize impairments, activity limitations and participation restrictions through a holistic multidisciplinary approach that focuses on what is truly important to the woman being cared for and never losing sight of the person behind the diagnosis. It is important to be open and receptive to learning her goals and the physical limitations that are preventing her from living her life to its fullest. This requires an understanding of the complex interactions described earlier and can serve as a foundation of a treatment plan that ideally prevents impairments from occurring in the first place or minimizes them once they occur.

The successful rehabilitation of the breast and gynecologic cancer patients should ideally start even before the beginning of cancer treatment. A prerehabilitation program emphasizing exercise, nutrition, smoking cessation as well as assessment and treatment of preexisting physical impairments such as shoulder dysfunction, joint pain, and psychosocial distress is paramount. The rehabilitation team should work on improving the breast and gynecologic cancer patients' physical and mental strength for the treatment that is about to start.

During active treatment, prioritization of rehabilitation interventions is important as cancer-related impairments often start to develop at this time. Interventions that can minimize loss of function to the shoulder for example can help the patient complete cancer treatments such as radiation therapy, where adequate shoulder range of motion is essential to position the patient for the treatment sessions. Psychosocial support, massage therapy, and acupuncture can be useful interventions as are judicious general conditioning exercises to maintain general strength and endurance.

Creative Art Therapies (art, music, and dance) can help patients explore and express difficult feelings and thoughts related to their diagnosis and experience as a cancer patient. Patients may appreciate the chance to create, reflect, and share their personal stories regarding their illness. This can take many forms, including drawing, painting, photography, sculpture, collage, craftwork, and design with technology. It can be a meaningful way to connect with others and gain strength and understanding from fellow patients. Art therapy can increase self-esteem and serve as a therapeutic distraction from the illness and side effects. It can also help a person adjust to a changing body image and can be beneficial to those who are dealing with serious physical challenges as well and may prefer this creative outlet as part of their treatment plan or when they feel ready to return to work.

In the postcancer treatment and survivorship stage, it is important to identify physical impairments, activity limitations, and participation restrictions and introduce interventions to minimize functional loss as early as possible. At this stage, there can be several disciplines called upon to assist the individual. Return to work issues can require the services of physical therapy, lymphedema therapist, occupational therapy, physiatrist, psychology, driver training, and even a pelvic floor therapist if there are bowel or bladder dysfunction issues.

CONCLUSION

By understanding the layers of impairments and how they contribute to a cascade of disability, the rehabilitation team can work to address them at several levels before, during, and after cancer treatment. A proactive approach employed by rehabilitation clinicians with timely and early interventions as the needs arise and surveillance for cancer-related impairments at regularly scheduled outpatient clinic visits are recommended. Integrating standardized functional outcome tools using both self-reported and objective testing can provide measurable benchmarks to assess the success of rehabilitative interventions.

REFERENCES

1. Surveillance, Epidemiology and End Results (SEER) program of the National Cancer Institute. <http://seer.cancer.gov/statfacts/html/cervix.html> Accessed 21820.
2. Surveillance, Epidemiology and End Results (SEER) program of the National Cancer Institute. <http://seer.cancer.gov/statfacts/html/corp.html> Accessed 21820.
3. Surveillance, Epidemiology and End Results (SEER) program of the National Cancer Institute. <http://seer.cancer.gov/statfacts/html/ovary.html> Accessed 21820.
4. Mehnert A. Employment and work related issues in cancer survivors. *Crit Rev Oncol Hematol*. 2011;77:109–130.
5. DeBoer AG, et al. Cancer survivors and unemployment: a meta-analysis and meta regression. *JAMA*. 2009;301:753–762.
6. Noeres D, Park-Simon TW, Grabow J, et al. Return to work after treatment for primary breast cancer over a six year period: results from a prospective study comparing patients with the general population. *Support Care Cancer*. 2013;(7)1901–1909.
7. Schmidt M, Scherer S, Wiskermann J, Steindorf K. Return to work after breast cancer: the role of treatment related side effects and potential impact on quality of life. *Eur J Cancer Care (Engl)*. 2019;28(4). N. PAG-N. PAG.
8. Jensen LS, Overgaard C, Game JP, Bogglid H, Fonager K. The impact of prior psychiatric medical treatment on return to work after a diagnosis of breast cancer: a registry based study. *Scand J Public Health*. 2019;47 (5):519–527.
9. Stergiou-Kita M, Pritlove C, Holness DL, et al. Am I ready to go back to work? Assisting cancer survivors to determine work readiness. *J Cancer Survivorship*. 2016;10 (4):699–710.
10. Nakamura K, Masuyama H, Nishida T, et al. Return to work after cancer treatment of gynecologic cancer in Japan. *BMC Cancer*. 2016;16:1–9.

CHAPTER 2

Practice Implementation, Clinical Assessment, and Outcomes Measurement

NICOLE L. STOUT, DPT, CLT-LANA, FAPTA • SHANA E. HARRINGTON, PT, PHD • MERYL J. ALAPPATTU, PT, PHD

INTRODUCTION

The cancer care continuum is a protracted time period with multiple medical treatments introduced at varying time points through that continuum. Each medical treatment brings with it the risk for different side effects that impact various body systems.[1] Implementing a model of care that optimally serves women during and after cancer treatment requires an understanding of the timing of onset of common impairments through the continuum of care and recognition of the measurement tools that are most appropriate for screening and assessment to identify impairment and ensure that evidence-based interventions are then introduced.[2] This chapter will present the framework of the prospective surveillance model (PSM) as a construct for rehabilitation of patients with breast and gynecological cancers and will review the evidence for screening and assessment measures most appropriate for these populations.

PROSPECTIVE SURVEILLANCE MODEL

Breast and gynecological cancer treatments–related impairments are prevalent and commonly incite functional morbidity. Due to the high risk of impairment throughout the continuum of cancer care, it is reasonable that a rehabilitation model of care should parallel medically directed treatment. The PSM encourages the implementation of rehabilitation services into the cancer care continuum from the point of diagnosis to encourage ongoing interval surveillance of function, identify impairment early, and introduce intervention to ameliorate functional decline.[3] Fig. 2.1 illustrates the PSM and its natural parallel with the cancer continuum.

Prior to the onset of cancer treatments, the PSM encourages the assessment of an individual's baseline level of function. Assessing comorbidities also provides insight on functional capabilities at baseline. For some populations a prehabilitation plan of care may be indicated.[4] Prehabilitation provides targeted interventions to prepare an individual for cancer treatments with the goal of optimizing physical function prior to the initiation of treatment.[5] The PSM then proceeds with follow-up assessments at intervals throughout the care continuum. The premise of the PSM is that repeated interval assessment will enable early identification of clinically meaningful changes in functional measures, compared to the baseline, that will promote early identification of emerging impairments and enables introduction of rehabilitation services proactively.[6,7]

Upon completion of cancer therapies, ongoing follow-up, screening, and monitoring for emerging late effects of treatment is warranted.[4] Late effects may present months or years following the completion of medical treatments and incite functional decline. The PSM is a highly regarded, evidence-based model that provides a clinical pathway for optimal integration of rehabilitation services into the cancer care continuum.[8] Use of proactive rehabilitation services, as enabled by the PSM, is considered to be an important component of high-quality cancer care.

Screening and Assessment Measures

Inherent in a surveillance model is the need for ongoing interval screening for treatment-related symptoms indicative of emerging impairment and assessment of various domains of physical function. These measures

Breast Cancer and Gynecologic Cancer Rehabilitation DOI: https://doi.org/10.1016/B978-0-323-72166-0.00002-5

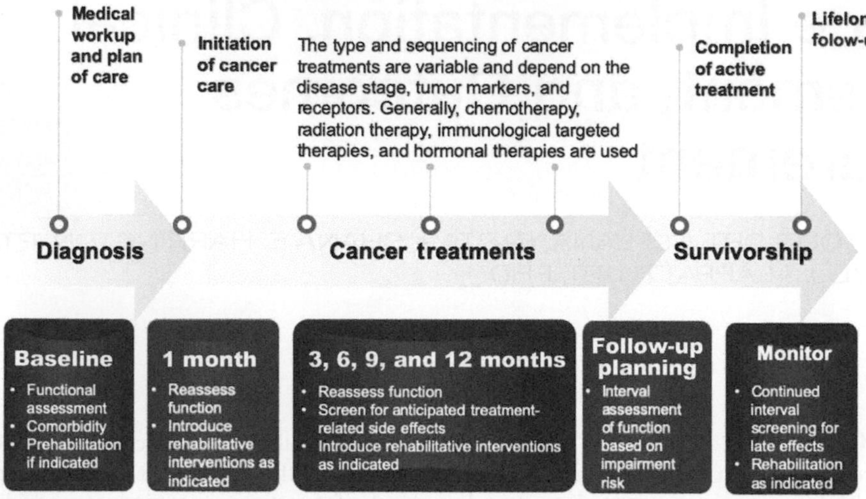

FIGURE 2.1 The prospective surveillance model for functional assessment throughout cancer treatment.

promote identification of clinically meaningful change and provide important insights to functional status. Screening tests are used when a high-risk population is identified, a variety of tests and measures exist that can identify important and meaningful changes that indicate a disease state or condition.[9] Screening typically is quick, unidimensional, easy to perform, and easy to interpret.[9] In contrast, assessments provide a richer understanding of impairments in order to drive rehabilitation strategies.[10] An assessment is conducted once symptoms consistent with impairment are identified and evaluates their severity and impact on function and quality of life. Assessments are multidimensional, and more comprehensive to identify not just that a problem exists but, more importantly, the extent to which it exists, and what the source of the problem may be.[9] Assessment findings are the basis for the rehabilitation plan of care. Assessment findings are also the baseline from which outcomes of intervention can be evaluated, providing insight on overall effectiveness of a rehabilitation plan of care.

The PSM uses screening and repeat assessment to drive the referral to rehabilitation services and to inform the plan of care. Whether screens or more detailed assessments are conducted depend on a variety of factors, including setting of cancer care delivery, timing of assessments, and access to specific providers as well as burden to the patient. Screening for cancer treatment–related impairments will commonly be symptom based and undertaken by oncology health-care professionals (i.e., nurse navigators) and ideally occur prior to and during active treatments.[10]

Implementing the PSM for breast and gynecological cancers may follow the basic framework as described previously; however, there are specific nuances to each of these populations that should be further contextualized to optimize rehabilitation interventions.

BREAST

Breast cancer treatment–related impairments occur based on the timing and type of cancer treatments. Most commonly, the upper quadrant is at risk for functional loss throughout the duration of cancer care and may result from surgical interventions and is often further exacerbated by radiation therapy. For the majority of individuals with breast cancer, surgery is the first intervention in the continuum of care. Breast surgery and lymph node removal may result in postoperative impairments affecting soft tissue and joint structure and function surrounding the surgical site.[11] These sequelae may lead to upper limb impairments, such as local postoperative pain and a subsequent decrease in range of motion.[12,13] In the postoperative subacute period, pain and impaired shoulder mobility may be due to adhesive capsulitis, myofascial dysfunctions, and/or nerve dysfunctions.[14]

In later phases of cancer treatments, radiation therapy introduces further upper quadrant impairment

TABLE 2.1
Breast Cancer Measures

Domain	Recommendations
Range of Motion[19]	Goniometry—passive range of motion At minimum: shoulder flexion and 90 degrees of external rotation
Volume[20]	Circumferential measures with volume calculation
Upper Extremity Strength[21]	Handheld dynamometry At minimum: shoulder horizontal adduction, internal and external rotators, and scaption
Upper Extremity Function[22]	*Patient-reported outcomes* DASH or University of PSS
Fatigue[23]	*Screening measures* Ten-point rating scale for fatigue *Patient-reported outcomes:* PROMIS Cancer Fatigue Short Form or PROMIS Cancer Fatigue
Functional Mobility[24]	*Clinical measures* 6MWT, TUG *Patient-reported outcomes:* AMPAC

6MWT, 6-Minute walk test; *AMPAC*, activity measure for post–acute care; *DASH*, disabilities of arm, shoulder, hand; *PSS*, Pennsylvania Shoulder Score; *TUG*, Timed Up and Go.

risk due to scar tissue formation, wound development, fibrosis, as well as shortening of soft tissues on the anterolateral chest wall, such as the pectoral muscles.[14] Shortened pectoral muscles, often exacerbated by forward shoulder position, may cause narrowing of the subacromial space leading to rotator cuff diseases that can be painful and may limit upper limb movements.[13] In addition, a history of previous shoulder pathology is a risk factor for developing shoulder and arm–shoulder morbidity.[15]

In addition to the upper quadrant impairments fatigue, chemotherapy-induced peripheral neuropathy (CIPN), joint arthralgia, cognitive dysfunction, anxiety, depression, and bone density loss are prevalent throughout the continuum of care due to chemotherapy, hormonal therapy, and radiation therapy. Evidence indicates that many women with breast cancer will experience ≥ 1 of these physical impairments and suffer from the cumulative burden of impairments, disease treatment, and comorbidities.[12,16] These impairments lead to difficulties in performing activities of daily living and negatively affect quality of life.[13] In addition, women often report being uninformed regarding the side effects related to their breast cancer treatment and are often surprised that they do not resolve after treatment.[17] Side effects of many of these treatments are amenable to rehabilitation interventions when identified *early* during treatment for breast cancer.[6,7,18]

Specific recommendations regarding impairments that should be assessed at baseline can be viewed in Table 2.1.

Along with conducting a baseline assessment, timing of future assessments depends on a variety of factors, including, but not limited to, stage of cancer; type of surgery, including reconstruction, chemotherapy, radiation, adjuvant hormone therapy such as aromatase inhibitor use; and a new onset of lymphedema.[15] The interval time points along the PSM trajectory enable providers to evaluate the impact of newly introduced antineoplastic therapies and assess for symptom impact on function.

PELVIC FLOOR

Patients with urogynecologic cancers experience higher rates of urinary and fecal incontinence as a result of their cancer treatment, and up to 50% report some level of incontinence prior to treatment,[25] with age and body mass index as identifiable risk factors for preexisting incontinence. Urinary incontinence, fecal incontinence, and painful intercourse are prevalent in women with cervical, uterine, vulvar, and ovarian cancers.[26] Pelvic pain and sexual dysfunction are also common sequelae of gynecological cancer treatments. Pelvic pain refers to pain in any structures of the pelvis, and when this pain persists, it can be associated with negative behavioral side effects. Sexual dysfunction represents a heterogeneous group of disorders characterized by a clinically significant disturbance in an individual's ability to respond sexually or to experience sexual pleasure. These disorders may include both arousal/interest disorders and/or sexual pain.[27]

The prevalence of sexual dysfunction in women with gynecologic cancers is estimated at up to 90%,[28,29] compared to 40% in the general population.[30] Sexual pain is associated with higher levels of depression and anxiety and lower levels of sexual enjoyment and satisfaction.[31] Additional impairments identified during and after treatment include increased vaginal dryness, decreased sexual desire and arousability, and dyspareunia associated with decreased vaginal diameter after surgical and radiation therapy.[32,33]

Collectively, the onset of these impairments negatively impacts functioning throughout the trajectory of cancer treatments, warranting a prospective approach to screening and assessment. Furthermore, the persistent nature of these issues requires ongoing long-term surveillance and management through rehabilitative interventions. In the preoperative period, pelvic floor functional assessment should be conducted to understand baseline level of function and to introduce interventions designed to optimize preexisting pelvic floor strength and continence deficits through supervised rehabilitation interventions as indicated. Prehabilitaiton for pelvic floor strengthening improves postoperative return to continence and overall pelvic function.[34]

Despite the high prevalence of sexual dysfunction and pelvic floor disorders in women following cancer treatments, these issues are infrequently addressed until they become substantially disabling to the individual. Sixty percent of gynecologic cancer survivors report that physicians did not discuss the impacts of cancer treatments on sexual function.[35]

While these side effects commonly present or worsen during active cancer treatments, they may persist for several years after the immediate posttreatment phase.[36] Furthermore, these impairments typically cooccur suggesting that multimorbidity should be considered and assessed. The delay of treatment occurs for many reasons: individuals may be embarrassed or uncomfortable initiating discussion on issues such as painful sex or incontinence with their providers, providers may be focused on the urgent, medically specific treatment-related issues rather than on supportive care. Therefore it is imperative for ongoing prospective surveillance at intervals during treatment to allow for a dialogue that provides the individual with an opportunity to discuss these issues as well as to enable a clinical assessment of pelvic floor function and to assess change since baseline.

Beyond the completion of cancer treatments, providers should be aware that these issues may be present given the cancer history and should ask important screening questions and use standardized, validated questionnaires to (1) assess the presence of symptoms and (2) refer to appropriately trained providers who can deliver treatment aimed at pelvic floor dysfunction.

The PSM is the gold standard for multidisciplinary, patient-centered care that involves regular assessment of potential impairments during and after cancer treatment in order to detect issues and intervene early.[3] Providers should consider administering evidence-based screening and assessment measures to evaluate the presence and impact of urinary and fecal incontinence and sexual dysfunction before, during, and after treatment. Table 2.2 outlines the recommended measures assessing gynecological cancer treatment–related impairments.

COMMON CANCER TREATMENT–RELATED IMPAIRMENTS

Cancer treatments are accompanied by a myriad of side effects that present based on the treatment rendered and may not necessarily be disease specific. For example, women with breast cancer as well as those with some gynecological cancers will receive neurotoxic chemotherapy agents leading to CIPN, gait deviations, and falls. Fatigue is a prevalent symptom across all antineoplastic therapies. Lymphedema commonly occurs across all solid tumor types when lymph nodes are dissected or irradiated as a part of the medical treatment plan. Distress, anxiety, and depression also occur commonly across these cancers. Recommendations for additional assessments will depend on the treatments received. An overview of the clinical measures recommended to assess these common impairments is described in Table 2.3.

PRACTICE IMPLEMENTATION

The abovementioned recommendations reflect the culmination of existing evidence for an optimal clinical model. However, each institution and clinic will

TABLE 2.2
Gynecological Cancer Measures

Domain	Recommendation
Urinary and Fecal Incontinence[37,38]	*Screening:* "Have you leaked any [urine or feces], even a small amount, in the last three months?" This screening question is adapted from the 3IQ measure[39] providing a general indication if incontinence has occurred in the last 3 months *Interval:* Baseline, pretreatment, and at regular intervals (every 4–6 weeks) to assess pre, during, and posttreatment severity and impact of incontinence
	Patient-reported outcomes: • *AUA-SI*: The AUA-SI assesses the severity of urinary urgency, frequency, and voiding symptoms. The AUA-SI is a 7-item self-report measure with scores ranging from 0 to 35 with higher scores indicating greater severity of symptoms (less than 8: mild symptoms, 8–19: moderate symptoms, 19 + : severe symptoms). • *IQOL questionnaire*: The IQOL is a 22-item quality of life questionnaire with subscales that assess behavior, psychosocial impact, and social embarrassment of UI in women and men. Each item is scored using a 1–5 Likert scale with 1 being "extremely" and 5 being "not at all" with higher scores corresponding to higher quality of life. • *ICIQ-SF*: The ICIQ-SF is a 5-item self-report questionnaire that assesses incontinence-related severity and impact on quality of life. A score between 1 and 5 is slight impact, 6 and 12 is moderate impact, 13 and 18 is severe impact, and 19 and 21 is very severe impact
	Patient-reported outcomes for combined urinary and fecal incontinence: • *Pelvic Floor Distress Inventory—Short Form (PFDI-20)*: The PFDI-20 contains 20 questions that assess the impact of pelvic floor disorders on the HRQoL in women. The PFDI-20 evaluates three domains of distress: pelvic organ prolapse distress, colorectal anal distress, and urinary distress. • *Pelvic Floor Impact Questionnaire—Short Form (PFIQ-7)*: The 7-item PFIQ-7 assesses the extent to which bladder, bowel, and vaginal symptoms affect activities, relationships, and feelings. Each subscale score is added to form the PFIQ-7 summary score ranging from 0 to 300 with higher scores indicating worse health status
	Patient-reported outcomes for fecal incontinence: • *ICIQ-B module*: This 21-item self-report measure assesses the domains of bowel patterns, bowel control, and quality of life. This measure also includes the Bristol Stool Scale, a standardized measure used to classify stool type. The ICIQ-B is able to distinguish between solid and stool incontinence, liquid/soft stool incontinence, and flatus incontinence
Pelvic Pain and Sexual Dysfunction[40]	*Screening:* A single screening question: "Do you experience pain with intercourse?" Patients who endorse sexual pain may then require a more in-depth assessment of their sexual function and pain experience
	Patient-reported outcomes: • *NPRS*: Current, least, worst, and average pelvic and/or intercourse pain intensity over the last 7 days may be assessed using the valid and reliable 11-point pain rating scale with 0 representing no pain and 10 representing the worst pain imaginable. • *SVQ*: The 20-item SVQ evaluates sexual and vaginal dysfunction in patients with gynecological cancer, including sexual interest, lubrication, orgasm, dyspareunia, vaginal dimensions, intimacy, partner sexual problems, sexual activity, sexual satisfaction, and body image. • *FSDS-R*: The FSDS is a 13-item questionnaire that evaluates negative emotions about sexuality and sexual relations. • *Sexual Interest and Desire Inventory*

3IQ, 3 Incontinence Questions; *AUA-SI*, American Urological Association Symptom Index; *FSDS-R*, Female Sexual Distress Scale-Revised; *HRQoL*, health-related quality of life; *ICIQ-B*, International Consultation on Incontinence Questionnaire-Bowels; *ICIQ-SF*, International Consultation on Incontinence Questionnaire—Short Form; *IQOL*, Incontinence Quality of Life; *NPRS*, Numerical Pain Rating Scale; *SVQ*, Sexual Function—Vaginal Changes Questionnaire.

TABLE 2.3
Functional Impairment Measures

Domain	Recommendations
Pain[41,42]	*Screening* VAS Numerical pain rating scale *Patient-reported outcomes*: McGill Pain Questionnaire—Short Form Brief Pain Inventory—Short Form Pain Disability Index
QOL[43–45]	*Breast cancer specific*: EORTC QLQ Breast 23 FACT—Breast + 4 *Cervical cancer specific*: EORTC QLQ Cervical cancer 24 AND a general QOL tool *Ovarian cancer specific:* EORTC QLQ Ovarian cancer 28 FACT Ovarian *General cancer:* EORTC QLQ—Cancer 30 FACT—General
Balance[46]	*Clinical measures*: Fullerton Advanced Balance Scale Gait speed Balance Evaluation Systems Test Timed Up and Go Five time sit to stand
CIPN[47,48]	*Patient-reported outcomes:* FACT–Gynecologic Oncology Group-Neurotoxicity Scale version 4 Participant Neurotoxicity Questionnaire *Clinical measures*: Total Neuropathy Score clinical version
Secondary Lymphedema[19,49]	*Patient-reported outcomes*: Functional Assessment of Cancer Therapies—Breast Disability of arm, shoulder, and hand Norman Questionnaire[a] Morbidity Screening Tool[a] *Clinical assessment*: Water displacement Circumferential measures and calculated volume Optoelectronic perometry Bioelectrical impedance analysis
Cancer-Related Fatigue[23]	*Patient-reported outcomes*: Modified Brief Fatigue Inventory Cancer-Related Fatigue Distress Scale 10-point VAS rating scale for fatigue MD Anderson Symptom Inventory Wu Cancer Fatigue Scale Patient-Reported Outcomes Measurement Information System—Fatigue
Cognitive Dysfunction[50]	*Screening*: Montreal Cognitive Assessment Clock Draw Test *Patient-reported outcomes*: Functional Assessment of Cancer Therapy—Cognitive Function

(*Continued*)

TABLE 2.3(Continued)

Domain	Recommendations
Distress[51]	*Screening*: Distress Thermometer and Problem List Patient Health Questionnaire 2 *Assessment*: Hospital Anxiety and Depression Scale Stress Scale-21

[a]Recommended for patients "at risk" for developing lymphedema.
EORTC QLQ, European Organization for Research and Treatment of Cancer Quality of Life Questionnaire; *FACT*, Functional Assessment of Cancer Therapy; *QOL*, quality of life; *VAS*, visual analog scale.

need to consider its own available resources and unique constraints in optimizing implementation of rehabilitation services. Issues for consideration include the following:

- *Workforce:* Cancer rehabilitation is an emerging area of practice, and rehabilitation providers in the system of care may not have specialty training in oncology care and may lack awareness of the common functional impairments and evidence-based rehabilitation interventions for individuals with cancer. Successful integration of rehabilitation services into oncology care will require staff and provider training to achieve competency in managing this complex population.[52]
- *Workflow:* Ideally, rehabilitation services should be integrated into the existing workflow of a cancer treatment center or oncology clinic. This can be achieved in many ways, including, but not limited to, preoperative education classes, embedded referrals in electronic health records and decision support tools, symptom-specific navigation pathways, and supportive care clinics.[8,53]
- *Physical location of services*: Integrated delivery models, where rehabilitation providers work within cancer centers and clinics, are identified as the optimal approach to aligning services and optimizing care.[54]

Furthermore, implementation may be challenged by overcoming cultural issues and long-standing paradigms of reactive rehabilitative care models. Promoting awareness of the effectiveness of the PSM along with enhancing knowledge of the benefit of rehabilitation services is also the responsibility of the oncology rehabilitation specialist. This requires relationship building with all providers on the cancer care team, engaging in tumor board meetings, and encouraging colocated clinical services to enable greater provider to provider contact as well as provider to patient contact.

SUMMARY

Breast and gynecological cancers commonly result in functional impairment for the majority of women with these diagnoses. Using standardized methodology for clinical assessment, through the framework of the PSM, and valid clinical measurement tools enables early identification of many symptom-related functional impairments and can optimize the introduction of rehabilitation services to promote optimal outcomes in cancer care.

KEY RESEARCH QUESTIONS

1. What is the optimal timing for rehabilitative interventions to prevent sequelae from cancer-related treatments in the short and long term?
2. What is the impact of early rehabilitative interventions on disease-specific endpoints such as progression-free survival and overall survival?
3. What is the impact of rehabilitation interventions on health service utilization during and after cancer treatments?
4. How do rehabilitation interventions influence the severity of toxicity from disease treatments?

REFERENCES

1. Silver JK, Baima J, Mayer RS. Impairment-driven cancer rehabilitation: an essential component of quality care and survivorship. *CA Cancer J Clin.* 2013;63(5):295–317.
2. Alfano CM, Cheville AL, Mustian K. Developing high-quality cancer rehabilitation programs: a timely need. *Am Soc Clin Oncol Educ Book.* 2016;35:241–249.
3. Stout NL, Binkley JM, Schmitz KH, et al. A prospective surveillance model for rehabilitation for women with breast cancer. *Cancer.* 2012;118(8 suppl):2191–2200.
4. National CPF. *Long-Term Survivorship Care After Cancer Treatment: Proceedings of a Workshop,* National Academies Press, Washington, DC. 2018.

5. Silver JK, Baima J. Cancer prehabilitation: an opportunity to decrease treatment-related morbidity, increase cancer treatment options, and improve physical and psychological health outcomes. *Am J Phys Med Rehabil.* 2013;92 (8):715–727.
6. Stout Gergich NL, Pfalzer LA, McGarvey C, Springer B, Gerber LH, Soballe P. Preoperative assessment enables the early diagnosis and successful treatment of lymphedema. *Cancer.* 2008;112(12):2809–2819.
7. Springer BA, Levy E, McGarvey C, et al. Pre-operative assessment enables early diagnosis and recovery of shoulder function in patients with breast cancer. *Breast Cancer Res Treat.* 2010;120(1):135–147.
8. Silver JK. Integrating rehabilitation into the cancer care continuum. *PM R.* 2017;9(9S2):S291–S296.
9. Richard KR. *Studying a Study and Testing a Test.* Wolters Kluwer Medical; 2020.
10. Fisher MI, Harrington S. Research roundup from the research committee. *Rehabil Oncol.* 2015;33(1).
11. Cheville A, Basford J. Multi-stakeholder attitudes regarding risk-based thresholds for initiating impairment-directed interventions among patients with breast cancer. *Ann Phys Rehabil Med.* 2018;61:e289.
12. Schmitz KH, Speck RM, Rye SA, DiSipio T, Hayes SC. Prevalence of breast cancer treatment sequelae over 6 years of follow-up: the Pulling Through Study. *Cancer.* 2012;118(8 suppl):2217–2225.
13. Stubblefield MD, Keole N. Upper body pain and functional disorders in patients with breast cancer. *PM R.* 2014;6(2):170–183.
14. Ewertz M, Jensen AB. Late effects of breast cancer treatment and potentials for rehabilitation. *Acta Oncol.* 2011;50(2):187–193.
15. de Carlos-Iriarte E, Mosquera-González M, Alonso-García M, et al. Upper-limb morbidity in patients undergoing a rehabilitation program after breast cancer surgery. *Rehabil Oncol.* 2019;37(2):70–76.
16. Kjaer TK, Johansen C, Ibfelt E, et al. Impact of symptom burden on health related quality of life of cancer survivors in a Danish cancer rehabilitation program: a longitudinal study. *Acta Oncol.* 2011;50(2):223–232.
17. Binkley JM, Harris SR, Levangie PK, et al. Patient perspectives on breast cancer treatment side effects and the prospective surveillance model for physical rehabilitation for women with breast cancer. *Cancer.* 2012;118(8 suppl):2207–2216.
18. Runowicz CD, Leach CR, Henry NL, et al. American Cancer Society/American Society of Clinical Oncology breast cancer survivorship care guideline. *CA Cancer J Clin.* 2016;66(1):43–73.
19. Perdomo M, Davies C, Levenhagen K, Ryans K. Breast cancer edge task force outcomes: assessment measures of secondary lymphedema in breast cancer survivors. *Rehabil Oncol.* 2014;32(1):22–35.
20. Levenhagen K, Davies C, Perdomo M, Ryans K, Gilchrist L. Diagnosis of upper quadrant lymphedema secondary to cancer: clinical practice guideline from the Oncology Section of the American Physical Therapy Association. *Phys Ther.* 2017;97(7):729–745.
21. Fisher MI, Levangie PK. Oncology Section Task Force on Breast Cancer Outcomes: scapular assessment. *Rehabil Oncol.* 2013;31(1):11–18.
22. Miale S, Harrington S, Kendig T. Oncology Section Task Force on Breast Cancer Outcomes: clinical measures of upper extremity function. *Rehabil Oncol.* 2013;31(1):27–34.
23. Fisher MI, Davies C, Lacy H, Doherty D. Oncology Section EDGE Task Force on Cancer: measures of cancer-related fatigue—a systematic review. *Rehabil Oncol.* 2018;36(2):93–105.
24. Fisher MI, Lee J, Davies CC, Geyer H, Colon G, Pfalzer L. Oncology Section EDGE Task Force on Breast Cancer Outcomes: a systematic review of outcome measures for functional mobility. *Rehabil Oncol.* 2015;33(3):19–31.
25. Thomas SG, Sato HR, Glantz JC, Doyle PJ, Buchsbaum GM. Prevalence of symptomatic pelvic floor disorders among gynecologic oncology patients. *Obstet Gynecol.* 2013;122(5):976–980.
26. Ramaseshan AS, Felton J, Roque D, Rao G, Shipper AG, Sanses TVD. Pelvic floor disorders in women with gynecologic malignancies: a systematic review. *Int Urogynecol J.* 2018;29(4):459–476.
27. Association AP. *Sexual dysfunctions. Diagnostic and Statistical Manual of Mental Disorders.* Fifth ed. Arlington, VA: American Psychiatric Association; 2013.
28. Onujiogu N, Johnson T, Seo S, et al. Survivors of endometrial cancer: who is at risk for sexual dysfunction? *Gynecol Oncol.* 2011;123(2):356–359.
29. Everhov AH, Floter Radestad A, Nyberg T, Smedby KE, Bergmark K, Linden Hirschberg A. Serum androgen levels and sexual function before and one year after treatment of uterine cervical cancer: a pilot study. *J Sex Med.* 2016;13(3):413–424.
30. Lindau ST, Schumm LP, Laumann EO, Levinson W, O'Muircheartaigh CA, Waite LJ. A study of sexuality and health among older adults in the United States. *N Engl J Med.* 2007;357(8):762–774.
31. De Graaff AA, Van Lankveld J, Smits LJ, Van Beek JJ, Dunselman GA. Dyspareunia and depressive symptoms are associated with impaired sexual functioning in women with endometriosis, whereas sexual functioning in their male partners is not affected. *Hum Reprod.* 2016;31(11):2577–2586.
32. Aerts L, Enzlin P, Verhaeghe J, Vergote I, Amant F. Sexual and psychological functioning in women after pelvic surgery for gynaecological cancer. *Eur J Gynaecol Oncol.* 2009;30(6):652–656.
33. Vaz AF, Pinto-Neto AM, Conde DM, et al. Quality of life and menopausal and sexual symptoms in gynecologic cancer survivors: a cohort study. *Menopause.* 2011;18 (6):662–669.
34. Singh F, Newton RU, Galvao DA, Spry N, Baker MK. A systematic review of pre-surgical exercise intervention studies with cancer patients. *Surg Oncol.* 2013;22 (2):92–104.
35. Lindau ST, Gavrilova N, Anderson D. Sexual morbidity in very long term survivors of vaginal and cervical cancer: a comparison to national norms. *Gynecol Oncol.* 2007;106(2):413–418.

36. Vistad I, Cvancarova M, Kristensen GB, Fossa SD. A study of chronic pelvic pain after radiotherapy in survivors of locally advanced cervical cancer. *J Cancer Surviv.* 2011;5(2):208–216.
37. Jeffrey A, Harrington SE, Hill A, Roscow A, Alappattu M. Oncology Section EDGE Task Force on Urogenital Cancer: a systematic review of clinical measures for incontinence. *Rehabil Oncol.* 2017;35(3):130.
38. Cotterill N, Norton C, Avery KN, Abrams P, Donovan JL. Psychometric evaluation of a new patient-completed questionnaire for evaluating anal incontinence symptoms and impact on quality of life: the ICIQ-B. *Dis Colon Rectum.* 2011;54(10):1235–1250.
39. Brown JS, Bradley CS, Subak LL, et al. The sensitivity and specificity of a simple test to distinguish between urge and stress urinary incontinence. *Ann Intern Med.* 2006;144(10):715–723.
40. Alappattu M, Harrington SE, Hill A, Roscow A, Jeffrey A. Oncology Section EDGE Task Force on Cancer: a systematic review of patient-reported measures for sexual dysfunction. *Rehabil Oncol.* 2017;35(3):137.
41. Harrington S, Gilchrist L, Sander A. Breast Cancer EDGE Task Force Outcomes: clinical measures of pain. *Rehabil Oncol.* 2014;32(1):13.
42. Harrington SE, Gilchrist L, Lee J, Westlake FL, Baker A. Oncology Section EDGE Task Force on Cancer: a systematic review of clinical measures for pain. *Rehabil Oncol.* 2018;36(2):83–92.
43. Harrington S, Miale S, Ebaugh D. Breast Cancer EDGE Task Force Outcomes: clinical measures of health related quality of life. *Rehabil Oncol.* 2015;33(1):5–17.
44. Tax C, Steenbergen ME, Zusterzeel PL, Bekkers RL, Rovers MM. Measuring health-related quality of life in cervical cancer patients: a systematic review of the most used questionnaires and their validity. *BMC Med Res Methodol.* 2017;17(1):15.
45. Ahmed-Lecheheb D, Joly F. Ovarian cancer survivors' quality of life: a systematic review. *J Cancer Survivorship.* 2016;10(5):789–801.
46. Huang M, Hile E, Croarkin E, et al. Academy of Oncologic Physical Therapy EDGE Task Force: a systematic review of measures of balance in adult cancer survivors. *Rehabil Oncol.* 2019;37(3):92–103.
47. Hile E, Levangie P, Ryans K, Gilchrist L. Oncology Section Task Force on Breast Cancer Outcomes: clinical measures of chemotherapy-induced peripheral neuropathy—a systematic review. *Rehabil Oncol.* 2015;33 (3):32–41.
48. McCrary JM, Goldstein D, Boyle F, et al. Optimal clinical assessment strategies for chemotherapy-induced peripheral neuropathy (CIPN): a systematic review and Delphi survey. *Supportive Care Cancer.* 2017;25 (11):3485–3493.
49. Cohn JC, Geyer H, Lee J, Fisher MI. Oncology Section EDGE Task Force on Urogenital Cancer Outcomes: clinical measures of lymphedema—a systematic review. *Rehabil Oncol.* 2017;35(3):119–129.
50. Isenberg-Grzeda E, Huband H, Lam H. A review of cognitive screening tools in cancer. *Curr Opin Support Palliat Care.* 2017;11(1):24–31.
51. Riba MB, Donovan KA, Andersen B, et al. Distress Management, Version 3.2019, NCCN clinical practice guidelines in oncology. *J Natl Compr Cancer Netw.* 2019;17(10):1229–1249.
52. Stout NL, Silver JK, Alfano CM, Ness KK, Gilchrist LS. Long-term survivorship care after cancer treatment: a new emphasis on the role of rehabilitation services. *Phys Ther.* 2019;99(1):10–13.
53. Stout NL, Sleight A, Pfeiffer D, Galantino ML, deSouza B. Promoting assessment and management of function through navigation: opportunities to bridge oncology and rehabilitation systems of care. *Support Care Cancer.* 2019;27(12):4497–4505.
54. Cheville AL, Mustian K, Winters-Stone K, Zucker DS, Gamble GL, Alfano CM. Cancer rehabilitation: an overview of current need, delivery models, and levels of care. *Phys Med Rehabil Clin N Am.* 2017;28 (1):1–17.

CHAPTER 3

Exercise While Living With Breast and Gynecological Cancers

CARLY ROTHMAN, DO • SUSAN MALTSER, DO

INTRODUCTION

Historically, cancer patients were advised to "take it easy" while they underwent treatment and recovery. Now, there is overwhelming evidence that we should encourage our patients to do the opposite. By increasing physical fitness, patients can better tolerate cancer treatment, maximize their functional independence, improve survival, and increase their quality of life.[1–3] Although there is no single exercise protocol or dose that has shown to be superior for breast and gynecological cancer patients as of yet, we can comfortably state that staying active in a variety of ways is vital for cancer treatment and recovery.[4] A collaborative team-based approach is essential to the success of an exercise program for patients with breast and gynecological cancer. Typically, patients will received primary treatment from oncologists, radiation oncologists, and surgeons. Referral to a physiatrist, particularly one who specializes in cancer rehabilitation, can ensure a patient starts an appropriate and safe exercise program that takes into account their individual needs. Teaching, training, and supervision from experienced physical therapists, fitness trainers, and exercise physiologists specializing in cancer rehabilitation allow patients to safely increase their physical fitness and adherence to their exercise program. Family and friends are a vital support system for patients with breast cancer and should be involved in medical/surgical treatment, as well as rehabilitation efforts.[5,6] This chapter will discuss the exercise recommendations and disease–specific modifications important for patients living with breast and gynecological cancers, highlighting the evidence of benefits and safety considerations. Compared to breast cancer, there is a significantly smaller body of literature exploring gynecological cancer and exercise, and therefore the majority of evidence presented in this chapter is derived from research examining breast cancer patients. When available, evidence pertaining to specific issues of patients with gynecological cancer will be presented.

TYPES OF EXERCISE

Exercise regimens for breast cancer patients should include a variety of activities that cause different primary physiological effects: aerobic, anaerobic, muscle strengthening, bone strengthening, balance training, and flexibility training. Yoga, tai chi, and qigong comprise an exercise category that combines many of the previous categories while "emphasizing relaxation, meditation and spirituality."[7] The absolute and relative intensity of exercise is important to consider when prescribing an exercise regimen. The absolute intensity, commonly measured in metabolic equivalents, is the "rate of energy expenditure required to perform any physical activity" (see Table 3.1).[7,8] Relative intensity can be measured objectively by VO_{2max} or the sing-talk test, or subjectively rated by the participant with a scale such as the rate of perceived exertion (see Table 3.2).[7,9] The term physical activity generally refers to a wide range of occupational, recreational, and household activities, while exercise refers to dedicated time to endurance, strengthening, or sport activities.[7] In this chapter the terms physical activity and exercise will be used interchangeably.

EXERCISE POSITIVELY INFLUENCES BREAST AND GYNECOLOGICAL CANCER PREVENTION, TREATMENT, SURVIVAL AND RECURRENCE

Exercise, in addition to being beneficial to general health, may prevent the development of breast cancer in a dose-dependent manner.[7,10,11] The main proposed mechanisms of how exercise decreases the risk of developing breast cancer are via decreased adiposity,

Breast Cancer and Gynecologic Cancer Rehabilitation DOI: https://doi.org/10.1016/B978-0-323-72166-0.00003-7

TABLE 3.1
Metabolic Equivalents (METs)

METs (Approximate)	Activity
1.0	Sleeping, sitting quietly, meditating
2.0	Cooking, folding laundry, light gardening, playing musical instrument
3.0	Walking, child care (moderate), occupational standing tasks, Tai Chi
4.0	Bicycling (leisure), power yoga, raking leaves
5.0	Elliptical trainer, resistance training, dancing
6.0	Power lifting, rowing (vigorous), shoveling snow
7.0	Running (13 min/mi), racquetball, soccer (casual), backpacking
8.0	Running (12 min/mi), calisthenics, circuit training, rock climbing
9.0	Running (11.5 min/mi), stair treadmill, cross-country skiing (moderate)
10.0	Running (9 min/mi), soccer (competitive), swimming (vigorous)
11.0	Running (8.5 min/mi), stationary bike (vigorous), rope jumping (moderate)
12.0	Running (7 min/mi), rowing (competitive), bicycling (racing)

Metabolic Equivalents (METs), a measure of absolute intensity of exercise.

TABLE 3.2
Rate of Perceived Exertion (RPE)

Numerical Rating	Qualitative Rating
6	
7	Very, very light
8	
9	Very light
10	
11	Fairly light
12	
13	Somewhat hard
14	
15	Hard
16	
17	Very hard
18	
19	Very, very hard
20	

Rate of Perceived Exertion (RPE), a measure of relative intensity of exercise.

improvement of metabolic and hormonal abnormalities, and immunomodulation[12–14] (Fig. 3.1). Adiposity promotes a chronic inflammatory and hypoxic state, coupled with excessive hormone production, and should be viewed as a "preventable and reversible risk factor" for breast cancer.[15] It is important to note that exercise has a greater impact on reducing obesity when combined with dietary modifications.[15] Higher intensity exercise correlates with increased risk reduction up to a certain point, as exhaustive exercise can have detrimental effects on the muscular microenvironment.[15] Current evidence is limited on whether the preventative effect of exercise is modified by age, race, or socioeconomic status, although some evidence points to a greater effect for postmenopausal women compared to premenopausal women.[7,10] It is also unclear whether patients with a family history of breast cancer receive the same risk reduction benefit from exercise compared to those without genetic predisposition.[11,16] There is strong evidence that increasing physical activity and limiting sedentary behavior lower the risk of endometrial cancer, with more limited evidence for ovarian cancer. It is important to note that there is a significant linear correlation between physical activity and melanoma risk, and therefore patients engaging in outdoor physical activity should be educated on sun-safe practices.[17]

Treatment

The National Comprehensive Cancer Network (NCCN) and the American College of Sports Medicine (ACSM) recommend physical activity, including aerobic exercise and resistance training, for cancer patients undergoing active cancer treatment and posttreatment.[4,18] Exercise can help patients better tolerate treatment, decrease treatment complications, and increase chemotherapy completion rates, translating to improved treatment outcomes.[1,19,20] Exercise may have these effects by increasing perfusion and oxygenation of tumor cells by normalizing tumor blood vessels and by promoting

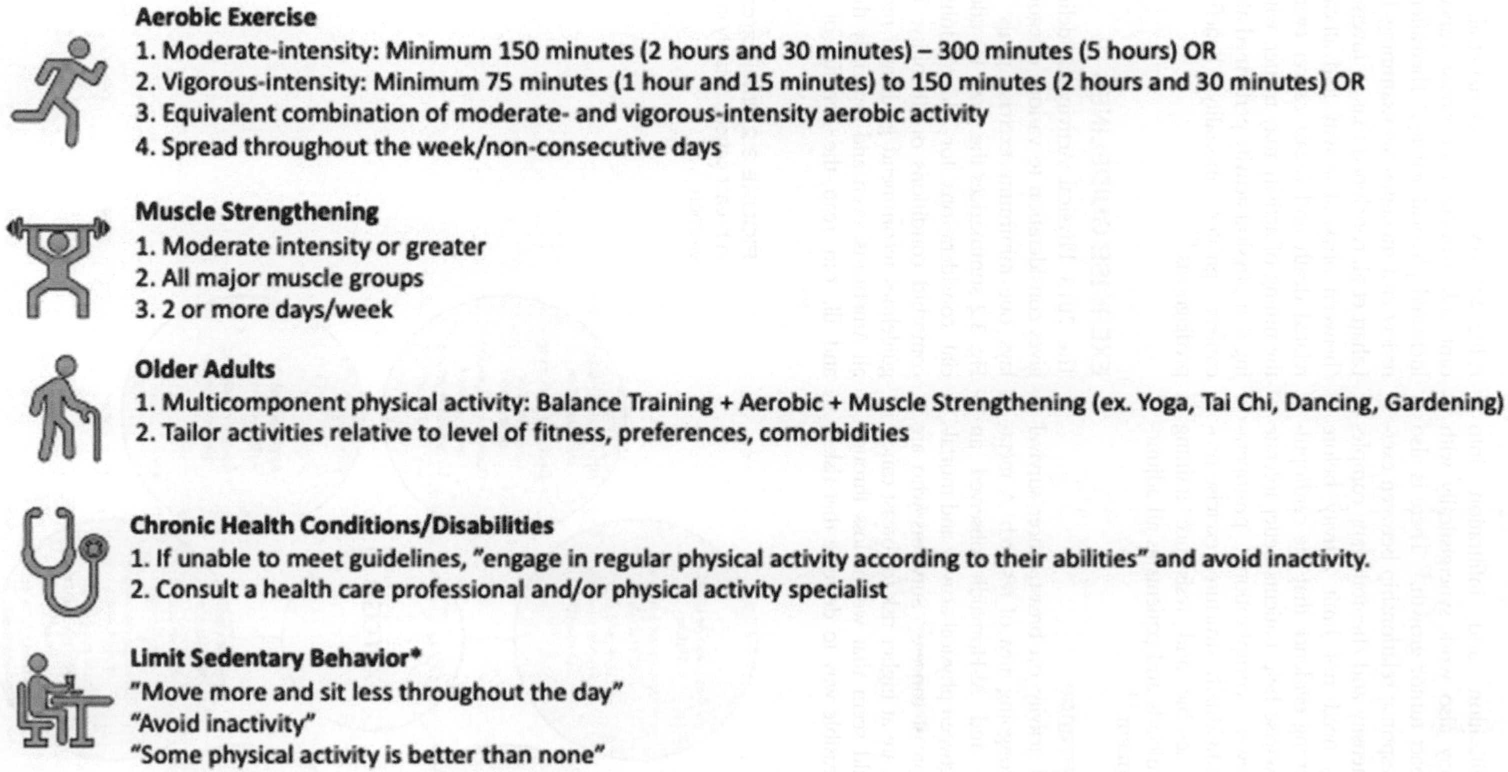

FIGURE 3.1 Suggested Exercise Guidelines for Adults.

immune cell mobilization and infiltration into tumors.[17] Exercise may also work synergistically with chemotherapy to impact tumor growth.[17] There is also evidence of a dose–response relationship between exercise frequency and intensity and chemotherapy completion rates.[21] Patients need not limit activity before surgery, as there is strong evidence that the cardiopulmonary benefits of exercise help patients better tolerate anesthesia, with fewer complications postoperatively.[19,22] Thus an individually structured exercise program consisting of aerobic and resistance training should be seen by clinicians and patients as an adjunctive breast cancer treatment.[14]

Survival and Recurrence

The effect of physical activity on breast cancer survival and recurrence is an ongoing area of research. A meta-analysis by Ibrahim and Al-Homaidh observed an inverse relationship between physical activity and mortality in patients with breast cancer.[23] Survivors who are overweight and obese are at higher risk for breast cancer recurrence, so it would seem that weight loss through exercise might be a feasible way to decrease that risk.[21] A literature review by Loprinzi et al. found a nonsignificant risk reduction of breast cancer recurrence with increased physical activity.[3] Thereafter, a robust systemic review and metaanalysis examining 123,574 patients by Lahart et al. concluded that an inverse relationship exists "between physical activity and all-cause, breast cancer-related death and breast cancer events."[24] In addition, the timing of activity may matter, with evidence suggesting that physical activity performed after cancer diagnosis confers greater mortality benefits compared to prediagnosis.[17]

EXERCISE GUIDELINES

The 2018 Physical Activity Guidelines for Americans gives consideration to various categories of exercise and lays out minimum exercise goals for all Americans. Fig. 3.2 summarizes the goals for adults, as well as special considerations for older adults and those with comorbid conditions or disability. The evidence-based guidelines recommend goals and modifications so that all Americans, even and especially the elderly, disabled, and ill, can reap the benefits of increased physical

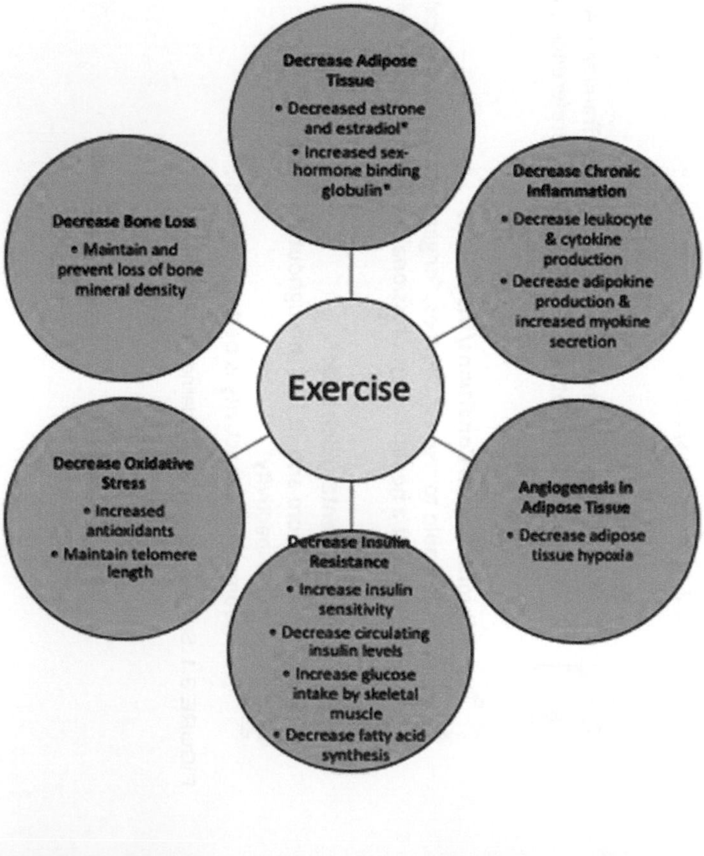
Decrease Adipose Tissue
• Decreased estrone and estradiol*
• Increased sex-hormone binding globulin*
Decrease Bone Loss
• Maintain and prevent loss of bone mineral density
Decrease Chronic Inflammation
• Decrease leukocyte & cytokine production
• Decrease adipokine production & increased myokine secretion
Exercise
Decrease Oxidative Stress
• Increased antioxidants
• Maintain telomere length
Angiogenesis in Adipose Tissue
• Decrease adipose tissue hypoxia
Decrease Insulin Resistance
• Increase insulin sensitivity
• Decrease circulating insulin levels
• Increase glucose intake by skeletal muscle
• Decrease fatty acid synthesis

FIGURE 3.2 Physiological effects of exercise in breast cancer. *Mainly in post-menopaulsal women.

activity.[9] It is encouraged that physicians use this information to help patients create an individualized exercise program based on their fitness level and interests, to help them meet the minimum requirements.[4] The guidelines emphasize minimizing total and interval duration of sedentary behavior, defined as "any waking behavior characterized by an energy expenditure ≤ 1.5 metabolic equivalents (METs), while in a sitting, reclining or lying posture," and encourage increasing activity through daily tasks such as walking or cycling. Inactivity should be avoided, with patients returning to regular daily activities as soon as possible.[7,9]

GENERAL SAFETY CONSIDERATIONS

Prior to starting an exercise regimen, patients should have a full history and physical by a physician to identify any safety considerations or contraindications to exercise. Relative and absolute contraindications to exercise can be found in Table 3.3. If a patient does have a contraindication to exercise, they should be referred for immediate treatment and reevaluated after their condition has been treated and/or stabilized.[19] Further testing may be necessary to assess patient tolerance and starting intensities for exercise. Pretesting for endurance exercise may include measuring VO_{2max} or the 6-minute walk test. Strength testing can be measured with one-repetition maximum testing and has been proven safe for patients with or at risk of lymphedema.[4] Baseline testing should always be performed so that progress, failure to progress, or regression can be tracked. An individualized program should then be created based on the patient's interests, exercise restrictions, and fitness level.[19]

Overall, exercise prior to, during and after chemotherapy, radiation, and surgery has been shown to be safe and is recommended for breast cancer patients.[4,6,19] Physicians may consider starting certain high-risk and/or deconditioned patients in a supervised program to ensure proper technique and improve adherence.[6] Once the patient has completed active treatment and has shown competency with their exercise program, they may continue on their own with regular medical follow-up.[19] A safe exercise "dose" for breast cancer patients and survivors has not been elucidated as of yet. However, there is robust evidence that aerobic and resistance training, either alone or in combination, are safe and feasible in this population. There is currently no upper limit on training for patients participating in a supervised, slowly progressive aerobic and resistance regimen.[25] In an ideal world, patients would undergo a formal functional assessment prior to any surgical, radiation, or chemotherapeutic interventions to more accurately monitor declines in function and progress in therapy; this information would also help further research in this field.[26]

The most common comorbid medical conditions that may affect the safety of an exercise routine for cancer patients and survivors are type II diabetes mellitus, coronary artery disease, heart failure, chronic obstructive pulmonary disease, obesity, hypertension, and osteoarthritis. Monitoring of blood glucose, heart rate, blood pressure, and oxygen saturation before, during, and after exercise may be warranted in patients who are

TABLE 3.3
Relative and Absolute Contraindications to Exercise

Absolute Contraindications to Exercise	Relative Contraindications to Exercise
Platelet count < 20,000 per μL[a]	Hemoglobin < 6 g/dL
Fever[a]	Severe nausea vomiting or diarrhea[b]
New onset "unusual or unexplained severe tiredness or unusual weakness"	Cardiovascular impairment (e.g., coronary ischemia, heart failure)
New-onset neurological deficits:	Arrhythmia with symptoms of dyspnea, anxiety, or fatigue
– Ataxia or changes in coordination	
– Muscle weakness	
– Changes in vision or hearing	
– Paresthesia or anesthesia in any dermatome	
Resting SBP > 180 mmHg or DBP > 110 mmHg	
Uncompensated heart failure, unstable angina	
COPD with superimposed pneumonia or exceptional involuntary loss of body weight (10% in the past half year of > 5% in the past month)	

Relative and Absolute Contraindications to Exercise.
[a]Activity restricted to walking and activities of daily living.
[b]May be able to tolerate low intensity; maintain hydration; monitor body weight.
SBP, Systolic Blood Pressure; DBP, diastolic blood pressure; COPD, chronic obstructive pulmonary disease.

frail, deconditioned, or have active medical issues. Modifications to an exercise protocol may be necessary due to complications and/or symptoms of these conditions, such as neuropathy, foot ulcers, dyspnea, edema, elevated blood pressure, and joint pain.[19]

BARRIERS TO EXERCISE/ADHERENCE

Breast cancer patients encounter many barriers to participating in physical activity and exercise, so not surprisingly they tend to be more sedentary than the general population.[27] Logistical barriers include time constraints due to frequent doctors' visits and treatments, financial strain due to medical bills and inability to work, and lack of transportation and childcare.[17] Physiological barriers include pain, fatigue, and neuropathy and will be further explored in subsequent sections of this chapter. Psychological barriers such as anxiety, depression, poor motivation, poor self-esteem, and cognitive deficits will also be discussed. Efforts to make physical activity more accessible and attainable for these patients are crucial, as emerging evidence continues to show that increased physical activity during cancer treatment results in better outcomes.[6]

Support from physicians, therapists, other patients, family, and friends can help motivate patients to begin and continue an exercise program and stay physically active. Supervised and group exercises have consistently shown to increase exercise adherence in patients with nonmetastatic breast cancer.[6,14,20,28,29] Patients with advanced disease tend to have more significant barriers to exercise and should be given alternatives such as home-based programs.[14] Incorporating behavioral techniques such as goal setting and activity diaries may also be helpful.[20] Making activities more fun, such as tailoring programs to patient's interests, adding music, and avoiding monotony can also increase adherence.[6]

With recent research supporting the role of technology in promoting physical activity, physical fitness, and weight loss, its potential to positively impact patients with cancer is now being explored.[30,31] eHealth is defined as the use of information and communication technologies for health and can include the use of email, text messaging, push notifications, websites, and mobile-based applications; mHealth is the specific use of mobile-based applications to deliver eHealth.[32] A mixed-methods study by Phillips et al explored breast cancer survivors' preferences for mHealth physical activity interventions, finding that while survivors are interested in these interventions, their "preferences varied around themes of relevance, ease of use, and enhancing personal motivation."[33] Studies have shown improved physical functioning in cancer patients with the use of a smartphone app; however, it is unclear if results are superior to the use of a pedometer alone, a brochure, or other eHealth such as web- or email-based interventions.[31,34,35] mHealth and eHealth for cancer survivors offer a promising new way to motivate and connect patients, but more research is needed to determine feasibility and effectiveness.[30,33,34]

MEDICAL AND SURGICAL COMPLICATIONS OF BREAST CANCER: EXERCISE BENEFITS, SAFETY CONSIDERATIONS, AND BARRIERS

Breast cancer treatment will generally include some combination of surgery, radiation, and chemotherapy, all of which can pose limitations to exercise and rehabilitation. In this section, we will review evidence-based safety considerations and benefits of various forms of exercise in relation to specific issues regarding surgical and medical treatments of breast cancer. Table 3.4 summarizes exercise modifications for specific complications of chemotherapy. Table 3.5 summarizes exercises that have been deemed safe and possibly beneficial for breast cancer-related complications.

Cancer-Related Fatigue

The NCCN defines cancer-related fatigue (CRF) as "a distressing, persistent, subjective sense of physical, emotional and/or cognitive tiredness or exhaustion related to cancer or cancer treatment that is not proportional to recent activity and interferes with usual functioning."[18] CRF is a prevalent issue among patients with cancer before, during, and after active treatment.[36] Fatigue tends to worsen both with progression of cancer and with subsequent chemotherapy and radiation, affecting quality of life, mood, pain tolerance, cognition, and sleep. Patients suffering from CRF are more likely to be sedentary, accelerating deconditioning.[37] While the exact pathophysiologic mechanism for CRF is unknown and is likely multifactorial, there is evidence that a concurrent, yet independent, parasympathetic underactivity and sympathetic overactivity contributes to the development and persistence of fatigue by inducing an inflammatory cascade, triggering production of proinflammatory cytokines.[37,38] It is important to keep in mind that the cause of CRF is often multifactorial, and cancer patients may have other noncancer factors contributing to fatigue so an individualized approach to treatment is critical. Evaluation into and treatment of medical causes of fatigue such as anemia, psychological causes such as "catastrophizing" and depression, and sleep disorders are

TABLE 3.4
Exercise Modifications for Patients Undergoing Chemotherapy

Complication	Modification
Leukopenia	Sanitize equipment, frequent hand washing May prefer home exercises over group setting
Thrombocytopenia	Low impact, low-intensity exercise Avoid large increases in blood pressure Monitor for bleeding
Anemia	Lower intensity of exercise
Fatigue	Avoid inactivity, avoid overtraining Decrease intensity and duration Relaxation exercises
Nausea/vomiting/ diarrhea	Ensure adequate hydration Avoid high-intensity exercise, rest when needed
Dizziness	Decrease intensity and duration Supervision to ensure safety Change positions slowly to avoid orthostasis
Pain	May need to decrease intensity of aerobic and resistance exercises Judicious use of analgesics
Dyspnea	Adjust exercise intensity as needed Monitor oxygen saturation
Tachycardia/ arrhythmia	Monitor heart rate before, during and after exercise Reassurance if no other symptoms, can be due to chemotherapy Adjust training intensity as needed Monitor symptoms, discontinue exercise, and refer to physician if associated with dyspnea and anxiety or fatigue
Numbness/ neuropathy	Caution with free weights in upper extremities (increased risk to drop weights) Supervision with balance exercises (increased risk of falls) Wear appropriate footwear with good grip
Skin/nail changes	Protect skin and nails, may need to use soft gloves in severe cases Avoid swimming and vigorous arm movement for patients with ports or catheters

Suggested Exercise Modifications for Patients Undergoing Chemotherapy.

necessary.[37] Overtraining and poor nutritional status can also contribute to fatigue and should be monitored on a regular basis.[19]

Exercise alone, or combined with psychological interventions, is recommended as a first-line option for treating CRF.[39,40] Many types of exercise have been shown to be safe and beneficial for slowing the progression of CRF, even in patients with advanced metastatic disease, including aerobic exercises, anaerobic exercises, and seated exercises.[18,39,41] Supervised aerobic and resistance training, in comparison to self-administered regimens, appear more effective at improving CRF and quality of life.[39,42] Patients who have completed primary treatment appear to benefit from a combination of exercise and psychological interventions, whereas patients receiving primary treatment can benefit from exercise alone.[39]

It has been proposed, with some promising initial evidence, that mindful and relaxing exercises such as yoga may improve CRF by calming sympathetic overactivity and stimulating parasympathetic responses, thereby reducing inflammatory activity.[36,37,43] Along similar reasoning, increasing physical activity in general and reducing body mass index (BMI) have been shown to reduce inflammation that may help improve fatigue[37,32] Yoga has been proven safe for patients with CRF undergoing active treatment and posttreatment and is listed as a category 1 recommendation by the NCCN.[18] Sprod et al. demonstrated safety, feasibility, and significant improvements in elderly, nonmetastatic cancer patients with CRF with a 4-week cancer-specific yoga intervention. Although any cancer type was eligible for the study, the majority were breast cancer survivors.[44] Patients with greater adherence to a regular yoga practice of two to three

TABLE 3.5
Overview of Safe and Beneficial Exercises for Specific Complications of Breast Cancer

Complication	Safe Exercises	Possibly Beneficial Exercises	Precautions/Modifications
Breast cancer-related lymphedema (BCRL)	Aerobic Strength Yoga/flexibility Aquatic	Lymphedema remedial exercises Strength Flexibility Aquatic	Wear compression garment during exercise Stop arm exercises and seek professional evaluation for new arm or shoulder heaviness, pain, and/or swelling Clean equipment prior to use Protect skin Avoid disuse of the limb
Cancer-related fatigue (CRF)	Aerobic Strength Yoga, Thai Chi, Qigong	Aerobic Strength Mixed training programs Yoga, Thai Chi	Avoid overtraining
Bone loss/disease	Aerobic Strength (pain free) Flexibility	Aerobic Strength Maintenance of previous levels of physical activity (prevent further bone loss)	Avoid painful resistance or weight-bearing exercises, seek medical care if pain develops during previously pain-free exercises Avoid heavy-lifting and high-impact activities Hip precautions for proximal femur and/or pelvic metastases Spinal precautions for spinal metastases Metastatic spinal cord compression: Follow spinal precautions, if new pain or neurological symptoms, stop activity immediately, assume a spinal protective position that reverses the symptoms
Chemotherapy-induced peripheral neuropathy (CIPN)	Aerobic Strength Balance training	Strength Balance training Sensorimotor exercises Task-specific exercises	High risk of falls due to numbness and proprioceptive deficits Avoid free weights if hands are affected Wear proper fitting, close-toed shoes
Cognitive impairment	Aerobic Strength Balance training Flexibility	Yoga	May need supervision for safety awareness
Axillary web syndrome (AWS)	Flexibility	Flexibility	Avoid disuse of the limb

sessions per week were more likely to report significant reductions of fatigue.[43,45,46] Studies examining the effect of yoga on CRF used various types and styles of yoga; however, all were tailored specifically to reduce fatigue, and patients with functional limitations were given modifications and/or props as needed.[43,47]

Altered Body Composition: Obesity and Cachexia

Breast cancer patients are at a higher risk of adiposity than the general population. This may be due to effects of breast cancer treatment, tendency toward more sedentary behavior, eating habits, hormone imbalances, metabolic changes, and menopausal status.[15] Chemotherapy-induced amenorrhea causes menopause that increases the likelihood of weight gain.[15] Chemotherapy regimens of cyclophosphamide, methotrexate, and fluorouracil cause an average weight gain of 2–6 kg.[48] Additional risks for increased weight gain include premenopausal status, prolonged chemotherapy regimens, and receiving steroids.[48]

There is now robust evidence that obesity and weight gain affect breast cancer development, progression, and recurrence via multiple biochemical pathways, including insulin resistance, chronic inflammation, endocrine fluctuations, and tissue hypoxia.[15] In fact, obesity has been linked to as many as 15%–20% of cancer deaths.[49] The link between excess weight gain and breast cancer development is stronger for postmenopausal women when compared to premenopausal women. Fortunately, adiposity is a reversible risk factor, and exercise has been shown to favorably affect breast cancer evolution in both pre- and postmenopausal women. Specifically, exercise has been shown to affect pathways that shift the body into an antiinflammatory, antimitotic and well-perfused state that is less likely to nurture the growth of a tumor. One of the most prominent risk factors for breast cancer recurrence is exposure to prolonged and elevated levels of estrogen. As adipose tissue is the main source of estrogens in postmenopausal women, reducing adipose tissue will invariably reduce estrogen exposure, thereby decreasing risk of breast cancer development. It is important to note that a combined program of exercise and dietary modifications was shown to reduce estrone and estradiol levels, as well as increase levels of sex hormone–binding globulin, more than an exercise program alone.[15]

Patients who are overweight or obese can decrease adipose tissue and increase lean muscle mass with aerobic and resistance exercises, which may result in overall weight loss or maintenance of body weight. However, weight loss is not always a positive sign in breast cancer patients, as it may be due to muscle wasting, sarcopenia, and/or cachexia. Muscle wasting can occur due to the tumor itself, host responses, and effects of cancer treatments.[50] Cancer cachexia is a distinct syndrome caused by inflammation and metabolic derangements that cannot be completely reversed by aggressive treatment of chemotherapy side effects and nutritional support.[6] Sarcopenia is a separate entity that may present as a component of cachexia and is defined by low muscle mass and reduced gait speed.[26] Patients with muscle wasting may not necessarily lose body weight, as loss of muscle mass is often coupled with increased fat mass, insulin resistance, and overall weight gain.[6] Side effects of chemotherapy such as nausea, vomiting, diarrhea, and anorexia can also contribute to weight loss.[15,13] Measurements of body weight alone may not give the full clinical picture, therefore monitoring of body composition parameters such as body fat and lean mass is recommended.[51] Skeletal muscle wasting in cancer patients worsens prognosis, and endurance and resistance exercise have been shown to help maintain muscle mass and decrease inflammation in this population.[52,53] Nutritional monitoring and support is essential for these patients while participating in an exercise program.[26]

BONE HEALTH

Bone Metastases

Bone is the most frequent site for metastatic disease in breast cancer, and while it carries a more favorable overall prognosis compared to visceral metastases, it can negatively affect functional capacity, fatigue, and quality of life.[5,54,55] Clinicians and patients alike may be fearful of an increased risk for falls, fractures, and pain, although there have been multiple randomized controlled trials showing that individualized exercise programs that "avoid loading bones and minimize shear forces on areas of the body with metastatic lesions" are feasible, safe, and well tolerated in this population.[5,56,57] According to the 2010 ACSM exercise guidelines for cancer survivors, patients with bone metastases should aim for the same minimum activity targets as cancer patients without metastases.[4] Reaching these targets can prove especially challenging in this population, and the majority of patients with bone metastases do not meet the guidelines. Physiatrists, physical and occupational therapists trained in cancer rehabilitation can be a vital resource in developing a safe and effective program for these patients.

Palliative treatment of bone metastases, such as radiation and chemotherapy, can further impact physical functioning due to negative impacts on muscle strength, fatigue, and skin integrity.[5] The Metastatic Exercise Training Trial examined the impact of a supervised exercise program for patients with metastatic disease. They determined that a moderate-intensity exercise program in this population is feasible; however, the study was limited by poor adherence, more-so in patients receiving chemotherapy.[57] Clinicians should therefore be aware that patients undergoing chemotherapy may need additional modifications, often on a day-to-day basis based on symptoms, to improve adherence to exercise. Patients should also be monitored for new or worsening neurologic deficits, as bone metastases may cause nerve root or spinal cord compression requiring urgent neurosurgical evaluation.[6] More studies are needed to elucidate if physical activity has an impact on treatment outcomes in this population. However, patients with metastatic disease are still encouraged to stay active to reap the cardiovascular and metabolic benefits of exercise.[9,57] A few animal studies do show some promising evidence that weight-bearing exercises may in fact inhibit the spread of bony metastatic disease.[5]

While the majority of patients with bone metastases will report bone pain, only bone pain associated with functional activity has been linked to an increased risk for pathologic fracture. Therefore it is recommended to encourage patients to start or continue an exercise regimen of aerobic and resistance exercises, unless they have or develop pain during activity. If pain develops, they should be assessed for pathologic fractures before returning to activity.

Prompt referral to orthopedic surgery when there is a concern for an impending fracture is critical, as elective prophylactic fixation can avoid serious complications associated with acute pathologic fractures such as "extreme pain, urgent hospitalization, and the risk of emergency surgery with compromised outcome."[5] Postoperative exercise may need to be modified to accommodate weight-bearing restrictions. Fracture risk screening tools, such as Mirels' Classification Scoring System and the World Health Organization screening tool (FRAX), may help clinicians identify patients that require exercise modifications.[5,26] Clinicians and patients should be aware that one randomized controlled trial demonstrated bisphosphonates to be superior compared to exercise alone in preventing bone loss during breast cancer treatment.[58] However, a subsequent study comparing a combination of guided paravertebral muscle resistance training, bisphosphonate, and radiation therapy to bisphosphonates and radiation therapy without resistance exercise showed significantly increased bone density in the area of stable spinal osteolytic metastases in the resistance exercise group, with no increased risk of fracture or disease progression.[59]

OSTEOPENIA/OSTEOPOROSIS

Osteopenia and osteoporosis in breast cancer patients can be caused by the cancer itself, as a separate disease process or a side effect of treatments such as chemotherapy, aromatase inhibitors, and steroids.[5,15] Chemotherapy regimens, especially those including cyclophosphamide, methotrexate, and fluorouracil, can lead to bone loss by causing premature ovarian failure.[48] The use of steroids alone significantly increases the risk for fractures.[5] Tamoxifen, while preserving bone mineral density in postmenopausal women, can act as an estrogen antagonist in premenopausal women and actually increase bone loss. Severe decreases in bone mineral density may require dose reduction of drug therapy, potentially affecting survival.[6] Research supports both aerobic and resistance exercises having beneficial effects on bone mineral density.[4] It is recommended that all women with osteoporosis perform both impact and resistance exercises regularly to maintain bone integrity.[4,40,48] Patients are encouraged to, at minimum, continue their current daily and functional activities to preserve bone mass, as bone loss occurs rapidly with unloading and is difficult to regain.[5]

Cardiovascular Health

Breast cancer patients are at increased risk of cardiovascular dysfunction due to effects of chemotherapy, radiation, weight gain, and inactivity. Some of the most commonly used chemotherapeutic agents to treat breast cancer, Doxorubicin (DOX) and trastuzumab, cause dose-dependent cardiotoxicity, especially when given concurrently or sequentially.[48,60] Cardiotoxicity is a common reason for dose reduction or discontinuation of chemotherapy, and there are currently no preventative treatments. Manifestation of cardiotoxicity from DOX and/or trastuzumab may be delayed for many years so it is important for clinicians and therapists to be aware of a patient's treatment history in order to identify symptoms such as dyspnea, shortness of breath, and edema promptly.[26,60] Animal studies show that exercise offers cardioprotection in animals receiving DOX; however, there are few studies examining animals given both DOX and trastuzumab.[60] The REHAB trial showed initial evidence that aerobic exercise training can improve cardiopulmonary function in postmenopausal breast cancer survivors.[40] Another trial by van Waart et al. showed that patients in a high-intensity exercise program better tolerate trastuzumab treatment, indicating a possible cardioprotective effect of exercise on trastuzumab cardiotoxicity.[20]

Cytopenias

Cytopenias due to breast cancer treatment will be monitored and treated by the patient's oncologist; however, it is important for patients, therapists, and trainers to be aware of safety precautions and exercise modifications in order to prevent injuries and adverse events. Patients with anemia should be monitored for symptoms such as dyspnea, fatigue, palpitations, and dizziness. Exercise intensity should be adjusted so that patients are symptom free. Severe anemia, defined as a hemoglobin less than 6 g/dL, is a relative contraindication to exercise and may require treatment with a blood transfusion prior to resuming activity. Patients with leukopenia are at increased risk for infection and should therefore follow strict hygiene precautions. Some may prefer to exercise at home so as not to expose themselves to contaminants at a public facility.[26] Patients who receive granulocyte-colony-stimulating factor injections to prevent leukopenia may develop musculoskeletal and bone pain within 2 days after injection and may need intensity reduction or rest during this time.[19] Lastly, thrombocytopenia puts patients at increased risk for bleeding. Patients should avoid high-impact, high-intensity exercise and be monitored for bruising or bleeding. A platelet count of <20,000/μL is a contraindication for exercise; however, patients may tolerate light walking and activities of daily living.[19,26]

Chemotherapy-Related Neurotoxicity

Patients undergoing treatment for cancer may receive chemotherapeutic agents that cause significant neurotoxicity, both in the central and peripheral nervous systems. The most common neurotoxic chemotherapeutic agents used to treat breast cancer include cisplatin, carboplatin, paclitaxel, fluorouracil, and cyclophosphamide[61] (see Table 3.6). Many neurotoxic effects of chemotherapy are seen in the immediate treatment period, are dose-dependent, and can resolve. However, with more patients participating in rehabilitation and exercise during treatment, it is important to be aware of them so that they can be identified and treated promptly.[62] These symptoms can be debilitating and often require dose reduction and/or cessation of chemotherapy, potentially limiting the possibility for cure.[48]

The most prevalent long-term neurotoxic effect of chemotherapy is chemotherapy-induced peripheral neuropathy (CIPN). Cisplatin, carboplatin, and paclitaxel are the most likely to cause peripheral neuropathy that can manifest as paresthesias, numbness, pain, and muscle cramps or weakness.[61] Patients with CIPN may also exhibit gait dysfunction caused by decreased proprioceptive sensory feedback, characterized by shorter, slower steps, and shorter strides.[63] CIPN symptoms lead to functional deficits, increased risk of falls and reduced quality of life.[61,63] Two-thirds of women undergoing chemotherapy will experience CIPN within the first month of treatment, and nearly half of women who develop CIPN will continue to report symptoms for an average of 6 years.[6,63] Modifiable risk factors for developing CIPN, including obesity and sedentary lifestyle, have potential to be improved with a regular exercise regimen.[63] While there are currently no drugs to prevent CIPN, animal and human studies provide evidence that exercise is a viable and safe nonpharmacologic therapy that can mitigate some of the neurotoxic effects of chemotherapy.[6,48,61,64] Mechanisms of the neuroprotective effect of exercise may be related to improved muscle strength, muscle reinnervation, and axonal regeneration.[6] Compared to aerobic and resistance exercises, balance training during static and dynamic movement has been shown to be the most beneficial for CIPN and should be incorporated into exercise routines for these patients.[65,66] Winters-Stone et al. support a functional approach to CIPN, emphasizing early recognition and referral to rehabilitation, teaching compensatory strategies, and engaging in task-specific exercises in order to preserve independence and reduce falls.[63] Paclitaxel acute pain syndrome (PAPS) is a distinct neuropathy from CIPN, causing predominantly sensory symptoms during paclitaxel treatment. Although symptoms of PAPS generally resolve within a week, patients may need exercise modifications in the interim.[67]

Cognitive impairments due to chemotherapy, the so-called chemo brain, can negatively impact breast cancer patients participating in an exercise program before, during, or after treatment. Cognitive impairment occurs in 10%–50% of women undergoing treatment for breast cancer but is also frequently observed before patients have received any systemic chemotherapy.[68,69]

TABLE 3.6
Commonly Used Neurotoxic Chemotherapies in Primary Breast Cancer

Drug	Central Nervous System	Peripheral Nervous System
Cisplatin	Rare: encephalopathy, headache, stroke seizures	Sensory peripheral neuropathy (off-therapy worsening): numbness, paresthesia, decreased vibratory sensation and loss of proprioception Lhermitte's sign Muscle cramps
Carboplatin	Rare: cortical blindness	Sensory peripheral neuropathy
Paclitaxel	Rare: acute encephalopathy, seizures	Sensorimotor peripheral neuropathy: paresthesia, numbness, neuropathic pain in hands and/or feet, myalgia, proximal muscle weakness
Fluorouracil (5-FU)	Rare: cerebellar dysfunction, inflammatory leukoencephalopathy	Rare: peripheral neuropathy
Cyclophosphamide	Rare: blurred vision, confusion	None

Rehabilitation professionals should screen patients for cognitive impairment prior to prescribing unsupervised exercise regimens to breast cancer patients, as oftentimes cognitive impairment goes undiagnosed. Appropriate referral for neuropsychological testing is warranted if cognitive impairment is suspected.[69] Although a systemic review by Zimmer et al. concluded that yoga-based interventions may improve self-perceived cognition after chemotherapy for breast cancer patients, there are currently no forms of physical activity definitively shown to mitigate the development of or improve cancer-related cognitive impairment.[14,70] Patients with cognitive impairment should be taught coping strategies, such as practical reminders.[71]

Postsurgical Limitations

Surgical interventions, such as lumpectomy, mastectomy, sentinel and axillary lymph node dissection, and breast reconstruction, are integral parts of the treatment protocol for breast cancer and can impact participation in exercise programs. Gynecological cancer patients also frequently undergo surgical intervention, including lymph node dissections. Common postoperative limitations to exercise include pain, drain placement, surgical site infections, and activity restrictions due to muscle flap reconstruction.[19] Patients need adequate time for healing after surgery before safely starting an exercise program; however, gentle breathing and mobilization exercises should start in the immediate postoperative period to prevent shoulder immobility, protective posturing, and functional decline.[72–74] Wound drains may need to be kept in for longer periods of time if shoulder and arm exercises are started within the first few days of surgery.[75] For patients undergoing latissimus dorsi flaps, contraction or stretching of the latissimus dorsi or pectoralis major muscle should be avoided until complete wound healing has occurred.[76] Patients who undergo breast reconstruction with tissue expanders will need exercise modifications due to limited range of motion of the shoulder. They should initially avoid exercises that stress the pectoral muscles, such as overhead lifting. In general, patients should avoid extreme shoulder flexion and abduction, heavy weight lifting, and jumping/jogging activities until cleared by their surgical team.[73]

Medical Devices

Peripherally inserted central catheters (PICCs) and port-a-catheters are commonly inserted venous access devices used for administration of chemotherapy, antibiotics, artificial nutrition, and other medical therapies. These devices need to be monitored regularly while patients are participating in exercise. Standard of care hygiene precautions should be maintained with regular dressing changes and appropriate securement. Patients with port-a-catheters should avoid heavy lifting and swimming for about 2 weeks after placement to ensure proper healing and prevent infection. Contact sports should also be avoided so as not to injure the site. For PICCs, patients may need to modify exercises in order to prevent migration of the catheter.[19] Generally, patients with PICCs are advised to avoid lifting heavy objects or weights, excessive movement of the arm, and getting the site wet or soiled. These precautions are intended to decrease the rate of catheter migration, breakage, or infection; however, there are no studies that examine the rate of these complications when adult patients engage in exercise.

ARM AND SHOULDER DYSFUNCTION

Lymphedema

Lymphedema is a chronic, painful, and disabling complication of breast and gynecological cancer treatments that can negatively impact function and quality of life.[6] It is characterized by abnormal accumulation of protein-rich fluid in tissues due to damage or inefficiency of the lymphatic system. The old dogma of lymphedema management was to limit use of the affected limb as this was believed to protect from injury or exacerbation. Conversely, we now know that disuse of the limb can lead to worsening pain, swelling, weakness, and disability. Unfortunately, patients today continue to receive inaccurate information, leading to fear of using the affected limb. It is the job of the medical and rehabilitation team to educate patients about lymphedema and encourage participation in safe and beneficial exercise.[77]

A slowly progressive weight lifting program has been proven safe for patients with stable breast cancer–related lymphedema of all grades and may lessen the incidence of exacerbations.[78] Even high-load, moderate-to-high intensity upper body resistance training has been shown to be safe, well tolerated and may improve symptoms of arm tightness in patients with stable lymphedema.[79,80] Resistance exercise has been proven safe in women at risk for lymphedema, and there is also preliminary evidence that it may improve and/or prevent upper extremity lymphedema.[81,82] Lacomba et al. found that a program of early physiotherapy with manual lymph drainage initiated in the immediate postoperative period may prevent lymphedema from developing.[83] The mechanism proposed is by improving both functional capacity and lymph flow via the muscle pumping effect.[84] Based on available data, it is recommended that a weight lifting program be initiated under the guidance of a trained fitness professional, with close medical follow-up to monitor for signs or symptoms of exacerbations.[51] Patients should receive medical clearance prior to starting a resistance exercise program, with considerations, including patient motivation, recent treatment for lymphedema exacerbation (antibiotics or decongestive therapy), and other medical/neurologic conditions that may limit participation.[78] After undergoing initial instruction regarding proper exercise technique, patients may continue their resistance training program unsupervised.[84] For patients with a history of lymphedema, it is recommended that compression garments be worn during resistance training; however, more research is needed to investigate if these garments are truly necessary to prevent worsening of lymphedema.[84–86] Patients who are at risk or who currently have stable breast cancer–related lymphedema should be encouraged to engage in an exercise program that includes upper body resistance training. Statistically, significant improvements in muscular strength, muscular endurance, and quality of life have been observed in as little as 3 months of twice weekly, 60-minute exercise sessions.[56] While an optimal and standardized protocol of resistance training for those with breast cancer–related lymphedema does not currently exist, there have been multiple variations studied that have been proven safe and effective.[84] The protocol from The Physical Activity and Lymphedema Trial by Schmitz et al. is provided to patients for free via the LIVESTRONG program in YMCAs across the United States.[81]

In addition to resistance training, the National Lymphedema Network states that patients with lymphedema can participate in any type of exercise as long as general safety precautions are followed and patients have regular medical follow-up.[86] Aerobic exercise has been proven feasible and safe in patients with or at risk for lymphedema, although whether it too can affect the course of lymphedema remains to be determined.[4,86] Lymphedema remedial exercises are rhythmic muscle and breathing exercises that are a component of the primary treatment for lymphedema, complex decongestive therapy, and can be integrated into exercise routines.[86] Flexibility exercises are important to preserve range of motion and reduce adhesions from surgery or radiation.[6,73] Pilates is another feasible form of exercise for breast cancer survivors and may improve symptoms of lymphedema and self-reported upper extremity function; however, more research is needed to determine if it is superior to other forms of exercise.[87]

Secondary lower extremity lymphedema is a progressive and debilitating condition that is distinct from upper extremity lymphedema in a number of ways. First, there are significant differences in functional anatomy between the lymphatic systems of arms and legs that must be considered. Second, patients undergoing treatment for gynecological cancer and subsequently developing secondary lower extremity lymphedema tend to be older than breast cancer patients who develop upper extremity lymphedema. And finally, losing use of one or both lower extremities have a considerably greater impact on completing activities of daily living compared to losing use of one arm.[88] A conservative estimate is that one out of every five patients who undergo chemotherapy, radiation, and/or surgical treatment for gynecological cancer will develop secondary lower extremity lymphedema.[89,90] Risk factors for its development include receiving adjuvant radiation, being obese, and having a greater number of lymph nodes removed.[90] Efforts should be made for prevention, early recognition, and regular monitoring for progression and/or flares.[89] A pilot study by Katz et al. provided evidence that weight lifting in patients with secondary lower extremity lymphedema to cancer is feasible and can improve lower body strength and endurance, although 2 out of 10 participants developed cellulitis during the study, limiting conclusions regarding safety. Of note, participants showed significant improvements in balance and dorsiflexion of the affected limb.[88] A randomized controlled crossover trial by Fukushima et al. compared high-load active exercise with compression therapy (AECT), low-load AECT, and compression-only therapy (CT) in patients with International Society of Lymphology stage II and late-stage II lymphedema secondary to gynecological cancer treatment. They found that high-load AECT significantly reduced lower limb volume compared to after CT. And although there was no significant difference between improvement of symptoms such as pain and skin tightness between the groups, there was evidence that patients with more marked pitting edema and/or harder skin may benefit more from AECT compared to those with milder skin signs.[89] Subsequently, a 6-month randomized controlled trial of 95 ovarian cancer survivors showed no difference in risk of developing lower extremity lymphedema with moderate-intensity aerobic exercise and no adverse events of participating in the intervention.[90] A specific aqua-lymphatic therapy protocol that consisted of breathing exercises, self-massage, and remedial exercises in warm water was shown to be safe for patients with both primary and secondary lower extremity lymphedema, with significantly greater improvements in edema, functional level, quality of life, and concern about the future compared to controls.[91] These preliminary studies highlight the need for further investigation to clarify the safety, potential benefits, and activity guidelines of exercise for patients with or at risk for secondary lower extremity lymphedema.

AXILLARY WEB SYNDROME

Axillary web syndrome (AWS) is a distressing, poorly understood, and often overlooked and underreported postoperative complication of both axillary lymph node dissection and sentinel lymph node biopsy. The hallmark of this condition is the presence of tight, painful cord(s) within the subcutaneous tissue of the axilla, which can radiate down the medial ipsilateral arm and/or over the ipsilateral chest wall. Shoulder abduction will cause painful tightening of the cord(s).[92] Not only do these cords cause pain but also functional limitations, altered cosmesis, psychological distress, and impaired quality of life.[93] Risk factors include lower BMI, younger age, greater number of lymph nodes removed, more extensive surgery, and receiving adjunctive chemotherapy and radiation. Classically, the condition was thought to occur in the early postoperative period (2–8 weeks) but resolve spontaneously within 3 months after surgery and without any long-term impairment. However, more recent literature has indicated that the condition can develop, recur, and continue to impair function for months to years after surgery.[93,94] The incidence and prevalence are likely higher than previously thought, estimated at around 50%. While the condition itself can limit participation in exercise, there is quality evidence indicating that early rehabilitative interventions can reduce both duration and morbidity. The primary treatment for AWS is a physical therapy program that includes patient education, range of motion exercises, and gentle manual therapies such as myofascial release, soft tissue mobilization, cord manipulation, and stretching. Exercises focusing on joint mobilization of the shoulder, scapula, rib, clavicle, and upper back are encouraged. Manual lymphatic drainage (MLD) can also be helpful if there is comorbid lymphedema.[94] One large, randomized controlled trial concluded that a gradually progressive exercise regimen plus MLD was more effective at preventing AWS than MLD alone; however, the study did not mention if incidence of lymphedema was assessed.[95]

Radiation Related

Patients undergoing radiation therapy for breast cancer should be aware of possible complications such as skin changes, brachial plexopathy, lymphedema, cardiovascular changes, and fatigue. The safety considerations and specific beneficial exercises for lymphedema, cardiotoxicity, and fatigue are covered elsewhere in this chapter. For patients with skin-related changes from radiation therapy, general hygiene precautions should be followed to avoid infection.[19] Due to wide ranges of severity, precautions for exercise will vary. Radiation-induced cutaneous reactions can be acute or chronic, with some chemotherapeutic agents causing an acute inflammatory reaction in an area of previous radiation. It may take months to years after radiation therapy until chronic radiation dermatitis will appear. Those with open wounds, ulcerations, or burns should avoid swimming. For patients with radiation-induced fibrosis, physical therapy, including active and passive range of motion, may help to prevent contracture.[96] Patients may need to avoid activities that put pressure or constrict the treated region.[19] Brachial plexopathy is a rare side effect of radiation that can present with paresthesia, hypesthesia, weakness, decreased muscle stretch reflexes, and pain. These patients may need referral to specialized neurorehabilitation.[48,97]

Psychosocial

Receiving a breast cancer diagnosis is a devastating life event and can have numerous psychological effects on a patient, not limited to anxiety, depression, sleep disturbance, poor body image, poor self-esteem, and reduced quality of life.[6,98,99] Physical effects of cancer and its treatment such as pain and fatigue can worsen these conditions. Socioeconomic factors such as loss of employment, financial hardship due to medical costs and childcare difficulties also contribute.[6] Not surprisingly, exercise has been shown to have a positive impact on symptoms of depression and anxiety in breast cancer patients. Supervised, higher frequency and longer duration exercise had a greater impact on these symptoms. Exercise, especially resistance training, is also an excellent way to improve self-esteem and body image.[6] Aerobic exercise has numerous effects on sleep and has been shown to improve sleep duration, architecture, and quality.[100] The physiological effects of exercise on sleep are via antiinflammatory effects and temperature regulation.[6,15] There is also evidence that yoga can promote better sleep in cancer patients.[6]

Returning to work has numerous benefits for cancer patients, both financially and psychologically.[101] Patients' likelihood of returning to work can depend on nonmodifiable factors such as their cancer site and invasiveness of their cancer treatment.[102] Modifiable positive prognostic factors include lower fatigue levels, higher value of work, workability, and job self-efficacy.[103] Unfortunately, there is currently a lack of high-quality interventional studies regarding the impact of rehabilitation and exercise interventions on the outcome of return to work for breast and gynecological cancer patients.[104] Leensen et al. demonstrated feasibility of a multidisciplinary intervention to improve return to work rates for cancer survivors, consisting of occupational counseling and physical exercise. However, the patients who participated were all highly motivated prior to any intervention.[103]

CONCLUSION

With new and improved therapies for breast and gynecological cancers increasing survival, research efforts are now directed at addressing the management of long-term treatment sequelae and maximizing functional independence in these patients. As described in this chapter, exercise has been shown to positively impact nearly every stage and complication of cancer. Therefore cancer patients should engage in a regular exercise program consisting of aerobic, resistance, bone strengthening, and flexibility and balance training (Table 3.7). Exercise is safe in this population, and patients should aim for the same intensities and frequencies recommended of the general public, with modifications as needed based on their specific needs. Physicians, other health-care providers, community programs, and family support are crucial to minimizing the many barriers to exercise adherence that cancer patients encounter. Patients should have regular medical follow-up while participating in an exercise program, to promptly identify and treat the numerous medical and surgical complications that may arise from cancer itself and its treatment. Research to elucidate an exact exercise "prescription" to address each patient's individual needs is ongoing. In the interim, patients should be educated on evidence-based and common-sense guidelines for exercise, encouraged and

TABLE 3.7
Sample Supervised Exercise Protocol for Patients with Breast Cancer

Type of exercise	Examples	Frequency	Intensity	Duration
 Aerobic exercise	Walking jogging cycling rowing	2–3x/wk	50%–80% VO2max Borg score 12–16	20–30 min
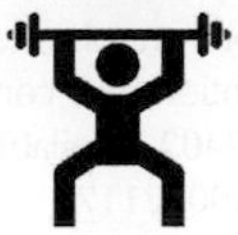 Muscle strengthening	Free weights body weight machines	2–3x/wk	60%–80% of 1RM	Two sets of 8–12 repetitions Major upper and lower limb muscle groups
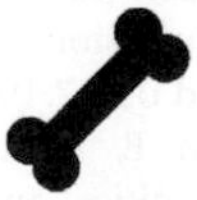 Bone strengthening	Resistance exercise weight bearing (e.g., running, jumping)	At least 2 days a week	The same as for aerobic and muscle strengthening	Can be combined with aerobic/muscle strengthening
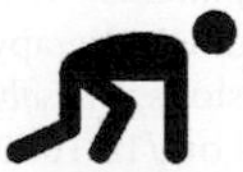 Balance training	Tai Chi Yoga	At least 2 days a week	Will vary depending on individual needs	Will vary depending on individual needs
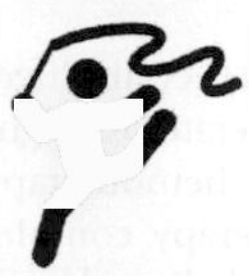 Flexibility training	Stretching Yoga	At minimum, on days that other exercises are performed	Will vary depending on individual needs	Stretch all major muscle groups

RM, Repetition Maximum; wk, week.

supported through all cancer stages, and referred to community resources and cancer rehabilitation specialists when warranted.

PATIENT RESOURCES

- National Lymphedema Network: https://lymphnet.org/
- LIVESTRONG at the YMCA: 12 week physical activity program for cancer survivors: https://www.livestrong.org/what-we-do/program/livestrong-at-the-ymca
- The Physical Activity Guidelines for Americans: https://www.hhs.gov/fitness/be-active/physical-activity-guidelines-for-americans/index.html
- National Comprehensive Cancer Network (NCCN) Patient Guides for Cancer App: https://www.nccn.org/apps/

REFERENCES

1. Courneya KS, Segal RJ, Mackey JR, et al. Effects of aerobic and resistance exercise in breast cancer patients receiving adjuvant chemotherapy: a multicenter randomized controlled trial. *J Clin Oncol*. 2007;25(28):4396–4404. Available from: https://doi.org/10.1200/JCO.2006.08.2024.
2. McNeely ML, Campbell KL, Rowe BH, Klassen TP, Mackey JR, Courneya KS. Effects of exercise on breast cancer patients and survivors: a systematic review and meta-analysis. *Can Med Assoc J*. 2006;175(1):34–41. Available from: https://doi.org/10.1503/cmaj.051073.
3. Loprinzi PD, Cardinal BJ, Winters-Stone K, Smit E, Loprinzi CL. Physical activity and the risk of breast cancer recurrence: a literature review. *Oncol Nurs Forum*. 2012;39(3):269–274. Available from: https://doi.org/10.1188/12.ONF.269-274.
4. Schmitz KH, Courneya KS, Matthews C, et al. American College of Sports Medicine roundtable on exercise guidelines for cancer survivors. *Med Sci Sports Exerc*. 2010;42(7):1409–1426. Available from: https://doi.org/10.1249/MSS.0b013e3181e0c112.
5. Sheill G, Guinan EM, Peat N, Hussey J. Considerations for exercise prescription in patients with bone metastases: a comprehensive narrative review. *PM R*. 2018;843–864. Available from: https://doi.org/10.1016/j.pmrj.2018.02.006.
6. Ferioli M, Zauli G, Martelli AM, et al. Impact of physical exercise in cancer survivors during and after antineoplastic treatments. *Oncotarget*. 2018;9(17):14005–14034. Available from: https://doi.org/10.18632/oncotarget.24456.
7. Department of Health & Human Services. *Physical Activity Guidelines Advisory Committee Scientific Report*; 2018. Available from: https://doi.org/10.1111/j.1753-4887.2008.00136.x>.
8. Byrne NM, Hills AP, Hunter GR, Weinsier RL, Schutz Y. Metabolic equivalent: one size does not fit all. *J Appl Physiol*. 2005;99(3):1112–1119. Available from: https://doi.org/10.1152/japplphysiol.00023.2004.
9. Piercy KL, Troiano RP, Ballard RM, et al. The physical activity guidelines for Americans. *JAMA*. 2013;202:56–63. Available from: https://doi.org/10.1001/jama.2018.14854.
10. Monninkhof EM, Elias SG, Vlems FA, et al. Physical activity and breast cancer: a systematic review. *Epidemiology*. 2007;18(1):137–157. Available from: https://doi.org/10.1097/01.ede.0000251167.75581.98.
11. Friedenreich CM. The role of physical activity in breast cancer etiology. *Semin Oncol*. 2010. Available from: https://doi.org/10.1053/j.seminoncol.2010.05.008.
12. Esfahbodi A, Fathi M, Rahimi GR. Changes of CEA and CA15-3 biomarkers in the breast cancer patients following eight weeks of aerobic exercise. *Basic Clin Cancer Res J*. 2018;9:4–12.
13. Kang DW, Lee J, Suh SH, Ligibel J, Courneya KS, Jeon JY. Effects of exercise on insulin, IGF axis, adipocytokines, and inflammatory markers in breast cancer survivors: a systematic review and meta-analysis. *Cancer Epidemiol Biomarkers Prev*. 2017;26(3):355–365. Available from: https://doi.org/10.1158/1055-9965.EPI-16-0602.
14. Wirtz P, Baumann FT. Physical activity, exercise and breast cancer—what is the evidence for rehabilitation, aftercare, and survival? A review. *Breast Care*. 2018;13(2):93–101. Available from: https://doi.org/10.1159/000488717.
15. Adraskela K, Veisaki E, Koutsilieris M, Philippou A. Physical exercise positively influences breast cancer evolution. *Clin Breast Cancer*. 2017;17(6):408–417. Available from: https://doi.org/10.1016/j.clbc.2017.05.003.
16. Lynch BM, Neilson HK. Physical activity and breast cancer prevention. *Phys Act Cancer*. 2011;186:13–42. Available from: https://doi.org/10.1007/978-3-642-04231-7_2.
17. Patel AV, Friedenreich CM, Moore SC, et al. American College of Sports Medicine roundtable report on physical activity, sedentary behavior, and cancer prevention and control. *Med Sci Sports Exerc*. 2019;51(11):2391–2402. Available from: https://doi.org/10.1249/MSS.0000000000002117.
18. *NCCN*. NCCN guidelines for supportive care: cancer-related fatigue. <https://www.nccn.org/professionals/physician_gls/pdf/fatigue.pdf>; 2019 Accessed 03.07.19.
19. van der Leeden M, Huijsmans RJ, Geleijn E, et al. Tailoring exercise interventions to comorbidities and treatment-induced adverse effects in patients with early stage breast cancer undergoing chemotherapy: a framework to support clinical decisions. *Disabil Rehabil*. 2018. Available from: https://doi.org/10.1080/09638288.2016.1260647.
20. Van Waart H, Stuiver MM, Van Harten WH, et al. Effect of low-intensity physical activity and moderate- to high-intensity physical exercise during adjuvant chemotherapy on physical fitness, fatigue, and chemotherapy completion rates: results of the PACES randomized clinical trial.

J Clin Oncol. 2015. Available from: https://doi.org/10.1200/JCO.2014.59.1081.
21. Biganzoli E, Desmedt C, Fornili M, et al. Recurrence dynamics of breast cancer according to baseline body mass index. *Eur J Cancer*. 2017. Available from: https://doi.org/10.1016/j.ejca.2017.10.007.
22. Cheville AL, McLaughlin SA, Haddad TC, Lyons KD, Newman R, Ruddy KJ. Integrated rehabilitation for breast cancer survivors. *Am J Phys Med Rehabil*. 2019;98(2):154–164. Available from: https://doi.org/10.1097/PHM.0000000000001017.
23. Ibrahim EM, Al-Homaidh A. Physical activity and survival after breast cancer diagnosis: meta-analysis of published studies. *Med Oncol*. 2011. Available from: https://doi.org/10.1007/s12032-010-9536-x.
24. Lahart IM, Metsios GS, Nevill AM, Carmichael AR. Physical activity, risk of death and recurrence in breast cancer survivors: a systematic review and meta-analysis of epidemiological studies. *Acta Oncol (Madr)*. 2015. Available from: https://doi.org/10.3109/0284186X.2014.998275.
25. Courneya KS, McKenzie DC, Mackey JR, et al. Effects of exercise dose and type during breast cancer chemotherapy: multicenter randomized trial. *J Natl Cancer Inst*. 2013. Available from: https://doi.org/10.1093/jnci/djt297.
26. Maltser S, Cristian A, Silver JK, Morris GS, Stout NL. A focused review of safety considerations in cancer rehabilitation. *PM R*. 2017. Available from: https://doi.org/10.1016/j.pmrj.2017.08.403.
27. Phillips SM, Dodd KW, Steeves J, McClain J, Alfano CM, McAuley E. Physical activity and sedentary behavior in breast cancer survivors: new insight into activity patterns and potential intervention targets. *Gynecol Oncol*. 2015. Available from: https://doi.org/10.1016/j.ygyno.2015.05.026.
28. Kolden GG, Strauman TJ, Ward A, et al. A pilot study of group exercise training (GET) for women with primary breast cancer: feasibility and health benefits. *Psychooncology*. 2002;11(5):447–456. Available from: https://doi.org/10.1002/pon.591.
29. Park JH, Lee J, Oh M, et al. The effect of oncologists' exercise recommendations on the level of exercise and quality of life in survivors of breast and colorectal cancer: a randomized controlled trial. *Cancer*. 2015. Available from: https://doi.org/10.1002/cncr.29400.
30. Mateo GF, Granado-Font E, Ferré-Grau C, Montaña-Carreras X. Mobile phone apps to promote weight loss and increase physical activity: a systematic review and meta-analysis. *J Med Internet Res*. 2015;17(11):1–11. Available from: https://doi.org/10.2196/jmir.4836.
31. Haberlin C, O'Dwyer T, Mockler D, Moran J, O'Donnell DM, Broderick J. The use of eHealth to promote physical activity in cancer survivors: a systematic review. *Support Care Cancer*. 2018;26(10):3323–3336. Available from: https://doi.org/10.1007/s00520-018-4305-z.
32. Organization WH. mHealth: new horizons for health through mobile technologies. *Observatory*. 2011. Available from: https://doi.org/10.4258/hir.2012.18.3.231.
33. Phillips SM, Courneya KS, Welch WA, et al. Breast cancer survivors' preferences for mHealth physical activity interventions: findings from a mixed methods study. *J Cancer Surviv*. 2019;13(2):292–305. Available from: https://doi.org/10.1007/s11764-019-00751-3.
34. Uhm KE, Yoo JS, Chung SH, et al. Effects of exercise intervention in breast cancer patients: is mobile health (mHealth) with pedometer more effective than conventional program using brochure? *Breast Cancer Res Treat*. 2017;161(3):443–452. Available from: https://doi.org/10.1007/s10549-016-4065-8.
35. Lee BJ, Park YH, Lee JY, Kim SJ, Jang Y, Lee JI. Smartphone application versus pedometer to promote physical activity in prostate cancer patients. *Telemed J E Health*. 2019;25(12):1231–1236. Available from: https://doi.org/10.1089/tmj.2018.0233.
36. Bower JE, Lamkin DM. Inflammation and cancer-related fatigue: mechanisms, contributing factors, and treatment implications. *Brain Behav Immun*. 2013. Available from: https://doi.org/10.1016/j.bbi.2012.06.011.
37. Bower JE. Cancer-related fatigue—mechanisms, risk factors, and treatments. *Nat Rev Clin Oncol*. 2014. Available from: https://doi.org/10.1038/nrclinonc.2014.127.
38. Fagundes CP, Murray DM, Hwang BS, et al. Sympathetic and parasympathetic activity in cancer-related fatigue: more evidence for a physiological substrate in cancer survivors. *Psychoneuroendocrinology*. 2011. Available from: https://doi.org/10.1016/j.psyneuen.2011.02.005.
39. Mustian KM, Alfano CM, Heckler C, et al. Comparison of pharmaceutical, psychological, and exercise treatments for cancer-related fatigue: a meta-analysis. *JAMA Oncol*. 2017. Available from: https://doi.org/10.1001/jamaoncol.2016.6914.
40. Courneya KS, Mackey JR, Bell GJ, Jones LW, Field CJ, Fairey AS. Randomized controlled trial of exercise training in postmenopausal breast cancer survivors: cardiopulmonary and quality of life outcomes. *J Clin Oncol*. 2003. Available from: https://doi.org/10.1200/JCO.2003.04.093.
41. Headley JA, Ownby KK, John LD. The effect of seated exercise on fatigue and quality of life in women with advanced breast cancer. *Oncol Nurs Forum*. 2004;31(5):977–983. Available from: https://doi.org/10.1188/04.ONF.977-983.
42. Meneses-Echávez JF, González-Jiménez E, Ramírez-Vélez R. Effects of supervised exercise on cancer-related fatigue in breast cancer survivors: a systematic review and meta-analysis. *BMC Cancer*. 2015;15(1):1–13. Available from: https://doi.org/10.1186/s12885-015-1069-4.
43. Kiecolt-Glaser JK, Bennett JM, Andridge R, et al. Yoga's impact on inflammation, mood, and fatigue in breast cancer survivors: a randomized controlled trial. *J Clin Oncol*. 2014. Available from: https://doi.org/10.1200/JCO.2013.51.8860.
44. Sprod LK, Fernandez ID, Janelsins MC, et al. Effects of yoga on cancer-related fatigue and global side-effect burden in older cancer survivors. *J Geriatr Oncol*. 2015. Available from: https://doi.org/10.1016/j.jgo.2014.09.184.

45. Sadja J, Mills PJ. Effects of yoga interventions on fatigue in cancer patients and survivors: a systematic review of randomized controlled trials. *Explor J Sci Heal*. 2013. Available from: https://doi.org/10.1016/j.explore.2013.04.005.
46. Stan DL, Croghan KA, Croghan IT, Jenkins SM, Sutherland SJ, Cheville AL. Randomized pilot trial of yoga versus strengthening exercises in breast cancer survivors with cancer-related fatigue. *Support Care Cancer*. 2016;24.
47. Bower JE, Garet D, Sternlieb B, et al. Yoga for persistent fatigue in breast cancer survivors: a randomized controlled trial. *Cancer*. 2012. Available from: https://doi.org/10.1002/cncr.26702.
48. Shapiro CL, Recht A. Side effects of adjuvant treatment of breast cancer. *N Engl J Med*. 2001. Available from: https://doi.org/10.1056/NEJM200106283442607.
49. Calle EE, Kaaks R. Overweight, obesity and cancer: epidemiological evidence and proposed mechanisms. *Nat Rev Cancer*. 2004. Available from: https://doi.org/10.1038/nrc1408.
50. Melstrom LG, Melstrom KA, Ding XZ, Adrian TE. Mechanisms of skeletal muscle degradation and its therapy in cancer cachexia. *Histol Histopathol*. 2007. Available from: https://doi.org/10.14670/HH-22.805.
51. Schmitz KH, Ahmed RL, Hannan PJ, Yee D. Safety and efficacy of weight training in recent breast cancer survivors to alter body composition, insulin, and insulin-like growth factor axis proteins. *Cancer Epidemiol Biomarkers Prev*. 2005;14(7):1672–1680. Available from: https://doi.org/10.1158/1055-9965.EPI-04-0736.
52. Montalvo RN, Counts BR, Carson JA. Understanding sex differences in the regulation of cancer-induced muscle wasting. *Curr Opin Support Palliat Care*. 2018;12(4):394–403. Available from: https://doi.org/10.1097/SPC.0000000000000380.
53. Lira FS, Rosa JC, Zanchi NE, et al. Regulation of inflammation in the adipose tissue in cancer cachexia: effect of exercise. *Cell Biochem Funct*. 2009. Available from: https://doi.org/10.1002/cbf.1540.
54. Pulido C, Vendrell I, Ferreira AR, et al. Bone metastasis risk factors in breast cancer. *Ecancermedicalscience*. 2017. Available from: https://doi.org/10.3332/ecancer.2017.715.
55. Kennecke H, Yerushalmi R, Woods R, et al. Metastatic behavior of breast cancer subtypes. *J Clin Oncol*. 2010. Available from: https://doi.org/10.1200/JCO.2009.25.9820.
56. Cormie P, Newton RU, Spry N, Joseph D, Taaffe DR, Galvão DA. Safety and efficacy of resistance exercise in prostate cancer patients with bone metastases. *Prostate Cancer Prostatic Dis*. 2013. Available from: https://doi.org/10.1038/pcan.2013.22.
57. Ligibel JA, Giobbie-Hurder A, Shockro L, et al. Randomized trial of a physical activity intervention in women with metastatic breast cancer. *Cancer*. 2016. Available from: https://doi.org/10.1002/cncr.29899.
58. Swenson KK, Nissen MJ, Anderson E, Shapiro A, Schouboe J, Leach J. Effects of exercise vs bisphosphonates on bone mineral density in breast cancer patients receiving chemotherapy. *J Support Oncol*. 2009;7.
59. Rief H, Petersen LC, Omlor G, et al. The effect of resistance training during radiotherapy on spinal bone metastases in cancer patients—a randomized trial. *Radiother Oncol*. 2014. Available from: https://doi.org/10.1016/j.radonc.2014.06.008.
60. Wonders KY, Reigle BS. Trastuzumab and doxorubicin-related cardiotoxicity and the cardioprotective role of exercise. *Integr Cancer Ther*. 2009. Available from: https://doi.org/10.1177/1534735408330717.
61. Verstappen CCP, Heimans JJ, Hoekman K, Postma TJ. Neurotoxic complications of chemotherapy in patients with cancer: clinical signs and optimal management. *Drugs*. 2003. Available from: https://doi.org/10.2165/00003495-200363150-00003.
62. Taillibert S, Le Rhun E, Chamberlain MC. Chemotherapy-related neurotoxicity. *Curr Neurol Neurosci Rep*. 2016. Available from: https://doi.org/10.1007/s11910-016-0686-x.
63. Winters-Stone KM, Horak F, Jacobs PG, et al. Falls, functioning, and disability among women with persistent symptoms of chemotherapy-induced peripheral neuropathy. *J Clin Oncol*. 2017;35(23):2604–2612. Available from: https://doi.org/10.1200/JCO.2016.71.3552.
64. Hensley ML, Hagerty KL, Kewalramani T, et al. American society of clinical oncology 2008 clinical practice guideline update: use of chemotherapy and radiation therapy protectants. *J Clin Oncol*. 2009;27(1):127–145. Available from: https://doi.org/10.1200/JCO.2008.17.2627.
65. Vollmers PL, Mundhenke C, Maass N, et al. Evaluation of the effects of sensorimotor exercise on physical and psychological parameters in breast cancer patients undergoing neurotoxic chemotherapy. *J Cancer Res Clin Oncol*. 2018;144(9):1785–1792. Available from: https://doi.org/10.1007/s00432-018-2686-5.
66. Streckmann F, Zopf EM, Lehmann HC, et al. Exercise intervention studies in patients with peripheral neuropathy: a systematic review. *Sports Med*. 2014. Available from: https://doi.org/10.1007/s40279-014-0207-5.
67. Loprinzi CL, Reeves BN, Dakhil SR, et al. Natural history of paclitaxel-associated acute pain syndrome: prospective cohort study NCCTG N08C1. *J Clin Oncol*. 2011;29(11):1472–1478. Available from: https://doi.org/10.1200/JCO.2010.33.0308.
68. Loh SY, Musa AN. Methods to improve rehabilitation of patients following breast cancer surgery: a review of systematic reviews. *Breast Cancer Targets Ther*. 2015. Available from: https://doi.org/10.2147/BCTT.S47012.
69. Wefel JS, Lenzi R, Theriault R, Buzdar AU, Cruickshank S, Meyers CA. "Chemobrain" in breast carcinoma? A prologue. *Cancer*. 2004;101(3):466–475. Available from: https://doi.org/10.1002/cncr.20393.
70. Zimmer P, Baumann FT, Oberste M, et al. Effects of exercise interventions and physical activity behavior on cancer related cognitive impairments: a systematic review. *Biomed Res Int*. 2016;2016. Available from: https://doi.org/10.1155/2016/1820954.
71. Fisher B, Anderson S, Bryant J, et al. Twenty-year follow-up of a randomized trial comparing total mastectomy, lumpectomy, and lumpectomy plus irradiation for the

treatment of invasive breast cancer. *N Engl J Med.* 2002;347(16):1233–1241. Available from: https://doi.org/10.1056/NEJMoa022152.

72. Scaffidi M, Vulpiani MC, Vetrano M, et al. Early Rehabilitation reduces the onset of complications in the upper limb following breast cancer surgery. *Eur J Phys Rehabil Med.* 2012;48.
73. Wilson DJ. Exercise for the patient after breast cancer surgery. *Semin Oncol Nurs.* 2017. Available from: https://doi.org/10.1016/j.soncn.2016.11.010.
74. Kim M, Lee M, Kim M, Oh S, Jung SP, Yoon B. Effectiveness of therapeutic inflatable ball self-exercises for improving shoulder function and quality of life in breast cancer survivors after sentinel lymph node dissection. *Support Care Cancer.* 2019. Available from: https://doi.org/10.1007/s00520-019-4656-0.
75. McNeely ML, Campbell K, Ospina M, et al. Exercise interventions for upper-limb dysfunction due to breast cancer treatment. *Cochrane Database Syst Rev.* 2010. Available from: https://doi.org/10.1002/14651858.cd005211.pub2.
76. Blackburn NE, Mc Veigh JG, Mc Caughan E, Wilson IM. The musculoskeletal consequences of breast reconstruction using the latissimus dorsi muscle for women following mastectomy for breast cancer: a critical review. *Eur J Cancer Care (Engl).* 2018. Available from: https://doi.org/10.1111/ecc.12664.
77. National Lymphedema Network Medical Advisory Committee. Position Statement of the National Lymphedema Network: Risk Reduction. In: *National Lymphedema Network Position Paper.* 2012:1–7. <https://lymphnet.org/position-papers>.
78. Schmitz KH, Ahmed RL, Troxel A, et al. Weight lifting in women with breast-cancer-related lymphedema. *N Engl J Med.* 2009. Available from: https://doi.org/10.1056/NEJMoa0810118.
79. Cormie P, Pumpa K, Galvão DA, et al. Is it safe and efficacious for women with lymphedema secondary to breast cancer to lift heavy weights during exercise: a randomised controlled trial. *J Cancer Surviv.* 2013;7(3):413–424. Available from: https://doi.org/10.1007/s11764-013-0284-8.
80. Cormie P, Singh B, Hayes S, et al. Acute inflammatory response to low-, moderate-, and high-load resistance exercise in women with breast cancer-related lymphedema. *Integr Cancer Ther.* 2016. Available from: https://doi.org/10.1177/1534735415617283.
81. Schmitz KH, Ahmed RL, Troxel AB, et al. Weight lifting for women at risk for breast cancer-related lymphedema: a randomized trial. *JAMA.* 2010;304(24):2699–2705. Available from: https://doi.org/10.1001/jama.2010.1837.
82. Baumann FT, Reike A, Hallek M, Wiskemann J, Reimer V. Does exercise have a preventive effect on secondary lymphedema in breast cancer patients following local treatment?—a systematic review. *Breast Care.* 2018. Available from: https://doi.org/10.1159/000487428.
83. Lacomba MT, Sánchez MJY, Goñi ÁZ, et al. Effectiveness of early physiotherapy to prevent lymphoedema after surgery for breast cancer: randomised, single blinded, clinical trial. *BMJ.* 2010. Available from: https://doi.org/10.1136/bmj.b5396.
84. Nelson NL. Breast cancer-related lymphedema and resistance exercise: a systematic review. *J Strength Cond Res.* 2016. Available from: https://doi.org/10.1519/JSC.0000000000001355.
85. Singh B, DiSipio T, Peake J, Hayes SC. Systematic review and meta-analysis of the effects of exercise for those with cancer-related lymphedema. *Arch Phys Med Rehabil.* 2016. Available from: https://doi.org/10.1016/j.apmr.2015.09.012.
86. *National Lymphedema Network Medical Advisory Committee.* Position statement of the National Lymphedema Network: exercise. <https://lymphnet.org/position-papers>; 2011.
87. Pinto-Carral A, Molina AJ, Pedro Á, Ayán C. Pilates for women with breast cancer: a systematic review and meta-analysis. *Complement Ther Med.* 2018;41:130–140. Available from: https://doi.org/10.1016/j.ctim.2018.09.011.
88. Katz E, Dugan NL, Cohn JC, Chu C, Smith RG, Schmitz KH. Weight lifting in patients with lower-extremity lymphedema secondary to cancer: a pilot and feasibility study. *Arch Phys Med Rehabil.* 2010;91(7):1070–1076. Available from: https://doi.org/10.1016/j.apmr.2010.03.021.
89. Fukushima T, Tsuji T, Sano Y, et al. Immediate effects of active exercise with compression therapy on lower-limb lymphedema. *Support Care Cancer.* 2017;25(8):2603–2610. Available from: https://doi.org/10.1007/s00520-017-3671-2.
90. Iyer NS, Cartmel B, Friedman L, et al. Lymphedema in ovarian cancer survivors: assessing diagnostic methods and the effects of physical activity. *Cancer.* 2018;124(9):1929–1937. Available from: https://doi.org/10.1002/cncr.31239.
91. Ergin G, Karadibak D, Sener HO, Gurpinar B. Effects of aqua-lymphatic therapy on lower extremity lymphedema: a randomized controlled study. *Lymphat Res Biol.* 2017;15(3):284–291. Available from: https://doi.org/10.1089/lrb.2017.0017.
92. Koehler LA, Haddad TC, Hunter DW, Tuttle TM. Axillary web syndrome following breast cancer surgery: symptoms, complications, and management strategies. *Breast Cancer Targets Ther.* 2019;11:13–19. Available from: https://doi.org/10.2147/BCTT.S146635.
93. Piper M, Guajardo I, Denkler K, Sbitany H. Axillary web syndrome: current understanding and new directions for treatment. *Ann Plast Surg.* 2016;76:S227–S231. Available from: https://doi.org/10.1097/SAP.0000000000000767.
94. Koehler LA, Hunter DW, Blaes AH, Haddad TC. Function, shoulder motion, pain and lymphedema in breast cancer with and without axillary web syndrome: an 18-month follow-up. *Phys Ther.* 2018;98(6):518–527. Available from: https://doi.org/10.1097/01.numa.0000435373.80608.40.

95. Xin M, Zhang H, Zhong Q, et al. Combining manual lymph drainage with physical exercise after modified radical mastectomy effectively prevents axillary web syndrome. *J Phlebol Lymphol*. 2017;10(1):15–18. <http://search.ebscohost.com/login.aspx?direct = true &db = a9h&AN = 127795562&site = ehost-live>.
96. Bray FN, Simmons BJ, Wolfson AH, Nouri K. Acute and chronic cutaneous reactions to ionizing radiation therapy. *Dermatol Ther (Heidelb)*. 2016;6(2):185–206. Available from: https://doi.org/10.1007/s13555-016-0120-y.
97. Olsen NK, Pfeiffer P, Johannsen L, Schrøder H, Rose C. Radiation-induced brachial plexopathy: neurological follow-up in 161 recurrence-free breast cancer patients. *Int J Radiat Oncol Biol Phys*. 1993;26(1):43–49. Available from: https://doi.org/10.1016/0360-3016(93)90171-Q.
98. Ribeiro FE, Vanderlei LCM, Palma MR, et al. Body dissatisfaction and its relationship with overweight, sedentary behavior and physical activity in survivors of breast cancer. *Eur J Obstet Gynecol Reprod Biol*. 2018;229:153–158. Available from: https://doi.org/10.1016/j.ejogrb.2018.08.581.
99. Mustian KM, Sprod LK, Palesh OG, et al. Exercise for the management of side effects and quality of life among cancer survivors. *Curr Sports Med Rep*. 2009;8(6):325–330. Available from: https://doi.org/10.1249/JSR.0b013e3181c22324.
100. Roveda E, Vitale JA, Bruno E, et al. Protective effect of aerobic physical activity on sleep behavior in breast cancer survivors. *Integr Cancer Ther*. 2017;16(1):21–31. Available from: https://doi.org/10.1177/1534735416651719.
101. Banning M. Employment and breast cancer: a meta-ethnography. *Eur J Cancer Care (Engl)*. 2011. Available from: https://doi.org/10.1111/j.1365-2354.2011.01291.x.
102. Van Muijen P, Weevers NLEC, Snels IAK, et al. Predictors of return to work and employment in cancer survivors: a systematic review. *Eur J Cancer Care (Engl)*. 2013. Available from: https://doi.org/10.1111/ecc.12033.
103. Wolvers MDJ, Leensen MCJ, Groeneveld IF, Frings-Dresen MHW, De Boer AGEM. Predictors for earlier return to work of cancer patients. *J Cancer Surviv*. 2018;12:169–177. doi:10.1007/s11764-017-0655-7.
104. Hoving JL, Broekhuizen MLA, Frings-Dresen MHW. Return to work of breast cancer survivors: a systematic review of intervention studies. *BMC Cancer*. 2009;9:1–10. Available from: https://doi.org/10.1186/1471-2407-9-117.

CHAPTER 4

Cancer-Related Fatigue in Breast and Gynecologic Cancers

JASMINE ZHENG, MD • BETTY CHERNACK, MD

INTRODUCTION

Patients with cancer experience a multitude of bodily changes and symptoms during cancer survivorship. Fatigue is common during the entire course of cancer treatment and has been reported to persist 10 years after cancer diagnosis in breast and gynecologic cancer patients.[1,2] For patients and their families, this can be a devastating barrier to participation in all aspects of one's day-to-day experiences, including at work and home. In addition, usual approaches to treating fatigue with self-regulation, such as getting additional rest, may not be entirely effective in pathological fatigue. For providers, cancer-related fatigue (CRF) can also be frustrating to treat given the overall limited understanding of its pathophysiology, treatment options, and prognosis over time.

The American Society of Clinical Oncology (ASCO) endorses CRF to be very common among those treated for cancer, and the majority will experience some amount of fatigue during their treatment course.[3] Prevalence is reported to range from 25% to 99%.[4] Not surprisingly, fatigue has a negative impact on patients' mood, sleep, and quality of life.[4] In one telephone interview of cancer patients, fatigue was reported to be worse than pain and disrupted day-to-day activity more than nausea, pain, or depression.[5]

Several studies examining fatigue in the general population have found a higher incidence of fatigue in women, which may be in part due to physiologic changes, including menopausal symptoms associated with lower estrogen levels, loss of bone density, and increased atherogenic risk factors. These physiological changes can lead to fatigue.[6] This has certain implications for the breast and gynecologic patient population, as the majority are women, and many undergo treatments that affect estrogen levels or lead to premature menopause.

Thirty percent of breast cancer survivors are estimated to experience CRF up to 5 years after treatment.[7] Others estimate the number to be as high as 50%.[8] Less is known about the amount of fatigue prior to treatment.[9] Numbers of CRF in gynecologic cancer populations were similar. Thirty percent of patients with invasive epithelial ovarian, peritoneal, or fallopian tube cancer reported fatigue in one study.[10] In another study of cervical cancer survivors, 23% of them reported chronic fatigue 11 years after their initial cancer diagnosis.[2] This was double that of an age-related normative sample, estimated at 11.4%.[11]

DEFINITIONS

Historically, there is a lack of consensus about the definition of CRF and the method of measurement in research.[12] This, along with heterogeneity of fatigue assessment tools, variation in treatment types, timing of assessments, and when the study was performed, impacts the differences in prevalence of fatigue cited in the cancer population.

The National Comprehensive Cancer Network (NCCN) defines CRF as "an unusual, persistent, subjective sense of tiredness related to cancer or cancer treatment that interferes with usual functioning."[13] Other descriptors of fatigue include lack of energy, malaise, exhaustion, impaired concentration, and amotivation.[14] Some also suggest making the distinction between central and peripheral fatigue. Central fatigue is defined as the failure to initiate or sustain tasks and activities requiring motivation. Patients may describe themselves as feeling "foggy," endorse changes in memory or concentration, or experience symptoms akin to depression. Peripheral fatigue, on the other hand, is independent of the central nervous system and is due to neuromuscular fatigue, for example, from cardiopulmonary deficits.[15]

Breast Cancer and Gynecologic Cancer Rehabilitation DOI: https://doi.org/10.1016/B978-0-323-72166-0.00004-9

MECHANISMS

Despite the pervasiveness of CRF, the mechanisms behind it are not entirely understood. The development and persistence of CRF are multifactorial and at this time can largely be divided into inflammatory, cellular, hormonal, genetic, and metabolic pathways (Fig. 4.1).

Inflammatory

Cytokines are chemical signaling molecules that play a critical role in inflammatory processes in the body. They can induce behaviors associated with sickness, including fatigue, and changes have been noted in those suffering from chronic fatigue syndrome and depression.[16,17] Multiple cytokines implicated to play roles in CRF may in part explain the persistence of fatigue in patients even after cancer treatment and in those who are devoid of disease. Breast cancer survivors with ongoing fatigue 3–5 years out from treatment were found to have higher than normal levels of proinflammatory cytokines.[18,19] Fatigue also correlated with increased proinflammatory markers prior to treatment.

Interleukin-6 (IL-6) is a cytokine heavily implicated in immune function, as it is a crucial component to the development and function of lymphocytes. It can act as an activator or inhibitor of T-cell responses, frequently elevated during infections, autoimmune diseases, and in cancer.[20] IL-6 has interesting significance in the ovarian cancer population, as levels are increased compared to patients with other types of gynecologic cancers and may play a critical role in cellular metastasis.[21] IL-6, in addition to other cytokines, including IL-1 and TNF-alpha, contributes to symptoms of anorexia, nausea and vomiting, weight loss, and changes in energy metabolism in ovarian cancer patients.[20] High levels of IL-6 are also associated with stress and depression, while social support appeared to have a protective effect.[21] In patients with ovarian cancer who were to undergo surgery, there were higher levels of IL-6 in those experiencing fatigue.[22,23] In a separate study, those with higher levels of IL-6 also had worse physical and functional well-being.[24]

Not surprisingly, proinflammatory markers are also noted to increase during cancer treatment. In radiation treatment for early-stage breast cancer, C-reactive protein and IL-1 receptor antagonist level increases were associated with increased levels of fatigue.[25] Similar findings were seen in levels of IL-6 during chemotherapy in breast[26] and ovarian cancers. In ovarian cancer patients, positive associations between levels of IL-6 and fatigue were found.[22,23]

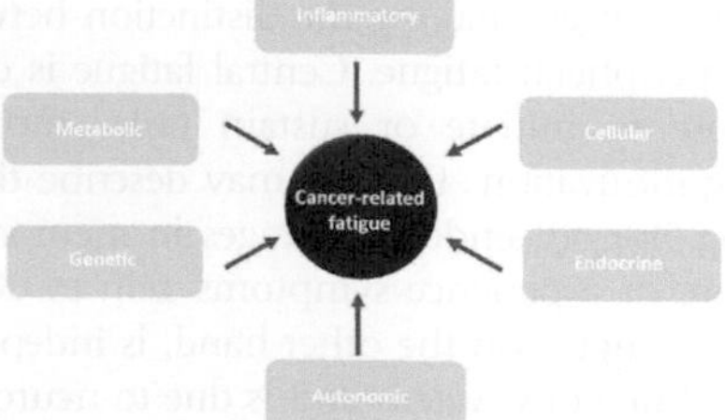

FIGURE 4.1 Mechanisms for the development of cancer-related fatigue.

Cellular

Cellular changes such as alterations in T-cell populations are correlated with inflammatory processes.[19,27,28] Elevated leukocyte numbers have been noted in breast cancer survivors with persistent fatigue, though this has not been consistently seen among studies.[4]

Endocrine

In addition to cytokine and cellular mechanisms, disruption of the hypothalamic–pituitary–adrenal (HPA) axis has also been implicated in CRF. Proinflammatory cytokines are stimulators of the HPA axis. In addition, cancer and its treatments can alter endocrine pathways.[20]

IL-6, as discussed earlier, is secreted when the HPA is activated. HPA activity and glucocorticoid levels are associated with social support, suggesting that IL-6 is mediated through HPA activity.[24] Cortisol plays a critical role in mediating inflammation and energy. Breast cancer survivors suffering from fatigue appear to have a less robust cortisol response to psychological stress.[29] In ovarian cancer patients before treatment, higher levels of nocturnal cortisol and reduced cortisol variability were associated with fatigue, in addition to higher functional impairments and depression.[30]

Additional Factors

Autonomic, genetic, and metabolic changes have also been implicated in fatigue in cancer patients. The sympathetic nervous system has proinflammatory associations, with higher levels of norepinephrine and decreased heart rate variability seen in breast cancer survivors with fatigue.[31] In one study, homozygous alleles of IL-6 were associated with higher evening and morning fatigue symptoms, and homozygous alleles of the TNF-alpha gene were associated with higher morning fatigue.[32] From a metabolic perspective, those with metabolic dysfunction such as diabetes had higher levels of fatigue. Interestingly, diabetes is one of the most common comorbidities in breast cancer.[33]

RISK FACTORS

Studies have looked at various contributors to CRF. Here, we will divide them into psychosocial and behavioral, medical, and other factors.

Psychosocial and Behavioral

Higher levels of stress and impaired coping are associated with fatigue. In one study that examined diurnal cortisol patterns in ovarian cancer survivors, those with greater lifetime stress exposure and severity were more likely to have circadian rhythm disruption that was associated with fatigue. In contrast, those with high social attachment had characteristic changes in their cortisol rhythms that suggest social support to be a buffer against stress or release of cortisol from the HPA axis.[34] A metaanalysis that examined risk factors for fatigue in breast cancer patients demonstrated that survivors who had a partner had a lower risk of severe fatigue than those without a partner.[35] Other studies have shown that those who expected to experience fatigue or catastrophized, or frequently engaged in negative thoughts about fatigue, had higher levels of fatigue.[36,37]

The relationship between depression and fatigue is not unidirectional, but it is clear that both depression and fatigue are correlated in cancer populations.[4] These relationships between anxiety, depression, and CRF are seen during active treatment and also after completion of treatment.[38] In Prue's study that looked at the gynecological population, psychological distress level was the only independent predictor of CRF during treatment.[38] In cervical cancer survivors, those with chronic fatigue have also reported higher levels of anxiety and depression and showed poorer self-reported health and less healthy lifestyle indicators.[2] Psychological distress is also associated with chronic fatigue in breast cancer survivors.[39] Breast cancer patients with a history of mental disorder prior to their cancer diagnosis appear to be at risk for posttreatment fatigue.[36,40] To that effect, stress reduction via mindfulness has shown improvement in distress and fatigue,[41] and this will be explored in more detail later in this chapter.

Medical and Treatment-Related Characteristics

There is conflicting data on whether sociodemographic variables, age at diagnosis, and treatment-related factors are associated with CRF.[35,38] For example, mixed findings exist on whether age, marital status, disease stage, and treatment characteristics are associated with fatigue in breast cancer patients; most of these studies included small numbers of patients. In a metaanalysis of over 12,000 breast cancer survivors, those with more advanced disease had increased risk of posttreatment fatigue. Risk was also higher in those treated with chemotherapy than those without. Isolated radiotherapy, hormone therapy, and targeted therapy were not significant risk factors. Those treated with combination surgery, chemotherapy, and radiotherapy were at higher risk than other treatment combinations; additional hormone therapy increased the risk.[35] In studies of women with gynecologic cancers, single chemotherapy and combination chemotherapies have been associated with higher levels of fatigue.[14]

It is important to remember that even in survivorship, patients can experience effects from original treatment, such as peripheral neuropathy, lymphedema, sexual dysfunction, GI distress, and urinary problems. All of these conditions have been shown to have an association with chronic fatigue.[2] In a case–control study, epithelial ovarian cancer survivors, neurotoxicity, depression, and sleep disturbance were significant predictors of severe, long-term fatigue.[42] This emphasizes the importance of performing a thorough review of systems throughout the care continuum, including in survivorship, and to treat symptoms that may contribute to CRF.

Other Risk Factors

Variations in genes associated with inflammatory markers have been suggested to play a role in the development of CRF. There are inconsistent findings of polymorphisms in TNF-alpha, IL-6, and IL-1B associated with higher levels of fatigue in breast cancer patients. Physical activity levels have also been implicated to affect CRF, with inactivity, impaired cardiopulmonary status, and high BMI correlating with the presence of CRF in breast cancer patients.[4]

SCREENING

In an effort to identify patients who have CRF, those who are at risk and provide efficient treatment, screening of most patients who have a diagnosis of cancer or have completed cancer treatment should be performed. There is a lack of consensus on a primary fatigue screening tool.[15] The NCCN recommends that once fatigue is identified, then determine the degree of fatigue on a numeric scale (0–10) or by discerning

TABLE 4.1
Common Fatigue Screening Tools

Instrument	Type of Instrument	Comments
FSI	11-Point Likert	Studied in breast and mixed cancers that included ovarian and endometrial cancers
BFI	11-Point Likert	Studied in mixed cancers that included breast and gynecologic
EORTC-QLQ-C30	4-Point Likert	Studied in mixed cancers, including breast and gynecologic
MFSI-SF	5-Point Likert	Studied in breast and mixed cancers, including ovarian, endometrial, and cervical cancers
PROMIS Cancer Fatigue	1 (never) to 5 (always)	Studied in mixed cancers, including breast and gynecologic

BFI, Brief Fatigue Inventory; *FSI*, Fatigue Symptom Inventory; *MFSI-SF*, Multidimensional Fatigue Symptom Inventory-Short Form; *PROMIS Cancer Fatigue*, Patient-Reported Outcomes Measurement Information System; *VAS*, Visual Analog Score.

among mild (1–3), moderate (4–6), or severe fatigue (7–10).[43] Those with no fatigue or mild fatigue can be provided with education and basic management tips with ongoing evaluation at routine clinic visits; patients with "red flags" such as new or worsening fatigue should be encouraged to reach out to their healthcare provider. Those who rate higher levels of fatigue or with moderate–severe fatigue should trigger a more extensive and thorough workup of fatigue in addition to being provided with basic educational and management information. A multitude of fatigue screening tools have been identified; some common fatigue scales used in breast and gynecologic CRF screening are included in Table 4.1.[43]

APPROACH TO PATIENT WITH CANCER-RELATED FATIGUE

Assessment

Patients with moderate-to-severe fatigue determined by the aforementioned systematic screening approaches require a comprehensive clinical assessment, including a focused physical examination, select laboratory studies, and pertinent imaging to best direct treatment. When gathering the history, clinicians should focus on onset, duration, temporal pattern throughout the day, alleviating/aggravating factors, and trajectory (i.e., whether the fatigue is getting worse or better over time). Particular attention should be devoted to ruling out medical- and substance-related causes of fatigue. A thorough review of current medications, including supplements, substance use, sleep pattern, and nutrition, is warranted. Table 4.2 outlines medical and substance use causes of fatigue.

TABLE 4.2
Medical and Substance Use Causes of Fatigue

Sleep disturbance
Hypothyroidism
Depression
Anxiety
Pain
Dyspnea
Dehydration
Infection
Anemia
Electrolyte abnormality (hyponatremia, hypokalemia, hypomagnesemia, hypercalcemia)
Progression of disease
Malnutrition
Medications
Alcohol
Marijuana medicinal or recreational

Finally, one of the most important aspects of the patient assessment is to determine how fatigue is affecting a patient's quality of life and function, including mobility, ability to perform activities of daily living, social, leisure, and vocational pursuits.[44]

PHYSICAL EXAM

After obtaining a detailed history a focused physical exam should be completed. For general appearance, clinicians should note any apparent distress, frailty, or cachexia. A focused exam should include evaluation for dry mucous membranes (dehydration), conjunctival pallor (anemia), and angular cheilosis (vitamin deficiencies). Cardiopulmonary exam should note any arrhythmias, cyanosis, tachypnea, or accessory muscle use. A musculoskeletal exam should note any atrophy and include evaluation of overall strength with manual muscle testing. Neurological exam can assess for polyneuropathy that may be contributing to fatigue. A flat or withdrawn affect noted on psychiatric exam may indicate underlying depression.

LABORATORY STUDIES

Initial diagnostic workup should include specific laboratory studies to help determine underlying contributors to fatigue. A complete metabolic panel can show disturbances in sodium, calcium, potassium, magnesium, and glucose that can all worsen energy levels. Blood urea nitrogen and creatinine are important to rule out dehydration and renal insufficiency. Underlying hepatic dysfunction as noted by transaminitis and hyperbilirubinemia can also contribute to a patient's presentation. Albumin and total protein are markers of nutritional status. Studies such as HgbA1C and thyroid-stimulating hormone can rule out endocrine dysfunction. Complete blood count with differential can assess for factors related to fatigue such as underlying infection or anemia.[44]

OTHER DIAGNOSTIC TESTING

Imaging can be important to look for progression of disease, overall disease burden, and infection that all could be contributing to fatigue. Conversely, stable imaging may lead to looking for alternative causes of worsened fatigue. Electromyography and nerve conduction studies can assess for underlying neuromuscular disorders that can possibly contribute to fatigue. Finally, an echocardiogram and electrocardiogram can determine if poor cardiopulmonary reserve or arrhythmias are involved.

Ultimately, a comprehensive history, physical examination, and diagnostic workup are crucial to determining appropriate patient-centered treatment plans (Fig. 4.2).

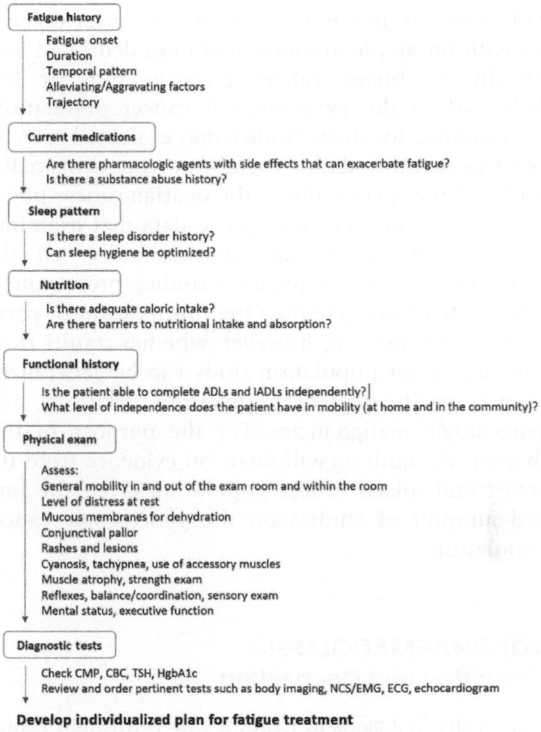

FIGURE 4.2 Suggested step-wise approach for patients presenting with fatigue.

TREATMENT

For cancer patients with moderate-to-severe fatigue, the first-line approach to treatment is to address any reversible contributing factors.[45] It is important to stop or at least reduce sedating medications. Common culprits in the cancer population include opioids and benzodiazepines. Untreated or undertreated depression, anxiety, and pain can worsen fatigue and thus addressing these contributing factors both nonpharmacologically and pharmacologically is necessary. After careful review of laboratory studies, providers can correct endocrine and fluid/electrolyte abnormalities with medication, supplements, and appropriate specialist consultation. In those patients who have anemia, erythropoietin-stimulating agents may provide some improvement to fatigue although come with risk of adverse events.[46] A nutritionist may need to be seen for any dietary deficiencies. Finally, if poor sleep is an issue, strategies to improve sleep hygiene and potentially pharmacologic treatment may be warranted.

If fatigue remains moderate-to-severe despite adequately treating all contributing factors, nonpharmacologic and pharmacologic management may be indicated. Before reviewing the evidence for a variety of CRF treatment interventions, it is important to note that most robust evidence for the treatment of

CRF comes from studies with mixed cancer diagnoses with an ample amount of studies dedicated specifically to breast cancer patients and far less dedicated to the gynecological cancer population. For example, for those studies that evaluated exercise as a treatment modality, there were only two smaller studies done specifically in the ovarian cancer population,[47,48] and there was sparse data that examines cervical and uterine cancers specifically. Of the many mixed cancer population studies, breast cancer patients tend to make up a high proportion of participants. It is unclear, however, whether results from a mixed cancer population study can be generalized to the specific patient populations of breast and gynecologic malignancies. For the purpose of this chapter, the authors will focus on evidence from the breast and mixed cancer population given the limited amount of studies on the gynecologic cancer population.

NONPHARMACOLOGIC

Education and Counseling

One of the first steps to treating CRF is through educational interventions. Several patient-friendly resources for CRF can be found on the websites of the NCCN, National Cancer Institute, American Cancer Society, and the ASCO's patient information website *Cancer.Net*. The NCCN Clinical Practice Guidelines in Oncology for cancer-related fatigue recommends education and counseling as the key management strategy.[43] Patients should be taught how to recognize CRF, including its natural history and temporal relation to specific cancer treatments. In addition, education on how best to manage the condition through energy conservation techniques, optimal sleep hygiene, diet, exercise, and mindfulness should be provided. Patients should be instructed to monitor their fatigue levels throughout the day with the use of a fatigue diary. Energy conservation techniques such as task delegation, adequate pacing of activities and avoiding multitasking are another key component of a fatigue education session. In a systematic review of 14 randomized controlled trials with 2213 participants who had mixed cancer diagnoses, educational interventions had a moderate effect in reduction of CRF distress and a small effect on reduction of fatigue intensity and fatigue's interference with daily life. Finally, there is substantial high-quality evidence to support cognitive behavioral therapy as an effective treatment tool for CRF.[49]

EXERCISE

Many randomized controlled trials and metaanalyses have demonstrated the effectiveness of exercise in the treatment of CRF among various cancer types.[50–52] The breast cancer population in particular has some of the most robust research in support of exercise as an effective treatment strategy for CRF.[53] In a systematic review of nine high-quality studies ($n = 1156$), supervised resistance and aerobic exercise was found to be more effective than conventional care for treatment of CRF in breast cancer survivors. This review not only showed efficacy but also safety of exercise, even at high volumes for this patient population.[52] Exercise as a treatment for CRF in the breast cancer population is not just beneficial to survivors but also those undergoing chemotherapy.[53]

While there is some evidence that aerobic versus resistive exercise programs show similar benefit in their effect on CRF[54] and that supervised exercise programs may have additional benefit when compared to unsupervised programs,[55] determination of specific exercise prescription and intensity has yet to be determined for our patients with breast and gynecologic malignancies.[56]

While it is widely accepted that exercise is an effective treatment for CRF, it is important to note that this modality may be contraindicated in certain patients. Precautions should be taken for patients with extensive lytic bone metastases, severe thrombocytopenia, active infections, and other safety concerns.[3]

NUTRITION

As CRF has been linked to chronic inflammation,[57] there is some evidence to suggest that a diet high in antioxidant nutrients may provide benefit for breast cancer patents.[58] Increased intake of omega-3 fatty acid–rich foods, known for their antioxidant effects, has been correlated with decreased physical aspects of fatigue among breast cancer survivors. In their pilot randomized clinical trial, Zick et al. utilized a fatigue reduction diet that consisted of fruit, vegetables, whole grains, and foods with high omega-3 fatty acid content. Over the course of 3 months, breast cancer survivors who followed the fatigue reduction diet demonstrated significantly less fatigue than the control group.[59]

Carnitine deficiency is also thought to play a role in the development of CRF and while a few nonrandomized and open-label studies showed improvement in fatigue with carnitine supplementation, a metaanalysis failed to show a significant reduction in CRF.[60]

Ginseng, ginger, guarana extract, and probiotics have similarly been studied in CRF treatment with promising results.[57,58]

COMPLEMENTARY AND ALTERNATIVE MEDICINE

Of the variety of complementary and alternative medicine (CAM) approaches to CRF, acupuncture is perhaps the most studied and has some robust evidence for efficacy, particularly among the breast cancer population. In their metaanalysis, Zhang et al. found that in the 10 randomized controlled trials that met inclusion criteria, there was a marked effect on CRF in patients with mixed cancer diagnoses who were and were not receiving concurrent chemotherapy or radiation. Furthermore, they found that acupuncture could reduce CRF when compared to sham procedure or usual care. This effect was seen with a variety of treatment timing and durations, from 20- to 30-minute sessions multiple times per week for as short as 2 weeks to once weekly sessions for 6 weeks. Effect size was particularly high among breast cancer patients.[61] An earlier metaanalysis also showed favorable results in support of acupuncture in terms of reduction in CRF from baseline to follow-up; however, the majority of pooled comparisons did not show statistically significant differences.[62] Results from yet another metaanalysis of seven RCTs were inconclusive with authors citing low quality and quantity of trials.[63] While there may be mixed results for acupuncture, there appears to be a clear understanding that this modality, when performed by experienced practitioners, is safe and well tolerated.[64] The overall safety of this therapy, along with the most recent metaanalysis' positive findings, makes acupuncture a promising treatment approach for CRF.

A modality of traditional acupuncture, infrared laser moxibustion, is another exciting potential treatment for CRF. A randomized, double-blind, placebo-controlled trial showed improved Brief Fatigue Inventory scores following 4 weeks of 10.6 μm of infrared laser moxibustion on the ST36 (bilateral), CV4, and CV6 acupoints compared to control group who received sham procedure to the same acupoints.[65] While this study's patient population consisted of mixed cancer types, breast (25.6%) and ovarian/endometrial/cervical (10.3%) cancer accounted for over a third of the diagnoses. A randomized controlled trial looking specifically at moxibustion's effects on CRF in breast cancer survivors is ongoing.[66]

Yoga, another popular CAM modality, may provide some benefit to those with CRF especially in the short-term period among breast cancer survivors. There was moderate-to-large effect of yoga on CRF among posttreatment breast cancer patients in a metaanalysis of 17 qualified studies with positive results also noted among intratreatment patients though, with only small effect size.[67] In their review of 11 studies, including a total of 883 patients with breast cancer that compared yoga versus no therapy, Cramer et al. demonstrated moderate-quality evidence showing that yoga reduced fatigue in the short term (6–12 weeks), but only low-quality evidence of longer lasting effects (30–40 weeks). When compared with more traditional forms of exercise, yoga had only very low-quality evidence to suggest similar efficacy.[68] Yoga, thus, appears beneficial, at least in the short term, in reduction of CRF but should not necessarily replace a more traditional exercise program.

Mindfulness-based approaches may be an effective tool to reduce fatigue in cancer patients. In a systematic review of 245 studies, relaxation exercise or meditation was the highest ranked intervention when compared to CBT, aerobic exercise, resistance exercise, and yoga among patients concurrently receiving cancer treatment.[69] In the breast cancer population specifically, a review of 14 studies revealed statistically significant reduction in fatigue following a mindfulness-based stress reduction intervention.[70]

PHARMACOLOGIC

Exercise and psychological interventions for the treatment of CRF have been found to be significantly better than pharmacologic options overall.[71] Some clinical guidelines even recommend strongly against the use of pharmacologic agents.[44] While nonpharmacologic approaches may be first-line, pharmacologic interventions may have a role in specific patient groups such as those at the end of life.

Methylphenidate, the central nervous system stimulant used for attention-deficit/hyperactivity disorder, has the most evidence for reducing CRF.[72] However, risks of anorexia and sleep disturbance, issues of great concern in a cancer patient population, may not outweigh the potential benefits. In those patients with advanced disease and limited life expectancy, those risks may not be as important to achieve a good quality of life and thus methylphenidate and other stimulants may be indicated.

Modafinil, another central nervous system stimulant used in the treatment of fatigue related to

TABLE 4.3
Pharmacologic Treatment of CRF With Typical Dosing, and Side Effects

Medication	Dose	Side Effects
Methylphenidate	5 mg twice daily (at 8 a.m. and 1 p.m.)	Weight loss, insomnia
Modafinil	200 mg daily	Headache, decreased appetite
Dexamethasone	2–4 mg daily	Agitation, weight gain, hyperglycemia, avascular necrosis, infection

narcolepsy and shift work sleep disorder, has had mixed results in its treatment of CRF. While at least one randomized, placebo-controlled, double-blind clinical trial of 631 patients with mixed cancer types on active chemotherapy showed a significant interaction between treatment condition and baseline fatigue in a subgroup of those with severe fatigue levels, those with mild-to-moderate fatigue had no significant effect.[73] Modafinil is thus likely best utilized for patients with severe fatigue currently undergoing active treatment.

Glucocorticoids such as dexamethasone are not currently recommended by the ASCO but are commonly prescribed by hospice providers for patients with advanced cancer and at least one double-blind, randomized, placebo-controlled trial showed greater efficacy than placebo[74] (Table 4.3).

CANCER-RELATED FATIGUE AND PREHABILITATION

The model of rehabilitation has generally been focused on the time period during and after cancer treatment. Prehabilitation is defined as the "process on the continuum of care that occurs between the time of cancer diagnosis and the beginning of acute treatment, includes physical and psychological assessments that establish a baseline function, identifies impairments, and provides targeted interventions that improve a patient's health to reduce the incidence and the severity of current and future impairments."[75] Studies that look at earlier rehabilitation interventions in breast cancer patients show faster return to baseline function,[76] supporting the idea that tackling functional issues prior to cancer treatment is a worthwhile endeavor, prior to the development of additional physical and cognitive stressors in the setting of chemotherapy, radiation, surgery, and associated side effects. Stress management preoperatively in patients with breast cancer showed successful reductions in depression and fatigue immediately postoperatively.[77] Yoga, breathing, muscle relaxation, meditation interventions prior to surgery resulted in less anxiety, depression, and fatigue after surgery.[78] There is little data on prehabilitation in the gynecologic cancer population. Recently, Miralpeix et al. created a multimodal prehabilitation program for gynecologic oncology patients that includes physical therapy, psychological support, in addition to other patient-tailored optimization in an effort to improve surgical outcomes.[79] It will be interesting to see whether prehabilitation models in the gynecologic population affect fatigue and function in similar ways to that seen in the breast cancer population. Given the link between premorbid fatigue and persistent fatigue during the cancer continuum, prehabilitation may be an underutilized opportunity to treat fatigue.

CANCER-RELATED FATIGUE AND HOSPICE/END OF LIFE

Even during the final days of life, patients with terminal cancer desire functional independence.[80] Uncontrolled symptoms of fatigue can limit mobility and can contribute to declining functional status. Effective treatment of fatigue in patients with advanced cancer can thus be critical in ensuring those with terminal disease can have the best quality of life possible. For the very debilitated, chair exercise programs can be helpful in the treatment of fatigue.[81] Home-based programs have been successful in treating fatigue and are especially suited for those enrolled in hospice care as transporting patients at late stages of disease can be especially burdensome.[82] The use of corticosteroids such as dexamethasone can improve a variety of symptoms at the end of life, including fatigue and over a short time course, has no significant difference in adverse effects when compared with placebo.[74] Megestrol acetate has also shown reduction of fatigue in those with advanced stages of cancer.[83] In terms of neurostimulants, methylphenidate has been studied in hospice patients with significantly lower fatigue scores reported after two weeks. In addition, the ASCO guidelines recommend the use of methylphenidate and modafinil in patients with advanced disease.

PROPOSED MULTIDIMENSIONAL APPROACH

The ASCO recommends a multimodal approach to the treatment of CRF. This expert group recommends addressing all medical and treatable contributing factors as the first-line treatment strategy. Another mainstay treatment approach includes counseling and education in regards to fatigue, including general strategies in fatigue management. ASCO guidelines strongly encourage patients to engage in 150 minutes of moderate aerobic activity per week with resistance training two to three times per week. For those at higher risk for injury a supervised exercise program is preferred. Psychosocial interventions such as CBT, mindfulness-based practice, yoga, and acupuncture are also suggested. Finally, the judicial use of methylphenidate or modafinil is noted for those with advanced disease or those currently receiving cancer treatment, but not recommended in cancer survivors.[4]

Another expert group, the Canadian Association of Psychosocial Oncology (CAPO), offers a more minimalist treatment approach that also includes addressing contributing factors, providing general fatigue education and counseling, physical exercise, and mindfulness-based interventions. CAPO, however, does not recommend any pharmacologic management, herbal supplements, or CAM such as acupuncture. CAPO's exercise program differs from ASCO guidelines with specific recommendations for supervised moderate-intensity physical activity of any type, including yoga and walking, at least five times per week.[44]

Given the new evidence from RCTs and metaanalyses published after the CAPO guidelines were established as well as anecdotally from clinical practice, the authors recommend a more holistic treatment approach, including both nonpharmacologic and pharmacologic strategies. These recommendations are outlined in Table 4.4.

TABLE 4.4
Multidimensional Approach to Treatment of Cancer-Related Fatigue

Address potential reversible contributing factors
Educational sessions on energy conservation and general fatigue management
Moderate-intensity physical activity of any type, including yoga and walking
Supervised exercise program for those with higher safety concerns
Acupuncture with or without moxibustion
Diet with high omega-3 fatty acid content
Cognitive behavioral therapy
Judicious use of methylphenidate and dexamethasone (patients with advanced disease, hospice population) and modafinil (patients currently receiving active treatment with severe fatigue)

CONCLUSION

CRF is a distressing experience that can last for months to years, impacting a patient's quality of life. Assessing for CRF in the breast and gynecologic cancer population along the care continuum is critical to provide appropriate and timely education and treatment options. There is opportunity for CRF treatment in the prehabilitation period and also at the end of life. Treatment requires a multimodal approach, and reassessment of CRF over time and adjustment to treatment is important due to the dynamic nature of patients' cancer trajectories.

REFERENCES

1. Bower JE, Ganz PA, Desmond KA, et al. Fatigue in long-term breast carcinoma survivors: a longitudinal investigation. *Cancer*. 2006;106(4):751–758.
2. Steen R, Dahl AA, Hess SL, Kiserud CE. A study of chronic fatigue in Norwegian cervical cancer survivors. *Gynecol Oncol*. 2017;146(3):630–635.
3. Bower JE, Bak K, Berger A, et al. Screening, assessment, and management of fatigue in adult survivors of cancer: an American Society of Clinical Oncology clinical practice guideline adaptation. *J Clin Oncol*. 2014;32(17):1840.
4. Bower JE. Cancer-related fatigue—mechanisms, risk factors, and treatments. *Nat Rev Clin Oncol*. 2014;11 (10):597.
5. Curt GA, Breitbart W, Cella D, et al. Impact of cancer-related fatigue on the lives of patients: new findings from the fatigue coalition. *Oncologist*. 2000;5(5):353–360.
6. Jing M, Wang J, Lin W, Lei Y, Wang P. A community-based cross-sectional study of fatigue in middle-aged and elderly women. *J Psychosom Res*. 2015;79(4):288–294.
7. Bower JE, Ganz PA, Desmond KA, Rowland JH, Meyerowitz BE, Belin TR. Fatigue in breast cancer survivors: occurrence, correlates, and impact on quality of life. *J Clin Oncol*. 2000;18(4):743.

8. Minton O, Stone P. How common is fatigue in disease-free breast cancer survivors? A systematic review of the literature. *Breast Cancer Res Treat*. 2008;112(1):5–13.
9. Jacobsen PB, Hann DM, Azzarello LM, Horton J, Balducci L, Lyman GH. Fatigue in women receiving adjuvant chemotherapy for breast cancer: characteristics, course, and correlates. *J Pain Symptom Manage*. 1999;18(4):233–242.
10. Sailors MH, Bodurka DC, Gning I, et al. Validating the MD Anderson symptom inventory (MDASI) for use in patients with ovarian cancer. *Gynecol Oncol*. 2013;130 (2):323–328.
11. Loge JH, Ekeberg Ø, Kaasa S. Fatigue in the general Norwegian population: normative data and associations. *J Psychosom Res*. 1998;45(1):53–65.
12. Barsevick AM, Cleeland CS, Manning DC, et al. ASCPRO recommendations for the assessment of fatigue as an outcome in clinical trials. *J Pain Symptom Manage*. 2010;39(6):1086–1099.
13. Mock V, Atkinson A, Barsevick A, et al. NCCN practice guidelines for cancer-related fatigue. *Oncol (Williston Park, NY)*. 2000;14(11A):151–161.
14. Anderson NJ, Hacker ED. Fatigue in women receiving intraperitoneal chemotherapy for ovarian cancer: a review of contributing factors. *Clin J Oncol Nurs*. 2008;12(3).
15. Gerber LH. Cancer-related fatigue: persistent, pervasive, and problematic. *Phys Med Rehabilitation Clin*. 2017;28 (1):65–88.
16. Dantzer R, Bluthé R, Gheusi G, et al. Molecular basis of sickness behavior. *Ann N Y Acad Sci*. 1998;856(1):132–138.
17. Kelley KW, Bluthé R, Dantzer R, et al. Cytokine-induced sickness behavior. *Brain Behav Immun*. 2003;17(1):112–118.
18. Bower JE, Ganz PA, Aziz N, Fahey JL. Fatigue and proinflammatory cytokine activity in breast cancer survivors. *Psychosom Med*. 2002;64(4):604–611.
19. Bower JE, Ganz PA, Aziz N, Fahey JL, Cole SW. T-cell homeostasis in breast cancer survivors with persistent fatigue. *J Natl Cancer Inst*. 2003;95(15):1165–1168.
20. Macciò A, Madeddu C. Inflammation and ovarian cancer. *Cytokine*. 2012;58(2):133–147.
21. Lutgendorf SK, Anderson B, Sorosky JI, Buller RE, Lubaroff DM. Interleukin-6 and use of social support in gynecologic cancer patients. *Int J Behav Med*. 2000;7 (2):127–142.
22. Clevenger L, Schrepf A, Christensen D, et al. Sleep disturbance, cytokines, and fatigue in women with ovarian cancer. *Brain Behav Immun*. 2012;26(7):1037–1044.
23. Lutgendorf SK, Weinrib AZ, Penedo F, et al. Interleukin-6, cortisol, and depressive symptoms in ovarian cancer patients. *J Clin Oncol*. 2008;26(29):4820.
24. Costanzo ES, Lutgendorf SK, Sood AK, Anderson B, Sorosky J, Lubaroff DM. Psychosocial factors and interleukin-6 among women with advanced ovarian cancer. *Cancer: Interdiscip Int J Am Cancer Soc*. 2005;104(2):305–313.
25. Bower JE, Ganz PA, Tao ML, et al. Inflammatory biomarkers and fatigue during radiation therapy for breast and prostate cancer. *Clin Cancer Res*. 2009;15(17):5534–5540.
26. Liu L, Mills PJ, Rissling M, et al. Fatigue and sleep quality are associated with changes in inflammatory markers in breast cancer patients undergoing chemotherapy. *Brain Behav Immun*. 2012;26(5):706–713.
27. Gerber LH, Stout N, McGarvey C, et al. Factors predicting clinically significant fatigue in women following treatment for primary breast cancer. *Supportive Care Cancer*. 2011;19(10):1581–1591.
28. Collado-Hidalgo A, Bower JE, Ganz PA, Cole SW, Irwin MR. Inflammatory biomarkers for persistent fatigue in breast cancer survivors. *Clin cancer Res*. 2006;12 (9):2759–2766.
29. Bower JE, Ganz PA, Aziz N. Altered cortisol response to psychologic stress in breast cancer survivors with persistent fatigue. *Psychosom Med*. 2005;67(2):277–280.
30. Weinrib AZ, Sephton SE, DeGeest K, et al. Diurnal cortisol dysregulation, functional disability, and depression in women with ovarian cancer. *Cancer.*. 2010;116 (18):4410–4419.
31. Fagundes CP, Murray DM, Hwang BS, et al. Sympathetic and parasympathetic activity in cancer-related fatigue: more evidence for a physiological substrate in cancer survivors. *Psychoneuroendocrinology*. 2011;36 (8):1137–1147.
32. Saligan LN, Kim HS. A systematic review of the association between immunogenomic markers and cancer-related fatigue. *Brain Behav Immun*. 2012;26 (6):830–848.
33. Tang Z, Wang J, Zhang H, et al. Associations between diabetes and quality of life among breast cancer survivors. *PLoS One*. 2016;11(6):e0157791.
34. Cuneo MG, Schrepf A, Slavich GM, et al. Diurnal cortisol rhythms, fatigue and psychosocial factors in five-year survivors of ovarian cancer. *Psychoneuroendocrinology*. 2017;84:139–142. Available from: https://doi.org/10.1016/j.psyneuen.2017.06.019. Available from: https://www.sciencedirect.com/science/article/pii/S0306453017300458.
35. Abrahams H, Gielissen M, Schmits IC, Verhagen C, Rovers MM, Knoop H. Risk factors, prevalence, and course of severe fatigue after breast cancer treatment: a meta-analysis involving 12,327 breast cancer survivors. *Ann Oncol*. 2016;27(6):965–974.
36. Andrykowski MA, Schmidt JE, Salsman JM, Beacham AO, Jacobsen PB. Use of a case definition approach to identify cancer-related fatigue in women undergoing adjuvant therapy for breast cancer. *J Clin Oncol*. 2005;23 (27):6613.
37. Jacobsen PB, Andrykowski MA, Thors CL. Relationship of catastrophizing to fatigue among women receiving treatment for breast cancer. *J Consult Clin Psychol*. 2004;72(2):355.
38. Prue G, Allen J, Gracey J, Rankin J, Cramp F. Fatigue in gynecological cancer patients during and after anticancer treatment. *J Pain Symptom Manage*. 2010;39(2):197–210.
39. Reinertsen KV, Engebraaten O, Loge JH, et al. Fatigue during and after breast cancer therapy—a prospective study. *J Pain Symptom Manage*. 2017;53(3):551–560.

40. Reinertsen KV, Cvancarova M, Loge JH, Edvardsen H, Wist E, Fosså SD. Predictors and course of chronic fatigue in long-term breast cancer survivors. *J Cancer Survivorship*. 2010;4(4):405–414.
41. Lengacher CA, Reich RR, Paterson CL, et al. Examination of broad symptom improvement resulting from mindfulness-based stress reduction in breast cancer survivors: a randomized controlled trial. *J Clin Oncol*. 2016;34(24):2827.
42. Joly F, Ahmed-Lecheheb D, Kalbacher E, et al. Long-term fatigue and quality of life among epithelial ovarian cancer survivors: a GINECO case/control VIVROVAIRE I study. *Ann Oncol*. 2019;30(5):845–852.
43. Berger AM, Mooney K, Alvarez-Perez A, et al. Cancer-related fatigue, version 2.2015. *J Natl Compr Canc Netw*. 2015;13(8):1012–1039. doi: 13/8/1012 [pii].
44. Howell D, Keller-Olaman S, Oliver TK, et al. A pan-Canadian practice guideline and algorithm: screening, assessment, and supportive care of adults with cancer-related fatigue. *Curr Oncol*. 2013;20(3):233–246. Available from: https://doi.org/10.3747/co.20.1302.
45. Mohandas H, Jaganathan SK, Mani MP, Ayyar M, Rohini Thevi GV. Cancer-related fatigue treatment: an overview. *J Cancer Res Ther*. 2017;13(6):916–929. Available from: https://doi.org/10.4103/jcrt.JCRT_50_17.
46. Minton O, Richardson A, Sharpe M, Hotopf M, Stone P. Drug therapy for the management of cancer-related fatigue. *Cochrane Database Syst Rev*. 2010;(7). Available from: https://doi.org/10.1002/14651858.CD006704.pub3.
47. Donnelly CM, Blaney JM, Lowe-Strong A, et al. A randomised controlled trial testing the feasibility and efficacy of a physical activity behavioural change intervention in managing fatigue with gynaecological cancer survivors. *Gynecol Oncol*. 2011;122(3):618–624. Available from: https://doi.org/10.1016/j.ygyno.2011.05.029.
48. Zhou Y, Cartmel B, Gottlieb L, et al. Randomized trial of exercise on quality of life in women with ovarian cancer: women's activity and lifestyle study in Connecticut (WALC). *J Natl Cancer Inst*. 2017;109(12). Available from: https://doi.org/10.1093/jnci/djx072.
49. Bennett S, Pigott A, Beller EM, Haines T, Meredith P, Delaney C. Educational interventions for the management of cancer-related fatigue in adults. *Cochrane Database Syst Rev*. 2016;11. Available from: https://doi.org/10.1002/14651858.CD008144.pub2.
50. Tian L, Lu HJ, Lin L, Hu Y. Effects of aerobic exercise on cancer-related fatigue: a meta-analysis of randomized controlled trials. *Support Care Cancer*. 2016;24(2):969–983. Available from: https://doi.org/10.1007/s00520-015-2953-9.
51. Meneses-Echavez JF, Gonzalez-Jimenez E, Ramirez-Velez R. Effects of supervised exercise on cancer-related fatigue in breast cancer survivors: a systematic review and meta-analysis. *BMC Cancer*. 2015;15:01–04. Available from: https://doi.org/10.1186/s12885-015-1069-4.
52. McNeely ML, Campbell KL, Rowe BH, Klassen TP, Mackey JR, Courneya KS. Effects of exercise on breast cancer patients and survivors: a systematic review and meta-analysis. *CMAJ*. 2006;175(1):34–41. doi: 175/1/34 [pii].
53. Cramp F, Byron-Daniel J. Exercise for the management of cancer-related fatigue in adults. *Cochrane Database Syst Rev*. 2012;11. Available from: https://doi.org/10.1002/14651858.CD006145.pub3.
54. Litterini AJ, Fieler VK, Cavanaugh JT, Lee JQ. Differential effects of cardiovascular and resistance exercise on functional mobility in individuals with advanced cancer: a randomized trial. *Arch Phys Med Rehabil*. 2013;94(12):2329–2335. Available from: https://doi.org/10.1016/j.apmr.2013.06.008.
55. Velthuis MJ, Agasi-Idenburg SC, Aufdemkampe G, Wittink HM. The effect of physical exercise on cancer-related fatigue during cancer treatment: a meta-analysis of randomised controlled trials. *Clin Oncol (R Coll Radiol)*. 2010;22(3):208–221. Available from: https://doi.org/10.1016/j.clon.2009.12.005.
56. Berntsen S, Aaronson NK, Buffart L, et al. Design of a randomized controlled trial of physical training and cancer (Phys-Can) – the impact of exercise intensity on cancer related fatigue, quality of life and disease outcome. *BMC Cancer*. 2017;17(1):01–05. Available from: https://doi.org/10.1186/s12885-017-3197-5.
57. Inglis JE, Lin PJ, Kerns SL, et al. Nutritional interventions for treating cancer-related fatigue: a qualitative review. *Nutr Cancer*. 2019;71(1):21–40. Available from: https://doi.org/10.1080/01635581.2018.1513046.
58. Pereira PTVT, Reis AD, Diniz RR, et al. Dietary supplements and fatigue in patients with breast cancer: a systematic review. *Breast Cancer Res Treat*. 2018;171(3):515–526. Available from: https://doi.org/10.1007/s10549-018-4857-0.
59. Zick SM, Colacino J, Cornellier M, Khabir T, Surnow K, Djuric Z. Fatigue reduction diet in breast cancer survivors: a pilot randomized clinical trial. *Breast Cancer Res Treat*. 2017;161(2):299–310. Available from: https://doi.org/10.1007/s10549-016-4070-y.
60. Marx W, Teleni L, Opie RS, et al. Efficacy and effectiveness of carnitine supplementation for cancer-related fatigue: a systematic literature review and meta-analysis. *Nutrients*. 2017;9(11). doi: E1224 [pii].
61. Zhang Y, Lin L, Li H, Hu Y, Tian L. Effects of acupuncture on cancer-related fatigue: a meta-analysis. *Support Care Cancer*. 2018;26(2):415–425. Available from: https://doi.org/10.1007/s00520-017-3955-6.
62. Zeng Y, Luo T, Finnegan-John J, Cheng AS. Meta-analysis of randomized controlled trials of acupuncture for cancer-related fatigue. *Integr Cancer Ther*. 2014;13(3):193–200. Available from: https://doi.org/10.1177/1534735413510024.
63. Posadzki P, Moon TW, Choi TY, Park TY, Lee MS, Ernst E. Acupuncture for cancer-related fatigue: a systematic review of randomized clinical trials. *Support Care Cancer*. 2013;21(7):2067–2073. Available from: https://doi.org/10.1007/s00520-013-1765-z.
64. Birch S, Lee MS, Alraek T, Kim TH. Evidence, safety and recommendations for when to use acupuncture for treating cancer related symptoms: a narrative review. *Integr Med Res*. 2019;8(3):160–166. Available from: https://doi.org/10.1016/j.imr.2019.05.002.

65. Mao H, Mao JJ, Guo M, et al. Effects of infrared laser moxibustion on cancer-related fatigue: a randomized, double-blind, placebo-controlled trial. *Cancer..* 2016;122 (23):3667–3672. Available from: https://doi.org/10.1002/cncr.30189.
66. Mao H, Mao JJ, Chen J, et al. Effects of infrared laser moxibustion on cancer-related fatigue in breast cancer survivors: study protocol for a randomized controlled trial. *Med (Baltim)*. 2019;98(34). Available from: https://doi.org/10.1097/MD.0000000000016882.
67. Dong B, Xie C, Jing X, Lin L, Tian L. Yoga has a solid effect on cancer-related fatigue in patients with breast cancer: a meta-analysis. *Breast Cancer Res Treat*. 2019;177 (1):5–16. Available from: https://doi.org/10.1007/s10549-019-05278-w.
68. Cramer H, Lauche R, Klose P, Lange S, Langhorst J, Dobos GJ. Yoga for improving health-related quality of life, mental health and cancer-related symptoms in women diagnosed with breast cancer. *Cochrane Database Syst Rev*. 2017;1. Available from: https://doi.org/10.1002/14651858.CD010802.pub2.
69. Hilfiker R, Meichtry A, Eicher M, et al. Exercise and other non-pharmaceutical interventions for cancer-related fatigue in patients during or after cancer treatment: a systematic review incorporating an indirect-comparisons meta-analysis. *Br J Sports Med*. 2018;52(10):651–658. Available from: https://doi.org/10.1136/bjsports-2016-096422.
70. Zhang Q, Zhao H, Zheng Y. Effectiveness of mindfulness-based stress reduction (MBSR) on symptom variables and health-related quality of life in breast cancer patients-a systematic review and meta-analysis. *Support Care Cancer*. 2019;27(3):771–781. Available from: https://doi.org/10.1007/s00520-018-4570-x.
71. Mustian KM, Alfano CM, Heckler C, et al. Comparison of pharmaceutical, psychological, and exercise treatments for cancer-related fatigue: a meta-analysis. *JAMA Oncol*. 2017;3(7):961–968. Available from: https://doi.org/10.1001/jamaoncol.2016.6914.
72. Tomlinson D, Robinson PD, Oberoi S, et al. Pharmacologic interventions for fatigue in cancer and transplantation: a meta-analysis. *Curr Oncol*. 2018;25(2): e152–e167. Available from: https://doi.org/10.3747/co.25.3883.
73. Jean-Pierre P, Morrow GR, Roscoe JA, et al. A phase 3 randomized, placebo-controlled, double-blind, clinical trial of the effect of modafinil on cancer-related fatigue among 631 patients receiving chemotherapy: a University of Rochester cancer center community clinical oncology program research base study. *Cancer*. 2010;116 (14):3513–3520. Available from: https://doi.org/10.1002/cncr.25083.
74. Yennurajalingam S, Frisbee-Hume S, Palmer JL, et al. Reduction of cancer-related fatigue with dexamethasone: a double-blind, randomized, placebo-controlled trial in patients with advanced cancer. *J Clin Oncol*. 2013;31 (25):3076–3082. Available from: https://doi.org/10.1200/JCO.2012.44.4661.
75. Silver JK, Baima J. Cancer prehabilitation: an opportunity to decrease treatment-related morbidity, increase cancer treatment options, and improve physical and psychological health outcomes. *Am J Phys Med Rehabil*. 2013;92(8):715–727.
76. Cinar N, Seckin Ü, Keskin D, Bodur H, Bozkurt B, Cengiz Ö. The effectiveness of early rehabilitation in patients with modified radical mastectomy. *Cancer Nurs*. 2008;31(2):160–165.
77. Garssen B, Boomsma MF, de Jager Meezenbroek E, et al. Stress management training for breast cancer surgery patients. *Psycho-Oncology*. 2013;22(3):572–580.
78. Tsimopoulou I, Pasquali S, Howard R, et al. Psychological prehabilitation before cancer surgery: a systematic review. *Ann surgical Oncol*. 2015;22 (13):4117–4123.
79. Miralpeix E, Mancebo G, Gayete S, Corcoy M, Solé-Sedeño J. Role and impact of multimodal prehabilitation for gynecologic oncology patients in an enhanced recovery after surgery (ERAS) program. *Int J Gynecologic Cancer*. 2019;29. ijg-000597.
80. Yoshioka H. Rehabilitation for the terminal cancer patient. *Am J Phys Med Rehabil*. 1994;73(3):199–206.
81. Headley JA, Ownby KK, John LD. The effect of seated exercise on fatigue and quality of life in women with advanced breast cancer. *Oncol Nurs Forum*. 2004;31 (5):977–983. Available from: https://doi.org/10.1188/04.ONF.977-983.
82. Cheville AL, Kollasch J, Vandenberg J, et al. A home--based exercise program to improve function, fatigue, and sleep quality in patients with stage IV lung and colorectal cancer: a randomized controlled trial. *J Pain Symptom Manage*. 2013;45(5):811–821. Available from: https://doi.org/10.1016/j.jpainsymman.2012.05.006.
83. Bruera E, Ernst S, Hagen N, et al. Effectiveness of megestrol acetate in patients with advanced cancer: a randomized, double-blind, crossover study. *Cancer Prev Control*. 1998;2(2):74–78.

CHAPTER 5

Nutritional Rehabilitation of Breast and Gynecologic Cancer Patients

KARLA OTERO, MS, RDN, LDN, CSO, CDE • CLAUDIA FERRI, MS, RD, CSO, LDN • CARLA ARAYA, MPH, RDN, LDN

NUTRITION SCREENING AND ASSESSMENT IN BREAST AND GYNECOLOGICAL CANCERS

Facing a cancer diagnosis is always detrimental. Many cancer patients have to deal with the physiological burden that cancer treatments may cause. Optimal nutrition during cancer treatment is essential in order to meet the increased nutritional demands needed to support healing and recovery. By achieving optimal nutrition, we assure that our patients are more prepared to tolerate a full treatment with fewer complications and better quality of life.[1]

Nutritional screening is the first step in determining nutritional problems. The purpose of nutrition screening and assessment is the early identification of malnutrition. As many as 40% of cancer patients experience anorexia prior to diagnosis, and 40%–80% will experience malnutrition during their treatment.[1] The Academy of Nutrition and Dietetics defines nutrition screening as the process of identifying characteristics known to be associated with nutrition problems, with a goal of identifying individuals who are malnourished or at nutritional risk and are in need of intervention and/or counseling from a registered dietitian nutritionist (RDN). Patients at nutritional risk should undergo a more detailed nutritional assessment to identify and quantify those nutritional problems.[1]

Malnutrition is an independent risk factor that adversely affects a patient's clinical outcomes, quality of life, body function, and autonomy. The early identification of patients at risk of malnutrition or who are malnourished is extremely important in order to start nutritional interventions in a timely manner.[2] Ovarian cancer patients have the highest rate of disease-related malnutrition among all gynecological (GYN) cancers. Malnutrition among ovarian cancer patients is an important predictor of mortality. In advanced ovarian cancer the involvement of the intraabdominal area is common. These patients present with multiple symptoms (dyspepsia, nausea, lack of appetite, fatigue, abdominal pain) that lead to inadequate caloric intake and impaired nutritional status.[3]

The use of a validated malnutrition screening tool (MST) has been associated with better nutritional care and outcome.[4] It is essential to have sensitive and appropriate screening parameters to make the best use of the RDN. At Miami Cancer Institute the clinical nutrition team is utilizing the MST to identify patients at nutritional risk. The MST is a validated evidence-based tool used in inpatient and ambulatory/outpatient care settings with adult patients who have cancer. It was selected for use based on its simplicity. It is a three-question tool with both high sensitivity and specificity. The presence of unintentional weight loss, amount of weight loss, and decreased appetite is used to identify malnutrition risk. The answers to the questions are electronically computed and referred to as the RDN for action.

The RDN then follows the Nutrition Care Process (NCP) model established by the Academy of Nutrition and Dietetics in 2003.[5] The NCP is a systematic method that the RDN uses to provide nutritional care. The NCP is a road map that consists of four separate yet interconnected steps: Nutrition Assessment and Reassessment, Nutrition Diagnosis, Nutrition Intervention, and Nutrition Monitoring and Evaluation.[6] Each step of NCP model is important to complete before advancing to the next step.

The NCP model is dynamic and multidirectional allowing the RDN to revisit previous steps of the NCP to reassess, update nutrition diagnosis, adapt interventions, and modify goals. The NCP is evolving to become the international standard for the delivery of nutritional care. Nutritional assessment and evidenced-based nutrition interventions by the oncology RDN allow cancer patients to achieve optimal nutrition during cancer treatment in order to have a better tolerance of treatment.

Breast Cancer and Gynecologic Cancer Rehabilitation DOI: https://doi.org/10.1016/B978-0-323-72166-0.00005-0

ESTIMATING ENERGY NEEDS FOR CANCER PATIENTS

Energy metabolism can vary significantly among cancer patients. When determining energy needs, best practice indicates that estimates should be individualized and based on clinical judgment. RDNs in clinical practice may quickly calculate energy needs from formulas that suggest that a certain number of kilocalories are required per kilogram of body weight.[7] These methods are useful as initial estimates and need to be adjusted based on an individual's nutritional status and activity level. Factors to consider when assessing calorie requirements include age, physical activity level, cancer treatment modality with anticipated side effects, and current nutritional status (e.g., involuntary weight loss).

In patients who are at a desirable body weight range (BMI 18.5–24.9 kg/m^2), the goal is to maintain weight during and after treatment. Most breast cancer patients may be either overweight or obese at the time of diagnosis, and many of them gain weight during treatment. However, some GYN cancer patients (e.g., ovarian) may present with unintentional weight loss and their energy needs may be higher. In patients who are underweight (BMI < 18.5 kg/m^2), calorie needs range between 30 and 35 cal/kg. For weight maintenance an acceptable caloric range is between 25 and 30 cal/kg of body weight. For overweight (BMI ≥ 25 kg/m^2) and obese (BMI ≥ 30 kg/m^2) breast/GYN cancer patients, an acceptable caloric level is around 20–25 cal/kg.[8]

OBESITY AND CANCER RISK

Obesity is associated with changes in the physiology and hormonal environment of the body, and these changes can promote the development of a number of chronic diseases, including diabetes and cardiovascular disease. Obesity is also associated with an increased risk of developing some types of cancer (e.g., endometrial, colorectal, esophageal, and breast cancer among others) and with a poorer survival outcome for patients with those cancers.[9]

At the time of diagnosis the majority of women with breast/GYN cancer are overweight or obese.[10] Obesity is associated with a 35%–40% increased risk for breast cancer recurrence and poorer survival outcomes.[5] This is most evidently recognized in postmenopausal women with estrogen-positive (ER+) breast cancer. This association can be attributed to the prevalence of higher estrogen levels in overweight, postmenopausal women. Conversely, in premenopausal hormone with receptor-positive breast cancer women, being overweight or obese has been associated with a lower risk.[11] On the other hand, recent evidence shows an increased risk of triple-negative breast cancers in obese premenopausal women.[12]

Evidence indicates that endometrial cancer, which is one the most common GYN cancers, is often associated with the metabolic syndrome (caused by obesity, diabetes, and hypertension). Furthermore, metabolic syndrome is closely associated with the incidence and poor prognosis of endometrial cancer.[13] Recent data suggest that high insulin levels in overweight women may also play a role in this association as insulin has mitogenic and antiapoptotic activity.[14] Some studies have shown that obese patients present with larger tumors, increased lymph node metastasis, and higher grade tumors.[15] This finding may reflect more aggressive biology in obesity that may lead to a higher risk of recurrence.

Weight gain is commonly reported by breast/GYN cancer patients who are receiving chemotherapy, as well as by patients on tamoxifen or aromatase inhibitors. The average weight gain for patients undergoing chemotherapy is between 3 and 7 kg[16] and for patients on endocrine therapy is between 1 and 2 kg.[17] Unfortunately, evidence indicates that excess weight at diagnosis and weight gain during treatment are associated with an increased relapse rate and poorer survival rate.[18] During chemotherapy, involuntary weight gain may be attributed to the use of corticosteroids as well as to the more frequent intake of food to prevent nausea. However, there is not enough evidence to confirm that the use of endocrine therapy such as tamoxifen or aromatase inhibitors can cause any significant involuntary weight gain in breast cancer patients. Indeed, in some of the studies reviewed, weight gain was also observed in those randomized to placebo as compared to the treatment group who were on tamoxifen or anastrozole.[19]

DIETARY INTERVENTIONS FOR OVERWEIGHT AND OBESE CANCER PATIENT AND SURVIVORS

Weight management plays an important role in the treatment, rehabilitation, and recovery of breast cancer. Obesity and/or weight gain during treatment may lead to poor prognosis as well as an increase of the prevalence of comorbid conditions, poor surgical outcomes, lymphedema, fatigue, functional decline, and decrease in the quality of life.[20] Weight management interventions at all phases of cancer care are important to possibly avoid adverse effects, to improve overall health and possibly survival. Thus it is imperative for health-care professionals to encourage breast and GYN cancer survivors to achieve and maintain a healthy weight that is within the ideal range in an effort to promote overall health.

Maintaining adequate energy balance is important for preventing chronic diseases that are associated with excess body weight. Regulation of body weight encompasses a balance between energy intake and energy expenditure. As previously mentioned, many cancer patients are overweight or obese at the time of diagnosis, and thus the recommendations on how to manage these patients have been changed. In the past, any weight loss during cancer treatment was not recommended due to its association with cachexia and poor survival. The 2012 American Cancer Society (ACS) Nutrition and Physical Activity Guidelines for Cancer Survivors state that intentional weight loss during treatment may not be contraindicated for those who are overweight or obese.[21] A controlled weight loss of up to 2 lb/week may be safe by following a healthy diet with regular physical activity as long as it does not interfere with treatment. However, it is important to identify the etiology of unintended weight loss that occurs during treatment. If weight loss is due to nutrition impact symptoms associated with treatment toxicities then the appropriate intervention is to control and minimize symptoms. Therefore weight loss recommendations for cancer patients should be individualized and based on patient's health status, goals, and physicians and RDNs.

RDNs are challenged to implement appropriate dietary interventions for breast/GYN cancer patients, whether it is before, during, or after treatment, with the ultimate goal being the preservation of lean muscle mass while promoting gradual loss of excess body fat. Controlling the amount and rate of weight loss along with regular physical activity is a strategy that can help achieve this. Further, regular nutritional assessments and reassessments conducted by the RDN while modifying the nutrition care plan will help to continue to meet the nutritional needs of the patient.

The RDN addresses different issues while treating breast/GYN cancer patients, whether they are in treatment or survivorship. First issue is to promote a healthy balanced diet for optimal nutrition and weight management. Second issue is to enhance the quality of life while undergoing cancer treatment. The RDN assists patients in managing nutrition impact symptoms while receiving radiation and chemotherapy. Third issue is to promote postsurgery recovery. The RDN provides nutritional recommendations to promote wound healing through a balance intake of macro- and micronutrients that are important to enhance the healing process. Last issue is to promote posttreatment recovery and a healthy survivorship that focuses on achieving a healthy weight with emphasis on a diet that is high on nutrients that have a protective effect on breast cancer.[19]

DIET COMPOSITION

In breast/GYN cancer survivors, low-fat diets rich in vegetables and fruits are generally recommended. However, in metabolic syndrome patients with central obesity, diets are often aimed at reducing glucose and insulin levels. In these patients, reduction of refined carbohydrates and controlled total carbohydrate intake may be more effective.[1] Multiple studies are being conducted on the effects of diet on breast cancer survivors. Two large studies tested whether diet modifications after breast cancer diagnosis affected their outcomes. The Women's Intervention Nutrition Study tested low-fat diets in postmenopausal women diagnosed with early stages of breast cancer. The women in the study reduced their fat intake to 20% of their total calories, which resulted in a 24% reduction of new breast cancer events.[22] The Women's Healthy Eating and Living Study looked at the effects of a low-fat diet high in vegetables, fruits, and fiber and its effect on cancer outcomes on pre- and postmenopausal women. The study did not find a significant difference between the recurrences of breast cancer, but it did find a protective effect of diet and decrease in hot flashes in the subgroup studied.[23]

A variety of dietary approaches can promote weight loss if a reduction of dietary intake is achieved. Multiple studies have looked at the macronutrient makeup and its effect on weight loss on overweight and obese individuals in a variety of populations. The ones that get the most attention are the diets that are low in carbohydrates and low in fat. Ultimately, weight loss is achieved when you create an energy deficit, and the best diet is the one that the patient will follow and incorporate into their daily life.

COUNSELING STRATEGIES

Healthy diet and regular physical activity are important factors in reducing cancer recurrence risk, mortality, and lifestyle-related chronic conditions. Counseling on weight control and physical activity is not currently used in all practices of the cancer care continuum. Clinicians typically advise their patients to change their lifestyle in a more prescriptive and impersonal approach. However, this is often ineffective. Patients often seem confused or unmotivated with these messages and can bring about resistance or indifference to make changes. When a patient does not follow the recommendations of the health-care practitioner, it is perceived as a lack of motivation. However, these assumptions are false. How a practitioner talks to patients about their health can affect their motivation to change behaviors.[24] Motivational interviewing (MI) is a way to get patients to adhere to healthy behavior changes. It elicits the patient's own interest in making these changes. It is usually described as a "dance rather than a wrestling match." MI is collaborative, evocative and honors the patient's autonomy.[25]

MI is an effective alternative approach to address behavior changes that promote a constructive patient—clinician relationship that leads to better results. This type of intervention is directed to encourage a positive health behavioral change and can help improve adherence to diet and other lifestyle modifications within a clinical setting (see Table 5.1). Furthermore, MI has been shown to be a highly effective counseling strategy, especially when combined with cognitive behavioral therapy (CBT). CBT is based on the assumption that all behavior is learned and that environmental and internal factors are related to one's behavior.[26] Some additional strategies used to promote behavior change are self-monitoring, problem-solving, goal setting, cognitive restructuring, stimulus control, stress management, and relapse prevention. These strategies make a person more aware of internal and external cues and how they respond to them. Nutrition counseling conducted by an RDN is a supportive process that is set to establish goals, individualize action plans, and promote behavior change. It uses both cognitive behavioral therapies and MI to foster positive healthy behavior changes.

A successful weight loss program encompasses a variety of successful strategies. Frequent follow-ups and encounters with the RDN help facilitate weight loss and keep the patient motivated and engaged in weight loss program. Self-monitoring, although challenging, has been identified as a successful tool to use when facilitating weight loss. With the use of technology, there are many tools that can be used such as cell phones, applications, computers, and activity trackers. Frequent contact with the clinician and self-monitoring helps with accountability. Social support is also an important part of the process.[27]

THE ROLE OF BARIATRIC SURGERY IN WEIGHT MANAGEMENT FOR BREAST AND GYNECOLOGICAL CANCERS

Over one-third of the adult population in the United States is classified as obese ($BMI \geq 30\ kg/m^2$). Evidence shows that obesity is associated with an increased risk for certain breast and GYN cancers, more specifically, postmenopausal breast and endometrial cancer. Therefore aggressive weight management seems a necessary intervention to help prevent breast and other GYN cancers and cancer recurrence.

The biggest challenge found in weight management is the maintenance of weight loss. Many patients are successful at losing weight but most gain the weight back. According to some studies, bariatric surgery is one of the few weight loss interventions where significant weight loss is maintained.[28] In addition, a recent retrospective cohort study that examined whether bariatric surgery is associated with reduced risk of breast cancer among pre- and post-menopausal women concluded that bariatric surgery

TABLE 5.1
Guiding Principles of Motivational Interviewing.

Guiding Principles	Definition
1. Resist the righting reflex	Resist telling the patient what they are doing wrong and what they need to do to fix it
2. Understand your patient's motivation	Patient's own reason for change is more likely to trigger change. Be interested in the concerns and motivations of the patient. Ask reasons why they want to change and how they may do it instead of telling them what to do
3. Listen to your patient	Listen as much as you educate and inform the patient
4. Empower your patient	Guide a patient through their own ideas on how they can make positive changes in health. The patient is more likely to make a change if they are engaged in the consultation and are able to think out loud of how and why they should make a change

was associated with a reduced risk of breast cancer among severely obese women (BMI $\geq$ 35 kg/m^2).[29]

The benefit of bariatric surgery in severely obese patients needs to be evaluated on a case-by-case basis. Patients at high risk for breast and other GYN cancer recurrence and who have been unsuccessful at reaching an acceptable weight after intensive nutritional counseling may benefit from this aggressive and more permanent weight loss intervention. Nutritional counseling needs to continue after bariatric surgery to ensure success. Even after bariatric surgery, there is a risk of gaining some of the weight back if healthy eating habits are not practiced on a consistent basis.

DIET AND INFLAMMATION

The immune system is the first line of defense that our bodies have against internal and external stressors (food, chemicals, virus, bacteria, psychological stress, etc.). Inflammation is a physiological way the body uses to repair itself. In normal condition of homeostasis the body controls the inflammatory responses necessary to fight infection or improve tissue repair. However, with aging, the load of internal and external stressors turns into a silent chronic inflammatory state that is associated with increased risk of many chronic diseases such as cardiovascular diseases, dementia, arthritis, depression, and cancer.[30] Chronic inflammation increases cancer risk and affects all cancer stages.

The way we eat can improve or worsen the state of inflammation. Nutrition has a strong power that modulates inflammation. The Western diet, characterized by high sugar intake, fried foods, and refined grains, is associated with higher levels of inflammatory biomarkers, such as C-reactive protein (CRP), tumor necrosis factor-alfa (TNF-α), and interleukin-6 (IL-6). The chronic state of hyperglycemia due to the intake of carbohydrates with high glycemic load promotes increased free radicals and proinflammatory cytokines, as well as insulin and insulin growth factor-1 (IGF-1).[31] Moreover, high intake of food sources of linoleic acid (LA) such as corn oil, sunflower oil, or safflower oil induces the conversion to arachidonic acid (AA) that is an omega-6 fatty acid, a highly inflammatory compound; naturally occurring food sources of AA are eggs, grain-fed poultry, and meat. Intake of *trans*-fatty acids (TFA) derived from hydrogenated fatty acids found in baked goods is also linked to high inflammation. The standard Western diet is considered to be high in omega-6 fatty acids and TFA. Intake of TFA has been associated with increased levels of IL-6 and CRP in women with high BMI.[32] High caloric intake has also been associated with chronic inflammation due to increased adiposity; adipose tissue releases proinflammatory cytokines, TNF-α and IL-6.[33]

HOW CAN WE FIGHT INFLAMMATION THROUGH FOOD?

The constituents of an antiinflammatory diet are described in the following sections.

Phytochemicals

Phytochemicals are plant chemicals with nonnutritive characteristics that have a strong antiinflammatory function due to their powerful antioxidant and antitumor role via the modulation of signaling pathways.[34] They are found in fruits, vegetables, legumes, nuts, seeds, herbs, and spices. They have a major role in preventing and fighting disease. The more studied phytochemicals are quercetin, polyphenols (flavonoids, catechins, resveratrol, and anthocyanins), carotenoids, and phytosterols. The best way to increase them in the diet is by eating a variety of colorful vegetables, fruits, and spices in every meal. Table 5.2 shows the more common phytochemicals and their related food source.

Omega-3 Polyunsaturated Fatty Acids

Omega-3 polyunsaturated fatty acids (PUFA) are essential fatty acids that the body does not make on its own. The two omega-3 fatty acids are eicosapentaenoic acid (EPA) and docosahexaenoic acid (DHA) mainly found in cold-water fish such as sardines, salmon, halibut, herring, and anchovies. Alpha-linolenic acid is also a PUFA and is found in plant-based fats such as flaxseeds, chia seeds, and walnuts.[26] These fatty acids have an antiinflammatory effect. A randomized clinical trial with healthy individuals using different dosages of EPA + DHA ranging from 0 to 1800 mg/day for 5 months demonstrated a reduction in TNF-α.[35] Case–control studies have shown a positive association between increase intake of EPA and DHA and decrease incidence of breast cancer in premenopausal women.[36,37] Furthermore, postmenopausal women with higher intake of omega-3 fatty acids from cold-water fish when compared with lower omega-3 consumers have reduced incidence of breast cancer.[38] As mentioned previously, AA (omega-6) has a proinflammatory effect in the body; however, the ratio between omega-3 and omega-6 in the diet controls inflammation levels and demonstrates that

TABLE 5.2
Common Phytochemicals Food Sources.

Color	Phytochemicals	Food Sources
Red	Lycopene, capsaicin	Tomatoes, watermelon, sweet bell peppers, chili peppers
Orange-yellow	Alpha and Beta carotenes Beta-cryptoxanthin and flavonoids, curcumin	Pumpkin, carrots, sweet potato, peaches, papaya, oranges, cantaloupe, turmeric, mustard
Red-purple	Anthocyanins and polyphenols	Grapes, blackberries, raspberries, blueberries, red cabbage, pomegranate
Yellow-green	Lutein, zeaxanthin, glucosinolates, indoles, epigallocatechin-3-gallate	Brussel sprouts, watercress, kale, spinach, broccoli, bok choi, green tea
White-green	Allyl sulfides	Leeks, garlic, onions, chives

higher omega-6 to omega-3 ratio promotes inflammation.[39] In vivo studies have shown that by increasing the ratio of omega-3 to omega-6 fatty acids in the diet of rodents, there is a decrease in the incidence of ER+ and ER− breast cancers.[40] The recommended ratio has not been determined; however, a ratio 1:1 or 1:2 has been associated with lower inflammation, whereas it is believed that in the United States the average ratio intake is 1:10.[41]

Vegetables and Fruits

This group of foods includes a variety of plant foods rich in fiber, phytochemicals, antioxidants, and vitamins and minerals, which have an antiinflammatory effect in the body. Intake of vegetables and fruits of 7–7.5 servings/day (550–600 g/day) has shown a reduction of cancer risk with the most significant association found in cruciferous vegetables and green–yellow vegetables.[42] Moreover, intake of 10 servings/day (800 g/day) has shown a reduction in all-cause mortality with the most significant association found in apples/pears, berries, citrus fruits, cooked vegetables, cruciferous vegetables, potatoes, and green leafy vegetables.[43] It is recommended that two-thirds of the total volume *of food should come* from vegetables and fruits.[43]

- Cruciferous vegetables (cabbage, broccoli, kale, Brussel sprouts, cauliflower, bok choy, collard greens, Chinese cabbage, asparagus)
- Salad greens (romaine lettuce, iceberg lettuce, spinach, Swiss chard, arugula, watercress, dandelion greens)
- Other nonstarchy vegetables (bell peppers, radish, eggplant, zucchini, mushrooms, garlic, onions, cucumbers, tomatoes, parsley, and green beans)
- Starchy vegetables [carrots, pumpkin, beets, green peas, organic corn, potatoes (all colors)]
- All fruits (with the highest antioxidant content being strawberries, raspberries, blueberries, pomegranate, kiwi, plum, orange/citrus, cherries)

What Does a Proinflammatory Diet Versus an Antiinflammatory Diet Looks Like?

	Proinflammatory Diet	Antiinflammatory Diet
Breakfast	One bacon One white flour biscuit or four crackers One egg Coffee with creamer and 2 tbsp of white sugar	3/4 c of berries of choice 1 c of Greek yogurt 1/2 tbsp powder cinnamon 1/4 c of raw nuts of choice 1 tbsp of honey 1 c of herbal tea
Lunch	Ham and cheese sandwich on white bread with mayonnaise Small bag of potato chips 1 can of soda	2–3 c of salad greens with a combination of mixed greens, cucumbers, tomatoes, olives, radish, and celery 1/2 c of chickpeas or hummus 2 tbsp sunflower seeds 1/2 small avocado (Hass type) *Salad dressing* 1 tbsp of extra virgin olive oil The juice of 1/2 squeezed lemon Touch of minced fresh ginger One apple or pear
Dinner	3 oz fried chicken leg and thigh 1 c of white rice with beans One bread roll with margarine 8 oz of iced tea	3–4 oz of oven grilled salmon 1 tbsp of extra virgin olive oil 1/2 garlic clove 1 1/2 c of sautéed bell peppers with mushrooms and asparagus One medium oven-baked sweet potato (no butter added) with cinnamon if desired 1 c of herbal tea

MEDITERRANEAN DIET AS AN ANTIINFLAMMATORY DIET

The Mediterranean diet (MD) is a well-studied dietary pattern in the literature.[44] The MD has the characteristics of an antiinflammatory eating pattern; however, there is no consensus on the definition with established macronutrients (proteins, carbohydrates, and fats) distribution.

The MD was based on the eating habits of Southern European countries around the 1960s. The diet is characterized by the consistent intake of monounsaturated fatty acids (MUFA) and PUFA from tree nuts and extra virgin olive oil, fiber derived from vegetables, fruits, whole grains, and beans and moderate intake of low-fat dairy, eggs, lean meats such as fish and red wine (usually during meals).

Research shows that the MD has many characteristics that promote the intake of antiinflammatory foods. The combination of PUFA and MUFA, dietary fiber, and a wide variety of antioxidants and phytonutrients makes the MD diet an optimal diet.[35] Moreover, it has been shown that its high content of antioxidants and vitamins increases the potential of reducing endogenic estrogen.[45]

Toledo et al. conducted a randomized controlled trial where it showed that MD had a strong protective effect on the incidence of breast cancer in postmenopausal women.[46] Moreover, in a meta-analysis of cohort studies conducted for a total of 20.3 years researchers in the Netherlands measured the adherence of the MD and risk of postmenopausal breast cancer, they found an increased risk of ER− breast cancer with poor adherence to MD in postmenopausal women.[47] In the study, alcohol intake was eliminated from the MD dietary pattern.

The MD has also been studied in endometrial cancer patients. In a case–control study from Northern Italy with 297 cases of biopsy-proven endometrial cancer and 307 controls, researchers found that high vegetable intake along with a good adherence to an MD has a protective effect to reduce the risk of endometrial cancer.[48]

DIETARY RECOMMENDATIONS FOR CANCER PATIENTS AND SURVIVORS

- Increase your intake of nonstarchy vegetables and try to incorporate leafy greens to every meal if possible. There is no limit in the intake of nonstarchy vegetables, follow the colors of the rainbow when choosing vegetables to add variety to your daily meals. Aim for no less than 5–6 servings/day (1 c for raw vegetables and 1/2 c cooked vegetables).
- Eat a variety of fresh fruits (emphasis on high antioxidant and dark red/purple color fruits such as berries, pomegranate, as well as high vitamin C

fruits such as kiwi and oranges/citrus family). Aim for 2–3 servings/day (serving varies depending on the type of fruit). For most fruits the serving equals 1/2 c or a small whole fruit.

- Choose whole grains (wild rice, quinoa, barley, multigrain bread, whole oats, and whole rye) rather than processed refined grains (white flour, white rice, pasta, white bread).
- Eat at least 25–30 g of fiber/day (good sources include beans, whole grains, fruit, and fresh vegetables).
- Limit the intake of red meat to no more than once a week and avoid intake of high fat and processed meats (hot dogs, bacon, sausage, ham, lunch meats).
- Choose healthy cooking methods, such as baking, steaming, grilling, and broiling rather than frying or charbroiling.
- Try a meatless meal one to two times a week. Eat beans or lentils as your plant-based source of protein.
- Limit the intake of added sugars (candies, cakes, pastries, and cookies) and limit empty calories, such as sodas and sweetened beverages.
- Increase intake of polyunsaturated and monounsaturated fats. Good sources are cold-pressed extra virgin olive oil, cold-pressed avocado oil, salmon, tree nuts (almonds, seeds, hazelnuts, walnuts, pistachios, and cashews), and olives and avocado. If cooking with oils, aim for 1–2 tbsp of oil per meal.
- Limit the intake of saturated fats, solid at room temperature, for example, butter, lard, coconut oil, palm oil, and full-fat dairy. Avoid the intake of *trans* fats, also known as hydrogenated and partially hydrogenated oils, examples are margarines and processed foods prepared with margarine or vegetable shortening (bagels, baked goods, pastries).
- When you are eating out, choose foods lower in calories, fat, and sugar. Share your meals and do not be afraid to have special requests (dressing on the side, no bread, change French fries for a side salad, steamed instead of fried).

THE LINK BETWEEN ETHANOL AND BREAST CANCER

The association between alcohol intake and breast cancer incidence and risk of recurrence has been well studied. According to the American Institute for Cancer Research, Continuous Update Project (AICR/CUP), diet, nutrition, physical activity, and breast cancer publication last revised in 2018, there is a strong evidence that consuming alcoholic drinks increases breast cancer risk and risk of recurrence with intakes above 15 g/day that is the equivalent of one standard alcoholic drink (5 oz wine, 12 oz beer, and 1.5 oz liquor) in pre- and postmenopausal women, specially ER + and PR + breast cancer subtypes.[49–51] There are different mechanisms that can explain this. It is not unusual that heavy drinkers tend to have a poor diet limited in antiinflammatory nutrients such as essential omega-3 fatty acids, vitamins such as folate, minerals, and antioxidants. This poor quality diet reduces the ability of the body to protect itself thus increasing the susceptibility to carcinogenesis. Alcohol consumption also produces more reactive oxygen species (ROS) contributing to DNA damage. It is also believed that alcohol consumption increases circulating levels of estrogen.[52] Furthermore, the National Institute of Health classifies ethanol as a known human carcinogen.[53] The Dietary Guidelines for Americans 2015–20 recommend that individuals who do not drink alcohol should not start drinking.[54] There are no established guidelines in regards of alcohol consumption for women with increased risk of breast cancer or risk of recurrence; however, regular consumption of alcoholic beverages of one to two drinks per day may contribute to an increase in risk.[52]

CONCLUSION

The nutritional management of breast and GYN cancer patients may be a multifaceted one that requires an early nutritional intervention not only to address and correct possible nutritional deficiencies related to cancer treatment but also to help these patients achieve a healthy weight through behavioral changes and dietary modifications.

There is convincing evidence that obesity is associated with an increased risk for cancer development and recurrence and poor survival, thus early dietary interventions such as calorie restriction, increased physical activity, and promotion of healthy eating habits may improve patient's outcomes. Counseling strategies such as MI has shown to be an effective approach to promote behavior change with diet adherence.

It has been shown that eating a more inflammatory diet consisting of refined grains, high sugar content, TFA, and reduced fiber intake from nonstarchy vegetables, fruits, legumes, and whole grains creates a negative impact on our health with increased risk for many chronic diseases, including cancer.

The MD has all the constituents of an antiinflammatory diet. Studies have shown that the MD reduces endogenic estrogen and in postmenopausal women has a protective effect on the incidence of breast cancer. Moreover, patients that adherence to the MD have a low risk of endometrial cancer.

Every cancer center should have available nutrition counseling for all cancer patients before, during, and after cancer treatment. The RDN plays a crucial role in helping patients make dietary changes that will have a positive impact on their overall health.

REFERENCES

1. Leser M, Ledesma N, Bergerson S, Trujillo EB. *Oncology Nutrition for Clinical Practice*. Chicago, IL: Academy of Nutrition and Dietetics; 2018.
2. Reber E, Gomes F, Vasiloglou MF, Schuetz P, Stanga Z. Nutritional risk screening and assessment. *J Clin Med*. 2019;8(7):1065. Available from: https://doi.org/10.3390/jcm8071065.
3. Rinninella E, Fagotti A, Cintoni M, et al. Nutritional interventions to improve clinical outcomes in ovarian cancer: a systematic review of randomized controlled trials. *Nutrients*. 2019;11(6):1404. Available from: https://doi.org/10.3390/nu11061404.
4. Eglseer D, Halfens RJ, Lohrmann C. Is the presence of a validated malnutrition screening tool associated with better nutritional care in hospitalized patients? *Nutrition*. 2017;37:104–111. Available from: https://doi.org/10.1016/j.nut.2016.12.016.
5. Lacey K, Pritchett E. Nutrition care process and model: ADA adopts road map to quality care and outcomes management. *J Am Dietetic Assoc*. 2003;103(8):1061–1072. Available from: https://doi.org/10.1016/s0002-8223(03)00971-4.
6. Swan WI, Vivanti A, Hakel-Smith NA, et al. Nutrition care process and model update: toward realizing people-centered care and outcomes management. *J Acad Nutr Dietetics*. 2017;117(12):2003–2014. Available from: https://doi.org/10.1016/j.jand.2017.07.015.
7. Reeves MM, Capra S. Predicting energy requirements in the clinical setting: are current methods evidence based? *Nutr Rev*. 2003;61(4):143–151. Available from: https://doi.org/10.1301/nr.2003.apr.143-151.
8. Grant BL. *Academy of Nutrition and Dietetics Pocket Guide to the Nutrition Care Process and Cancer*. Chicago, IL: Academy of Nutrition and Dietetics; 2015.
9. Jiralerspong S, Goodwin PJ. Obesity and breast cancer prognosis: evidence, challenges, and opportunities. *J Clin Oncol*. 2016;34(35):4203–4216. Available from: https://doi.org/10.1200/jco.2016.68.4480.
10. Harvie M. The importance of controlling body weight after a diagnosis of breast cancer: the role of diet and exercise in breast cancer patient management. *Exerc Cancer Survivorship*. 2009;73–96. Available from: https://doi.org/10.1007/978-1-4419-1173-5_5.
11. Suzuki R, Orsini N, Saji S, Key TJ, Wolk A. Body weight and incidence of breast cancer defined by estrogen and progesterone receptor status—a meta-analysis. *Int J Cancer*. 2009;124(3):698–712. Available from: https://doi.org/10.1002/ijc.23943.
12. Pierobon M, Frankenfeld CL. Obesity as a risk factor for triple-negative breast cancers: a systematic review and meta-analysis. *Breast Cancer Res Treat*. 2012;137(1):307–314. Available from: https://doi.org/10.1007/s10549-012-2339-3.
13. Yang X, Wang J. The role of metabolic syndrome in endometrial cancer: a review. *Front Oncol*. 2019;9. Available from: https://doi.org/10.3389/fonc.2019.00744.
14. Gunter MJ, Xie X, Xue X, et al. Breast cancer risk in metabolically healthy but overweight postmenopausal women. *Cancer Res*. 2015;75(2):270–274. Available from: https://doi.org/10.1158/0008-5472.can-14-2317.
15. Majed B, Moreau T, Senouci K, Salmon RJ, Fourquet A, Asselain B. Is obesity an independent prognosis factor in woman breast cancer? *Breast Cancer Res Treat*. 2007;111(2):329–342. Available from: https://doi.org/10.1007/s10549-007-9785-3.
16. Saquib N, Flatt SW, Natarajan L, et al. Weight gain and recovery of pre-cancer weight after breast cancer treatments: evidence from the women's healthy eating and living (WHEL) study. *Breast Cancer Res Treat*. 2006;105(2):177–186. Available from: https://doi.org/10.1007/s10549-006-9442-2.
17. Goodwin PJ, Ennis M, Pritchard KI, et al. Adjuvant treatment and onset of menopause predict weight gain after breast cancer diagnosis. *J Clin Oncol*. 1999;17(1):120. Available from: https://doi.org/10.1200/jco.1999.17.1.120.
18. Kroenke CH, Chen WY, Rosner B, Holmes MD. Weight, weight gain, and survival after breast cancer diagnosis. *J Clin Oncol*. 2005;23(7):1370–1378. Available from: https://doi.org/10.1200/jco.2005.01.079.
19. Sestak I, Harvie M, Howell A, Forbes JF, Dowsett M, Cuzick J. Weight change associated with anastrozole and tamoxifen treatment in postmenopausal women with or at high risk of developing breast cancer. *Breast Cancer Res Treat*. 2012;134(2):727–734. Available from: https://doi.org/10.1007/s10549-012-2085-6.
20. Demark-Wahnefried W, Campbell KL, Hayes SC. Weight management and its role in breast cancer rehabilitation. *Cancer*. 2012;118(S8):2277–2287. Available from: https://doi.org/10.1002/cncr.27466.
21. Rock CL, Doyle C, Demark-Wahnefried W, et al. Nutrition and physical activity guidelines for cancer survivors. *CA: Cancer J Clin*. 2012;62(4):275–276. Available from: https://doi.org/10.3322/caac.21146.
22. Robien K, Demark-Wahnefried W, Rock CL. Evidence-based nutrition guidelines for cancer survivors: current guidelines, knowledge gaps, and future research directions. *J Am Diet Assoc*. 2011;111(3):368–375. Available from: https://doi.org/10.1016/j.jada.2010.11.014.

23. Pierce JP, Stefanick ML, Flatt SW, et al. Greater survival after breast cancer in physically active women with high vegetable-fruit intake regardless of obesity. *J Clin Oncol.* 2007;25(17):2345–2351. Available from: https://doi.org/10.1200/jco.2006.08.6819.
24. Gnagnarella P, Dragà D, Baggi F, et al. Promoting weight loss through diet and exercise in overweight or obese breast cancer survivors (InForma): study protocol for a randomized controlled trial. *Trials.* 2016;17(1). Available from: https://doi.org/10.1186/s13063-016-1487-x.
25. Rollnick S, Miller WR, Butler CC. *Motivational Interviewing in Health Care: Helping Patients Change Behavior.* New York: The Guilford Press; 2008.
26. Spahn JM, Reeves RS, Keim KS, et al. State of the evidence regarding behavior change theories and strategies in nutrition counseling to facilitate health and food behavior change. *J Am Dietetic Assoc.* 2010;110(6):879–891. Available from: https://doi.org/10.1016/j.jada.2010.03.021.
27. Terranova CO, Lawler SP, Spathonis K, Eakin EG, Reeves MM. Breast cancer survivors' experience of making weight, dietary and physical activity changes during participation in a weight loss intervention. *Supportive Care Cancer.* 2016;25(5):1455–1463. Available from: https://doi.org/10.1007/s00520-016-3542-2.
28. Chang S-H, Stoll CRT, Song J, Varela JE, Eagon CJ, Colditz GA. The effectiveness and risks of bariatric surgery. *JAMA Surg.* 2014;149(3):275. Available from: https://doi.org/10.1001/jamasurg.2013.3654.
29. Feigelson HS, Caan B, Weinmann S, et al. Bariatric surgery is associated with reduced risk of breast cancer in both premenopausal and postmenopausal women. *Ann Surg.* 2019;1. Available from: https://doi.org/10.1097/sla.0000000000003331.
30. Martucci M, Ostan R, Biondi F, et al. Mediterranean diet and inflammaging within the hormesis paradigm. *Nutr Rev.* 2017;75(6):442–455. Available from: https://doi.org/10.1093/nutrit/nux013.
31. Ricker MA, Haas WC. Anti-inflammatory diet in clinical practice: a review. *Nutr Clin Pract.* 2017;32(3):318–325. Available from: https://doi.org/10.1177/0884533617700353.
32. Mozaffarian D, Pischon T, Hankinson SE, et al. Dietary intake of trans fatty acids and systemic inflammation in women. *Am J Clin Nutr.* 2004;79(4):606–612. Available from: https://doi.org/10.1093/ajcn/79.4.606.
33. Rajala MW, Scherer PE. Minireview: the adipocyte—at the crossroads of energy homeostasis, inflammation, and atherosclerosis. *Endocrinology.* 2003;144(9):3765–3773. Available from: https://doi.org/10.1210/en.2003-0580.
34. Ostan R, Lanzarini C, Pini E, et al. Inflammaging and cancer: a challenge for the Mediterranean diet. *Nutrients.* 2015;7(4):2589–2621. Available from: https://doi.org/10.3390/nu7042589.
35. Flock MR, Skulas-Ray AC, Harris WS, Gaugler TL, Fleming JA, Kris-Etherton PM. Effects of supplemental long-chain omega-3 fatty acids and erythrocyte membrane fatty acid content on circulating inflammatory markers in a randomized controlled trial of healthy adults. *Prostaglandins, Leukotrienes Essent Fat Acids.* 2014;91(4):161–168. Available from: https://doi.org/10.1016/j.plefa.2014.07.006.
36. Chajes V, Torres-Mejia G, Biessy C, et al. ω-3 and ω-6 Polyunsaturated fatty acid intakes and the risk of breast cancer in Mexican women: impact of obesity status. *Cancer Epidemiol Biomarkers Prev.* 2011;21(2):319–326. Available from: https://doi.org/10.1158/1055-9965.epi-11-0896.
37. Goodstine SL, Zheng T, Holford TR, et al. Dietary (n-3)/(n-6) fatty acid ratio: possible relationship to premenopausal but not postmenopausal breast cancer risk in U.S. women. *J Nutr.* 2003;133(5):1409–1414. Available from: https://doi.org/10.1093/jn/133.5.1409.
38. Zheng J-S, Hu X-J, Zhao Y-M, Yang J, Li D. Intake of fish and marine n-3 polyunsaturated fatty acids and risk of breast cancer: meta-analysis of data from 21 independent prospective cohort studies. *BMJ.* 2013;346(jun27 5). Available from: https://doi.org/10.1136/bmj.f3706.
39. Simopoulos AP. The importance of the omega-6/omega-3 fatty acid ratio in cardiovascular disease and other chronic diseases. *Exp Biol Med.* 2008;233(6):674–688. Available from: https://doi.org/10.3181/0711-mr-311.
40. Fabian CJ, Kimler BF, Hursting SD. Omega-3 fatty acids for breast cancer prevention and survivorship. *Breast Cancer Res.* 2015;17(1). Available from: https://doi.org/10.1186/s13058-015-0571-6.
41. Blasbalg TL, Hibbeln JR, Ramsden CE, Majchrzak SF, Rawlings RR. Changes in consumption of omega-3 and omega-6 fatty acids in the United States during the 20th century. *Am J Clin Nutr.* 2011;93(5):950–962. Available from: https://doi.org/10.3945/ajcn.110.006643.
42. Aune D, Giovannucci E, Boffetta P, et al. Fruit and vegetable intake and the risk of cardiovascular disease, total cancer and all-cause mortality—a systematic review and dose-response meta-analysis of prospective studies. *Int J Epidemiol.* 2017;46(3):1029–1056. Available from: https://doi.org/10.1093/ije/dyw319.
43. Sears B. Anti-inflammatory diets. *J Am Coll Nutr.* 2015;34(suppl 1):14–21. Available from: https://doi.org/10.1080/07315724.2015.1080105.
44. Sofi F, Abbate R, Gensini GF, Casini A. Accruing evidence on benefits of adherence to the Mediterranean diet on health: an updated systematic review and meta-analysis. *Am J Clin Nutr.* 2010;92(5):1189–1196. Available from: https://doi.org/10.3945/ajcn.2010.29673.
45. Carruba G, Granata OM, Pala V, et al. A traditional Mediterranean diet decreases endogenous estrogens in healthy postmenopausal women. *Nutr Cancer.* 2006;56(2):253–259. Available from: https://doi.org/10.1207/s15327914nc5602_18.
46. Toledo E, Salas-Salvadó J, Donat-Vargas C, et al. Mediterranean diet and invasive breast cancer risk among women at high cardiovascular risk in the PREDIMED

Trial. *JAMA Intern Med.* 2015;175(11):1752. Available from: https://doi.org/10.1001/jamainternmed.2015.4838.

47. Brandt PAVD, Schulpen M. Mediterranean diet adherence and risk of postmenopausal breast cancer: results of a cohort study and meta-analysis. *Int J Cancer.* 2017;140(10):2220–2231. Available from: https://doi.org/10.1002/ijc.30654.
48. Ricceri F, Giraudo MT, Fasanelli F, et al. Diet and endometrial cancer: a focus on the role of fruit and vegetable intake, Mediterranean diet and dietary inflammatory index in the endometrial cancer risk. *BMC Cancer.* 2017;17(1). Available from: https://doi.org/10.1186/s12885-017-3754-y.
49. World Cancer Research Fund International. *Diet, Nutrition, Physical Activity and Cancer: a Global Perspective: a Summary of the Third Expert Report.* London: World Cancer Research Fund International; 2018.
50. Fagherazzi G, Vilier A, Boutron-Ruault M-C, Mesrine S, Clavel-Chapelon F. Alcohol consumption and breast cancer risk subtypes in the E3N-EPIC cohort. *Eur J Cancer Prev.* 2015;24(3):209–214. Available from: https://doi.org/10.1097/cej.0000000000000031.
51. Chen WY, Rosner B, Hankinson SE, Colditz GA, Willett WC. Moderate alcohol consumption during adult life, drinking patterns, and breast cancer risk. *JAMA.* 2011;306(17):1884. Available from: https://doi.org/10.1001/jama.2011.1590.
52. Singletary KW, Gapstur SM. Alcohol and breast cancer. *JAMA.* 2001;286(17):2143. Available from: https://doi.org/10.1001/jama.286.17.2143.
53. National Cancer Institute. *Alcohol and Cancer Risk Fact Sheet.* National Cancer Institute. <https://www.cancer.gov/about-cancer/causes-prevention/risk/alcohol/alcohol-fact-sheet> Accessed 18.09.19.
54. Dietary Guidelines for Americans. *2015-2020 Dietary Guidelines: Dietary Guidelines for Americans.* 2015-2020 Dietary Guidelines | Dietary Guidelines for Americans. <http://www.dietaryguidelines.gov/current-dietary-guidelines/2015-2020-dietary-guidelines> Accessed 18.09.19.

CHAPTER 6

A Comprehensive Approach to Psychosocial Distress and Anxiety in Breast and Gynecological Cancers

LYNN KIM, OTD, OTR/L • VINITA KHANNA, LCSW, MPH, ACHP-SW, OSW-C • VANESSA YANEZ, MOT, OTR/L • SHERRY HITE, MOT, OTR/L

BACKGROUND

Cancer-related psychological distress and anxiety is widely reported side effect of cancer during and after treatment. Nearly one-third of cancer survivors, around 16.9 million in the United States, are diagnosed with mental health conditions.[1] Failure to recognize and address psychosocial concerns, such as distress and anxiety, have been associated with decreased immune function among cancer survivors,[2] resulting in more frequent infections[2] and lower adherence to cancer treatment.[3] Recent studies have also demonstrated that psychological stress can affect tumor emergence, progression, and metastasis.[2]

Addressing psychosocial distress and anxiety can result in improved health outcomes and quality of life. As the number of cancer survivors increase with long-term challenges impacting psychosocial well-being, there has been a growing awareness and prioritization of distress and anxiety management as part of standard care. National oncology organizations, such as the National Comprehensive Cancer Network (NCCN) and the American College of Surgeons (ACoS) Commission on Cancer (CoC), have established recommendations to integrate psychosocial care into standard practice.[4,5]

DEFINITION OF DISTRESS AND ANXIETY

Cancer-related distress and anxiety extends along a range of emotions and is a subjective experience that may fluctuate throughout an individual's disease course. Distress can range from normal feelings of nervousness to disabling emotions that can impact adherence to treatment, decrease satisfaction with medical care, increase health-care costs, lead to poor self-management of symptoms, and decreased quality of life. The NCCN defines distress as "a multifactorial unpleasant experience of a psychological (i.e., cognitive, behavioral, emotional), social, spiritual, and/or physical nature that may interfere with the ability to cope effectively with cancer, its physical symptoms, and its treatment."[4] Symptoms of anxiety are also normal feelings and can be a temporary and adaptive reaction to cancer and its treatment. However, when symptoms of anxiety, such as excessive worrying and fear, are prolonged, intense, and interfering with daily functioning, it might be classified as a psychological disorder.

Distinguishing normal symptoms of emotional distress and psychiatric disorders might present as a challenge to the primary cancer team due to multiple reasons, such as minimization of symptoms by patients or red flags being ignored by the medical team. Therefore it is important to identify and address symptoms of emotional distress and anxiety as early as possible with potential referral to mental health specialists available in one's facility or community. Addressing psychosocial distress is recommended during routine care with some concerns being managed or resolved by the primary team during visits or follow-ups, such as questions regarding treatments and long-term prognosis. To illustrate its critical importance within routine care, distress screening has been increasingly considered the "sixth vital sign," along with pain, temperature, pulse, respiration, and blood pressure.[4]

Breast Cancer and Gynecologic Cancer Rehabilitation DOI: https://doi.org/10.1016/B978-0-323-72166-0.00006-2

DISTRESS AND ANXIETY IN THE BREAST AND GYNECOLOGICAL CANCER POPULATIONS

The growing population of survivors of breast and gynecological cancers and the increased prevalence of distress and anxiety necessitate the pressing need for health-care professionals to address psychosocial issues throughout the continuum of cancer care. Advancements in cancer research and treatment are saving and prolonging the lives of many individuals diagnosed with breast and gynecological cancers. Survivors are now more likely to undergo treatments that may trigger distress and anxiety at various time points, including diagnostic workup, early-stage cancer, active treatment, advanced stage and metastatic disease, and end-of-life. Given the volume of triggers across both populations and the likelihood of encountering and managing these triggers during the rehabilitation process, it is imperative that health-care professionals are aware of the signs and symptoms of mental health concerns and provide support as appropriate. For many patients, effectively addressing these symptoms can alleviate some, if not all, of the psychosocial burden.

THE IMPORTANCE OF PSYCHOSOCIAL SCREENING AND INTERVENTION

In the last decade, there has been a growing awareness of the importance of psychosocial screening and intervention as part of comprehensive cancer care. The negative effects of distress and anxiety on health outcomes have been increasingly reported in the literature, and current research shows that survivors of cancer treatment are at elevated risk for mental health issues, fear of recurrence, and depression, which may persist many years after diagnosis.[4] To highlight the importance of integrated distress screening in standard cancer care, the ACoS CoC has mandated psychosocial distress screening and referral as a condition for cancer center accreditation beginning in 2015. In order to standardize care across cancer centers, several regulatory bodies have published guidelines for screening, assessment, and management of psychosocial concerns with the provision of clinical pathways to guide clinical practice in efforts to standardize care across oncology centers and equip health-care professionals with the tools necessary to implement these recommendations into everyday practice. The NCCN recommends routine screening and monitoring of emotional distress, as cancer diagnosis and treatment burden can impact an individual's functional performance and quality of life throughout treatment and into survivorship and end-of-life.[4]

PSYCHOSOCIAL NEEDS IN THE BREAST AND GYNECOLOGICAL CANCER POPULATIONS

While certain triggers for distress and anxiety may be more common or generalizable to the oncology population, such as receiving a cancer diagnosis or treatment-related fatigue, there are certain triggers specific to the breast and gynecological cancer populations, which must be considered in order to provide the most holistic and individualized care possible.

Distress and Anxiety in Early-Stage Disease

Due to increased awareness of disease and early screening methods, patients are being diagnosed with breast and gynecological cancer at earlier stages than in the past. In these scenarios, patients may be scheduled for treatment not long after diagnosis. Patients are at increased risk for distress during this initial stage, as they may be caught in the throes of processing the diagnosis itself while being required to make crucial decisions about their health care, preparing for treatment, and managing subsequent recovery. Improved survival rates of early-stage breast cancer and the opportunity for immediate breast reconstruction have been beneficial for health outcomes, but this group is at risk for being overlooked during psychosocial screening due to the curable nature of early-stage disease. It is crucial to recognize that distress is not dependent on prognosis and should be addressed despite the stage of disease or type of treatment.

Impact on Progress and Treatment Adherence

Studies have shown that underlying distress or anxiety can inhibit progress and even impact treatment adherence. For example, multiple studies have found associations between higher levels of distress and increased risk of intentional nonadherence to tamoxifen after breast cancer surgery, despite the known benefits of hormone treatments in preventing disease recurrence.[3] Furthermore, women with elevated levels of distress and anxiety were found to have increased persistent postmastectomy pain.[6] Health-care professionals should make efforts to identify predictors of intentional or unintentional nonadherence and sources of distress to ensure patient understanding of the necessity of such treatments. Research has shown inconclusive evidence for the relationship between side effects and nonadherence; rather, evidence suggests that belief systems around illness and treatment necessity have far more weight in decision-making around adherence.[3] This highlights the importance of investigation into psychological or psychosocial factors, which may contribute to nonadherence from early stages to later in the treatment pathway.

Fear of Recurrence

Fear of recurrence is a prevalent psychological burden that may manifest from a normal response to cancer to a pathological response. The potential ramifications of improved treatment methods and increased survival rates may lead to an increase in psychological burden over a prolonged period of time due to fear of disease recurrence despite having reached remission. Gynecological cancers have one of the highest cancer recurrence rates, with recurrence estimated in 70% of patients with ovarian cancer.[7] Type of breast cancer treatments can influence fear of cancer recurrence; breast conservation can lead to increased anxiety while double mastectomies can actually lead to nonadherence with adjuvant hormonal therapies.[3,8] Higher levels of fear of recurrence have been correlated with lower quality of life, anxiety, and functional impairment.[9] Long-term treatment and psychosocial care are warranted in order to ensure positive adjustment and improved quality of life after treatment.

Sexual Dysfunction and Altered Body Image

The sensitive nature of sexuality and cultural notions of sex as "taboo" may contribute to increased distress, as patients may feel that their needs are not being addressed appropriately. Patients themselves may also feel uncomfortable bringing up sexual concerns with their health-care provider. The neurotoxic side effects of chemotherapy may lead to estrogen deprivation, menopause, vaginal dryness, and fertility loss. Side effects of radiation include lymphedema, inflammation of tissues, and loss of organ function. Side effects of hormonal treatments include estrogen deprivation or decline with resulting side effects such as menopause, hair thinning, weight loss or gain, and hot flashes. Surgery can result in disfigurement, scarring, and resection of sexual organs.

Sexual dysfunction can be a source of significant distress depending on the type and location of treatment intervention. Women with breast cancer may experience alterations in body image perception and difficulty with body acceptance with partial or entire breast removal, breast reconstruction, appearance of scars, and/or postoperative side effects such as pain or lymphedema. Women with gynecological cancer warrant specialized attention in the area of sexual dysfunction, as surgery and radiation to the pelvic organs have direct impact on sexual functioning. Women have reported that after surgery, radiation, or a combination of both treatments, sexuality-related and bowel symptoms were most distressful, some of which include reduced orgasm frequency, overall intercourse dysfunction, reduced orgasms, vaginal changes, dyspareunia, and bowel dysfunction.[10]

Adolescent and Young Adult Survivors of Breast and Gynecological Cancers

Throughout the course of diagnosis and treatment, it is pertinent to be mindful of the age range of the breast and gynecological cancer patient in order to address distress levels and structure goals of treatment appropriately. The young adult population, defined as ages 18–39, with breast and gynecological cancers report significant levels of distress, as they may be less likely to anticipate the onset of cancer and have to confront the potential impact of the disease on developmental milestones.[11] Diagnosis and treatment may lead to decreased independence, treatment-induced infertility, loss of school or work, and increased social isolation. Younger age at diagnosis in of itself was found to be a predictor of psychological distress in gynecological cancer survivors.[12] Furthermore, when compared to their disease-free counterparts, young women diagnosed with breast or gynecological cancer were found to be four times more likely to have serious psychological distress.[12] A majority of young women with breast cancer reported distress at the end of treatment with concerns, including fertility-related distress, body image changes, and fear of recurrence.[12] A study comparing adolescent and young adult (AYA) breast cancer patients to adult breast cancer patients in their forties found that more aggressive therapy, specifically mastectomy, lymph node removal, and chemotherapy, was recommended or chosen for women in the AYA age-group.[13] More aggressive disease and treatment may result in greater functional limitations and distress later on in life.

Metastatic Breast Cancer

With advancements in metastatic breast cancer treatment, patients are now living longer than ever before. The unique aspect of this is the need for indefinite treatment due to the incurable nature of the disease. High levels of distress and increased symptom burden have been noted in this population due to the psychological impact of needing continuous treatment in order to survive.[8] In addition, many providers do not refer these patients to rehabilitation services due to prognosis and fear of increasing fracture risk in those with bone metastases.[14] However, this patient population would benefit greatly from continued rehabilitation efforts despite overall prognosis. For example, a physical therapy referral would inform appropriate physical activity within safety precautions, an occupational therapy referral would facilitate optimal engagement in meaningful occupations, and a psychosocial referral to a mental health specialist would address distress and anxiety. Health-care providers should advocate for early and continuous involvement of rehabilitation for those diagnosed with metastatic breast cancer in order to mitigate distress caused by symptom burden.

Men With Breast Cancer

Breast cancer in men is rare, consisting of only less than 1% of all breast cancers. However, this population requires special consideration because a decreased awareness of the disease in men may also result in diagnostic delays and poorer prognosis.[15] It is common for programs to tailor resources and materials to women, thus creating a less inclusive environment for men who are diagnosed. Men have oftentimes expressed hesitation while discussing their diagnosis with others, which can ultimately foster social isolation, as they may feel stigmatized by a diagnosis so strongly associated with women.[15] Men with breast cancer also reported worse health-related quality of life, particularly in role functioning, compared with their disease-free counterparts.[16] These effects may be minimized by proactively screening for distress and effectively providing support in this patient population.

Caregiver Needs

Caregivers play a pivotal role in the promotion of recovery and provision of support for these patients. In addition to providing instrumental care and support, caregivers are often tasked with clinical responsibilities as well, including postsurgical drain management, administration of medication, and assistance with activities of daily living. For male caregivers of postsurgical patients with gynecological cancer during hospitalization, the perceived preparedness of the caregiver was not related to emotional distress, indicating that even those who appear well prepared may have significant needs related to health and psychological problems.[17] Another study found that in 50 caregivers of patients with end-stage ovarian cancer, caregivers reported that they enjoyed and felt privileged to care for their loved one, but that this was independent from the burden of disrupted schedules and financial hardship.[18] It is important to consider that caregiver burden can be expected to increase due to increased disability and declining functional abilities in individuals with progressive or end-stage disease.[19]

SCREENING FOR DISTRESS AND ANXIETY

Screening as Preventative Medicine

"Preventive medicine is a medical specialty recognized by the American Board of Medical Specialties (ABMS), which focuses on the health of individuals and communities. The goal of preventive medicine is to promote health and well-being and prevent disease, disability and death."[20] Screening should be viewed as a powerful preventive medicine tool utilized in health care. It is also vital to be aware of further benefits of reducing distress, such as decreased visits to emergency or urgent care rooms, decreased hospital readmissions, decreased consumption of resources, and decreased length of stays during an inpatient admission.[21] The NCCN, the Institute of Medicine, and the American Society of Clinical Oncology (ASCO) have identified the screening, assessment, and follow-up as well as treatment of psychosocial distress as a quality care standard in routine cancer care.[4,5,22] The US Preventive Services Task Force recommends screening patients in clinical practices that have systems in place to ensure precise diagnosis, efficient treatment, and follow-up care.

Screening for distress near the time of diagnosis and rescreening throughout the treatment continuum serves as a preventative medicine tool to minimize the consequences of substantial psychosocial concerns. By preventing, addressing, and reducing distress and anxiety, health-care professionals can improve the quality of life of patients and "reduce the human cost of cancer" by addressing not only medical but also psychosocial, psychiatric, financial, emotional, and spiritual concerns.[23]

Oncology Stakeholders and Standards for Distress Screening

American College of Surgeons Commission on Cancer

The ACoS CoC is a consortium of professional organizations that publishes requirements for accreditation of cancer clinics and establishes standards to support high-quality, comprehensive cancer care. The CoC recently published *Optimal Resources for Cancer Care:*

2020 Standards that are effective as of January 2020 and provide accreditation requirements for psychosocial distress screening. The CoC requires that psychosocial services are available on-site or by referral, and that the findings of psychosocial distress screenings must be reported to the institution's cancer committee.[5]

It is recommended that all cancer programs implement a policy and procedure for distress screening in order to identify the psychological, social, financial, and behavioral issues, which may affect the patient's treatment plan and treatment outcomes.[5] The CoC provides a list of requirements necessary to support the implementation of comprehensive psychosocial distress screening in cancer programs and measure compliance with accreditation standards.[5] The feasibility of implementing these standards requires cancer programs to carefully consider their program's size, resources, location, and patient population.[5]

At least one distress screening during the first course of treatment is required, with additional screenings to be administered as necessary or at the discretion of the health-care provider.[5] The mode of administration is to be determined by the site, and medical staff who administer or interpret that the screening must be properly trained. Standardized and validated instruments or tools are recommended.[5] Upon identification of moderate or severe distress, it is crucial to follow up via direct contact in order to confirm the screening results and identify the appropriate referrals.[5]

The National Comprehensive Cancer Network

The NCCN's Guidelines for Distress Management provides an overview of the evidence in support of early and regular distress screening and a consensus of evidence-based screening and treatment methods.[4] The NCCN's Distress Management Panel has established Standards of Care for Distress Management with principles for implementation of these standards in-line with the recommendations of the ACoS CoC[4] (Fig. 6.1).

American Society of Clinical Oncology's Quality Oncology Practice Initiative

In 2002 the ASCO introduced the Quality Oncology Practice Initiative (QOPI) measure as a pilot project aimed at evaluating current practices and fostering performance improvement in the management of

- Distress should be recognized, monitored, documented, and treated promptly at all stages of disease and in all settings
- Screening should identify the level and nature of the distress
- Ideally, patients should be screened for distress at every medical visit as a hallmark of patient-centered care. At a minimum, patients should be screened to ascertain their level of distress at the initial visit, at appropriate intervals, and as clinically indicated, especially with changes in disease status
- Distress should be assessed and managed according to clinical practice guidelines
- Interdisciplinary institutional committees should be formed to implement standards for distress management
- Educational and training programs should be developed to ensure that health-care professionals and certified chaplains have knowledge and skills in the assessment and management of distress
- Licensed mental health professionals and certified chaplains experienced in the psychosocial aspects of cancer should be readily available as staff members or by referral
- Medical care contracts should include adequate reimbursement for services provided by mental health professionals
- Clinical health outcome measurements should include assessment of the psychosocial domain
- Patients, families, and treatment teams should be informed that distress management is an integral part of total medical care and includes appropriate information about psychosocial services in the treatment center and in the community
- The quality of distress management programs/services should be included in institutional continuous quality improvement projects

FIGURE 6.1 NCCN Standards of Care for Distress Management.[4] *NCCN*, The National Comprehensive Cancer Network. *Adapted with permission from the NCCN Guidelines® for Distress Management V.3.2019 © 2019 National Comprehensive Cancer Network, Inc. All rights reserved. The NCCN Guidelines and illustrations herein may not be reproduced in any form for any purpose without the express written permission of the NCCN.*

physical and psychological issues within outpatient oncology settings. The QOPI Program understands the essential nature of psychosocial screening and how cancer diagnosis and treatment can cause detrimental effects on well-being, functional outcomes, and quality of life. The QOPI Certification Program Standards requires documentation of initial psychosocial assessment in the medical record and subsequent action as indicated. Psychosocial documentation may include a distress or anxiety screening, patient self-report of distress or anxiety, or medical record documentation regarding patient's coping, adjustment, depression, distress, anxiety, emotional status, family support and caregiving, coping style, cultural background, and socioeconomic status.[22] In recognition of the fact that psychosocial considerations may change over time, it is recommended to conduct reassessments at regular intervals as well as establish policy or written procedure to describe the workflow and parameters for referral processes.[22] For example, reassessments may be conducted with each new cycle of chemotherapy, the start of a clinical trial, or a transition to the next level of care. These are all vital time points during which distress and anxiety screening and assessment are warranted.

IMPLEMENTATION OF PSYCHOSOCIAL SCREENING OF DISTRESS AND ANXIETY

Distress screening by health-care professionals can be performed periodically through various communication pathways such as face-to-face clinic appointments, phone calls, and electronic methods. Leveraging the functionality of institution electronic medical records (EMRs) could increase efficiency and the volume of patients screened. A key aspect of implementing a screening process is to include stakeholders throughout the institution, for example, physicians, nurses, patient navigators, and rehabilitation clinicians and schedulers.

The Association of Community Cancer Centers recommends the following to implement distress screening[24]:

1. Establish a point person for the screening program.
2. Create a psychosocial care network.
3. Design a standardized protocol.
4. Tailor the screening program to the patient population.

With an increase in distress screening comes the responsibility to create effective evaluation and treatment pathways to address the resulting increase in volume of needs and referrals. Identifying which team member is responsible for specific concerns on the screening tool is the key to directing patients to the appropriate provider. It is important that every team member involved in the screening and treatment process communicates their involvement within the medical record in order for the team to see that the patient was screened, assessed, and provided resources for their particular concerns. Once a process is set in place within an institution, it is recommended to then reassess the process to evaluate the effectiveness of the screening program.

Screening Tools

Prior to utilizing a screening tool, it is crucial to obtain a thorough understanding of the patient's biopsychosocial profile that may include the patient's medical history, social issues, psychiatric history, drug/alcohol history, faith system/spirituality, cognitive concerns, and physical issues. Ideally, multiple disciplines may contribute to the documentation of the patient's profile in order to ensure that complete and accurate information is obtained. Upon a review of the patient's history, validated screening tools (Table 6.1) may be utilized to further pinpoint areas of distress or anxiety and identify potential referral sources.

Suicide Risk

When screening or providing follow-up care, concerns such as suicidal ideations, depressive symptoms, or other mental health concerns may arise. Upon identification of such concerns, additional screening tools or assessments may be administered in order to further investigate risk factors, ensure patient's safety, and facilitate appropriate referrals to psychological or psychiatric care as warranted. For example, an individual may disclose or present at risk for suicidal concerns. An example of an assessment tool that may be administered at this time is the Columbia–Suicide Severity Rating Scale, which can quantify the severity of suicidal ideation as well as correlated behavior. This scale is also supported by the National Institute of Mental Health and is in 103 languages. It can be utilized in any setting, including inpatient, outpatient, private practice, and clinic settings.[25]

INTERVENTIONS FOR MANAGEMENT OF DISTRESS AND ANXIETY

The subsequent referral for the treatment of cancer-related distress is a crucial and mandated component in ensuring that individuals with cancer receive

TABLE 6.1
Screening Instruments for Distress and Anxiety

Screening Instruments for Distress and Anxiety			
Instrument	**Measures**	**Scales**	**Scoring**
NCCN Distress Thermometer[4]	General distress	1 Item, 11-point Likert scale	≥ 4 Indicates moderate-to-severe distress
Symptom Distress Scale	Symptom-related distress	13 Items, 5-point Likert scale	≥ 25 Moderate distress ≥ 33 Severe distress
Edmonton Symptom Severity Scale Revised (ESAS-r)	Symptom-related distress	9 Items, 10-point scale	3–4 Moderate/severe intensity of symptoms; 6–7 severe intensity of symptoms
The Patient Health Questionnaire-4 (PHQ-4)	Anxiety and depression	4 Items, 4-point Likert scale	3–5 Mild, 6–8 moderate, 9–12 severe; total score ≥ 3 for first two questions suggests anxiety
Hospital Anxiety and Depression Scale (HADS)	Anxiety and depression	14-Item scale	8–10 Borderline 11–21 Abnormal
Generalized Anxiety Disorder-7 (GAD-7)	Anxiety	7-Item questionnaire on 4-point scale	5 Mild anxiety 10 Moderate anxiety 15 Severe anxiety ≥ 10 Further evaluation recommended

comprehensive psychosocial support. Upon completion of a standardized screening and identification of sources of distress and anxiety, health-care providers within the multidisciplinary care team must interpret these results, determine when to refer to the appropriate professionals to address the source(s) of distress, and understand how to address the issues upon patient encountered at various time points along the continuum of care.

All members of the cancer rehabilitation team may address the various contributing factors of distress and anxiety specific to their subspecialties. For example, the distress of a woman with breast cancer experiencing high symptom burden due to tamoxifen may be addressed by a physician to maintain medication adherence, an occupational therapist to address symptom management strategies, or a psychologist for anxiety management. Recent research shows promising support for psychosocial interventions, which may target both distress and anxiety in the breast and gynecological cancer populations. Identification of the triggers for psychosocial concerns upon screening is a crucial step in ensuring the provision of appropriate referrals and care.

Pharmacological Management

The NCCN Guidelines for Distress Management recommend psychotherapy as first-line treatment for anxiety disorders and subsequent treatment with an antidepressant or an anxiolytic if necessary.[4] Best practices recommend thorough psychological or psychiatric assessment prior to administration of medication and a revisiting of any prescribed medications if the desired response is not achieved. The NCCN Guidelines propose that a response to first-line treatment warrants further follow-up with the primary oncology team, while no or partial response warrants a reevaluation of the patient and different medications with psychotherapy and further education.[4] If a complete response is not achieved, further evaluation for depression and other psychiatric comorbidity is warranted.[4]

Upon evaluation of the patient, it is recommended to conduct a thorough chart review to discern the potential impact that the type and dosage of a certain medication may have on an individual's functional status. A prime example of this is the use of antianxiety medications. The benefits include relief of muscle tension and promotion of relaxation, but the potential sedating effects may directly limit an individual's ability to fully participate in rehabilitation sessions. In order to ensure that the goals of the rehabilitation team are aligned with the care plan of the medical team, the potential benefits and side effects of medications should be weighed and considered by the primary oncology and psychiatric teams with frequent communication with first-line rehabilitation staff.

Psychological/Psychiatric Interventions

Cognitive–Behavioral Therapy

Cognitive–behavioral interventions are commonly referred to as the gold standard for psychosocial intervention in various patient populations. Benefits of cognitive–behavioral interventions in both nonmetastatic and metastatic breast cancer survivors include reduced anxiety, reduced depression, and improved quality of life.[26] Cognitive and Behavioral Cancer Stress Management (CBCSM) programs have been increasingly studied in the literature for breast cancer patients. CBCSM programs include instruction in approach-oriented coping, problem-solving, thought-reframing, interpersonal skills training, and relaxation skills training.[26] The results of a randomized controlled trial of nonmetastatic breast cancer patients found that a group-based cognitive–behavioral therapy (CBT) and relaxation training group were associated with improved survival upon 11-year follow-up.[27] The findings of this study suggest that a cognitive–behavioral stress management intervention post-surgery may provide long-term benefits.[27]

Health-care professionals trained to administer cognitive–behavioral interventions are encouraged to base their interventions on the individual psychosocial needs of their patients, rather than basing interventions on prognosis or medical status.[26] A systematic review analyzing psychosocial interventions in breast cancer suggested that cognitive–behavioral stress management interventions may be more appropriate for those patients seeking resources to live well with their cancer, while more meaning-based psychotherapy may be appropriate for those seeking to explore death trajectory and existential questions.[26]

Acceptance and Commitment Therapy

Acceptance and commitment therapy (ACT) is an intervention that can be administered by trained professionals, including psychologists, social workers, and mental health counselors, within psycho-oncology settings. The emphasis of ACT is an acceptance of distress with the goal of achieving healthy adjustment to current circumstances and thereby achieving greater life fulfillment. The foundational principle of ACT emphasizes "psychological flexibility" to manage suffering, which is viewed as an inevitable part of the human experience.[28]

ACT has overlapping processes with other psychosocial interventions, including CBT and mindfulness-based therapy. However, it differs from these other therapies in its emphasis on appraising and changing the relationship with one's thoughts rather than changing the thoughts themselves, which may be a great benefit to cancer patients who are faced with life-altering decisions and concerns upon diagnosis.[29] Strengths of the ACT model include opportunity for transdiagnostic application, flexibility in the delivery of the intervention based on individual patient needs, and use of experiential learning.[29] Research findings have shown strong support for ACT interventions in reducing psychological distress, increasing quality of life, and decreasing relapse-related fears in breast and gynecological cancer patients.[29,30]

Psychoeducation

The primary goal of psychoeducation is to provide guidance and education to patients and caregivers in order to empower them to manage their day-to-day disease, manage decision-making, relieve uncertainty, and facilitate psychosocial adaptation to illness.[31] Psychoeducation can be a primary or adjuvant intervention, and rehabilitation providers may choose to incorporate psychoeducation into treatments in order to improve functional performance and enhance patient empowerment in the management of their disease. Psychoeducation may be delivered in individual or group format and can be complemented with provision of resources (e.g., online, community programs, leaflets or brochures, handouts, books, and support groups).[31] Even a single psychoeducation session may be beneficial for addressing distressed patients and their caregivers,[32] and there is growing support for distance delivery of psychoeducation via telephone or Internet.[33]

Mind–Body Practices

By definition, mind–body practices are defined as techniques that elicit relaxation in order to decrease stress and distress as well as improve quality of life. There is a growing body of evidence in support of mindfulness-based interventions addressing distress in breast and gynecological cancer patients. The core components of mindfulness-based interventions include techniques to facilitate nonjudgmental awareness of both internal and external experiences in order to alleviate distress and improve psychological functioning.

Meditation

Meditation is an ancient practice, the common features of which include focused attention, open attitude, breathing regulation and control, and increased awareness of the dialogue between mind and body.

Techniques may also encompass mental training practices that involve self-regulation of attention toward a chosen object of awareness, such as the breath or a mantra.[34]

Mindfulness-Based Stress Reduction

Mindfulness-based stress reduction (MBSR) is a structured 8-week group program that combines meditative practices, yoga exercises, and mindful relaxation techniques. MBSR was shown to significantly reduce anxiety and depression in breast cancer survivors[35] and improve menopause-specific quality of life in women after risk-reductive salpingo-oophorectomy.[36]

Yoga

The NCCN Guidelines for Distress Management currently do not recommend yoga for patients for distress, citing lack of robust studies supporting this intervention.[4] Yoga was found at least to have short-term effects on reducing depression and anxiety in several systematic reviews and metaanalyses,[37] but the quality of study methodologies was deemed low.[4] However, it is worthy to note that the NCCN has incorporated yoga into its guidelines for fatigue,[38] and if this symptom is a primary source of distress, the appropriate disciplines may target symptom burden reduction in order to support the overall goals of rehabilitation by means of a yoga-based intervention. Further research in yoga is warranted to support its use exclusive to distress management, though existing evidence shows promising results that illustrate benefits in stress reduction and physical conditioning.

Other Considerations for Interventions

The interventions listed and described in this section have been included as noteworthy considerations for standard care in distress management in the breast and gynecological cancer populations. Considerations of various delivery methods of interventions, timing of interventions, and intervention topics have been addressed here.

Sexual Health Counseling

Health-care professionals are encouraged to discuss sexual health concerns with patients in order to decrease the stigma and taboo surrounding this topic and facilitate an open, nonjudgmental space for the discussion of sensitive issues. The integration of a designated sexual health specialist and/or pelvic floor therapist within the rehabilitation team may be beneficial to ensure adjustment after treatment and promote overall well-being. Examples of interventions that may be provided by a sexual health specialist include recommendations on vaginal moisturizers or lubricants for dryness, education on dilator therapy for vaginal stenosis, body positioning strategies to improve comfort, or medication management to cope with treatment side effects.[39]

Psychotropic medications, including selective serotonin reuptake inhibitors (SSRIs), may help relieve anxiety and distress, but it is important to weigh the cost–benefit ratio of these medications due to the known negative side effects on sexuality such as decreased libido, difficulty or inability to achieve orgasm, and decreased vaginal lubrication. The side effects of SSRIs may compound the already present deficits in sexual functioning due to surgical resection of pelvic organs or pelvic radiation, so it is pertinent for health-care providers to establish patient goals appropriately and establish open lines of communication with each other in order to prevent impedance of rehabilitative efforts.

Prehabilitation

"Prehabilitation" is defined as interventions that occur "between the time of cancer diagnosis and the beginning of acute treatment and includes a physical and psychological assessments that establish a baseline function level, identify impairments, and provide interventions that promote physical and psychological health to reduce the incidence and/or severity of future impairments."[40] Breast and gynecological cancer patients may benefit from comprehensive multimodal prehabilitation, as this preoperative time period is commonly associated with high levels of distress. At the time of evaluation a therapist may screen for psychosocial needs and gather useful baseline information, which may inform areas of rehabilitation and facilitate a quicker recovery. Prehabilitation programs may include interventions targeting not only physical treatments, such as exercise and smoking cessation, but also stress reduction and psychosocial support.[41] Health-care providers are encouraged to advocate for and implement prehabilitation programing to alleviate acute distress and promote improved psychosocial adjustment before and after treatment.

Telemedicine

Telemedicine, or telephone-delivered interventions, may provide more opportunities for health-care providers to serve larger geographical regions and access patients who may have limited community resources. Studies have shown patient's preference to receive or participate in interventions delivered over the telephone rather than in-person and when intervention is offered shortly after diagnosis.[42] The feasibility and cost-effectiveness of distance delivery of interventions via the telephone or Internet should be explored further in order to increase geographical scope of services and improve patient accessibility to resources.

For both breast and gynecological cancers, higher levels of depression and anxiety symptoms have been linked to unmet information needs and an unmet need for psychosocial support.[43] For this reason, exploring resources to address these impairments both within and outside of one's own institution is beneficial in expediting appropriate referrals and addressing distress in real time. Practitioners across the multidisciplinary team should be equipped with the knowledge and confidence to reinforce information regarding treatment and to provide support or resources to address psychosocial needs.

Caregiver Support and Education

It is crucial that all rehabilitation professionals recruit and train caregivers in order to equip them with the skills needed to effectively care for their loved ones in the hospital and at home. Efforts to meet caregiver needs must be made by involving them early in the patient's care and engaging them in hands-on training when appropriate, thereby increasing the caregiver's sense of self-efficacy with providing the appropriate level of care at home. Transitions of care, such as transitioning from hospital to home, are critical time points in which to prioritize caregiver education and training. Rehabilitation intervention may address caregiver education in transfers, mobility skills, and hygiene techniques.[19] With increasing caregiving burden due to increased disability as a result of progressive disease or end-of-life, rehabilitation may choose to address recommendations for durable medical equipment, symptom management strategies, referrals to financial assistance, and resources for respite care.[18,19]

Timing of Intervention

Prior to initiation of psychosocial treatment, it is pertinent to consider the timing of interventions. Studies have shown varied results in treatment outcomes based on timing of intervention, such as "prehabilitation," postsurgery, or posttreatment. In order to address patient needs, health-care providers are recommended to address distress at the earliest opportunity and then determine the timing of interventions based on patient need and readiness to receive the recommended interventions.

OVERCOMING CHALLENGES

Rescreening

Establishment of time points for rescreening is vital in ensuring that psychosocial needs are being addressed in a timely manner. Many institutions have implemented initial screening of distress and anxiety at initial intake or initiation of treatment cycles but have yet to determine concrete time points for rescreening. ASCO's QOPI measure provides standards for rescreening at every line of therapy and every new admission. The application of these standards is dependent on the treatment setting, type of cancer, and resources available in the institution.[24]

Resource Management

Health-care providers must be prepared to initiate and implement appropriate interventions based on the capabilities and feasibility within their respective oncology settings. Evaluation of one's clinical setting and conducting a review on available resources are essential to ensure that the recommended interventions are available and can be implemented accordingly. Improving efficiency in service delivery is also critical and can be achieved by embedding screenings and assessments into the EMR, creating clinical pathways to guide health-care professionals on referral processes, incorporating distress screening into daily rounds with the medical team, and optimizing communication flows among members of the multidisciplinary care team.

Within the rehabilitation setting, providers often build close rapport with their patients due to frequent follow-up and inquiries into personal life factors. These patients may be increasingly inclined to disclose psychosocial concerns with their rehabilitation provider during sessions. Rehabilitation team members are encouraged to maintain a sense of vigilance and sensitivity to psychosocial issues that may not only impede the goal progression in rehabilitation but also affect the individual's quality of life.

Institutions are recommended to utilize their resources to the highest potential. Community resources can be leveraged as additional support to effectively address patient needs and ensure continued follow-up in the outpatient setting. Such sources can include the Social Security Administration, the Leukemia and Lymphoma Society, and the American Cancer Society. In addition, some communities may offer community-based programs, which may provide classes, events, groups, or social support for cancer survivors. Furthermore, assisting patients with finding mental health providers in the community based on insurance coverage may help alleviate the need for additional resources within the institution and ensure that the patient has access to long-term support if needed.

CONCLUSION

No single distress screening program will be feasible for every cancer center or oncology practice given the variability in volume, resources, and site culture across practice settings. However, utilization of the standards established by the ACoS CoC and the National Comprehensive Cancer Center can assist cancer programs in establishing their own comprehensive distress screening programs and clinical pathways based on availability of resources.

In order to effectively implement a comprehensive, biopsychosocial approach to distress screening and management, all health-care professionals must identify themselves as part of the mental health-care team and designate responsibilities for the administration of screening tools, review of results, referral to appropriate providers, or provision of support and resources to patients and caregivers. Rehabilitation professionals are key members of this team as they often have consistent involvement in the patient's care and closely monitor progress toward functional goals. During this process, mental health needs may be identified as barriers to progress and appropriate referrals should be made. A vigilant health-care team must be acutely aware of the signs and symptoms of both distress and anxiety in order to optimize success in the integration of distress management throughout the continuum of cancer care.

REFERENCES

1. Miller KD, Nogueira L, Mariotto AB, et al. Cancer treatment and survivorship statistics. *CA Cancer J Clin.* 2019;69:363–385.
2. Antoni MH, Dhabhar FS. The impact of psychosocial stress and stress management on immune responses in patients with cancer. *Cancer.* 2019;125:1417–1431.
3. Moon Z, Moss-Morris R, Hunter MS, Hughes LD. More than just side-effects: the role of clinical and psychosocial factors in non-adherence to tamoxifen. *Br J Health Psychol.* 2017;22:998–1018.
4. National Comprehensive Cancer Network. Distress Management (Version 3.2019). <https://jnccn.org/view/journals/jnccn/17/10/article-p1229.xml>. Accessed 15.12.19.
5. American College of Surgeons Commission on Cancer. Optimal Resources for Cancer Care: 2020 Standards. American College of Surgeons Commission on Cancer, Chicago, IL, 2020. <https://www.facs.org/-/media/files/quality-programs/cancer/coc/optimal_resources_for_cancer_care_2020_standards.ashx>. Accessed 15.12.19.
6. Schreiber KL, Martel MO, Shnol H, et al. Persistent pain in postmastectomy patients: comparison of psychophysical, medical, surgical, and psychosocial characteristics between patients with and without pain. *Pain.* 2013;154(5):660–668.
7. Ovarian Cancer Research Alliance. Recurrence. <https://ocrahope.org/patients/about-ovarian-cancer/recurrence/>. Accessed 15.12.19.
8. Brandao T, Schultz MS, Matos PM. Psychological adjustment after breast cancer: a systematic review of longitudinal studies. *Psycho-Oncology.* 2017;26:917–926.
9. Hanprasertpong J, Geater A, Jiamset I, Padungkul L, Hirunkajonpan P, Sonhong N. Fear of cancer recurrence and its predictors among cervical cancer survivors. *J Gynecol Oncol.* 2017;28(6):e72.
10. Bergmark K, Avall-Lundqvist E, Dickman PW, Henningsohn L, Steineck G. Patient-rating of distressful symptoms after treatment for early cervical cancer. *Acta Obstet Gynecol Scand.* 2002;81(5):443–450.
11. Phillips-Salimi CR, Andrykowski MA. Physical and mental health status of female adolescent/young adult survivors of breast and gynecological cancer: a national, population-based, case-control study. *Support Care Cancer.* 2013;21(6):1597–1604.
12. Mattsson E, Einhorn K, Ljungman L, Sundstrom-Poromaa I, Stalberg K, Wikman A. Women treated for gynaecological cancer during young adulthood—a mixed-methods study of perceived psychological distress and experiences of support from health care following end-of-treatment. *Gynecol Oncol.* 2018;149:464–469.
13. Murphy BL, Day CN, Hoskin TL, Habermann EB, Boughey JC. Adolescents and young adults with breast cancer have more aggressive disease and treatment than patients in their forties. *Ann Surg Oncol.* 2019;26:3920–3930.
14. Sheill G, Guinan EM, Peat N, Hussey J. Considerations for exercise prescription in patients with bone metastases: a comprehensive narrative review. *PM R.* 2018;10:843–864.
15. Ruddy KJ, Winer EP. Male breast cancer: risk factors, biology, diagnosis, treatment, and survivorship. *Ann Oncol.* 2013;24:1434–1443.
16. Kowalski C, Steffen P, Ernstmann N, Wuerstlein R, Harbeck N, Pfaff H. Health-related quality of life in male breast cancer patients. *Breast Cancer Res Treat.* 2012;133:753–757.
17. Mazanec SR, Reichlin D, Gittleman G, Daly BJ. Perceived needs, preparedness, and emotional distress of male caregivers of postsurgical women with gynecologic cancer. *Oncol Nurs Forum.* 2018;45(2):197–205.

18. Hartnett J, Thom B, Kline N. Caregiver burden in end-stage ovarian cancer. *Clin J Oncol Nurs*. 2016;20(2):169–173.
19. Yadav R. Rehabilitation of surgical cancer patients at University of Texas M.D. Anderson Cancer Center. *J Surgical Oncol*. 2007;95:361–369.
20. About Preventive Medicine. Retrieved 20.12.19. <https://www.acpm.org/about-acpm/what-is-preventive-medicine/>; n.d.
21. Crawford K. Mental health conditions contribute to increased cancer care-related costs, hospital visits for patients with breast and prostate cancers. Retrieved from <https://www.asco.org/about-asco/press-center/news-releases/mental-health-conditions-contribute-increased-cancer-care>; 2017.
22. ASCO. *ASCO QOPI Certification Program Standards Manual: Required Processes and Documentation to Meet Certification Standards and Elements. Version 6.1.2018*. American Society of Clinical Oncology; 2018.
23. Andersen BL, DeRubeis RJ, Berman BS, et al. Screening, assessment, and care of anxiety and depressive symptoms in adults with cancer: an American Society of Clinical Oncology guideline adaptation. *J Clin Oncol*. 2014;32(15):1605–1619.
24. Buxton D, Lazenby M, Daugherty A, et al. Distress screening for oncology patients: practical steps for developing and implementing a comprehensive distress screening program. *Oncol Issues*. 2014;29.
25. Posner K, Brown GK, Stanley B, et al. The Columbia–Suicide Severity Rating Scale: initial validity and internal consistency findings from three multisite studies with adolescents and adults. *Am J Psychiatry*. 2011;168(12):1266–1277.
26. Gudenkauf LM, Ehlers SL. Psychosocial interventions in breast cancer survivorship care. *Breast*. 2018;38:1–6.
27. Stagl JM, Lechner SC, Carver CS, et al. A randomized controlled trial of cognitive-behavioral stress management in breast cancer: survival and recurrence at 11-year follow-up. *Breast Cancer Res Treat*. 2015;154(2):319–328.
28. Hayes SC, Strosahl KD, Wilson KG. *Acceptance and Commitment Therapy: The Process and Practice of Mindful Change*. New York: Guilford Press; 2011.
29. Fashler SR, Weinrib AZ, Azam MA, Katz J. The use of acceptance and commitment therapy in oncology settings: a narrative review. *Psychol Rep*. 2018;121(2):229–252.
30. Angiola JE, Bowen AM. Quality of life in advanced cancer: an acceptance and commitment therapy view. *Couns Psychol*. 2012;41(2):313–335.
31. Thompson AL, Young-Saleme TK. Anticipatory guidance and psychoeducation as a standard of care in pediatric oncology. *Pediatr Blood Cancer*. 2015;62:S684–S693.
32. Chambers S, Girgis A, Occhipinti S, et al. A randomized trial comparing two low-intensity psychological interventions for distressed patients with cancer and their caregivers. *Oncol Nurs Forum*. 2014;41(4):E256–E266.
33. Urech C, Grossert A, Alder J. Web-based stress management for newly diagnosed patients with cancer (STREAM): a randomized, wait-list controlled intervention study. *J Clin Oncol*. 2018;36:780–788.
34. Hall DL, Luberto CM, Philpotts LL, Song R, Park ER, Yeh GY. Mind-body interventions for fear of cancer recurrence: a systematic review and meta-analysis. *Psycho-Oncology*. 2018;27:2546–2558.
35. Wurtzen H, Dalton SO, Elsass P, et al. Mindfulness significantly reduces self-reported levels of anxiety and depression: results of a randomised controlled trial among 336 Danish women treated for stage I-III breast cancer. *Eur J Cancer*. 2013;49(6):1365–1373.
36. van Driel C, de Bock GH, Schroevers MJ, Mourits MJ. Mindfulness-based stress reduction for menopausal symptoms after risk-reducing salpingo-oophorectomy (PURSUE study): a randomised controlled trial. *BJOG*. 2019;126(3):402–411.
37. Pan Y, Yang K, Wang Y, et al. Could yoga practice improve treatment-related side effects and quality of life for women with breast cancer? A systematic review and meta-analysis. *Asia Pac J Clin Oncol*. 2017;13:e79–e95.
38. National Comprehensive Cancer Network. Cancer-Related Fatigue (Version 2.2015). <https://jnccn.org/view/journals/jnccn/13/8/article-p1012.xml?rskey = H3NiDk&result = 1>. Accessed 15.12.19.
39. Stabile C, Gunn A, Sonoda Y, Carter J. Emotional and sexual concerns in women undergoing pelvic surgery and associated treatment for gynecologic cancer. *Transl Androl Urol*. 2015;4(2):169–185.
40. Silver JK. Cancer rehabilitation and prehabilitation may reduce disability and early retirement. *Cancer*. 2014;120:2072–2076.
41. Santa Mina D, Brahmbhatt P, Lopez C, et al. The case for prehabilitation prior to breast cancer treatment. *PM R*. 2017;9(9):S305–S316.
42. Brebach R, Sharpe L, Costa DSJ, Rhodes P, Butow P. Psychological intervention targeting distress for cancer patients: a meta-analytic study investigating uptake and adherence. *Psycho-Oncology*. 2016;25:882–890.
43. Faller H, Brahler E, Harter M, et al. Unmet needs for information and psychosocial support in relation to quality of life and emotional distress: a comparison between gynecological and breast cancer patients. *Patient Educ Counseling*. 2017;100:1934–1942.

CHAPTER 7

Prehabilitation in Breast and Gynecologic Oncology

JULIA M. REILLY, MD • ALEXANDRA I. GUNDERSEN, MD • SASHA E. KNOWLTON, MD

INTRODUCTION

Prehabilitation has been defined in the literature as "a process on the cancer continuum of care that occurs between the time of cancer diagnosis and the beginning of acute treatment and includes physical and psychological assessments that establish a baseline functional level, identify impairments, and provide interventions that promote physical and psychological health to reduce the incidence and/or severity of future impairments."[1] At the time of cancer diagnosis, functional status among patients may vary significantly. While some patients may be functioning independently and routinely exercising, others may be requiring total assistance with activities of daily living. As a result, patients should be medically and functionally screened at the time of cancer diagnosis in order to properly assess needs for prehabilitation. The overall purpose of prehabilitation is to maximize patients'ahealth and functional status prior to undergoing treatment for cancer, which can include surgery, radiation, and/or systemic chemotherapy or other targeted medications. Ideally, participation in prehabilitation will enable patients to tolerate treatment better, improve function and health during and after treatment, and prevent deleterious complications.

GOALS OF PREHABILITATION

The goals of prehabilitation have been described in different ways in the literature; while there are different proposed models, multimodal interventions provide a comprehensive approach to treatment of patients with cancer.[2–4] Identification of functional impairments can allow for the design of individual exercise programs to improve functional outcomes and prevent injury.[3,4] However, while exercise itself is beneficial, it does not fully constitute a prehabilitation program. Additional components should include the assessment and optimization of nutrition, mental health, and smoking cessation.[3] Prior to participation in a prehabilitation program, patients should be screened for other medical comorbidities to prevent injury. Participation in a comprehensive prehabilitation program enables patients with cancer to maintain, if not improve, health, function, and quality of life during and after cancer treatment.

BREAST CANCER PREHABILITATION

Breast cancer is the most common cancer diagnosed in women in the United States, and survival has been improving for the past few decades.[5] Prognosis is largely based on the cancer stage and the estrogen, progesterone, and human epidermal growth factor receptor 2 receptor status. Increased survival in breast cancer is likely due to improve screening and enhancements in adjuvant therapy. The current overall 5-year survival rate for breast cancer is around 90%.[5] Breast cancer treatment can include neoadjuvant chemotherapy to reduce the size of the tumor prior to surgery, therefore increasing the potential of breast conservation. Postoperative chemotherapy along with endocrine therapy may be required as well. These interventions to treat breast cancer, while effective, may result in adverse effects that can negatively impact function. For example, radiation can result in fibrosis, while mastectomy and lymph node resection frequently lead to postmastectomy pain syndrome (PMPS), restricted range of motion (ROM), cording, and lymphedema. Knowledge of these common impairments can help design a prehabilitation program to prevent further morbidity posttreatment.

Breast Cancer and Gynecologic Cancer Rehabilitation DOI: https://doi.org/10.1016/B978-0-323-72166-0.00007-4

Neuropathy

Certain types of chemotherapy such as taxanes and platinum agents are often associated with neuropathy. Symptoms of neuropathy can be classified as positive or "presence" of symptoms in addition to negative or "absence" of symptoms. Positive symptoms can include paresthesia such as burning, tingling, and neuropathic pain while negative symptoms include numbness, weakness, and lack of proprioception.[6] As a result of neuropathy, patients can develop impaired balance and gait and experience frequent falls resulting in further morbidity.

Some of these adverse effects can be partially addressed with medications. Neuropathic oral pain medications such as duloxetine, gabapentin, and pregabalin, as well as topical agents such as lidocaine can be used to treat the positive symptoms of neuropathy. Other medications such as tricyclic antidepressants (TCAs) can also be tried, though these medications often cause more adverse effects. To address the functional impairments from neuropathy, physical and/or occupational therapy along with ambulatory aids can be used. At times, use of compression garments and proprioceptive bracing can assist with numbness and impaired gait.

Lymphedema

Lymphedema affects approximately 40% of women treated for breast cancer.[7] Lymphedema can occur after the removal of lymph nodes or radiation therapy and results from the blockage or disturbance of the lymphatic system. Patients with lymphedema experience a lower quality of life and increased psychosocial complications.[7] Despite increasing amounts of research, a large percentage of women continue to experience lymphedema, and management remains a major challenge. Complete decongestive therapy involves manual lymph drainage by a trained lymphedema therapist, who performs and instructs on compression bandaging; in addition, therapy sessions include exercise with focus on ROM, skin care, and patient education.[8] Intensive therapy can result in 50%–60% long-term volume reduction.[7] Effective treatment of lymphedema can prevent complications such as skin breakdown and cellulitis. Previously, patients were counseled to avoid exercise to prevent lymphedema or prevent worsening of symptoms. However, close evaluation of the available literature has demonstrated no association with the development or worsening of lymphedema with exercise.[9]

Axillary Web Syndrome

Axillary web syndrome (AWS) (also known as cording) is the development of a palpable, sometimes painful, rope-like cord in the axilla and/or in the ipsilateral arm after lymph node dissection.[10] The incidence of this phenomenon ranges 10%–85% and is not well defined.[11] AWS can result in significant discomfort along with decreased shoulder ROM. While AWS may resolve within a few months, a course of physical therapy focusing on ROM exercises, gentle stretching, and manual manipulation of the cord along with manual lymph drainage can be beneficial to improve the ROM along with function of the shoulder and arm and reduce pain.[10,12]

Postmastectomy Pain Syndrome

Unilateral or bilateral mastectomy is one of the main treatments for invasive breast cancer. Approximately 20%–68% of patients who undergo a mastectomy experience PMPS, which is pain described as neuropathic discomfort or aching in the anterior chest, arm, or axilla that persists more than 3 months after surgery.[13] Treatment strategies for PMPS include pharmacologic management with nonsteroidal anti-inflammatory drugs (NSAIDs), neuropathic agents (gabapentin, pregabalin, duloxetine, and TCAs), and topical lidocaine, along with physical therapy, acupuncture, and regional nerve blocks.[13] Physical therapy focusing on shoulder ROM and myofascial release has also been shown to have some benefits for PMPS.[13] Understanding the pathophysiology of PMPS along with early recognition and education of patients allows better pain management and improved function.

Mental and Physical Fatigue

Treatment for breast cancer can be extensive and may involve neoadjuvant chemotherapy, surgical intervention, radiation, and postoperative chemotherapy, and/or endocrine therapy. Fatigue is common in patients with breast cancer; between 60%–90% of patients report fatigue during treatment, and 30% of patients with breast cancer report ongoing fatigue after completion of treatment.[14] As discussed previously, in the past, patients were instructed to not participate in strenuous exercise out of safety concerns. However, research has found that not only is physical therapy safe but also is extremely important in patients with breast cancer to treat cancer-related fatigue well into survivorship.[14]

Prehabilitation Recommendations

Currently, rehabilitation for patients with breast cancer is commonly started after completion of treatment to address the previously listed impairments. Increasingly, studies demonstrate that earlier integration of postoperative rehabilitation significantly improves outcomes.[15] With this evidence demonstrating improved outcomes from rehabilitation, prehabilitation for patients with breast cancer is being studied more closely. Prehabilitation in patients with breast cancer includes pretreatment screening of physical function and psychosocial well-being with the intent to address any impairments that may exist before treatment, and to follow the patients closely throughout their treatment period to address any impairments that may occur throughout the duration of the treatment. The focus of prehabilitation in this population is on general conditioning exercise, targeted exercise, nutritional interventions, psychosocial well-being, smoking cessation, and patient education.[15] A meta-analysis of 33 randomized controlled trials examining exercise in breast cancer patients illustrated significant improvement in body composition, emotional well-being (including anxiety and depression), and quality of life in patients who exercised.[16] Studies have also shown that women with breast cancer who engage in physical activity preoperatively compared with sedentary women have an 85% greater chance of reporting improved return to baseline level of function 3 weeks postoperatively.[17] Patients with breast cancer who exercise prior to chemotherapy demonstrate improved cardiovascular health, and a higher likelihood of completing chemotherapy treatment.[18,19]

During breast cancer treatment the shoulder and upper quadrant are areas that are largely affected. Patients often lose shoulder ROM and function after surgical intervention and radiation treatment. Exercise focusing on shoulder abduction and external rotation can reduce pain and maintain ROM. Breast reconstruction through the use of an abdominal flap may result in reduced core strength and ROM along with lower back pain; as a result, specific exercise to the abdominal wall and postural muscles may lead to the prevention of these symptoms preoperatively.[15]

While exercise is important in breast cancer prehabilitation, patients should be assessed and counseled on adequate protein intake, good glycemic control, appropriate vitamin supplementation, and overall weight loss to reduce postoperative complications and improve functional outcomes.[15,20] Addressing psychological components of breast cancer is important during a prehabilitation program as well, and elements should include stress reduction, coping strategies, and overall psychological counseling to create long-term positive changes in health behaviors.[21]

The multimodal prehabilitation approach described previously, including exercise, nutritional and psychological interventions can improve functional outcomes of breast cancer patients; yet overall, prehabilitation is understudied and underutilized. Generally, patients are neither routinely educated on prehabilitation nor are they aware of the impact these interventions can have on their functional and overall health. In this setting, physiatrists and other rehabilitation providers should be encouraged to be involved with oncology patients'a-care to provide education and access to the multimodal strategies of prehabilitation. Ideally, prehabilitation in the breast cancer population would lead to less postoperative complications, higher completion rates of adjuvant treatment, and overall increased survival and functional outcomes for breast cancer patients.

GYNECOLOGIC CANCER PREHABILITATION

The most common types of gynecologic cancers are uterine, ovarian, and cervical, though cancer can occur in various locations along the reproductive tract.[5] Treatment of gynecologic cancer generally involves surgical management and adjuvant treatment based on multiple factors, including cancer stage and grade. In addition to shared symptoms seen with many different types of cancers such as fatigue, pain, and neuropathy, symptoms after treatment of gynecologic cancers may also include lower limb lymphedema (LLL), pelvic floor dysfunction, bowel/bladder impairment, and reduced quality of life.[22]

Lower Limb Lymphedema

The incidence and prevalence of lymphedema after treatment of gynecologic cancers vary in the literature, with certain studies noting 20%–30% incidence after treatment of all gynecologic cancer, 0%–50% prevalence after treatment of endometrial cancer, and 7%–47% incidence after treatment of uterine cancer.[22–24] Risk factors for developing lower extremity lymphedema from cancer treatment appear to include treatment-related factors such as extent of lymphadenectomy and use of radiation, as well as patient-related factors such as obesity and age.[22,24,25]

Lymphedema may be noticed immediately postoperatively, or may take several months to years to develop.[24] Women with LLL after treatment of endometrial cancer have been found to have lower health-related quality of life.[24]

As compared to upper limb lymphedema, LLL presents specific problems related to the dependent edema accrued from standing and walking. Patients who experience LLL may be more inclined to limit physical activity from the fear of worsening lymphedema.[22] Do et al. studied 40 patients with lymphedema after gynecologic cancer surgery, who were randomly assigned to either receive decongestive therapy alone or decongestive therapy and an exercise program consisting of aerobic exercise and strengthening.[22] After 4 weeks of treatment, physical function, leg volume, quality of life, pain, and fatigue were noted to improve in both groups; however, the exercise group was found to have significantly improved fatigue, physical function, and strength compared to those in the control group. Neither group was noted to have exacerbation of LLL.[22] Similarly, another study found that physical activity reduced risk of developing LLL, although this reduction was seen only in patients with a body mass index less than 30 kg/m^2.[23]

Sexual Dysfunction

Impairments in sexual function may be affected by several variables in the treatment of gynecologic cancers. A study of gynecological cancer patients and breast cancer patients revealed that nearly 42% of patients were interested in discussing sexual care needs, and yet only 7% had sought medical help for these issues.[26] After gynecologic cancer treatment, patients may be left with permanent physical impairments such as difficulty in experiencing orgasm, vaginal dryness, pelvic pain, and dyspareunia.[26] In addition, procedures such as vaginectomies and radical vulvectomies may remove tissues involved in sexual function. Physicians, treating patients with a history of gynecological cancer, should take time to discuss sexual health concerns with their patients. In 2018 Stabile et al. found that among 231 women with gynecological or breast cancer diagnoses, 70% preferred that their medical team raise the issue of sexual dysfunction.[27] In this study, 66% of women were found to prefer written educational material followed by discussion.[27]

Pelvic Floor, Urinary, and Fecal Dysfunction

Because of the closely intertwined anatomy, dysfunction of the pelvic floor related to treatment of gynecologic cancer with surgery and radiation may affect urologic and gastrointestinal function. Injury from surgery and radiation may directly injure the muscles of the pelvic floor, or indirectly affect the function of these muscles through damage to the nerves supplying them. Disruption of the pelvic floor may result in issues in pelvic organ prolapse, continence, and elimination. A recent systematic review article examined the prevalence of pelvic floor symptoms after treatment of cervical cancer and found the prevalence of stress urinary incontinence to range from 4% to 76%, urinary frequency 6% to 71%, and fecal incontinence 2% to 34%.[28] Similarly, among patients with endometrial cancer, prevalence of stress urinary incontinence ranged from 69% to 84%, fecal incontinence 11% to 24%, and pelvic organ prolapse 44%.[28] Urinary incontinence is more common after radical hysterectomies than nerve-sparing radical hysterectomies.[28] In the literature, pelvic floor therapy has been studied and found to improve urinary continence, pelvic pain, and sexual dysfunction. Yang et al. studied 24 patients with gynecologic cancer and randomly assigned them to participate in pelvic floor therapy or a control group without intervention. After 4 weeks of treatment the group that received pelvic floor therapy was noted to have improved pelvic floor strength, sexual, and physical function.[29] Similarly, Rutledge et al. studied women with urinary incontinence after treatment of gynecologic cancer and found that the women assigned to treatment with pelvic floor training noted significant improvement in urinary incontinence symptoms over patients assigned to "usual care."[30]

Pain

Pain in patients with gynecologic cancers is related to extent of disease and treatment of disease. Hacker et al. noted "gynecologic oncology patients frequently have higher rates of moderate to severe pain and opioid use than patients diagnosed with other cancers."[31] Though mechanisms behind cancer-related pain are poorly understood, cytokine secretion and local tissue invasion are thought to be important factors. Pain from treatment may be related to surgery (acute postoperative pain), chemotherapy, and radiation. Patients may develop pain after surgery, which may be nociceptive and related to incisional or myofascial pain, and/or neuropathic pain related to nerve dysfunction from treatment. In addition, with radiation patients may develop complications such as radiation cystitis and postradiation vaginal strictures/ atrophy.[31] Obtaining an accurate and detailed pain history is imperative for better pain management assessment and treatment.

Prehabilitation Recommendations

No studies on prehabilitation exist in the gynecologic oncology patient population. However, screening patients for the earlier listed and other impairments along with counseling patients about the importance of exercise should be part of a general prehabilitation program in this population. In addition, addressing nutrition, stress reduction, and smoking cessation should also be a part of a prehabilitation program for the gynecology oncology population.

RECOMMENDATIONS FOR PREHABILITATION AND FUTURE DIRECTIONS

There are no studies on prehabilitation in the gynecologic oncology population, and only a few studies conducted on the breast cancer population. In one breast cancer prehabilitation study, Baima et al. studied the feasibility of prehabilitation by providing upper extremity exercises to 60 patients with breast cancer via instructional videos or in-person training.[32] The patients were scheduled to have surgery within 1–4 weeks of the intervention. The study found no difference in adherence to exercises between groups, and no increased risk of seroma formation in the prehabilitation participants.[32] A systematic review by Tsimopoulou et al. examined preoperative psychological intervention in the cancer population, with four of the seven studies reviewed involving breast cancer patients.[33] The review noted improvement in several patient-reported outcomes such as quality of life, anxiety, and depression.[33]

Santa Mina et al. recommended five components for breast cancer prehabilitation, including "total body exercise, loco-regional exercise pertinent to treatment-related deficits, nutritional optimization, stress reduction/psychosocial support, and smoking cessation."[15] Cardiovascular fitness and conditioning are thought to improve surgical oncology outcomes by reducing perioperative complications, reducing length of stay, and improving postoperative pain and function.[15] By improving preintervention fitness a patient may be less affected by cardiotoxic effects of chemotherapy and better able to tolerate treatment. The goal of targeted exercise is to strengthen an area of particular vulnerability for patients with specific types of cancer. As described earlier in this chapter, upper extremity dysfunction is common after treatment of breast cancer. By understanding this tendency and treating any preexisting impairments in strength or ROM, a patient may experience less upper extremity morbidity after treatment.

Nutritional support for breast and gynecologic cancer patients is critical, as there are risks associated with being malnourished as well as being overweight or obese during and prior to treatment. Patients who are overweight are more likely to have poor prognoses, with reduced disease-free recurrence and increased mortality.[15,34] Similarly, patients with sarcopenia may be more prone to experiencing adverse side effects from cancer treatment.[15] As alluded to earlier, there is literature that suggests that psychological intervention prior to cancer treatment may reduce severity of several patient-reported outcomes. Smoking cessation counseling should be provided throughout all stages of prehabilitation, as patients who smoke throughout cancer treatment are at increased risk for surgical and postoperative complications, disease recurrence, development of second primary tumor, mortality, and reduced quality of life.[15,35]

Though there are several gaps in knowledge on the topics of breast cancer and gynecologic cancer prehabilitation, by drawing from prehabilitation studies on available cancer populations, multimodal approaches to prehabilitation appear to be feasible and appear to improve surgical and patient-reported outcomes. Further research is needed to better delineate the best time-frame, patient population, and interventions for prehabilitation.

REFERENCES

1. Silver JK, Baima J. Cancer prehabilitation: an opportunity to decrease treatment-related morbidity, increase cancer treatment options, and improve physical and psychological health outcomes. *Am J Phys Med Rehab*. 2013;92:715–727.
2. Maltser S, Cristian A, Silver JK, Morris GS, Stout NL. A focused review of safety considerations in cancer rehabilitation. *PMR*. 2018;9(suppl 2):S415–S428.
3. Carli F, Silver JK, Feldman LS, et al. Surgical prehabilitation in patients with cancer: state-of-the-science and recommendations for future research from a panel of subject matter experts. *Phys Med Rehabil Clin N Am*. 2017;28:49–64.
4. Cheville AL, McLaughlin SA, Haddad T, Lyons KD, Newman R, Ruddy KJ. Integrated rehabilitation for breast cancer survivors. *Am J Phys Med Rehabil [Internet]*. 2018. E.pub ahead of print. Available from: <http://insights.ovid.com/crossref?an = 00002060-900000000-98440>.
5. Siegel RL, Miller KD, Jemal A. Cancer statistics. *CA Cancer J*. 2019;69(1):7–34.
6. Zajaczkowska R, Kocot-Kepska M, Leppert W, Wrzosek A, Mika J, Wordliczek J. Mechanisms of chemotherapy-induced peripheral neuropathy. *Int J Mol Sci*. 2019;20 (6):1451.

7. Fu M. Breast cancer-related lymphedema: symptoms, diagnosis, risk reduction and management. *World J Clin Oncol*. 2014;5(3):241–247.
8. Gillespie TC, Sayegh HE, Brunelle CL, Daniell KM, Taghian AG. Breast cancer-related lymphedema: risk factors, precautionary measures, and treatments. *Gland Surg*. 2018;7(6):379–403.
9. Cemal Y, Pusic A, Mehrara B. Preventative measures for lymphedema: separating fact from fiction. *J Am Coll Surg*. 2011;213(4):543–551.
10. Tilley A, Thomas-MacLean R, Kwan W. Lymphatic cording or axillary web syndrome after breast cancer surgery. *Can J Surg*. 2009;52(4):105–106.
11. Harris SR. Axillary web syndrome in breast cancer: a prevalent but under-recognized postoperative complication. *Breast Care*. 2018;13:132–135.
12. Beurskens CHG, Van Uden CJ, Strobbe LJA, Oostendorp RAB, Wobbes T. The efficacy of physiotherapy upon shoulder function following axillary dissection in breast cancer, a randomized controlled study. *BMC Cancer*. 2007;7:1–6.
13. Cui L, Fan P, Qiu C, Hong Y. Single institution analysis of incidence and risk factors for post- mastectomy pain syndrome. *Sci Rep*. 2018;8:1–6.
14. Bardwell WA, Ancoli-Israel S. Breast cancer and fatigue. *Sleep Med Clin*. 2008;3(1):61–71.
15. Santa Mina D, Brahmbhatt P, Lopez C, et al. The case for prehabilitation prior to breast cancer treatment. *PM&R [Internet]*. 2017;9(9):S305–S316. Available from: https://doi.org/10.1016/j.pmrj.2017.08.402.
16. Zhu G, Zhang X, Wang Y, Ziong H, Zhao Y, Sun F. Effects of exercise intervention in breast cancer survivors: a meta-analysis of 33 randomized controlled trails. *Onco Targets Ther*. 2016;9:2153–2168.
17. Nilsson H, Angerås U, Bock D, et al. Is preoperative physical activity related to post-surgery recovery? A cohort study of patients with breast cancer. *BMJ Open*. 2016;6:1–9.
18. Kirkham AA, Shave RE, Bland KA, et al. Protective effects of acute exercise prior to doxorubicin on cardiac function of breast cancer patients: a proof-of-concept RCT. *Int J Cardiol*. 2017;245:263–270.
19. Courneya KS, Segal RJ, Mackey JR, et al. Effects of aerobic and resistance exercise in breast cancer patients receiving adjuvant chemotherapy: a multicenter randomized controlled trial. *J Clin Oncol*. 2007;25(28):4396–4404.
20. Demark-Wahnefried W, Campbell KL, Hayes SC. Weight management and its role in breast cancer rehabilitation. *Cancer*. 2012;118(8 suppl):2277–2287.
21. Garssen B, Boomsma MF, Meezenbroek EDJ, et al. Stress management training for breast cancer surgery patients. *Psychooncology*. 2013;22:572–580.
22. Do JH, Choi KH, Ahn JS, Jeon JY. Effects of a complex rehabilitation program on edema status, physical function, and quality of life in lower-limb lymphedema after gynecological cancer surgery. *Gynecol Oncol [Internet]*. 2017;147(2):450–455. Available from: https://doi.org/10.1016/j.ygyno.2017.09.003.
23. Brown JC, John GM, Segal S, Chu CS, Schmitz KH. Physical activity and lower limb lymphedema among uterine cancer survivors. *Med Sci Sport Exerc*. 2013;45(11):2091–2097.
24. Lindqvist E, Wedin M, Fredrikson M, Kjølhede P. Lymphedema after treatment for endometrial cancer – a review of prevalence and risk factors. *Eur J Obstet Gynecol [Internet]*. 2017;211:112–121. Available from: https://doi.org/10.1016/j.ejogrb.2017. 02.021.
25. Rowlands IJ, Beesley VL, Janda M, et al. Gynecologic oncology quality of life of women with lower limb swelling or lymphedema 3–5 years following endometrial cancer. *Gynecol Oncol [Internet]*. 2014;133(2):314–318. Available from: https://doi.org/10.1016/j.ygyno.2014.03.003.
26. Hill EK, Sandbo S, Abramsohn E, et al. Assessing gynecologic and breast cancer survivors' sexual health care needs (sexual care needs of cancer survivors). *Cancer*. 2012;117(12):2643–2651.
27. Stabile C, Goldfarb S, Baser RE, et al. Sexual health needs and educational intervention preference for women with cancer. *Breast Cancer Res Treat*. 2017;165(1):77–84.
28. Ramaseshan AS, Felton J, Roque D, Rao G, Shipper AG, Sanses TVD. Pelvic floor disorders in women with gynecologic malignancies: a systematic review. *Int Urogynecol J*. 2018;29:459–476.
29. Yang EJ, Lim J-Y, Rah UW, Kim YB. Gynecologic oncology effect of a pelvic floor muscle training program on gynecologic cancer survivors with pelvic floor dysfunction: a randomized controlled trial. *Gynecol Oncol [Internet]*. 2012;125(3):705–711. Available from: https://doi.org/10.1016/j.ygyno.2012.03.045.
30. Rutledge TL, Rogers R, Lee S, Muller CY. A pilot randomized control trial to evaluate pelvic floor muscle training for urinary incontinence among gynecologic cancer survivors. *Gynecol Oncol*. 2014;132(1):154–158.
31. Hacker KE, Reynolds RK, Uppal S. Ongoing strategies and updates on pain management in gynecologic oncology patients. *Gynecol Oncol [Internet]*. 2018;149(2):410–419. Available from: https://doi.org/10.1016/j.ygyno.2018.01.034.
32. Baima J, Reynolds S, Edmiston K, Larkin A, Ward BM, Connor AO. Teaching of independent exercises for prehabilitation in breast cancer. *J Cancer Educ*. 2017;32:252–256.
33. Tsimopoulou I, Pasquali S, Howard R, et al. Psychological prehabilitation before cancer surgery: a systematic review. *Ann Surg Oncol*. 2015;22:4117–4123.
34. Jiralerspong S, Goodwin PJ. Obesity and breast cancer prognosis: evidence, challenges, and opportunities. *J Clin Oncol*. 2016;34(35):4203–4216.
35. Schnoll RA, Martinez E, Langer C, Miyamoto C, Leone F. Predictors of smoking cessation among cancer patients enrolled in a smoking cessation program. *Acta Oncol (Madr)*. 2011;50(5):678–694.

CHAPTER 8

Systemic Therapy for the Treatment of Breast Cancer

ANA CRISTINA SANDOVAL LEON, MD • ANGELIQUE ELLERBEE RICHARDSON, MD, PHD

INTRODUCTION

Breast cancer is the most common type of cancer and the second leading cause of death in women.[1] Approximately one in eight women will develop breast cancer in their lifetime. The treatment of breast cancer requires a multidisciplinary approach and often includes a surgical, medical, and radiation oncologist. An extensive network of subspecialists is also needed, including pathologist, radiologist, physiatrist, physical therapist, occupational therapist, and pain management and palliative care physicians. Also, integrative services such as massage therapy and acupuncture are increasingly being utilized. Herein we will discuss the systemic treatment of breast cancer.

CLINICAL PRESENTATION AND DIAGNOSTIC WORKUP

The majority of breast cancers are diagnosed with mammogram. Over 90% of breast cancers are detected mammographically.[2] Only about 10% of patients present with a palpable breast mass, overlying skin breakdown, redness, nipple retraction, and/or discharge. Patients who have an abnormal screening mammogram undergo further diagnostic workup with a mammogram showing additional views and/or limited breast ultrasound. This information is used to determine if a biopsy of a concerning area is needed. A clinically suspicious mass is always biopsied. Once a tissue biopsy is obtained, it is reviewed by a pathologist to determine if it is cancer. After a diagnosis of breast cancer is made, it is important to determine the receptor status in order to assess the prognosis and plan the treatment. Additional images such as a magnetic resonance imaging might be needed to evaluate the extent of the disease. Only patients with signs or symptoms of systemic involvement, large tumors (≥5 cm), and/or multiple lymph nodes (≥3) require further staging with either a computed tomography (CT) of the chest–abdomen–pelvis and a bone scan or a positron emission tomography–CT. Head imaging is done if patients have concerning neurological symptoms. Patients diagnosed with metastatic cancer undergo routine scans and tumor markers to assess the response to therapy. Patients with metastatic breast cancer (MBC) present with symptoms such as fatigue, weight loss, changes in lab chemistries, new and persistent pain, or new masses. Common sites of breast cancer metastasis are lungs, bones, liver, and brain.

NONMETASTATIC VERSUS METASTATIC BREAST CANCER

Breast cancer is a heterogeneous disease. Systemic treatment refers to medications that work throughout the body, eliminating cancer cells. The treatment options include endocrine therapies (ETs), chemotherapy, and targeted therapies. Clinical trials should always be considered. Fortunately, there have been some meaningful improvements in survival due to the increasing availability of more effective systemic therapies.

The treatment options are based on the tumor type, receptor status, and extent or burden of disease. Patient's baseline functional status and comorbidities are also considered. The treatment differs widely in patients with nonmetastatic versus MBC. In patients with non-MBC the goal of treatment is curative. Systemic therapy can be given either before (neoadjuvant) or after (adjuvant)

Breast Cancer and Gynecologic Cancer Rehabilitation DOI: https://doi.org/10.1016/B978-0-323-72166-0.00008-6

surgery. For large tumors and tumors with positive lymph nodes, neoadjuvant systemic therapy is often preferred. One of the benefits of administering neoadjuvant chemotherapy is that it can downstage the tumor, permitting a less extensive surgery. In addition, it allows for the evaluation of the effectiveness of the systemic therapy, and in the case of a suboptimal response, it gives the opportunity for additional treatment after surgery. An Early Breast Cancer Trialist Collaborative Group (EBCTCG) metaanalysis of long-term outcomes of neoadjuvant versus adjuvant chemotherapy showed that neoadjuvant chemotherapy was associated with more breast-conserving therapy and similar rates of distant recurrence and overall survival.[3] The effectiveness of neoadjuvant therapy can be determined by assessing the complete pathologic response (pCR) that is defined as the absence of residual invasive cancer after neoadjuvant therapy. It has been used as a surrogate end point in many clinical trials. Patients who achieve a pCR have better disease-free survival and overall survival when compared to patients who have residual disease.[4]

The approach to the treatment of MBC differs from that of non-MBC because the goal of therapy is usually not curative. The goal of treatment is palliative and to extend life. However, a large focus is also placed on maintaining an acceptable quality of life and improving symptoms. The role of surgery and radiation is usually reserved for palliation of distressing symptoms. Systemic therapies are typically given sequentially to minimize toxicity. However, there are times when combination therapies are administered.

SYSTEMIC TREATMENT BY RECEPTOR STATUS

Depending on the receptor status, tumors can be categorized as hormone receptor (HR) positive, human epidermal growth factor receptor 2 (HER2) positive or triple negative.

HORMONE RECEPTOR–POSITIVE BREAST CANCER

The majority of breast cancers have estrogen and/or progesterone receptors. ET is the mainstay treatment, but chemotherapy can be given in a subset of patients.

Nonmetastatic

Adjuvant endocrine therapy is recommended for the majority of patients with HR-positive breast cancer and is administered after completing chemotherapy in patients who require it. ET is typically given for 5–10 years. Since HR-positive tumors grow with estrogen the aim is to decrease the estrogen levels and/or the estrogen activity. In premenopausal women, estrogen is primarily produced by the ovaries. In these women, estrogen can be depleted by ET alone or by using a combination therapy of ovarian function suppression (OFS) or ovarian ablation with ET. Tamoxifen, a selective estrogen receptor (ER) modulator, is the most widely used drug. It blocks the ER and decreases the activity of estrogen in the breasts. In young patients and/or patients with high risk of recurrence, the combination of OFS with an aromatase inhibitor (AI) or tamoxifen has shown a decrease in the risk of recurrence with a trade-off of more side effects.[5] OFS is done either surgically by removing the ovaries with an oophorectomy or chemically using luteinizing hormone-releasing hormone agonists and antagonists.

When the ovaries stop making estrogen, a woman enters menopause. In postmenopausal women, low levels of estrogen are still being made by conversion of adrenal precursors, testosterone, and androstenedione through aromatase activity in the body. AIs are used to block this production of estrogen in postmenopausal women. For postmenopausal women, AIs are the preferred treatment. They include letrozole, anastrozole, and exemestane. All of them have shown to improve outcomes when compared to tamoxifen in the adjuvant setting.

In general, patients with tumors of ≤ 1 cm do not require chemotherapy. Genomic testing to assess the benefit of chemotherapy should be considered in patients who have small tumors (≤ 5 cm) and three or less positive lymph nodes. The 21-gene expression assay (Oncotype DX) categorizes patients in three risk groups: low, intermediate, and high. Patients in the low-risk group are not offered chemotherapy, whereas patient in the high-risk group receive chemotherapy. The intermediate group was studied in the TAILORx trial. This study randomized patients with an intermediate score to chemotherapy versus no chemotherapy. The study only included patients with HR-positive and HER2-negative breast cancer who had negative lymph nodes and T1 (≤ 2 cm) or T2 (≤ 5 cm) tumors. This trial showed that ET alone was noninferior to the addition of chemotherapy.[6] Another genomic test that is widely used is the 70-gene signature test (MammaPrint). The MINDACT study demonstrated that the 70-gene signature test can be used to determine which patients benefit from adjuvant chemotherapy. They included patients with early node-negative disease or with one to three positive lymph nodes.[7]

Based on these results, chemotherapy is only offered to patients with high recurrence scores. Patients with large tumors and/or with multiple positive lymph nodes do not need to have genomic testing and receive chemotherapy upfront. The chemotherapy options are discussed in the triple negative section.

Metastatic

Patients with HR-positive MBC can be treated with ET only or in combination with targeted agents. Typically, ET is the first choice for the treatment of HR-positive MBC, unless a more rapid response is needed due to a patient's symptoms or tumor burden.[8] The choice of therapy depends on the degree of HR positivity, the use and timing of previous therapies, and the HER2 status. The use of ET alone or in combination with targeted agents is used to reduce cancer burden and cancer-related symptoms. These therapies have different side effects when compared to chemotherapy.

HR-positive MBC therapy is targeted at depleting estrogen. In premenopausal women, OFS is recommended.[9] The ET used in the combination with OS can be tamoxifen or AIs. The first choice is usually OFS in combination with an AI.[9] If ET is given alone in premenopausal women, then tamoxifen is typically used.

AIs should be offered as part of the first-line therapy in postmenopausal women.[9] As discussed before, there are three different AIs: letrozole, anastrozole, and exemestane. Since the clinical activity, side effects and toxicities of these medications are nearly identical, they can be used interchangeably.

Since the approval of the cyclin-dependent kinase (CDK) 4/6 inhibitors, their combination with ET is the preferred first-line endocrine treatment for MBC. CDK 4/6 inhibitors are targeted therapies that block cell growth by stopping the progression from G1 to S phase. CDK 4/6 inhibitors are typically used as first-line therapy, but they can also be used in subsequent lines of treatment.[9] Currently, there are three approved CDK 4/6 inhibitors for MBC treatment: palbociclib, ribociclib, and abemaciclib. They all have progression-free survival (PFS) benefit. Ribociclib and Abemaciclib have also shown an overall survival benefit.[10,11]

Fulvestrant, a selective ER degrader is another option. It can be given alone or in combination with a CDK 4/6 inhibitor or with alpelisib, a phosphatidylinositol-4,5-bisphosphate 3-kinase catalytic subunit alpha (PIK3CA) inhibitor.[9] In order to receive alpelisib, tumors must have a PIK3CA mutation and should have progressed after treatment with an AI. This combination has shown to improve PFS when compared with single-agent fulvestrant.[12]

Everolimus can be given in combination with an AI. Everolimus inhibits the mammalian target of rapamycin pathway. The combination of everolimus with an AI has a PFS benefit when used after progression on ET.[13]

In BRCA-associated breast cancer with prior exposure to chemotherapy, the polyadenosinediphosphate-ribose polymerase (PARP) inhibitors, olaparib and talazoparib can be used after ET.[14,15]

The presence of new metastatic lesions, worsening symptoms, or clinical deterioration is a sign concerning for disease progression. After progression on ET or a targeted therapy a decision is made to either proceed with another line of ET, with or without a targeted agent, or with chemotherapy. The patient's tolerance of therapy, the duration of response, and the extent of disease are all factored into the decision-making process. Most patients are given two or three lines of ET therapy, with or without targeted agents, before receiving chemotherapy. Chemotherapy is typically given as single-agent sequential therapy. The goal of therapy is to stabilize or reduce disease with the fewest side effects, and therapy is continued until the patient develops significant side effects or disease progression occurs.

Toxicities

Endocrine Therapy

Common side effects of tamoxifen include, but are not limited to, hot flashes, amenorrhea, decreased sex drive, vaginal dryness, and fatigue. Hot flashes can be managed with the use of medications such as venlafaxine or less commonly oxybutynin. Vaginal dryness can improve with the use of vaginal lubricants. Cancer and cancer therapy-related fatigue can be distressing for patients, and at times, it may be difficult to treat. This type of fatigue is persistent, and it affects the individual physically, emotionally, and cognitively, and it is not proportionally related to recent activity. It is recommended to first look for underlying medical causes for fatigue such as hypothyroidism, electrolyte imbalances, deconditioning, cardiac dysfunction, depression, anxiety, poor nutrition, or anemia as well as to evaluate the patient for obstructive sleep apnea or poor sleep hygiene. A nonpharmacologic approach may include yoga, massage therapy, cognitive behavioral therapy, and supportive therapies such as group therapy or counseling. The use of psychostimulants such as methylphenidate remains investigational. There is also an increased risk of thrombosis, stroke, cataracts and uterine hyperplasia, and uterine cancer due to the effects of tamoxifen in the uterus.

The side effects of AIs include, but are not limited to, fatigue, hot flashes, arthralgias, and decreased bone mineral density. AIs can lead to the loss of bone over time. Patients are encouraged to take vitamin D and calcium supplements. In the setting of osteopenia or osteoporosis, bisphosphonates or denosumab are used. The addition of ovarian suppression to ET has shown to increase the rate of adverse events, especially musculoskeletal symptoms, decreased bone density, dyspareunia, and vaginal dryness.[5] Common side effects with fulvestrant include injection site pain, musculoskeletal symptoms, and fatigue.

Targeted Therapy

CDK 4/6 inhibitors: The common side effects are neutropenia, anemia, thrombocytopenia, fatigue, and nausea. Diarrhea is seen with abemaciclib.

Everolimus: The side effects include, but are not limited to, hyperglycemia, stomatitis, pneumonitis, and risk of infection.

Alpelisib: Common side effects include hyperglycemia, sometimes requiring involvement of an endocrinologist, lymphopenia, anemia, nausea, rash, interstitial pneumonitis, and headaches.

HUMAN EPIDERMAL GROWTH FACTOR RECEPTOR 2–POSITIVE BREAST CANCER

Approximately 20% of breast cancers have HER2 amplification. Prior to HER2-targeted therapy, the prognosis was dismal. HER2-directed therapy greatly changed the outcomes in this patient population.

Nonmetastatic

Trastuzumab is a monoclonal antibody directed against the HER2 receptor. The combination of trastuzumab with different chemotherapy backbones has shown to improve both disease-free survival and overall survival in the adjuvant setting.[16] Most studies have shown that 1 year of trastuzumab is the optimal length of therapy.

In patients with small tumors (≤2 cm) and negative lymph nodes, the combination of trastuzumab with single-agent paclitaxel given weekly for 12 weeks in the adjuvant setting is appropriate. This is based on a phase 2 single-arm study that showed a 7-year disease-free survival of 93%.[17]

For patients with tumors larger than 2 cm and/or positive lymph nodes, neoadjuvant therapy is often preferred. Pertuzumab is a newer monoclonal antibody that binds to a different domain of the HER2 receptor that has been studied in combination with trastuzumab and different chemotherapy regimens. In the neoadjuvant setting, it improved the rate of pCR,[18] whereas in the adjuvant setting it showed a small but statistically significant improvement in invasive disease-free survival (IDFS), especially in patients with positive lymph nodes.[19]

Neratinib is an oral tyrosine kinase inhibitor that was studied in the ExteNET trial. The addition of neratinib for 1 year, after completing a year of adjuvant trastuzumab, showed a statistically significant improvement in IDFS. A prespecified subgroup analysis suggested that the benefit was greater in patients with HR-positive disease.[20]

Ado-trastuzumab emtansine (T-DM1) is an antibody–drug conjugate of trastuzumab with the cytotoxic agent DM1 that is approved for the adjuvant treatment of HER2-positive disease in patients who do not achieve a pathologic complete response after neoadjuvant therapy. This approval was based on the results of the Katherine trial.[21]

Metastatic

The combination of a taxane with trastuzumab and pertuzumab is the preferred first-line therapy for metastatic HER2-positive breast cancer. The pivotal trial that led to the approval of trastuzumab in 2001 showed a significant improvement of PFS and overall survival when it was added to chemotherapy in patients with metastatic HER2-positive breast cancer.[22] The addition of pertuzumab is supported by the results of the Cleopatra trial.[23] Chemotherapy is continued for 4–6 months or to the time of maximal response, and then HER2-targeted therapy is continued until progression.[24]

The preferred second-line agent is the antibody–drug conjugate T-DM1. It has shown to improve PFS and overall survival.[25] The treatment beyond second line often includes some form of HER2-directed therapy, in combination with chemotherapy. Lapatinib, an oral tyrosine kinase inhibitor, can be used in this setting.[26]

In patients with HER2-positive and HR-positive breast cancer, ET is usually added in combination with HER2-directed therapy once chemotherapy is completed.

Toxicities

Trastuzumab is associated with the increased risk of heart failure. Patients need to be monitored with routine echocardiograms while receiving trastuzumab. The incidence is higher in patients who receive anthracycline-based chemotherapy. Other side effects include infusion reactions and pulmonary toxicity. The addition of pertuzumab to trastuzumab-containing regimens increases the incidence of diarrhea and rash.[27]

In the Katherine trial, more patients in the T-DM1 arm had neuropathy, thrombocytopenia, and pneumonitis when compared to trastuzumab.[21] Diarrhea is a common side effect of lapatinib and neratinib. For this reason, antidiarrheal prophylaxis is often given with these medications.

TRIPLE-NEGATIVE BREAST CANCER

Triple-negative breast cancer (TNBC) lacks the expression of the ER, progesterone receptor, and HER2 receptor. TNBC is a very aggressive subtype of breast cancer. Chemotherapy is the mainstay treatment for TNBC.

Nonmetastatic

Chemotherapy is indicated for any tumor that is greater than 0.5 cm. Depending on the size of the tumor and the presence of lymph nodes, chemotherapy is given either prior to surgery (neoadjuvant) or after surgery (adjuvant).

There are a number of chemotherapy regimens that are active in breast cancer. The most widely used regimens include anthracyclines, alkylators, and taxanes. The preferred regimen is dose-dense adriamycin with cyclophosphamide followed by paclitaxel (dd AC-T).[28] Other regimens include the combination of cyclophosphamide, methotrexate and fluorouracil or the combination of docetaxel with cyclophosphamide.

The addition of taxanes is supported by many randomized trials. A metaanalysis of 13 trials, including 22,903 patients, showed that the addition of taxanes to an anthracycline-based regimen improved both disease-free survival and overall survival.[29] The benefit was independent of HR status.

A metaanalysis of three adjuvant trials, including 4242 women, showed that the addition of anthracyclines to a taxane-based regimen improved IDFS in patients with high-risk breast cancer. The 4-year IDFS was 90.7% for the anthracycline-containing regimen and 88.2% for the nonanthracycline-containing regimen. Exploratory analysis suggested that the benefit of adding anthracyclines was greater in patients with HR-negative breast cancer and in women with positive lymph nodes.[30]

Finally, shortening the interval between treatments (dose-dense regimens) has shown to improve disease-free survival and breast cancer mortality.[31]

The addition of carboplatin in the neoadjuvant setting has shown to improve the rates of pathologic complete response, but this has not translated into improvement in overall survival and is not widely used.[32]

In patients who received neoadjuvant chemotherapy and do not achieve a pathologic complete response, adjuvant capecitabine has shown to improve outcomes in patients with TNBC.[33]

Metastatic

Chemotherapy is the mainstay treatment for TNBC and is used first line with or without immunotherapy.

For patients who have programmed cell death-ligand 1 (PD-L1), positive immune cells in their tumor, the combination of atezolizumab with paclitaxel protein bound (nab-paclitaxel) as first-line treatment has shown to improve outcomes when compared with chemotherapy.[34]

For patients who lack PD-L1 positive immune cells and do not have progressive visceral disease, single-agent sequential chemotherapy is the preferred option. Combination chemotherapy can be considered in patients with progressive visceral disease who need a prompt response. The patient's preferences and overall health status are always taken into consideration when deciding on treatment. Common chemotherapy treatments are taxanes, anthracyclines, vinorelbine, gemcitabine, eribulin, and capecitabine. In individuals with BRCA mutations, carboplatin may be considered.

Poly (ADP-ribose) polymerase (PARP) inhibitors are an option for patients with germ line BRCA1 or BRCA2 mutations and MBC. Talazoparib and olaparib have shown to improve outcomes when compared to standard chemotherapy and are approved for patients with locally advanced or metastatic breast cancer with a BRCA1 or BRCA2 mutation who were treated with chemotherapy in the neoadjuvant, adjuvant or metastatic setting.[14,15]

Toxicities

Chemotherapy

Chemotherapy is associated with many toxicities. Many patients will have fatigue, nausea, vomiting, mucositis, and alopecia. Cytopenias are not uncommon. Prophylactic growth factor support is needed in some adjuvant and neoadjuvant regimens to decrease the risk of febrile neutropenia.

Depending on the type of chemotherapy and the risk of emesis, patients receive prophylactic medications. Some of the premedications include steroids, olanzapine, and neurokinin 1 receptor (NKR1) antagonists such as aprepitant and selective type three 5-hydroxytryptamine (5-HT3) receptor antagonists such as ondansetron or palonosetron. Patients may require additional medications to control the nausea and vomit after chemotherapy. Antiemetics such as ondansetron and prochlorperazine are often given. Anticipatory nausea and vomiting can be triggered by strong smells, taste, or emotions and may not have a direct relationship with the timing of chemotherapy. This can be controlled with cognitive behavioral therapy, acupuncture, or with anxiolytic medications such as lorazepam.

Anthracyclines are associated with cardiotoxicity. Prior to initiation of anthracyclines, patients need to have a baseline echocardiogram. Anthracyclines have also been associated with secondary acute myeloid leukemia and myelodysplastic syndrome. Taxanes can cause anaphylaxis, and patients need premedication with steroids and antihistamines prior to starting the infusion. Patients need to be monitored for peripheral neuropathy and fluid retention.

Atezolizumab

In patients receiving immunotherapy, it is important to monitor immune-mediated reactions such as pneumonitis, thyroiditis, and hepatitis.

PARP Inhibitors

The two approved PARP inhibitors for breast cancer are olaparib and talazoparib. Talazoparib is associated with more fatigue, nausea, and anemia when compared with chemotherapy.[15] Anemia, requiring transfusion, is more frequent with olaparib than in patients receiving chemotherapy.[35]

CONCLUSION

When treating breast cancer, it is always important to maximize efficacy and minimize toxicity. Patient's preferences should always guide the therapy that is given. The systemic treatment differs based on the stage of the disease (metastatic vs nonmetastatic) and the receptor status. Great advances have been made in the systemic treatment of breast cancer, and the outcomes have improved significantly with the discovery of new therapies. Unfortunately, there are still many patients that recur and die from the disease despite systemic therapy. For this reason, many clinical trials are evaluating new drugs and different combinations with the ultimate goal of reducing breast cancer mortality.

PATIENT RESOURCES

- American Cancer Society: https://www.cancer.org/cancer/breast-cancer.html
- American Society of Clinical Oncology (ASCO): https://www.cancer.net/sites/cancer.net/files/asco_answers_guide_breast.pdf
- Clinical Trials: https://clinicaltrials.gov
- NCCN guidelines for patients: https://www.nccn.org/patients/guidelines/breast-invasive/index.html
- Up To Date: https://www.uptodate.com/contents/search?search = BREAST%20CANCER&sp = 3&searchType = PLAIN_TEXT&source = USER_PREF&searchOffset = 1&language = en&max = 10&index = &autoCompleteTerm =

REFERENCES

1. USCS. USCS data visualizations. <https://gis.cdc.gov/grasp/USCS/DataViz.html>; 2019 (Accessed 10.09.19).
2. Smart CR, Hartmann WH, Beahrs OH, Garfinkel L. Insights into breast cancer screening of younger women. Evidence from the 14-year follow-up of the Breast Cancer Detection Demonstration Project. *Cancer*. 1993;72(4 suppl):1449–1456.
3. Alberro JA, Ballester B, Deulofeu P, et al. Long-term outcomes for neoadjuvant versus adjuvant chemotherapy in early breast cancer: meta-analysis of individual patient data from ten randomized trials. *Lancet Oncol*. 2018;19(1):27–39.
4. Spring L, Fell G, Arfe A, et al. Abstract GS2-03: pathological complete response after neoadjuvant chemotherapy and impact on breast cancer recurrence and mortality, stratified by breast cancer subtypes and adjuvant chemotherapy usage: Individual patient-level meta-analyses of over 27,000 patients. *Cancer Res*. 2019;79(4 suppl). GS2-03-GS02-03.
5. Francis PA, Pagani O, Fleming GF, et al. Tailoring adjuvant endocrine therapy for premenopausal breast cancer. *N Engl J Med*. 2018;379(2):122–137.
6. Sparano JA, Gray RJ, Makower DF, et al. Adjuvant chemotherapy guided by a 21-gene expression assay in breast cancer. *N Engl J Med*. 2018;379(2):111–121.
7. Cardoso F, van't Veer LJ, Bogaerts J, et al. 70-Gene signature as an aid to treatment decisions in early-stage breast cancer. *N Engl J Med*. 2016;375(8):717–729.
8. Wilcken N, Hornbuckle J, Ghersi D. Chemotherapy alone versus endocrine therapy alone for metastatic breast cancer. *Cochrane Database Syst Rev*. 2003;(2) Cd002747.
9. Rugo HS, Rumble RB, Macrae E, et al. Endocrine therapy for hormone receptor-positive metastatic breast cancer: American Society of Clinical Oncology Guideline. *J Clin Oncol*. 2016;34(25):3069–3103.
10. Sledge Jr. GW, Toi M, Neven P, et al. The effect of abemaciclib plus fulvestrant on overall survival in hormone

receptor-positive, ERBB2-negative breast cancer that progressed on endocrine therapy-MONARCH 2: a randomized clinical trial. *JAMA Oncol*. 2019. Available from: http://dx.doi.org/10.1001/jamaoncol.2019.4782.
11. Im SA, Lu YS, Bardia A, et al. Overall survival with ribociclib plus endocrine therapy in breast cancer. *N Engl J Med*. 2019;381(4):307–316.
12. Andre F, Ciruelos E, Rubovszky G, et al. Alpelisib for PIK3CA-mutated, hormone receptor-positive advanced breast cancer. *N Engl J Med*. 2019;380(20):1929–1940.
13. Baselga J, Campone M, Piccart M, et al. Everolimus in postmenopausal hormone-receptor-positive advanced breast cancer. *N Engl J Med*. 2012;366(6):520–529.
14. Robson ME, Tung N, Conte P, et al. OlympiAD final overall survival and tolerability results: olaparib versus chemotherapy treatment of physician's choice in patients with a germline BRCA mutation and HER2-negative metastatic breast cancer. *Ann Oncol*. 2019;30(4):558–566.
15. Litton JK, Rugo HS, Ettl J, et al. Talazoparib in patients with advanced breast cancer and a germline BRCA mutation. *N Engl J Med*. 2018;379(8):753–763.
16. Baselga J, Perez EA, Pienkowski T, Bell R. Adjuvant trastuzumab: a milestone in the treatment of HER-2-positive early breast cancer. *Oncologist*. 2006;11(suppl 1):4–12.
17. Tolaney SM, Guo H, Pernas S, et al. Seven-year follow-up analysis of adjuvant paclitaxel and trastuzumab trial for node-negative, human epidermal growth factor receptor 2-positive breast cancer. *J Clin Oncol*. 2019;37(22):1868–1875.
18. Gianni L, Pienkowski T, Im YH, et al. 5-Year analysis of neoadjuvant pertuzumab and trastuzumab in patients with locally advanced, inflammatory, or early-stage HER2-positive breast cancer (NeoSphere): a multicentre, open-label, phase 2 randomized trial. *Lancet Oncol*. 2016;17(6):791–800.
19. von Minckwitz G, Procter M, de Azambuja E, et al. Adjuvant pertuzumab and trastuzumab in early HER2-positive breast cancer. *N Engl J Med*. 2017;377(2):122–131.
20. Martin M, Holmes FA, Ejlertsen B, et al. Neratinib after trastuzumab-based adjuvant therapy in HER2-positive breast cancer (ExteNET): 5-year analysis of a randomized, double-blind, placebo-controlled, phase 3 trial. *Lancet Oncol*. 2017;18(12):1688–1700.
21. von Minckwitz G, Huang CS, Mano MS, et al. Trastuzumab emtansine for residual invasive HER2-positive breast cancer. *N Engl J Med*. 2019;380(7):617–628.
22. Slamon DJ, Leyland-Jones B, Shak S, et al. Use of chemotherapy plus a monoclonal antibody against HER2 for metastatic breast cancer that over expresses HER2. *N Engl J Med*. 2001;344(11):783–792.
23. Swain SM, Baselga J, Kim SB, et al. Pertuzumab, trastuzumab, and docetaxel in HER2-positive metastatic breast cancer. *N Engl J Med*. 2015;372(8):724–734.
24. Giordano SH, Temin S, Chandarlapaty S, et al. Systemic therapy for patients with advanced human epidermal growth factor receptor 2-positive breast cancer: ASCO clinical practice guideline update. *J Clin Oncol*. 2018;36(26):2736–2740.
25. Verma S, Miles D, Gianni L, et al. Trastuzumab emtansine for HER2-positive advanced breast cancer. *N Engl J Med*. 2012;367(19):1783–1791.
26. Blackwell KL, Burstein HJ, Storniolo AM, et al. Randomized study of Lapatinib alone or in combination with trastuzumab in women with ErbB2-positive, trastuzumab-refractory metastatic breast cancer. *J Clin Oncol*. 2010;28(7):1124–1130.
27. Baselga J, Cortes J, Kim SB, et al. Pertuzumab plus trastuzumab plus docetaxel for metastatic breast cancer. *N Engl J Med*. 2012;366(2):109–119.
28. National Comprehensive Cancer Network. *Breast cancer (version 3.2019)*. 2019. <https://www.nccn.org/professionals/physician_gls/pdf/breast.pdf>; 2019 Accessed 10.09.19.
29. De Laurentiis M, Cancello G, D'Agostino D, et al. Taxane-based combinations as adjuvant chemotherapy of early breast cancer: a meta-analysis of randomized trials. *J Clin Oncol*. 2008;26(1):44–53.
30. Blum JL, Flynn PJ, Yothers G, et al. Anthracyclines in early breast cancer: the ABC trials—USOR 06-090, NSABP B-46-I/USOR 07132, and NSABP B-49 (NRG Oncology). *J Clin Oncol*. 2017;35(23):2647–2655.
31. Early Breast Cancer Trialists' Collaborative Group (EBCTCG). Increasing the dose intensity of chemotherapy by more frequent administration or sequential scheduling: a patient-level meta-analysis of 37 298 women with early breast cancer in 26 randomized trials. *Lancet (London, Engl)*. 2019;393(10179):1440–1452.
32. von Minckwitz G, Schneeweiss A, Loibl S, et al. Neoadjuvant carboplatin in patients with triple-negative and HER2-positive early breast cancer (GeparSixto; GBG 66): a randomized phase 2 trial. *Lancet Oncol*. 2014;15(7):747–756.
33. Masuda N, Lee SJ, Ohtani S, et al. Adjuvant capecitabine for breast cancer after preoperative chemotherapy. *N Engl J Med*. 2017;376(22):2147–2159.
34. Schmid P, Adams S, Rugo HS, et al. Atezolizumab and nab-paclitaxel in advanced triple-negative breast cancer. *N Engl J Med*. 2018;379(22):2108–2121.
35. Robson M, Im SA, Senkus E, et al. Olaparib for metastatic breast cancer in patients with a germline BRCA mutation. *N Engl J Med*. 2017;377(6):523–533.

CHAPTER 9

Principles of Radiation Therapy in Breast Cancer

MARIA-AMELIA RODRIGUES, MD

INTRODUCTION

Breast cancer is a heterogeneous group of diseases in which cells originating most commonly from the ducts and lobules in the breast tissue, change and divide uncontrollably with the resulting formation of a lump or mass. Breast cancer is the most common cancer in women throughout the world, representing a major public health problem. In the United States, breast cancer is the most frequent cancer in women and the second most frequent cause of cancer death in females. The American Cancer Society estimates that in 2019 in the United States, there will be approximately 268,600 new cancer cases of invasive breast cancer diagnosed in women. An additional 2,670 cases will be diagnosed in men. Approximately 62,930 cases of in situ (pre-invasive) breast cancer will be diagnosed (ductal carcinoma in situ or lobular carcinoma in situ) in women. It is anticipated that 41,760 women and 500 men will die from breast cancer in 2019.[1]

RADIATION THERAPY IN THE TREATMENT OF BREAST CANCER

Breast cancer is most commonly a disease of women. In the United States, approximately 1 in 8 women (13%) will be diagnosed with invasive breast cancer in their lifetime and 1 in 39 women (3%) will die from the disease. The risk in men is significantly less. Most cases of breast cancer are sporadic. Despite an association between the BRCA 1 and 2 genes and breast cancer, genetically associated breast cancer comprises approximately 10% of all cases. However, with extended genetic testing, newer genes associated with breast cancer are emerging.

The use of screening mammography has greatly changed the outcome of patients with breast cancer where most women are now diagnosed with small, lymph node–negative disease. The cure rate for early stage breast cancer is above 95%.

Radiation is utilized to treat malignant neoplasms and some forms of benign disease marked by an excessive proliferation of cells. Radiation Therapy (RT) therefore is effective in killing cancer cells. Radiation kills cells by damaging DNA strands. There are two primary mechanisms of radiation damage. In the direct action the particle directly affects the clinical target (DNA) inside the cell. The indirect action of radiation is a result of the interaction of the radiation (primarily photons or electrons) with molecules in the cell producing free radicals, which in turn will cause DNA damage (Fig. 9.1). Contrary to normal cells, tumor cells lack repair mechanism that can correct the DNA damage caused by radiation and therefore cell death ensues.

RT is an integral component in the treatment of breast cancer. In patients with early stage disease, surgical options include a lumpectomy and sentinel lymph node biopsy also known as breast conservation. In this setting, RT reduces the local recurrence rates by 50%–70%. RT is also utilized in patients having positive lymph node disease at surgery either after lumpectomy and sentinel lymph node biopsy or

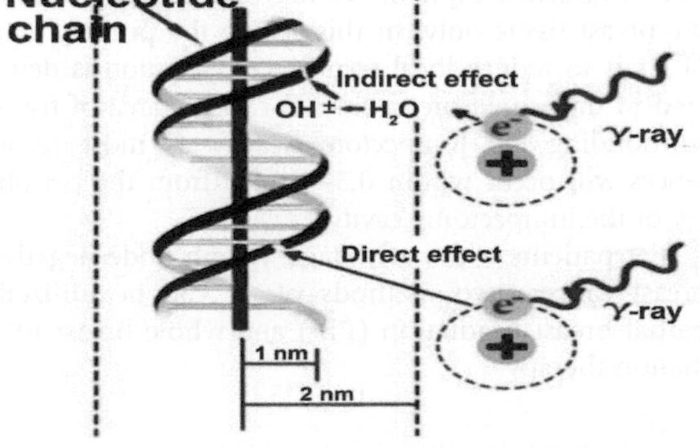

FIGURE 9.1 Mechanism of cellular damage by radiation.[2]

Breast Cancer and Gynecologic Cancer Rehabilitation DOI: https://doi.org/10.1016/B978-0-323-72166-0.00009-8

mastectomy. In this patient population, radiation is delivered not only to the breast and chest wall regions but also to the regional lymph node basins. In this setting, RT has been shown to not only decrease local recurrence but also improve overall survival.[3,4]

For breast cancer patients with locally advanced disease and patients with inoperable disease, RT is utilized in the palliative treatment of bleeding, chest wall pain and brachial plexus neuropathy, and for relief of symptoms in patients with metastatic disease. In this chapter, we will discuss primarily the role of RT in the curative setting.

RT is utilized in the majority of patients diagnosed with early stage breast cancer after lumpectomy and in patients with lymph node positive disease after lumpectomy or mastectomy. The majority of patients with breast cancer are eligible for RT. However, in patients who are entertaining the possibility of breast conservation, RT is not indicated for patients with collagen vascular disease, more specifically, scleroderma and patients with active, uncontrolled systemic lupus erythematosus. These patients are at risk for development of severe fibrosis after RT. Another group of patients for whom RT should be used with caution are patients with mutations in the ATM gene. Ataxia telangiectasia is a mostly neurological disease caused by a defect in the ATM gene, which is responsible for recognition of DNA damage and its repair. These patients are at risk of complications from radiation exposure.

TYPES OF RADIATION THERAPY FOR BREAST CANCER

Patients diagnosed with preinvasive (in situ) disease and those with invasive breast cancer with pathologically negative lymph nodes are candidates for RT to the breast tissue only. In this setting the primary goal of RT is to reduce local recurrence. Radiation is delivered to the whole breast tissue or to the area of tissue surrounding the lumpectomy cavity as most recurrences will occur within 0.5–0.8 cm from the periphery of the lumpectomy cavity.[5]

For patients with early stage, lymph node negative breast cancer, two methods of RT can be utilized-partial breast irradiation (PBI) and whole breast irradiation therapy.

PARTIAL BREAST IRRADIATION

A select group of patients with breast cancer who undergo a lumpectomy, are candidates for treatments to the lumpectomy area alone without the necessity of exposing the entire breast tissue to RT. Patients that qualify for PBI include

- age ≥ 40
- tumor ≤ 3 cm
- negative margins
- ductal carcinoma in situ, invasive ductal carcinoma and invasive lobular carcinoma
- any receptor status
- focal lymphovascular invasion
- negative lymph nodes

This type of radiation is called accelerated PBI (APBI). The early clinical trials that revealed equivalence between breast-conserving surgery followed by RT and mastectomy, utilized traditionally radiation regimens of 1.8–2 Gy per fraction to a total dose of 45–50 Gy to the whole breast and an additional 5–8 fractions to the lumpectomy cavity (usually called boost field). Therefore patients underwent radiation typically for 5–6.5 weeks of treatment. Many patients that underwent breast-conserving surgery ultimately did not receive the necessary RT due to the inconvenience of several weeks of radiation most notably in patients living in rural areas, elderly patients with transportation difficulties as well as younger women for whom the commitment to RT for several weeks created a burden on the daily living schedules with work and care of family and children. Currently, several single institution experiences as well as randomized trials in the United States and Europe have established the effectiveness, safety, and equivalent local control with the utilization of RT to the lumpectomy cavity only (PBI) in qualified patients.[6] In addition, the cosmetic result has been excellent, particularly in patients undergoing partial breast radiation with brachytherapy, which treats a smaller volume of breast tissue.

Brachytherapy is a technique by which RT is delivered to the tissue via radioactive seeds. The most common isotope utilized in brachytherapy for breast cancer is iridium 192 that delivers gamma rays. Usually, a device or several small hollow catheters are placed inside or around the lumpectomy cavity. The radioactive source then will reach the proper location via the catheters. Some methods of delivering this type of radiation are illustrated next (Fig. 9.2).

Radiation Dose in Accelerated Partial Breast Irradiation

From its early inception until recently, patients undergoing APBI would be treated twice a day at a dose of 3.4 Gy to the planning target volume (PTV) corresponding to the lumpectomy cavity with an added 1 cm margin deeming the PTV. This dose was delivered for a

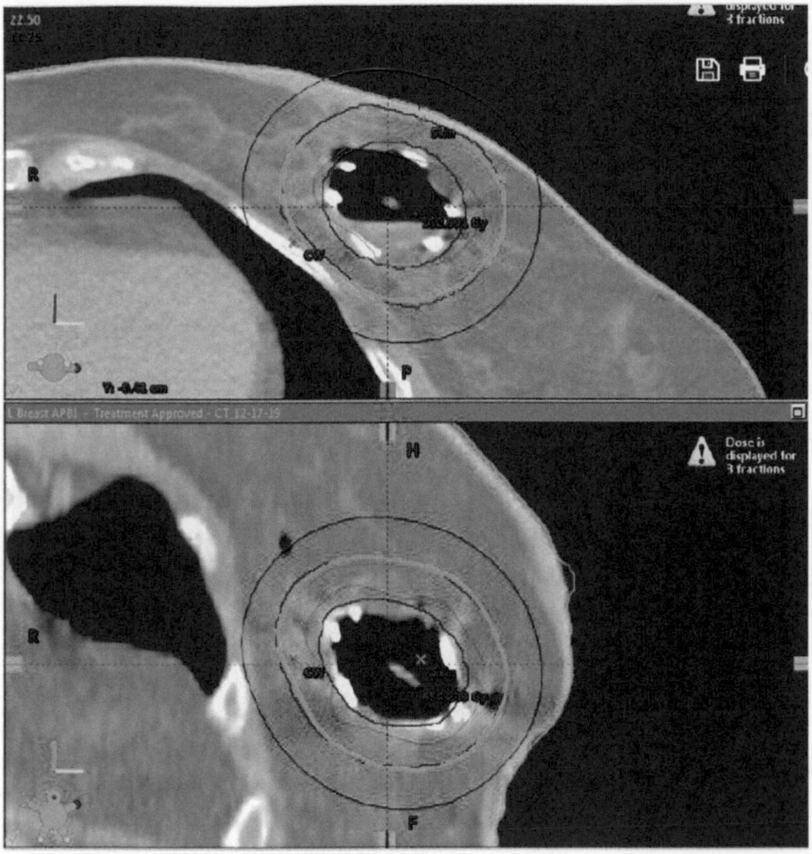

FIGURE 9.2 CT images illustrating a treatment plan for APBI with brachytherapy. A small volume of tissue is treated with this method. Constraints are placed on the skin and chest wall where recurrences rarely occur and late effects such as rib fracture, myositis, telangiectasias, and skin atrophy have been reported in earlier experiences. *APBI*, Accelerated partial breast irradiation.

total of 10 fractions culminating with a total dose of 34 Gy to the PCV and five treatment days. A recently multiinstitutional clinical trial was published reporting on a three fraction regimen of 7.5 Gy per fraction to a total dose of 22.5 Gy delivered over 2–3 days. The triumph–T trial reported excellent cosmetic outcomes and comparable recurrence rates to the experience with whole breast radiation and accelerated partial breast radiation from multiple single institutional trials, registry trials, and randomized phase 3 clinical trial.[7]

WHOLE BREAST IRRADIATION

The majority of patients with early stage breast cancer who may not be eligible for PBI receive RT to the whole breast tissue. Traditionally, patients have been treated in the supine position with the arms raised above the head. Merchant and McCormick[8] were pioneers in introducing prone positioning for patients receiving radiation to the whole breast. In their early experience, patient selection was limited to women who had large, pendulous breasts. Given the benefits of a reduced dose to the chest wall and to lungs and heart, most radiation oncology departments that treat a large volume of breast cancer patients have embraced prone positioning for early-stage breast cancer.

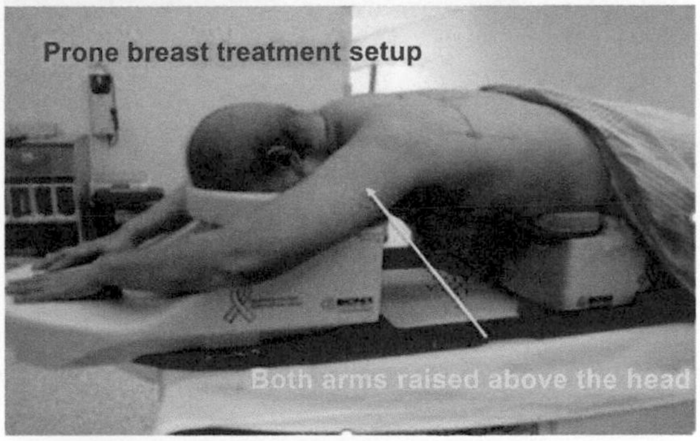

FIGURE 9.3 Prone position.

Fig. 9.3 demonstrates the prone breast radiation treatment setup. Fig. 9.4 illustrates the advantages of

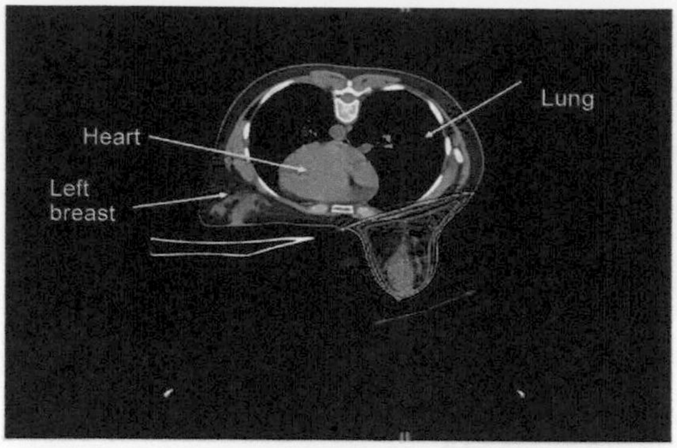

FIGURE 9.4 Prone position whole breast irradiation. The arrow indicates lung, heart, and the contralateral breast (left) effectively protected from radiation dose.

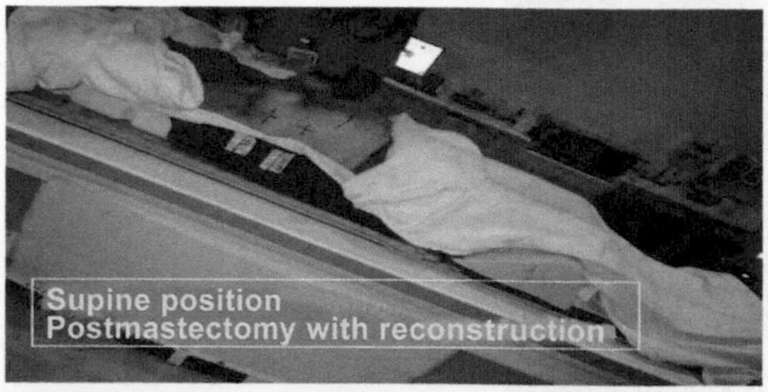

FIGURE 9.5 Supine position.

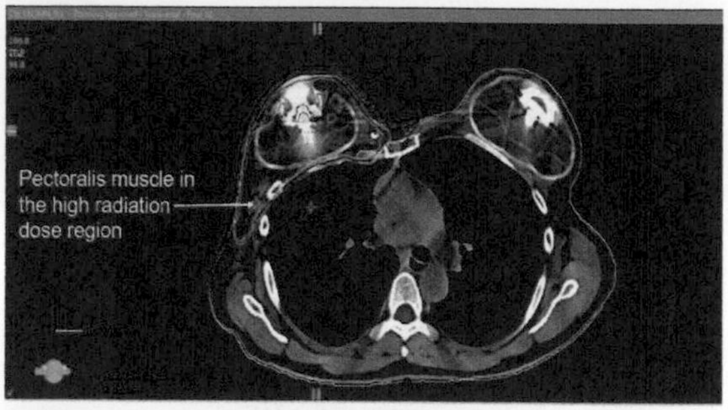

FIGURE 9.6 RT and pectoralis major. *RT*, Radiation therapy.

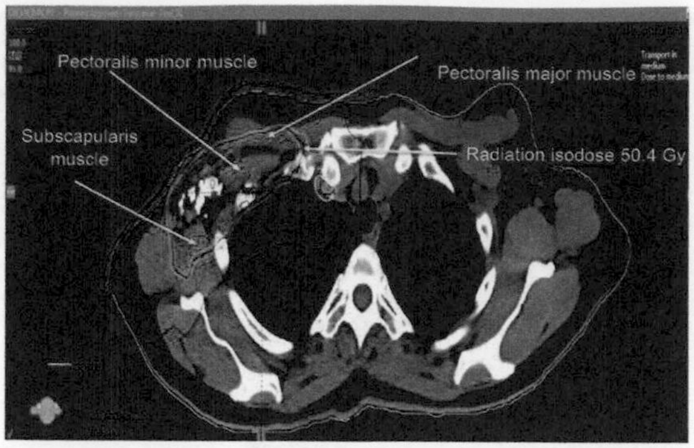

FIGURE 9.7 RT and pectoralis major, pectoralis minor, and subscapularis muscle. *RT*, Radiation therapy.

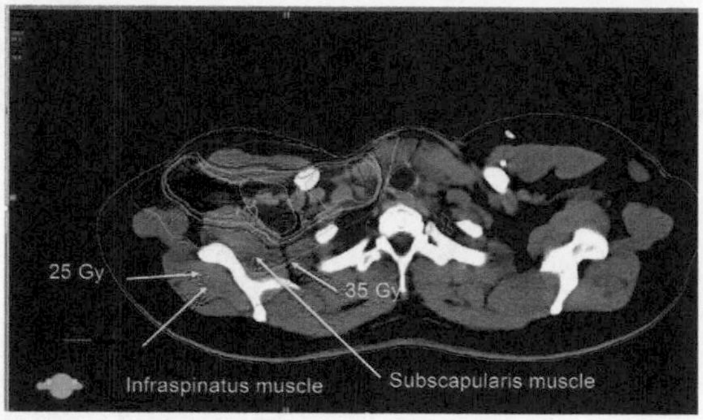

FIGURE 9.8 RT to regional lymph nodes. Shoulder girdle muscles and the relationship to radiation dose. *RT*, Radiation therapy.

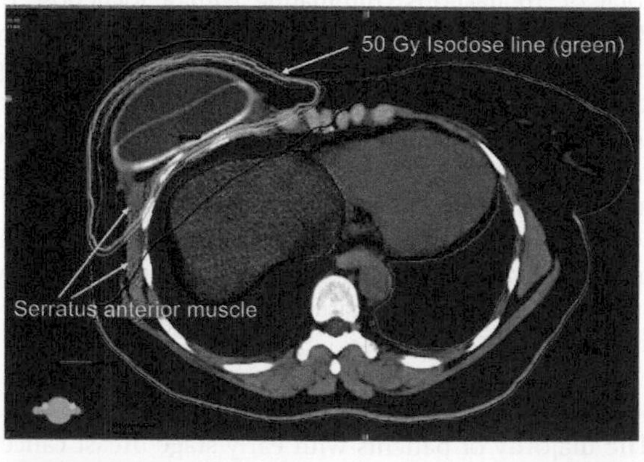

FIGURE 9.9 Serratus anterior muscle and the 50 Gy isodose line.

the prone position in minimizing the exposure to radiation dose to the lung, heart, and the contralateral breast. In Fig. 9.5 the supine position is demonstrated for comparison. It is important that for each of these positions, the patient needs to have an adequate range of motion for both shoulders to be able to tolerate lying in the required treatment position during the RT session. Figs. 9.6–9.9 demonstrate the radiation fields as they correlate with important muscles for shoulder function, including the pectoralis major, pectoralis minor, serratus anterior, infraspinatus and subscapularis, and brachial plexus (Fig. 9.10).

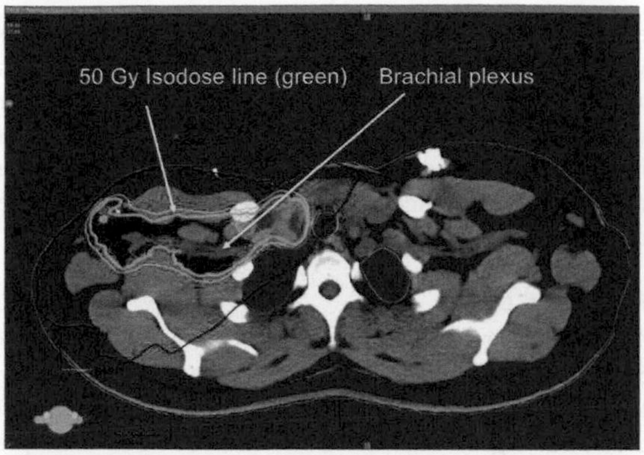

FIGURE 9.10 Location of the brachial plexus (neurovascular bundle) in relationship to the prescription dose. Special care is taken to avoid "hot spots"—higher doses than prescription—in this region.

BREAST OR CHEST WALL IRRADIATION, INCLUDING REGIONAL LYMPH NODES

Traditionally, RT to the breast tissue or chest wall, including the regional lymph nodes, has been utilized in patients with stage III, locally advanced breast cancer as defined by patients with T3–T4 (tumors that are typically greater than 5 cm and invade the chest wall, the skin), patients with inflammatory breast cancer, and patients with N2 or N3 disease (lymph node involvement in greater than 4 lymph nodes or extension to the supraclavicular lymph nodes or internal mammary lymph nodes).

Two seminal randomized clinical trials published in 1997 and 1999 changed the paradigm of treatment of patients with earlier stage disease and smaller volume of cancer in the lymph nodes. These clinical trials by Whelan and Overgaard[4,9] showed that in patients with T1–T2 tumors (tumors with size up to 5 cm) and 1–3 + lymph nodes derived not only a benefit in local recurrence but also had improved overall survival after mastectomy, adjuvant chemotherapy, and RT compared to the standard arm group, which did not receive RT after mastectomy. In both trials with currently over 15–20 years of follow-up, the improvement in local regional control and overall survival is still demonstrated.

The advances in plastic reconstructive surgery have impacted significantly on the psychological aspect of patients who undergo a mastectomy. In most centers today, women who undergo a mastectomy have immediate reconstruction with typically a two-stage procedure where a tissue expander is placed at the time of mastectomy and a completion of reconstruction follows several months later. For most women an excellent cosmetic outcome is achieved with patient satisfaction above 80%. However, in patients who undergo mastectomy with reconstruction who are candidates for postmastectomy RT, the rate of complications has risen.

In patients with breast cancer who have positive lymph nodes, RT is directed to the breast tissue and the regional lymph nodes. Most patients at risk for a local regional recurrence are those with large tumors (greater than 5 cm), tumors that involve the chest wall, the skin, patients with inflammatory breast cancer, and patients with more than 4 + lymph nodes in the axilla at the time of surgery.

THE PATIENT EXPERIENCE IN THE RADIATION ONCOLOGY DEPARTMENT

Current best practices in the care of a breast cancer patient include a multidisciplinary treatment team approach. This includes an evaluation by a team of health-care providers that includes diagnostic radiologist, breast surgeon, medical oncologist, radiation oncologist, and, in some cases, a plastic surgeon when a mastectomy with reconstruction is envisioned as well as early engagement of rehabilitative services.

The first encounter in the radiation oncology department by a patient with breast cancer will be the initial consultation that involves the evaluation by the radiation oncologist and advanced practice provider. In this initial evaluation the radiation oncologist reviews the pertinent images, the results of the initial breast biopsy, and all pertinent documentation by the surgeon, medical oncologist, and plastic surgeon if indicated. In many cases a patient's case may have been previously discussed in a multidisciplinary conference. With the patient's disease knowledge in hand, the radiation oncologist will proceed to collect additional history details such as history of previous radiation that could limit the ability of a new course of radiation, the presence of certain collagen vascular diseases, which preclude the utilization of RT, and breast conservation such as scleroderma and active, uncontrolled systemic lupus erythematosus.

After history taking a thorough physical examination is performed. In assessing the patient with breast cancer, special attention will be given to the examination of the breast and the regional lymph node stations. Focused attention is also directed to the patient's shoulder range of motion and the ability to hold the arms elevated for the purposes of positioning of the patient during radiation treatment.

At the end of the consultation a treatment plan recommendation is made. The process of RT, including the first treatment planning appointment (simulation), the daily radiation delivery process, and the side effects (both acute and late) of the proposed treatment are discussed with the patient and a consent form is signed.

Simulation

After the initial consultation the next appointment is called simulation. In this appointment the patient is placed in the appropriate position as illustrated next. A CT scan is performed in the treatment position. Small 3–5 tattoo dots are placed at the center of the treatment area, which will yield the daily treatment setup. The CT images are subsequently transferred to the treatment planning system for the physician and dosimetrist to work on outlining the treatment volumes, the normal tissues to be spared and avoided, ultimately creating the isodose lines and a dose volume histogram for plan evaluation.

In patients with breast cancer, depending on the patient's stage and surgery, treatment is directed to a partial volume in the breast, the whole breast or chest wall and the whole breast, chest wall, and regional lymph nodes.

Daily Treatment

The first day of treatment includes a verification of all the treatment parameters and the patient positioning. After this initial treatment day the patient will embark on his or her treatment. The patient should expect to be in the radiation department for daily treatments of about 30–40 minutes. The actual RT lasts for 6–7 minutes; however, the patient will be in the treatment room for approximately 20 minutes to allow for positioning, verification of setup by X-ray films, and final treatment delivery. Once a week or more often if needed, the patient will be evaluated on treatment progress by the radiation oncologist, the advanced practice provider, and the nurse. At completion of treatment the patient will see the radiation oncology nurse and will be given instructions on the management of any side effects and follow-up appointments.

RADIATION THERAPY ADVERSE EFFECTS

While RT is one of the main therapeutic components in the curative approach to breast cancer, normal tissues surrounding the volume of interest will react to radiation as well. Normal tissue radiation injury has been known to occur since the early days of RT. Different tissues in the body will react and demonstrate radiation injury over time. Generally, these effects are termed acute, subacute, and late effects. When these reactions occur, they are generally termed side effects of RT. Acute and late effects of RT in normal tissue are generally independent of each other; however, in some cases such as skin desquamation may lead to telangiectasias and skin fibrosis years after the acute reaction occurred.

Acute Effects

Acute reactions to RT develop during a standard 6- to 8-week course of RT. Acute reactions occur in tissues that typically multiply quickly such as the skin, the oral pharyngeal, and the bone marrow. For example, patients may experience changes in the breast such as breast swelling, skin erythema, and breast tenderness due to the radiation-induced inflammation. These side effects tend to subside and completely resolve in 2 weeks after completion of a radiation course. Given the nature of these reactions, changes in the dose and occasional treatment breaks of a few days can help in the management of these effects.

Subacute Effects

Subacute changes in tissues due to radiation effects are expressed several months after the treatment course is completed. These effects are associated with cell loss and inflammation and for most part are reversible although on occasion may progress to severe damage. In the treatment of patients with breast cancer, an example of such effect is radiation pneumonitis where there is loss of type I pneumocytes that leads to increased microvascular permeability, inflammatory reaction, and activation of cells producing cytokines. Most of the effect resolves clinically; however, at the cellular level it can progress into chronic pulmonary disease due to fibrosis.

Late Effects

These occur usually several months to years after RT has been completed and can be permanent. As these responses occur after radiation has been completed, dose modification, treatment breaks no longer apply in the management of these effects. Late effects of radiation are thought to result from the depletion of cells in slow with low proliferative index.

RADIATION EFFECTS ON THE SKIN AND BREAST

The most common acute side effect experienced during radiation for breast cancer is radiation-induced dermatitis. Clinical findings range from faint erythema to moist desquamation. In most patients brisk-to-modest erythema, hyperpigmentation, dry desquamation with pruritus and papular rash are commonly observed. Most of the experience with breast conservation has utilized a standard fractionation of one-point 8–2 Gy per fraction and has been utilized to a total dose of 45–50 Gy. Whelan et al. in the British Columbia Cancer Center randomized patients to standard fractionation compared to a shortened course of 2.66 Gy per fraction to 42.56 Gy total dose and observed equivalent local control rates and cosmetic outcome. However, the acute side effects of radiation were reduced with a significant decrease in acute dermatitis in the patients receiving hypofractionation treated in the affected arm. Initial concern regarding ultimate cosmetic results has been unfounded by solid randomized data from the experience in Canada, England, and currently this regimen has been widely adopted in the United States.[10]

Second to skin reaction, breast tissue changes are frequently experienced by patients undergoing whole breast radiation. Inflammatory changes cause breast edema and breast pain, which occurs in approximately a third of the patients. Effects on the skin occur later.

Lymphedema

Patients with breast cancer who undergo axillary surgery for staging procedures such as axillary lymph node dissection or sentinel lymph node biopsy are at risk for developing lymphedema. The consequences of surgery have been well reported and depend on the extent of axillary node dissection. Sentinel lymph node biopsy carries a lesser risk of development of lymphedema. McLoughlin et al. reported that series of 936 women who underwent sentinel lymph node biopsy alone versus sentinel lymph node biopsy followed by axillary node dissection. In their experience, 16% of patients that underwent sentinel lymph node biopsy followed by axillary node dissection had lymphedema compared to 5% of patients that underwent sentinel lymph node biopsy alone. Of the patients who underwent ipsilateral breast or chest wall radiation, a slightly higher incidence of lymphedema was found, however, not statistically significant (10% vs 8%; $P = .29$). Additional risk factors associated with a higher likelihood of lymphedema development were greater body weight, higher body mass, and the development of infection or injury in the ipsilateral arm since surgical procedure. RT can add to the incidence of lymphedema.[11]

Brachial Plexopathy

Brachial plexus dysfunction is a disabling syndrome. The incidence of brachial plexopathy from RT radiation to the regional lymph nodes is less than 1%. At standard doses, this is a rare complication in patients receiving RT. However, with doses over 50–56 Gy, the concomitant use of chemotherapy can increase the likelihood of brachioplexopathy.[12] At Miami Cancer Institute, patients that require higher than 50.4 Gy to the regional lymph nodes in the axilla or supraclavicular regions, special attention is paid to carefully outline the brachial plexus and to avoid hotspots (unintended higher doses of radiation) in this region.

MYOSITIS AND SHOULDER DYSFUNCTION

Radiation myositis is rare and seldom reported side effect of RT. In patients receiving RT, radiation-induced myositis is commonly reported in patients with sarcomas where a high dose of radiation, greater than 62.3 Gy are delivered directly to the affected muscle compartment. The cellular response to radiation injury to the muscle include edema, mild follow-up, filament disruption, and endothelial swelling, which can be seen after single doses of 11–13 Gy in animal models.[13] The onset of symptoms related to the radiation effect in the muscular skeletal symptoms stem is approximately 5–6 months after radiation and in many patients years later. Therefore little attention has been paid to this effect of RT. In patients with breast cancer, muscle pain can develop after 1–2 years of RT. In most patients, treatment with nonsteroidal antiinflammatory drugs is effective.

Shoulder dysfunction is a well-known morbidity after breast cancer. The etiology of shoulder dysfunction is multifactorial and includes surgery, radiation, and utilization of aromatase inhibitors in the adjuvant treatment of breast cancer. In the report by Andras et al.[14] showed decreased EMG activity in the upper trapezius and rhomboid muscles and shortening of the pectoralis major and minor muscles in patients treated for breast cancer. Most of the patients in the study had received radiation either to the breast only or to the breast, chest wall, and regional lymph nodes.[15]

Radiation Pneumonitis

Radiation pneumonitis a known sequelae of RT albeit is uncommon. Clinically significant radiation pneumonitis is observed in less than 2% of patients treated with radiation. Factors associated with the development of pneumonitis include radiation fields with higher likelihood of radiation pneumonitis when fields are extended to involve the regional lymph nodes, the use of concomitant chemotherapy.

Cardiac-Related Complications

It is well known that RT can lead to excess cardiovascular disease and potential mortality. The early experience of radiation in patients with Hodgkin's disease and non-Hodgkin's lymphoma has shown an increase risk of heart failure after a mean heart dose of 5–14 Gy. These late effects can manifest after a period in excess of 10 years in breast cancer patients where cardiotoxic chemotherapy is frequently utilized, so several strategies are utilized to reduce the dose to left coronary artery, left ventricular, and mean heart dose. Such techniques include deep inspiration breath hold, prone positioning, partial breast radiation, or proton therapy. A comprehensive review is cited in Ref. [2].

Other Late Effects of Radiation Therapy

Secondary breast cancer due to low dose of radiation is rarely observed, the risk is higher in younger patients receiving RT. Additional secondary malignancies such as lung cancer, esophageal cancer, leukemia, and sarcoma have been reported. Older series have reported a relative risk for all secondary nonbreast malignancies at 1.2, although this increased risk is likely driven by clinical trials using older techniques. An important second malignancy arising from RT in breast cancer patient is radiation-induced angiosarcoma. Unlike other secondary malignancies from radiation, angiosarcoma can occur within a short interval after completion of treatment. This is a particularly aggressive malignancy. Despite the fact that radiation is the cause of breast angiosarcoma, treatment for these tumors includes surgery and hyperfractionated RT. Prognosis is generally poor.

IMPLICATIONS FOR REHABILITATION MEDICINE

Rehabilitation medicine should be an integral part of the care of the breast cancer patient before, during, and after receiving RT. As noted earlier, RT affects numerous structures involved in the proper functioning of the arm that includes muscles, ligaments, tendons, and neurovascular structures. These effects can be exacerbated if the patient has a prior history of arm dysfunction. Prior to the start of radiation treatments, physiatrists can assess the patient for shoulder impairments and initiate treatment for persons at high risk for developing shoulder dysfunction or lymphedema post treatments. This is critical for the patient to have the adequate range of motion of the shoulder to be able to tolerate the prone or supine position during treatment sessions. Following the completion of treatments, surveillance for shoulder dysfunction, lymphedema, and early initiation of treatments as necessary can help to minimize impairments, activity limitations, and participation restrictions thereby ensuring that the person can resume life roles and work.

CONCLUSION

With 3.8 million breast cancer survivors in the United States, careful planning in radiation delivery as well as a coordinated team approach with breast surgeons, medical oncologists, plastic surgeons, and rehabilitative services is extremely important in the treatment of breast cancer and improving the quality of life of survivors.

REFERENCES

1. American Cancer Society. *Breast Cancer Fact & Figures 2019–2020*. Atlanta, GA: American Cancer Society, Inc.; 2019.
2. Hall EJ. *Radiobiology for the Radiologist*. 6th ed. Lippincott Williams; 2006.
3. Overgaard M, et al. Randomized trial evaluating postoperative radiotherapy in high risk postmenopausal breast cancer patients given adjuvant tamoxifen: results from the DBCG 82c trial. *Lancet*. 1999;353:1641–1648.
4. Ragaz J, Jackson SM, Le N, et al. Adjuvant radiotherapy and chemotherapy in node-positive premenopausal women with breast cancer. *N Engl J Med*. 1997;337(14):956–962.
5. Imamura H, Haga S, Shimizu T, et al. Relationship between the morphological and biological characteristics of intraductal components accompanying invasive ductal breast carcinoma and patient age. *Breast Cancer Res Treat*. 2000;62:177–184.
6. Correa C, Harris E, Leonardi M, et al. Accelerated partial breast irradiation: executive summary for the update of an ASTRO evidence-based consensus statement. *Pract Radiat Oncol*. 2017;7:73–79.
7. Khan A, Chen P, Yashar C, et al. Three-Fraction accelerated partial breast irradiation (APBI) Delivered with brachytherapy applicators is feasible and safe: first results from the TRIUMPH-T Trial. *Int J Radiat Oncol Biol Phys*. 2019;104(1):67–74.
8. Merchant TE, McCormick B. Prone position breast irradiation. *Int J Radiat Oncol Biol Phys*. 1994;30(1):197–203.
9. Whelan TJ, Julian J, Wright J, et al. Does locoregional radiation therapy improve survival in breast cancer? A meta-analysis. *J Clin Oncol*. 2000;18(6):1220–1229.

10. Whelan T, Pignol JP, Levine M, et al. Long-term results of hypofractionated radiation therapy for breast cancer. *N Engl J Med*. 2010;362(6).
11. Wu S, Huang S, Zhou J, et al. Dosimetric analysis of the brachial plexus among patients with breast cancer treated with post-mastectomy radiotherapy to the ipsilateral supraclavicular area: report of 3 cases of radiation-induced brachial plexus neuropathy. *Radiat Oncol*. 2014;9:292.
12. Welsh JS, Torre TG, DeWeese TL, et al. Radiation myositis. *Ann Oncol*. 1999;10:1105–1108.
13. Shamley D, Srinanaganathan R, Weatherall R, et al. Changes in shoulder muscle size and activity following treatment for breast cancer. *Breast Cancer Res Treat*. 2007;106:19–27. Available from: https://doi.org/10.1007/s10549-006-9466-7.
14. Andras C, Bodoki L, Nagy-Vincze M, et al. Retrospective analysis of cancer-associated myositis patients over the past 3 decades in a Hungarian myositis cohort. *Pathol Oncol Res*. 2019;. Available from: https://doi.org/10.1007/s12253-019-00756-4.
15. Armanious MA, Mohammadi H, Khodor S, et al. Cardiovascular effects of radiation therapy. *Curr Probl Cancer*. 2018;42:433–442.

FURTHER READING

Halperin E, Wazer D, Perez C, et al. *Principles and Practices of Radiation Oncology*. 7th ed. Philadelphia, PA: Wolters Kluwer; 2018.

START Trialists' Group, Bentzen SM, Agrawal RK, et al. The UK Standardization of Breast Radiotherapy (START) Trial A of radiotherapy hypofractionation for treatment of early breast cancer: a randomized trial. *Lancet Oncol*. 2008;9(4):331–341. Available from: https://doi.org/10.1016/S1470-2045(08)70077-9.

CHAPTER 10

Breast Cancer Surgery

JANE MENDEZ, MD

INTRODUCTION

Breast cancer is the most common cancer in women accounting for 266,000 new cancers in 2019 alone. It is the second most common cause of cancer-related mortality in women.[1] It has been estimated that 12% of American women will be diagnosed with breast cancer during their lifetime (1/8) and 3.5% will die of the disease. The incidence of breast cancer increases with age. Male breast cancer accounts for 1% of all breast cancers.[2]

Globally, breast cancer incidence rates are highest in North America and Northern Europe, and lowest in Asia and Africa. Studies of migration patterns to the United States are consistent with the importance of cultural and/or environmental changes. In general, incidence rates of breast cancer are greater in second-generation migrants and increase further in third- and fourth-generation migrants. Overall, breast cancer mortality rates have declined since 1975, attributable to the increased use of screening mammography and the aggressive use of adjuvant therapies. Despite having a lower incidence rate than white women, black women have a higher mortality rate that is attributable to both more advanced stage at diagnosis and higher stage-specific mortality.

Multiple risk factors have been associated with breast cancer. These include

- age and gender,
- family history and genetic factors,
- personal history of breast cancer,
- race and ethnicity,
- reproductive and hormonal factors,
- benign breast disease,
- lifestyle and dietary factors,
- exposure to ionizing radiation, and
- environmental factors.

Age and Gender

Both age and gender are among the strongest risk factors for breast cancer development. The female breast cancer incidence increases with age. Male breast cancer incidence is approximately 1%.[3]

Family History and Genetic Factors

Family history is an important risk factor for breast cancer. However, a positive family history is only reported by 10%–15% of women with breast cancer. Most breast cancers, 85% are sporadic in nature.[4]

The risk associated with having an affected first or second degree maternal or paternal relative is modulated by the age of both the case patient and the family member at diagnosis, and the number of female first-degree relatives with and without cancer. Specific genetic mutations that predispose to breast cancer are rare; only 5%–6% of all breast cancers are directly attributable to inheritance of a breast cancer susceptibility gene such as BRCA1, BRCA2, p53, ATM, PTEN, and other breast cancer–related actionable mutations. Once a patient is identified as a high risk for a genetic predisposition for breast cancer based on the personal history of cancer or the family history, the patient is referred for genetic counseling and possible genetic testing. Only about 5% of breast cancer patients will harbor an actionable breast cancer–related mutation. In this subset of patients, prophylactic surgical intervention might be indicated depending on the specific gene identified. The BRCA1 and BRCA2 are the most prevalent breast cancer–related genes and the following are considered "red flags" for the hereditary breast and ovarian cancer: breast cancer before age 50, ovarian cancer at any age, male breast cancer at any age, multiple primary cancers, and Ashkenazi Jewish ancestry.

Personal History of Breast Cancer

A personal history of invasive or in situ breast cancer increases the risk of developing an invasive breast cancer in the contralateral breast. With in situ lesions the 10-year risk of developing a contralateral invasive cancer is 5%. In women with invasive breast cancer the risk of developing contralateral breast cancer is 1% and 0.5% per year for premenopausal and postmenopausal women, respectively.

Breast Cancer and Gynecologic Cancer Rehabilitation DOI: https://doi.org/10.1016/B978-0-323-72166-0.00010-4

Benign Breast Disease

Nonproliferative breast lesions such as fibrocystic changes, solitary papilloma, and simple fibroadenoma are not associated with an increased risk for breast cancer. The more important precursors of noninvasive or invasive breast cancer are proliferative lesions, particularly those with cytologic atypia. The risk of invasive breast cancer is slightly increased (relative risk 1.3–2) for a proliferative lesion without atypia (complex fibroadenoma, moderate or florid hyperplasia, sclerosing adenosis, and intraductal papillomas). For a proliferative lesion with atypia (atypical lobular hyperplasia, atypical ductal hyperplasia, and atypical papillary lesion), the risk is higher (relative risk 4–6) and higher still (10-fold) when the atypia is multifocal.[5]

Race and Ethnicity

In the United States, breast cancer is the most common cancer among women of every major ethnic group, although there are interracial differences. Given data from the American Cancer Society, the highest rates occur in whites. The rates are lower in blacks, Asian Americans/Pacific Islanders, Hispanic/Latina women, and American Indians/Alaska natives.[6] These ethnic differences may be related to factors associated with lifestyle and socioeconomic status (e.g., access to diagnosis and treatment). Disparities in breast cancer survival may be attributed to race, genetic, and/or biologic factors.

Reproductive and Hormonal Factors

Prolonged exposure to and higher concentrations of endogenous estrogen increase the risk of breast cancer. The key reproductive factors that influence breast cancer risk are age at menarche, age at first live birth, age at menopause, and possibly parity and breastfeeding. Younger age at menarche and later age of menopause are associated with a higher risk of breast cancer (cumulative estrogen exposure). Nulliparous women are at increased risk for breast cancer compared with parous women; the relative risk ranges from 1.2 to 1.7. The younger a woman is at her first full-term pregnancy, the lower her breast cancer risk: A protective effect of breastfeeding has been shown in multiple case–control and cohort studies, the magnitude of which is dependent on the duration of breastfeeding and the confounding factor of parity. Other controversial areas include the risk of hormone replacement therapy, the use of oral contraceptives, and infertility treatments.

LIFESTYLE AND DIETARY FACTORS

Socioeconomic Status

Women of higher socioeconomic status are at greater risk for breast cancer, with as much as a two-fold increase in incidence from lowest to the highest strata. However, it does not appear that socioeconomic status is an independent risk factor. Instead, the influence of socioeconomic status (educational, occupational, and economic level) is thought to reflect differing reproductive patterns with respect to parity, age at first birth, age at menarche, and utilization of screening mammography.

Geographic Residence

There are marked variations in breast cancer incidence and mortality among countries.

Weight

Weight and body mass index have opposite influences on postmenopausal as compared to premenopausal breast cancer (higher circulating levels of estrogens in women who have more adipose tissue that increases peripheral conversion of estrogen precursors to estrogen).

Physical Activity

Regular physical exercise appears to provide modest protection against breast cancer, but the relationship is complex, particularly in premenopausal women. The reduction in breast cancer risk seen with exercise may be mediated in part through weight control.

Alcohol

Moderate alcohol intake is associated with an increased risk of hormone receptor-positive breast cancer, and the effect appears to be additive with hormone replacement therapy.[7]

Fat Intake

Several studies have shown a positive correlation between fat consumption and increased breast cancer risk. However, the results of case–control and prospective cohort studies have been mixed, possibly because of the limited range of dietary fat in the typical American diet and an interaction between reproductive variables, menopausal status, and fat intake.

Caffeine

A number of studies have failed to show any association between caffeine intake and breast cancer risk.

Smoking

The relationship between cigarette smoking and breast cancer is controversial and complicated by the interaction of smoking with alcohol and the endogenous hormonal influences that alter breast cancer risk. As part of a healthy lifestyle, patient should be advised to refrain from cigarette smoking as lung cancer the most common cause of cancer–related mortality in women.

Exposure to Ionizing Radiation

Exposure to ionizing radiation of the chest at a young age, as occurs with treatment of Hodgkin lymphoma or in survivors of atomic bomb or nuclear plant accidents, is associated with an increased risk of breast cancer. The most vulnerable ages appear to be between 10 and 14 years of age (the prepubertal years), but excess risk is seen in women exposed as late as 45 years of age. Whether there is a link between breast cancer and low levels of irradiation, such as those in diagnostic imaging tests, is controversial.

Environmental Factors

Organochlorines include polychlorinated biphenyls, dioxins, and organochlorine pesticides such as dichlorodiphenyltrichloroethane (DDT). These compounds are weak estrogens, highly lipophilic, and capable of persisting in body tissues for years. However, most large studies have failed to find an association.[8]

The best defense against breast cancer is early detection to the extent that for stage I breast cancer the 10-year survival is 98.5%. The multidisciplinary approach is critical to maximize the breast cancer cure, including surgical oncology, medical oncology, radiation oncology, plastic surgery, and rehab oncology. The optimal treatment needs to be individualized taking into consideration the breast tumor characteristics, breast cancer stage, and the patient's underlying comorbidities.

ROLE OF SURGERY IN THE TREATMENT OF BREAST CANCER

The role of surgery in the treatment of breast cancer has two main primary goals: extirpation of the breast tumor burden for local control and axillary lymph node assessment for staging purposes when indicated. As part of the multidisciplinary treatment, the role of chemotherapy or adjuvant endocrine therapy is systemic control and the role of adjuvant radiation therapy is local control. Each of the treatment strategies has associated side effects that need to be thoroughly discussed as part of the decision-making process. Though the most critical goal is to maximize the breast cancer cure and minimize the likelihood of local recurrence, quality of life issues need to be addressed. Given the state-of-the-art treatment available, active research, and increased breast cancer awareness, there are more than 3 million breast cancer survivors in the United States alone. The challenge for providers is to maximize the breast cancer cure while maintaining good quality of life.[9]

Surgical Management of Breast Cancer

Overall, there are two main types of surgery for the treatment of breast cancer: breast conservation treatment (BCT) that may be referred to as lumpectomy, wide excision, partial mastectomy followed by radiation therapy or a type of mastectomy. With both options the primary aim is to remove the tumor burden to pathologically negative margins. For the axillary lymph node assessment an axillary sentinel lymph node (SLN) biopsy or an axillary lymph node dissection (ALND) needs to be performed for the invasive breast cancers.

Breast Conservation

Determining which is the optimal surgical intervention requires a thorough discussion with the patient taking into consideration a multitude of factors, including tumor size, tumor location, extent of disease, tumor characteristics, ability to receive adjuvant radiation therapy, and genetic predisposition. Breast cancer patients with multicentric disease, unable to receive radiation therapy or persistently positive surgical margins despite multiple excisions, will not be candidates for breast conservation and will require a mastectomy. There is a relative contraindication to breast conservation in patients with large tumors relative to the native breast size. Often times, if these patients are interested in breast conservation neoadjuvant chemotherapy or neo-endocrine therapy might be offered to reduce the tumor burden and make the patient a better operable candidate.

Contraindications to BCT:

Absolute—There are few absolute contraindications to BCT. In most of these cases, attempts to preserve the breast have been fraught with very high rates of in-breast recurrence:

- Persistently positive resection margins after reasonable reexcision attempts.
- Multicentric disease in which there are two or more primary tumors in separate breast quadrants.
- Diffuse malignant-appearing mammographic microcalcifications, suggesting multicentricity.

- A history of prior radiation therapy (RT) to the breast or chest wall; this usually precludes further RT.
- Pregnancy, although it may be possible to perform breast-conserving surgery in the third trimester, deferring breast RT until after delivery.

Relative—Relative contraindications include the following:

- Patients with a history of scleroderma tolerate RT poorly and have a greater possibility of dermal complications. Whether other connective tissue diseases (e.g., rheumatoid arthritis, lupus) are associated with an increased risk of acute or late skin complications is controversial.
- Breast size is not in itself a contraindication to BCT. However, a large tumor in a small breast is a relative contraindication, as an adequate resection would result in significant cosmetic alteration.

Mastectomy

When a mastectomy needs to be performed or when it is the patient's personal choice issues pertaining to breast reconstruction options, different types of mastectomy and management of the contralateral breast need to be addressed. Provided all clinical factors are equal and there is no contraindication to breast preservation, the overall survival for the breast cancer patients is the same.[10,11] The main difference between breast conservation and mastectomy is the local recurrence. For breast conservation (lumpectomy followed by radiation) versus mastectomy, the local recurrence is 10% versus 2%–5%, respectively. Often times, the patients have unrealistic expectations, and these need to be clarified as part of the surgical planning.

Types of mastectomy include as follows:

- *Total mastectomy*. A total mastectomy, also known as a simple mastectomy, involves removal of the entire breast, including the breast tissue, areola, and nipple. A SLN biopsy may be done at the time of a total mastectomy.
- *Skin-sparing mastectomy*. A skin-sparing mastectomy involves removal of all the breast tissue, nipple, and areola but not the breast skin. A SLN biopsy also may be done. Breast reconstruction can be performed immediately after the mastectomy.
- *Nipple-sparing mastectomy*. A nipple- or areola-sparing mastectomy involves removal of only breast tissue, sparing the skin, nipple, and areola. A SLN biopsy also may be done. Breast reconstruction is performed immediately afterward.[12,13]
- *Modified radical mastectomy*. A modified radical mastectomy involves removal of the entire breast, areola, and nipple with a complete ALND.

Breast Reconstruction

Breast reconstruction has increased in popularity, largely due to changing attitudes among women with breast cancer and their doctors, and recognition of the psychosocial benefits gained by reconstruction. The type of breast surgery impacts on the need for breast reconstruction.

Patients who require a mastectomy or those who choose to proceed with a mastectomy need to be referred for plastic surgery consultation to further explore the reconstructive options. The two main types of reconstruction include implant based versus autologous tissue reconstruction. Both types of procedures may be performed at the time of the primary breast cancer surgery or deferred. With immediate reconstruction the surgical process is streamlined, since both tumor resection and reconstruction are performed in one operative setting. There appears to be no adverse oncologic impact for immediate compared to delayed reconstruction. In addition, the emotional benefit of having begun reconstruction at the time of extirpation may reduce the impact of the loss of a breast. On the negative side, surgical time is lengthened with immediate reconstruction, and potential complications of mastectomy (e.g., skin loss and infection) or postoperative RT can adversely affect the reconstruction.

A myriad of factors impacts the decision of the optimal recommendation. There are different types of mastectomy that may be performed, including total mastectomy, skin-sparing mastectomy, and nipple- and areola-sparing mastectomy. Determining the optimal type of mastectomy depends on the location of the tumor, breast and tumor size, breast ptosis, and any previous breast surgical procedures. It is important to know that not all patients are equally eligible for the different options. Often times, the reconstruction occurs in multiple stages, and the reconstructive surgeon has to work with the rest of the multidisciplinary team especially when adjuvant chemotherapy or postmastectomy radiation therapy is required.[14]

It is vitally important that the reconstructive surgeon be consulted before definitive breast cancer surgery takes place so that an in-depth discussion regarding options for reconstruction can be undertaken with the patient and her family.

Axillary Lymph Node Assessment

The status of the axillary nodes is the single most important prognostic factor in women with early-stage disease. Furthermore, axillary metastases are an important indicator of the need for adjuvant systemic therapy and postmastectomy RT.

Irrespective of the breast management, the axillary node assessment needs to occur for the invasive breast cancers. In patients with a clinically negative axilla at presentation, the state-of-the-art is to perform an axillary SLN biopsy. Depending on surgeon preference, there are three different techniques that may be used with the injection of isosulfan blue dye, sulfur colloid technetium 99, or a combination of both. By definition, the SLN biopsy will identify the first node that the breast cancer is draining to for staging purposes. In the event the axillary SLN has evidence of metastatic disease, then the need to proceed with a complete ALND will be discussed based on the pathological findings. If the patient presents with clinically palpable nodes, then further assessment with an axillary ultrasound and possible core biopsy might be recommended to exclude metastatic disease. If there is evidence of axillary biopsy-proven metastasis, neoadjuvant chemotherapy might be necessary to downstage the axilla and try to avoid an axillary dissection. In an attempt to avoid unnecessary morbidity associated with the axillary assessment, the Choosing Wisely campaign advocates to avoid axillary SLN biopsy in women 70 years of age or older with favorable tumor characteristics. If the axillary lymph node information is not going to change the overall management, why expose these patients to increased morbidity?[15,16]

DESCRIPTION OF HOW THE SURGERIES ARE PERFORMED

Lumpectomy

The lumpectomy procedure begins with locating the area of the breast that contains the abnormality. If the breast abnormality was detected on a mammogram or breast ultrasound and confirmed with a biopsy, the radiologist would have placed a marker or clip to allow for subsequent identification of the area. If this is the case, a thin wire, a reflector, or radioactive marker may be inserted just before surgery to identify the marker or clip. This allows the surgeon to use the wire/reflector or radioactive seed as a guide to the precise area that needs to be removed during surgery. In the case of a palpable mass that can be easily found, no localization will be necessary as the surgeon can easily find the abnormal area to be excised. The location of the lumpectomy scar depends the tumor location. All the breast tissue excised is sent for pathologic analysis. Key pathologic information will be the margin assessment as all margins need to be free of cancer in order to proceed with a successful lumpectomy. If there is evidence of residual carcinoma at any of the margins, then a breast reexcision or mastectomy will be necessary. The lumpectomy procedure is usually an outpatient surgery procedure and may be performed under monitored anesthesia care or general anesthesia depending on the surgeon's preference and the patient's comorbidities.

Mastectomy

A mastectomy is usually performed under general anesthesia. The breast tissue is removed, and depending on the procedure, other parts of the breast also may be removed, including the nipple and the areola. If an immediate breast reconstruction is planned, the breast surgeon will coordinate with the plastic surgeon to plan the surgery and the incisions. The mastectomy is an anatomic operation that requires removal of the breast tissue from the clavicle as the superior margin, the lateral border of the sternum medially, the inframammary fold inferiorly, the latissimus dorsi muscle laterally, and the pectoralis major muscle posteriorly. All these anatomic landmarks need to be identified to assure proper breast tissue removed. There needs to be close attention to the mastectomy flaps not to compromise the vascular supply. Issues pertaining to the preservation of the nipple–areolar complex are an important part of the discussion and presurgical planning. If the patient is deemed to be a candidate for preservation of the nipple–areolar complex, the nipple tissue needs to be sent for intraoperative frozen section analysis to assure that it is safe from the oncological standpoint. As the surgery is completed, the incision is closed with stitches (sutures) that either dissolve or are removed later. Given the size of the mastectomy wound, surgical drains are left in place and removed in the postoperative period.

One option for breast reconstruction involves placing temporary tissue expanders in the chest. These temporary expanders will form the new breast mound. For women who will have radiation therapy after surgery, one option is to place temporary tissue expanders in the chest to hold the breast skin in place. This allows you to delay final breast reconstruction until after radiation therapy.

Lymph Node Surgery

Lymph nodes are often removed during surgery to determine whether cancer has spread beyond the breast. Options may include the following:

- *Axillary node dissection.* It is usually reserved for patients with known axillary metastasis. This requires general anesthesia with anatomic removal of axillary nodes levels I and II that are lateral and deep to the pectoralis minor muscle. Intraoperatively will require identification of the long thoracic and thoracodorsal nerves, axillary artery, and vein and if possible preservation of the costobrachial sensory nerves. Patients will require a surgical drainage to avoid a postoperative fluid collection. Ideally, these patients should be evaluated preoperatively by the rehabilitation oncology service to have a baseline assessment prior to surgical intervention.

- *SLN biopsy*. The surgeon removes only the first one or two nodes into which a tumor drains (sentinel nodes). These are then tested for cancer. Before the surgery a radioactive substance or blue dye or both is injected into the area around the tumor or the skin above the tumor. The dye travels to the sentinel node or nodes, allowing the surgeon to identify which are the nodes that need to be removed. All the sentinel nodes removed are submitted for pathologic analysis. If the final pathology shows no evidence of cancer, no further lymph nodes need to be removed. If cancer is present, the surgeon will discuss options, such as receiving radiation to the axilla to treat the affected lymph node versus a complete ALND for local control and staging purposes.
- *Postoperative management*. Postoperatively, further recommendations will be dependent upon the final pathologic findings. Provided the surgical margins are negative for cancer and no further axillary surgery is necessary, the patients are then referred to the medical and radiation oncology services as needed for further evaluation and management to maximize the breast cancer cure.
- For those patients who underwent an immediate breast reconstruction coordination of care, the rest of the multidisciplinary team is very important.
- For patients with an ALND, follow-up with the rehabilitation service is critical for upper extremity lymphedema prevention.
- *Common postsurgery complications*. Most breast operations are categorized as low-morbidity procedures, but a variety of complications can occur in association with diagnostic and multidisciplinary management procedures. Some of these complications are related to the breast itself, and others are associated with axillary staging procedures.[17]
  - *General wound complications related to breast and axillary surgery* such as infection, bleeding/hematoma, seroma, paresthesias, sensory loss, tingling, and keloid formation.
  - *Complications specific to lumpectomy procedures* such as breast asymmetry, breast deformity, inability to lactate (central location), and compromised nipple sensation.
  - *Complications specific to mastectomy procedures* such as breast asymmetry, flap necrosis, phantom pain, reconstruction-related capsular contractures, reduced upper extremity range of motion, and right upper extremity limited range of motion.
- *Complications related to axillary staging procedures*
- Although major complications of ALND are infrequent (e.g., injury or thrombosis of the axillary vein, injury to the motor nerves, and severe lymphedema), minor complications are much more common (e.g., seroma formation, shoulder dysfunction, loss of sensation in the distribution of the intercostobrachial nerve, and mild edema of the arm and breast). Arm edema is more common in women who undergo more extensive ALND, especially when combined with postoperative RT to the axilla. SLN biopsy is associated with a significant reduction in arm morbidity compared to ALND.[18]
- *Axillary web syndrome (AWS)*. AWS is a common condition occurring in up to 86% of patients following breast cancer surgery with ipsilateral lymphadenectomy of one or more nodes. AWS presents as a single cord or multiple thin cords in the subcutaneous tissues of the ipsilateral axilla. The cords may extend variable distances "down" the ipsilateral arm and/or chest wall. The cords frequently result in painful shoulder abduction and limited shoulder range of motion. AWS most frequently becomes symptomatic between 2 and 8 weeks postoperatively but can also develop and recur months to years after surgery. Education about and increased awareness of AWS should be promoted for patients and caregivers. Physical therapy, which consists of manual therapy, exercise, education, and other rehabilitation modalities to improve range of motion and decrease pain, is recommended in the treatment of AWS.[19]
- *Lymphedema*. Lymphedema can develop in the breast cancer patient as a result of the interruption of lymphatic flow from postsurgical, postradiation, taxane-based chemotherapy, and infectious causes. It can present at various points after breast cancer treatment and may range from mild to a seriously disabling enlargement. Because lymphedema is permanent, the goal of treatment options is the control of edema, and a multidimensional approach to care is often needed. Early detection and intervention, including preoperative consultation in those patients

undergoing an ALND, is paramount to decrease the likelihood of this morbidity.[20,21]

Implications of Rehabilitation

Given that breast cancer patients are surviving their breast cancer, quality of life issues and maintenance of functional performance status have become very important. As such, prerehabilitation and postoperative rehabilitation are critical components of the multidisciplinary approach to breast cancer. Key areas to be addressed include

- lymphedema prevention and treatment,
- AWS, and
- shoulder.

Patient Education

As the options for the multidisciplinary approach to breast cancer treatment are so complex and diverse, the patients and their family members need to be well informed and educated about the different treatment options with the associated side effects, expected recurrence and breast cancer survival rates. It is not only important to educate the patients on their treatment options but also to have realistic expectations about the quality of life issues and potential side effects on their physical performance and mental health.

Areas of Future Research

One of the most challenging sequelae of the breast cancer treatment is the management of breast cancer–related lymphedema.

In 2017 the American Society of Breast Surgeons convened an international multidisciplinary consensus panel to discuss this important topic, and the manuscripts describe the recommendations from this panel and shed some light on the prevention, diagnosis, and new treatment strategies for this potentially debilitating condition. There is ongoing research to stratify the risk of lymphedema and identify patients who might benefit from techniques, such as axillary reverse mapping (ARM) and/or lymphatic microsurgical preventative healing approach (LYMPHA). ARM entails mapping upper extremity lymphatics with blue dye allowing for differentiation of lymphatics draining the breast (radioactive) and the upper extremity (blue). In the only prospective study, Yue et al. randomized 265 patients to undergo ALND versus ALND + ARM. With 20-month follow-up, lymphedema developed in 33% of patients in the ALND group and 6% of the ALND + ARM group.[22]

LYMPHA is a surgical approach for the primary prevention of arm lymphedema following axillary nodal dissection. The idea of LYMPHA was conceived 10 years ago, and the preliminary results were published a few years after. LYMPHA couples lymphovenous bypass with ALND performing an anastomosis dunking the transected main lymphatic trunk(s) into a lateral branch of the axillary vein distal to a competent valve. Furthermore, which patients with lymphedema refractory to physical therapy and compression garments would benefit from lymph node transfer surgery? With improved understanding of the underlying pathophysiology of lymphedema, newer strategies both in the prevention and treatment of lymphedema continue to emerge. Also, we need to acknowledge that lymphedema may be secondary to factors other than just axillary surgery, including radiation therapy and chemotherapy, especially taxanes-based chemotherapy.[23–25]

SLN surgery has been the standard of care for axillary staging of the clinically negative axilla since the late 1990s. It has decreased the likelihood of upper extremity lymphedema associated with axillary surgery from 20%–40% to 5%–7%. One could argue that for a staging procedure, albeit lower, this is still a significant risk. Hence, can we identify subsets of patients where axillary surgical staging can be avoided altogether? The recent Society of Surgical Oncology Choosing Wisely guidelines recommended against SLN surgery in women older than age 70 years with hormone receptor-positive breast cancer. There is a model to predict likelihood of nodal positivity that can be useful for patients and surgeons to identify those women age 70 + at low risk of nodal positivity where SLN surgery may be avoided, and also to identify those women at higher risk of nodal positivity where surgical staging of the axilla may alter treatment recommendations.[26,27]

Another ongoing, controversial debate in breast cancer is the appropriate treatment for ductal carcinoma in situ (DCIS). Currently, there are three randomized, controlled trials for low-risk DCIS underway in Europe and the United States designed to test the safety, efficacy, and trade-offs of active surveillance compared with usual care: LORIS (multicenter UK study), LORD (EORTC study), and COMET (comparison of operative to monitoring and endocrine therapy trial for low-risk DCIS—a cooperative group US study). All three trials seek to identify a subset of patients with DCIS with low risk of both occult invasive disease at initial presentation and subsequent progression to invasive disease.[28–30]

CONCLUSION

The field of breast cancer is extremely dynamic. Research, technology, and better understanding of biology continue to drive the needle forward to cure breast cancer with the ultimate goal to one day prevent and eliminate breast cancer. In the meantime, it is with a tailored individualized multidisciplinary approach to breast cancer treatment that we will continue to optimize the oncologic outcome with good quality of life.[31,32]

PATIENT RESOURCES

American Cancer Society Breast Cancer Facts and Figures

NCI breast cancer Website

REFERENCES

1. American Cancer Society. *Breast Cancer Facts and Figures 2019, 2019*.
2. Siegel RL, Miller KD, Jemal A. *Cancer statistics, CA Cancer J Clin*. 2015;65(1):5–29.
3. Howell A, Anderson A, et al. Risk determination and prevention of breast cancer. *Breast Cancer Res*. 2014;16:446.
4. Newman L., US Preventive Services Task Force breast cancer recommendation statement on risk assessment, genetic counseling, and genetic testing for BRCA-related cancer. *JAMA Surg*. 2019;154(10):895–896.
5. Rageth C, O'Flynn EAM, et al. Second international consensus conference on lesions of uncertain malignant potential in the breast (B3 lesions). *Breast Cancer Res Treat*. 2019;174(2):279–296.
6. Iqbal J, Ginsburg O, et al. Differences in breast cancer stage at diagnosis and cancer-specific survival by race and ethnicity in the United States. *JAMA*. 2015;313(2):165–173.
7. Ali A, Schmidt M, et al. Alcohol consumption and survival after a breast cancer diagnosis: a literature-based meta-analysis and collaborative analysis of data for 29,239 cases. *Cancer Epidemiol Biomarkers Prev*. 2014;23 (6):934–945.
8. Gray J, Rasanayagam A, et al. State of the evidence 2017: an update on the connection between breast cancer and the environment. *Environ Health*. 2017;16:94.
9. Curigliano G, Burstein HJ, Winer EP, et al. De-escalating and escalating treatments for early-stage breast cancer: the St. Gallen International Expert Consensus Conference on the Primary Therapy of Early Breast Cancer 2017. *Ann Oncol*. 2017;28(8):1700–1712.
10. Fisher B, Andersen S, Bryant J, et al. Twenty-year follow-up of a randomized trial comparing total mastectomy, lumpectomy, and lumpectomy plus irradiation for the treatment of invasive breast cancer. *N Engl J Med*. 2002;347(16):1233–1241.
11. Veronesi U, Cascinelli N, Mariani L, et al. Twenty-year follow-up of a randomized study comparing breast-conserving surgery with radical mastectomy for early breast cancer. *N Engl J Med*. 2002;347(16):1227–1232.
12. Agha RA, Omran Y, et al. Systematic review of therapeutic nipple-sparing versus skin-sparing mastectomy. *BJS Open*. 2019;3(2):135–145.
13. Tsousimis E, Haslinger M. Overview of indications for nipple sparing mastectomy. *Gland Surg*. 2018;7(3):288–300.
14. Billig J, Jagsi R, et al. Should immediate autologous breast reconstruction be considered in women who require post-mastectomy radiation therapy? A prospective analysis of outcomes. *Plast Reconstr Surg*. 2017;139 (6):1279–1288.
15. Caretta-Weyer H, Greenberg C, et al. Impact of the American College of Surgeons Oncology Group (ACOSOG) Z0011 trial on clinical management of the axilla in older breast cancer patients: a SEER-Medicare analysis. *Ann Surg Oncol*. 2013;20(13). 10.1245/s.
16. Giuliano A, Ballman K, et al. Effect of axillary dissection vs no axillary dissection on 10-year overall survival among women with invasive breast cancer and sentinel node metastasis: the ACOSOG Z0011 (Alliance) Randomized Clinical Trial. *JAMA*. 2017;318(10):918–926.
17. Newman L. Complications in breast surgery. *Surg Clin North Am*. 2007;87(2):431–451.
18. Sclafani L, Baron R. Sentinel lymph node biopsy and axillary dissection: added morbidity of the arm, shoulder and chest wall after mastectomy and reconstruction. *Cancer J*. 2008;14(4):216–222.
19. Koehler LA, Haddad TC, et al. Axillary web syndrome following breast cancer surgery: symptoms, complications, and management strategies. *Breast Cancer (Dove Med Press)*. 2019;11:13–19.
20. McLaughlin SA, Staley AC, Vicini F, et al. Considerations for clinicians in the diagnosis, prevention, and treatment of breast cancer-related lymphedema: recommendations from a multidisciplinary expert ASBrS panel. Part 1: Definitions, assessments, education, and future directions. *Ann Surg Oncol*. 2017;24.
21. McLaughlin SA, DeSnyder SM, Klimberg S, et al. Considerations for clinicians in the diagnosis, prevention, and treatment of breast cancer-related lymphedema, recommendations from an expert panel. Part 2: Preventive and therapeutic options. *Ann Surg Oncol*. 2017;24.
22. Ahmed M, Rubio IT, Kovacs T, Klimberg VS, Douek M. Systematic review of axillary reverse mapping in breast cancer. *Br J Surg*. 2016;103(3):170–178.
23. Yue T, Zhuang D, Zhou P, et al. A prospective study to assess the feasibility of axillary reverse mapping and evaluate its effect on preventing lymphedema in breast cancer patients. *Clin Breast Cancer*. 2015;15(4):301–306.
24. Nguyen TT, Hoskin TL, Habermann EB, Cheville AL, Boughey JC. Breast cancer-related lymphedema risk is related to multidisciplinary treatment and not surgery alone: results from a large cohort study. *Ann Surg Oncol*. 2017;24.
25. Shaitelman SF, Cromwell KD, Rasmussen JC, et al. Recent progress in the treatment and prevention of

cancer-related lymphedema. *CA Cancer J Clin.* 2015;65 (1):55–81.
26. Society of Surgical Oncology choosing wisely guidelines. <http://www.surgonc.org/docs/default-source/default-document-library/sso-five-things-physicians-and-patients-should-question-7-11-2016.pdf?sfvrsn = 2>.
27. Welsh JL, Hoskin TL, Day CN, Habermann EB, Goetz MP, Boughey JC. Predicting nodal positivity in women 70 years of age and older with hormone receptor-positive breast cancer to aid incorporation of a Society of Surgical Oncology choosing wisely guideline into clinical practice. *Ann Surg Oncol.* 2017;24.
28. Francis A, Thomas J, Fallowfield L, Wallis M, et al. Addressing overtreatment of screen detected DCIS; the LORIS trial. *Eur J Cancer.* 2015;51(16):2296–2303.
29. Elshof LE, Tryfonidis K, van Leeuwen-Stok AE, et al. Feasibility of a prospective, randomised, open-label, international multicentre, phase III, non-inferiority trial to assess the safety of active surveillance for low risk ductal carcinoma in situ—the LORD study. *Eur J Cancer.* 2015;51(12):1497–1510.
30. Comparison of Operative Monitoring and Endocrine Therapy (COMET) Trial for low risk DCIS. <https://clinicaltrials.gov/ct2/show/NCT02926911>.
31. Grimm LJ, Shelley Hwang E. Active surveillance for DCIS: the importance of selection criteria and monitoring. *Ann Surg Oncol.* 2016;23(13):4134–4136.
32. Chollet-Hinton L, Anders CK, Tse CK, et al. Breast cancer biologic and etiologic heterogeneity by young age and menopausal status in the Carolina Breast Cancer Study: a case–control study. *Breast Cancer Res.* 2016;18(1):79.

CHAPTER 11

Reconstructive Surgery and Postoperative Care for Breast Cancer

MIGUEL A. MEDINA, III, MD • AUSTIN J. POURMOUSSA • ERIN M. WOLFE, BS • HARRY M. SALINAS, MD

INTRODUCTION

Breast cancer is the most common cancer in women, with a reported prevalence of more than 3.8 million women in the United States as of January 1, 2019.[1] It is estimated that 268,600 women will be newly diagnosed with breast cancer by the end of 2019. For women with early stage (I or II) breast cancer, the most common treatments are breast-conserving surgery with adjuvant radiation (49%) and mastectomy (34%). For women with stage III disease, mastectomy is the most common surgical treatment (68%).[1]

Breast cancer patients are of great importance to Plastic and Reconstructive surgeons. A national study conducted at Memorial Sloan Kettering found that in 2013, 41% of women who underwent mastectomy received immediate breast reconstruction procedures.[2] That number increased further to 43.3% in 2014.[3] This current reconstruction rate is a significant increase from the previous rate of 18% in 2004. The benefits of breast reconstruction after mastectomy have been well documented, including improved quality of life, body image, psychosocial well-being, sexual well-being, and patient satisfaction.[4–10]

The two main routes of breast reconstruction involve utilization of either autologous tissue or prosthetic implants. Implant-based breast reconstruction is the most common method of breast reconstruction in the United States, with over 83,000 procedures performed in 2018.[11,12] This procedure is typically preceded by placement of a tissue expander, which may remain in the breast pocket for up to 3–18 months depending on the need for adjuvant therapies. In traditional breast reconstruction, tissue expanders are used to expand the skin of the breast thereby recreating a breast mound. In addition, a mature retropectoral capsule for the prosthetic implant placement in a second procedure is created. With the advent of the routine use of acellular dermal matrices (ADMs) and skin sparing, along with nipple-sparing mastectomies, the tissue expander allows for controlled recovery of ischemic tissue followed by rapid expansion recovering the soft tissue envelope of the breast. This is of particular importance for nipple-sparing procedures. Recently, advances have been made in a hybrid approach that incorporates both prosthetic implants and autologous tissue in patients who desire autologous reconstruction but lack the soft-tissue volume required.[13] These operations combine lipo-harvest fat for the uses of medium volume fat grafting to the breast in order to reconstruct the soft tissue envelope of the breast over an implant. These techniques are also powerful in targeted soft tissue reconstruction with flap.

The most popular autologous reconstructive options for flap reconstruction include the deep inferior epigastric perforator (DIEP) flap, transverse rectus abdominis myocutaneous (TRAM) flap, and the latissimus dorsi flap. Other autologous reconstructive options include the gluteal artery perforator flap and a novel approach utilizing a stacked perforator flaps from various donor sites.[14]

ANATOMY

Pertinent anatomy involved in breast reconstruction spans the entire thorax and abdomen. The breast is a mound of adipose, gland lobules, lactiferous ducts, and suspensory ligaments that sits atop the pectoralis major, serratus anterior, and intercostal muscles.[15] Breast tissue extends from the second to sixth or seventh rib, bordered superiorly by the axillary tail and inferiorly by the inframammary fold. The female breast is enveloped by the superficial fascia of the anterior chest wall that is continuous with the neck superiorly and Camper's abdominal fascia inferiorly. The base of the breast extends from the sternal border medially to the midaxillary line laterally (Fig. 11.1).[16]

Breast Cancer and Gynecologic Cancer Rehabilitation DOI: https://doi.org/10.1016/B978-0-323-72166-0.00011-6

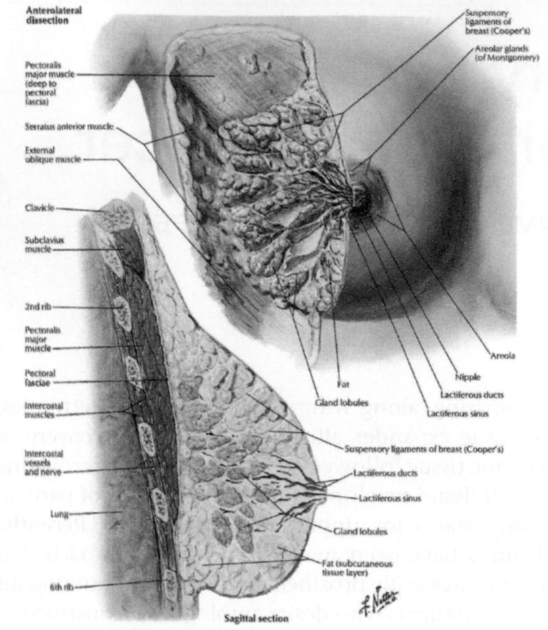

FIGURE 11.1 Anatomy of the breast.

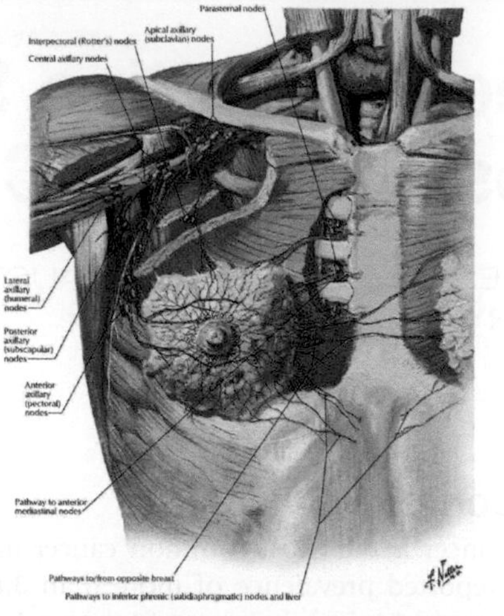

FIGURE 11.2 Vasculature and lymph nodes of the breast.

At least 50% of the blood supply to the breast comes from the internal mammary artery, a branch of the subclavian artery. The remainder of the blood supply to the breast comes from branches of the lateral thoracic artery, axillary artery, and intercostal perforators, forming a well-collateralized anastomotic network.[16,17] Venous return from the breast is primarily via the axillary vein, in addition to intercostal and internal mammary veins. Lymphatic drainage follows venous drainage.

The axilla is intimately connected with the breast, located between the upper extremity and thoracic wall. The lymph nodes in the axillary chain have important implications in breast cancer, as they receive about three quarters of all lymphatic drainage from the breast. The remaining one quarter of lymphatic drainage runs through lymph nodes in the internal mammary chain (Fig. 11.2).[18] Resection of lymph nodes during the treatment of breast cancer can result in secondary lymphedema due to interruption of the lymphatic network. This can cause swelling of the upper extremity, breast, or chest wall that may negatively impact patient quality of life.[19]

The nerve supply to the breast was first described in 1840 by Sir Astley Cooper who identified the second to sixth intercostal nerves as its primary innervation along with intercommunicating mammary branches.[20] Importantly, he described the innervation of the areola and nipple coming from mammary branches of the lateral cutaneous nerve at the T4 level, forming a plexus under the nipple. These branches provide sensation to the areola and nipple as well as motor supply to the smooth muscle of the nipple.[16] For patients undergoing mastectomy these nerves cannot be spared, leaving the patient without sensation in the breast and nipple–areolar complex.

Of importance to note, the long thoracic nerve may be invaded by cancer or interrupted during breast surgery, which may lead to a presentation of winged scapula due to loss of function in the serratus anterior. However, preservation of the nerve during axillary nodal dissection and latissimus dorsi flap operations is of more clinical significance.

Abdominal anatomy has relevance in the topic of breast reconstruction, as the majority of autologous tissue used for breast reconstruction comes from the lower abdomen. These flaps typically include the skin and subcutaneous fat, with variations on inclusion of recuts abdominis fascia or muscle. The rectus abdominis is a vertically positioned abdominal muscle that originates on the pubis and inserts into cartilages of the fifth, sixth, and seventh ribs.[21] The primary blood supply to the rectus abdominis includes the superior epigastric artery in the upper abdomen and the deep inferior epigastric artery in the lower abdomen. Of particular note for abdominal flaps, the deep inferior epigastric is the dominant blood supply, and the superior epigastric artery is typically variably collateralized in a zone above the umbilicus. The rectus abdominis receives its motor and sensory innervation primarily from the seventh to twelfth intercostal nerves. The nerves enter in variable segmental branches from lateral to medial; denervation of these nerves during abdominally based flaps results in a range of abdominal dysfunction secondary to segmental loss rectus motor function.

The posterior thorax is also relevant, as the latissimus dorsi may be used for breast reconstruction. The latissimus dorsi is a large, flat, triangular muscle that originates on the iliac crest, spinous processes of T7-L5, 10th–12th ribs, and inserts onto the bicipital groove of the humerus.[15,21] The muscle gains its blood supply from dual vascular beds—one a dominant pedicle and the other segmental: the thoracodorsal artery, and from segmental paraspinal perforators and perforators of the lumbar artery. Venous drainage is achieved by the accompanying thoracodorsal veins and paraspinal venous perforators. The latissimus dorsi receives motor innervation by the thoracodorsal nerve, and sensory innervation from cutaneous branches of the intercostal nerves.

PREOPERATIVE EVALUATION AND PATIENT ASSESSMENT

Breast reconstruction is a complicated and elective part of breast cancer care. Primary reconstruction should be offered to all reasonable candidates, but not all patients are candidates for primary breast reconstruction. A thorough preoperative assessment of risk factors is critical. General preoperative risk factors for mortality include the presence of disseminated cancer, weight loss >10% in the last 6 months, age, WBC >11,000/mm^3, and ASA classification and functional status.[17] Risk factors specific to breast reconstruction are obesity, smoking, diabetes, abdominal scarring, lupus, and vasculitis.[22] Patients undergoing surgery are strongly advised to stop smoking for at least 6–8 weeks before the procedures. Nicotine is a potent capillary level vasoconstrictor, and thus smokers are at a significantly elevated risk for mastectomy skin flap necrosis and may not be candidates for nipple-sparing procedures or even primary breast reconstruction. The surgeon can check carboxyhemoglobin levels prior to the operation in order to ensure that the patient was compliant with smoking cessation.[17]

Radiation therapy in the setting of breast reconstruction is the most significant complicating factor. Previous radiation therapy is a relative contraindication for tissue expansion and implant-based breast reconstruction without the use of additional autologous tissue. Radiation-related fibrosis decreases skin compliance resulting in a high rate of device failure. The placement of a tissue expander in a previously radiated field may result in device exposure, failed expansion, inadequate expansion with lack of projection, poor wound healing, and an inability to achieve the desired result.[22] Patients with implant-based breast reconstruction who receive postoperative radiation also face an increased risk of capsular contracture, with a reported incidence as high as 68%.[23] A large cohort study in 2012 showed that, among patients who received breast reconstruction with tissue expanders/implants followed by radiation, the rate of reconstruction failure (defined by loss of reconstruction) at 3-year follow-up was 25.5%.[24] This study showed that the remaining 75% of patients who did not experience failure were satisfied with their aesthetic outcome.

An alternative to tissue expander/implant reconstruction is autologous reconstruction. However, in general, patients at high risk for undergoing postmastectomy radiation should delay autologous breast reconstruction until after completion of radiation therapy. Radiation will significantly affect overlying skin. The internal mammary vessels are still suitable for microsurgical anastomosis.[22,25] Therefore microsurgical free-tissue transfers may serve as a favorable option for this patient population. In the postradiated nonreconstructed chest wall mastectomy defect, the DIEP flap is the preferred reconstructive operation. These procedures are more technically challenging and require close monitoring during the acute postoperative period to ensure flap viability. Autologous tissue transfers also require adequate volume of soft tissue available for harvest. This may become an issue in thin patients with minimal abdominal soft tissue, patients with previous abdominoplasties, or in patients who desire breasts larger than what can be created with the available tissue. In these cases, surgeons can achieve the desired result by performing a hybrid implant/autologous reconstruction or other variation.

PROCEDURES

In 2018 there was a total of 9497 DIEP flaps, 3799 TRAM flaps, and 4188 latissimus flaps performed.[12] The DIEP and TRAM flaps are abdominal flaps based on the deep inferior epigastric artery and vein. The TRAM flap typically includes rectus abdominis muscle and fascia, while the DIEP flap spares the muscle and

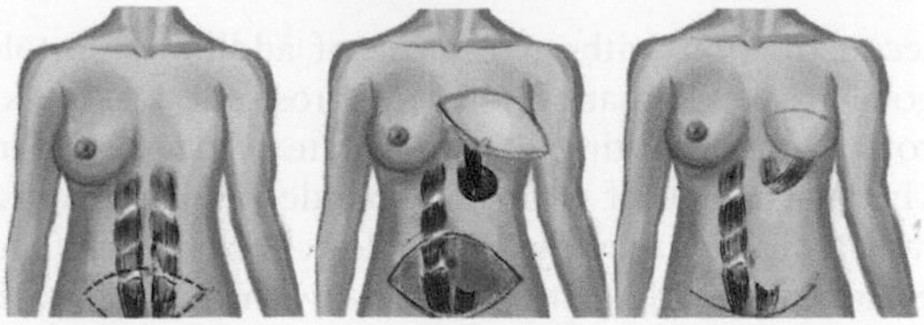

FIGURE 11.3 Illustration of TRAM flap dissection and transposition. *TRAM*, Transverse rectus abdominis myocutaneous.

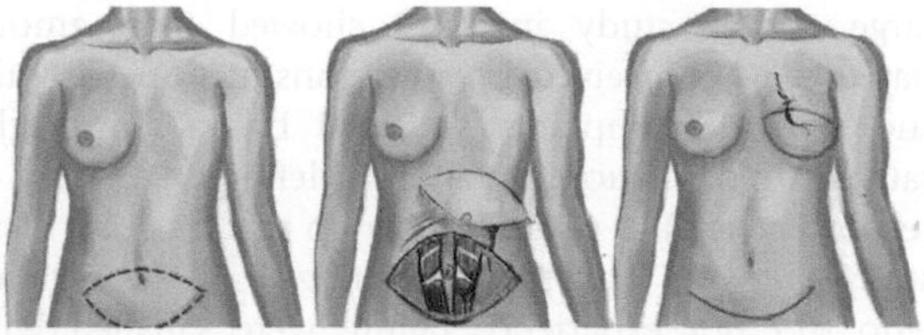

FIGURE 11.4 Illustration of DIEP flap harvest and anastomosis. *DIEP*, Deep inferior epigastric perforator.

fascia (Figs. 11.3 and 11.4). The DIEP flap is used as a free flap, meaning that the entire section of tissue and its blood supply are transplanted out of the abdomen on its vascular pedicle, shaped into a breast mound, and anastomosed to blood vessels in the chest (Fig. 11.5). The internal mammary vessels are the most typical recipients of the free-flap anastomosis. The TRAM flap may be used as a free flap and may also be used as a rotational flap wherein the vascular pedicle remains intact as the flap is rotated superiorly into the breast pocket through a subcutaneous tunnel.[21] Rotational TRAM flaps may also involve microsurgical anastomosis in the distal portion for additional venous outflow if the flap becomes congested. Free TRAM flaps may take small portions of muscle with minimal rectus dysfunction or may take all the rectus muscle. In TRAM flaps the rectus donor site requires repair. This is most frequently treated with the placement of prosthetic mesh, although biologic mesh/ADMs are rising in popularity.

Complications of the DIEP and TRAM flap include donor-site morbidity and flap morbidity. These include abdominal wound infection, bulge, hernia, partial flap necrosis, and total flap loss. New techniques are constantly being developed to address these issues. For example, in 2015 *Rietjens et al.* published their new technique for pedicled TRAM flap breast reconstruction, which achieved 0% abdominal hernia or bulge and 0% total flap loss at a median follow-up period of 13 months.[26] Nonetheless, expected bulge

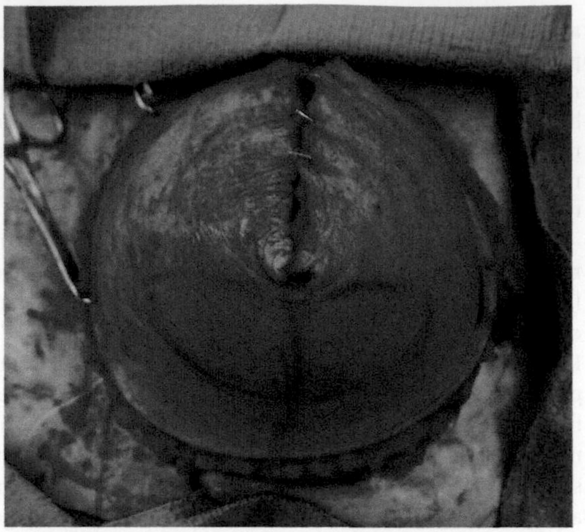

FIGURE 11.5 Creating the breast mound.

rates in TRAM flaps run between 20% and 30% of cases while DIEP flaps and highly selective muscle-sparing free TRAMs report bulge rates of 12%–20% of cases. In addition, a larger number of these patients experience some degree of weakness, subclinical chronic bulges, and chronic pain. The donor-site effects must always be remembered in autologous breast reconstruction patients.

Risk factors play an important role in complication rates. A study by *Chang et al.* at the MD Anderson Cancer Center showed that obese and overweight patients had significantly higher rates of overall flap complications, total flap loss, and mastectomy flap necrosis when compared with normal-weight patients.[27] Obese and overweight patients also had significantly higher rates of overall donor-site complications, infection, and hernia. A potential source of bias in this study is that the obese group had a significantly higher incidence of preoperative radiation and preoperative chemotherapy than the overweight or normal weight groups. Another study by *Chang et al.* showed that smokers undergoing free TRAM flap breast reconstruction experienced significantly higher rates of mastectomy flap necrosis (18.9% vs 9%, $P = .005$), donor-site complications (25.6% vs 14.2%, $P = .007$), abdominal flap necrosis (4.4% vs 0.8%, $P = .025$), and hernia (6.7% vs 2.1%, $P = .016$) when compared with nonsmokers.[28]

Functional deficits may arise postoperatively; these vary primarily based on the amount of muscle removed and/or number of nerves either stretched or transected during flap harvest. Studies have shown that muscle-sparing techniques can significantly reduce donor-site morbidity and preserve abdominal wall function.[29,30] Interestingly, it appears that patients with good preoperative abdominal muscle function may be better candidates for muscle-sparing procedures.[30] DIEP flaps have the lowest published rates of abdominal dysfunction, most significantly in bilateral procedures. This outcome is in contrast to what may be seen with single or bilateral TRAM flaps that incorporate the entire rectus muscle. *Petit et al.* showed that 50% of patients who underwent a single-pedicle TRAM flap and 60% of patients who underwent a double-pedicle TRAM flap experienced functional impairment of the abdominal muscles.[31] This study also showed that 30%–55% of patients undergoing single or bilateral TRAM flap breast reconstruction complained of back pain in the 6-month postoperative period. The degree of postoperative functional deficit is greater in patients receiving bilateral TRAM flaps compared with unilateral TRAM flaps. A study by *Fitoussi et al.* showed that, out of 12 patients receiving a double-pedicle TRAM flap breast reconstruction, none were able to sit up from a lying position without using their hands at an average of 28 months after the procedure. In contrast, 47% of patients receiving unilateral TRAM flaps were able to perform the task.[32]

The latissimus dorsi flap is versatile flap with in general low donor-site morbidity. The latissimus dorsi is a reliable, large thin, well-vascularized flap with a broad scope of application (Fig. 11.6). In the context of breast reconstruction, the latissimus flap comes with a caveat in that it most commonly requires tissue expansion and implant. It is thus a compromise flap, and not commonly utilized in primary breast reconstruction. In previously radiated patients who are not candidates for free-flap breast or for salvage of implant-based complications, the latissimus dorsi is an excellent option. It allows for replacement of lower pole breast skin and provides a large vascularized muscle for coverage of the implant.[22] Prosthetic implants are typically required in conjunction with the latissimus flap to provide adequate volume and projection. Functional deficit associated with the latissimus flap is controversial, with older studies stating negligible deficit and newer studies revealing a high incidence of significant shoulder dysfunction.[33–39] In patients receiving reconstruction with a latissimus flap, it is important to strengthen surrounding back and shoulder muscles to compensate for any potential loss of function. The most common complication of the latissimus flap is the formation of donor-site seroma.[22] Drains may remain in the back for up to 6 weeks after the operation, and outpatient aspiration of a seroma may be necessary after removal of the drain. Fat necrosis or vascular compromise is rare with the latissimus flap, but donor-site marginal skin necrosis may be seen in smokers. Latissimus flaps may also be used in patients with multiple recurrent capsular contractures. These patients are treated with a complete capsulectomy. The pectoralis major in retropectoral reconstructions is placed back in anatomic position, with the implant now placed in the prepectoral and retrolatissimus position.

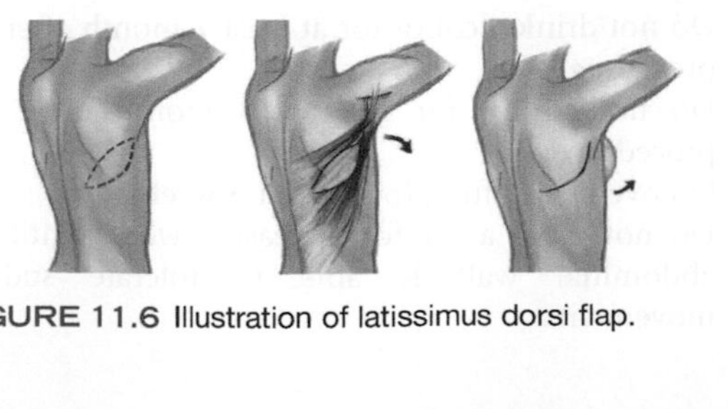

FIGURE 11.6 Illustration of latissimus dorsi flap.

Tissue expansion is the equivalent of placing a deflated water balloon under the skin. The expander is gradually inflated over a period of weeks to months, resulting in increased surface area and vascularity of the overlying skin and soft tissues. This technique was first described in 1957 in the context of ear reconstruction and has been used for breast reconstruction after mastectomy since the early 1980s.[40,41] Tissue expansion is advantageous in that it provides skin with perfect color match, texture match, intact innervation, and typically alleviates the need for creation of a donor site. With regards to breast reconstruction, tissue expanders may be placed in a prepectoral or subpectoral pocket. Subpectoral expanders are placed under the pectoralis muscle, while prepectoral expanders are placed above the muscle (Fig. 11.7).

The traditional approach to implant-based breast reconstruction has been the subpectoral technique. This approach provides ample coverage of the implant with vascularized soft tissue, minimizing rippling of the breast implant, and softening the superior pole of the breast transition from the chest wall to the implant. However, the subpectoral technique can be complicated by postoperative Breast Animation Deformity (BAD). BAD is a condition in which the shape of the breast becomes distorted during contraction of the pectoralis major muscle. This condition is very common among women receiving subpectoral implant-based breast reconstruction, with one study showing that 75.6% of patients reported some degree

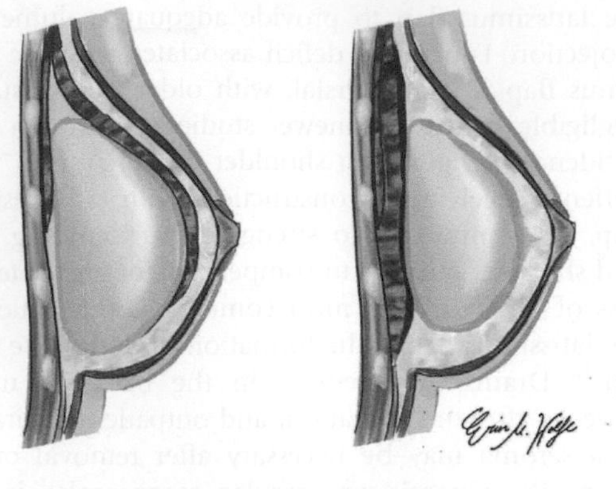

FIGURE 11.7 Illustration of subpectoral (left) and prepectoral (right) implant placement.

of BAD after the procedure.[42] BAD not only affects breast aesthetics but may also have an impact on muscle function; this condition may lead to pain, muscle twitching and could potentially impair shoulder function in physically active patients.[43,44] The degree of BAD appears to be proportional to the degree of muscle involvement.

The prepectoral approach was previously unpopular due to the high rate of complications, especially capsular contracture, and implant loss secondary to exposure or infections of the device.[45–48] However, with the recent advent of ADMs, there has been a revolution in implant-based breast reconstruction, particularly with the prepectoral approach. ADM can be wrapped around expanders, providing reinforcement and thus making tissue expansion possible in areas that were previously not feasible.[21,49] Importantly, the use of ADM in conjunction with prepectoral tissue expanders appears to attenuate complication rates, including capsular contracture.[50] This may be due to a decrease in myofibroblasts in breast capsules when ADM is incorporated in the prepectoral pocket.[51] Thus the prepectoral approach has seen an increase in popularity recently due to its potential to eliminate BAD and decrease postoperative pain.[52,53] Prepectoral reconstruction, however, is not for all patients. Patients with significant ptosis preoperatively may develop unacceptably ptotic reconstructions postoperatively because only the skin envelope supports the implant. In addition, prepectoral implants tend to develop high rates of implant-related rippling deformities. These patients in particular tend to benefit significantly from a hybrid technique of medium volume fat grafting for soft tissue reconstruction of the entire breast envelope.

POSTOPERATIVE CARE AND PATIENT EDUCATION

Enhanced Recovery after Surgery (ERAS) protocols have recently become a popular method to reduce postoperative hospital length of stay without increasing morbidity after breast reconstruction.[54–56] At our practice, we have employed an ERAS protocol that facilitates safe discharge on postoperative day (POD) 3 after microsurgical breast reconstruction. Our protocol is centered on a two-team approach to surgery to reduce operative time, a multimodal analgesic regimen with heavy reliance on NSAIDs, early resumption of diet, and early mobilization.[57] Our analgesic regimen includes an intraoperative transverse abdominis plane block, intraoperative ketorolac loading dose prior to emerging from anesthesia, around the clock Tylenol and/or ketorolac for the first 48 hours postoperatively, followed by ibuprofen 600 mg and cyclobenzaprine as needed, with narcotics only for breakthrough pain. Our postoperative goals for patients are as follows:

- POD 0
  - NPO, bed rest
- POD 1
  - Clear fluids in the morning, diet as tolerated in the evening
  - Out of bed to chair in the morning, ambulate in the evening
  - Foley out in the evening
- POD 2
  - Ambulate 3 × /day
  - Discontinue monitoring device in the evening
  - Transition to PRN Motrin in the evening after 48 hours of ketorolac are completed
- POD 3
  - Begin ASA 81 mg × 1 month
  - Shower in AM with help from nurse
  - Discharge home with cyclobenzaprine, ibuprofen, and oxycodone

In addition to the ERAS protocol, we advise the following precautions[58] to all patients after breast reconstruction:

- Plan to have someone who can drive you home after discharge and help you at home for a few days.
- Do not drink alcohol for at least 1 month after the procedure.
- Do not smoke for at least 3 months after the procedure.
- No overhead lifting for at least 3 weeks.
- Do not drive a car for at least 4 weeks until the abdominal wall is able to tolerate sudden movements.

- Do not lift anything heavier than a gallon of milk for 6–8 weeks.
- Do not submerge in water for 6–8 weeks.
- Minimize scar exposure to sunlight for at least 12 months. Always wear sunscreen (>SPF30) when anticipating sun exposure.
- Sleep with pillows under knees or in a recliner for 2 weeks to reduce tension on the abdomen.
- Call the doctor if you have severe pain not relieved by medications, temperature >100.4°F, any yellow or green discharge or drainage from incisions, numbness, persistent swelling, bruising, or redness.
- Be patient with the healing process. Surgery is only the beginning of a long road to recovery. Think positively and reflect on how you will become a stronger person by overcoming the challenges.

CONCLUSION

Breast reconstruction is a potentially life-changing procedure, affording women the opportunity to maintain their quality of life and feminine identity after enduring the tribulations of breast cancer (Figs. 11.8 and 11.9). As such, breast reconstruction is performed on nearly half of all women who undergo mastectomy. The two methods of breast reconstruction involve either tissue expanders/implants or autologous tissue. Implant-based breast reconstruction is the most commonly performed method in the United States. This may be in part due to the revolutionary changes brought about by the advent of ADMs. ADM has allowed plastic surgeons to utilize skin-sparing and nipple-sparing envelopes for preexpansion of

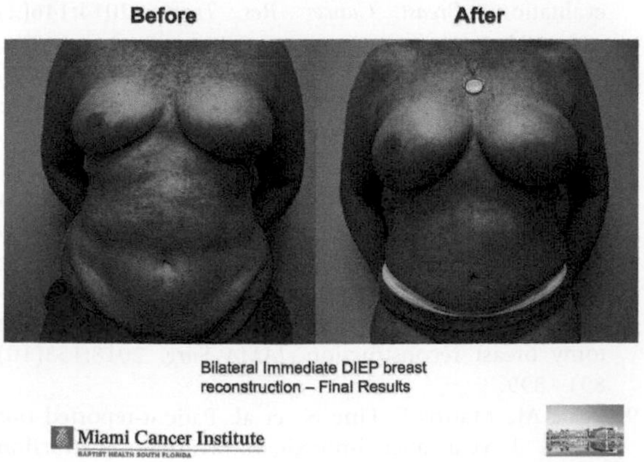

FIGURE 11.8 Before and after bilateral immediate DIEP breast reconstruction. *DIEP*, Deep inferior epigastric perforator.

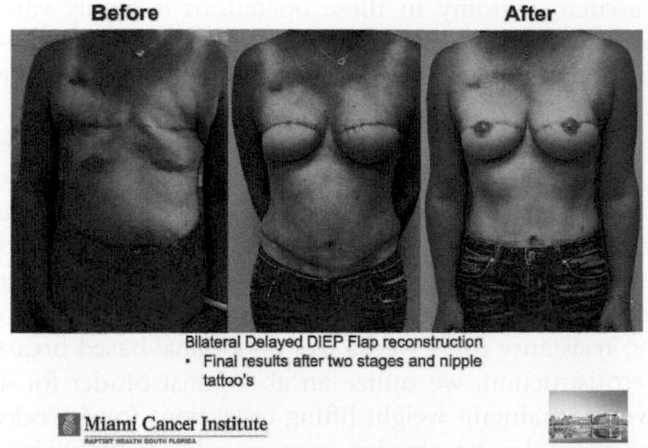

Before
After
Bilateral Delayed DIEP Flap reconstruction
• Final results after two stages and nipple tattoo's
Miami Cancer Institute

FIGURE 11.9 Before and after bilateral delayed DIEP flap reconstruction. *DIEP*, Deep inferior epigastric perforator.

expanders, use of direct to implant reconstruction (breast in a day), and prepectoral placement of implants. Nonetheless, autologous breast reconstruction techniques are powerful tools. For example, autologous breast reconstruction allows for aesthetic breast reconstruction even in patients with previous radiation and no prior reconstruction without the use of an implant (Fig. 11.9).

Plastic surgeons need to consider the entire scope of each breast cancer patient's condition, risk factors, and treatment. Risk factors for unsuccessful breast reconstruction include radiation, smoking, obesity, diabetes, rapid unintentional weight loss, and presence of disseminated cancer. Radiation poses significant challenges to successful reconstruction, particularly with implant-based breast reconstruction. In such cases, autologous reconstruction serves as a viable alternative. The most commonly performed autologous reconstruction methods include the DIEP flap, TRAM flap, and the latissimus dorsi flap. DIEP and TRAM flaps are typically performed immediately after mastectomy in one stage, but frequently benefit from a second stage revision, while the latissimus dorsi flap most often involves tissue expansion and implant placement programmed in two stages. Autologous reconstructions may involve rotational flaps or free flaps. Rotational flaps maintain the integrity of the vascular pedicle, as soft tissue is rotated to cover a defect. Free flaps involve complete dissection of tissue and its vascular pedicle out of the body, followed by microsurgical anastomosis to arteries and veins elsewhere on the body. Muscle-sparing techniques may significantly reduce donor-site morbidity and postoperative functional deficits. However, vascular anatomy in these operations is highly variable as is segmental nerve anatomy. All abdominal-based breast reconstruction patients benefit from core strengthening postoperatively.

Involvement of physical therapists throughout the pre- and postoperative process is important to ensure the best outcome. Patients are encouraged to ambulate early but should avoid heavy lifting and overhead movements. Once drains are removed, we allow upper extremity full active and passive range of motion with no resistance for 4 weeks. For abdominal-based breast reconstruction, we utilize an abdominal binder for 4 weeks, maintain weight lifting restrictions for 6 weeks followed by progressive core muscle strengthening. Patients with abdominal incisions should sleep with pillows under their knees for at least 2 weeks to avoid excess tension on the wound. The help of physical therapists is especially important in patients with donor sites involving muscle. With appropriate muscle strengthening, patients may enjoy minimal functional deficit and return to their baseline level of activity.

Finally, the importance of resilience and positive thinking cannot be understated. Breast cancer can be very frightening, and treatments such as mastectomy, radiation, chemotherapy, and breast reconstruction are not always easy to endure. Many patients will feel like they are faced with the most difficult challenge of their lives, rightfully so. As health-care providers, we must encourage patients to be strong during this process. We must shed light on the notion that these challenges pose great opportunity—that the patient may come out the other side stronger, healthier, and happier after overcoming adversity.

PATIENT RESOURCES

American Society of Plastic Surgeons—"Breast Reconstruction": https://www.plasticsurgery.org/reconstructive-procedures/breast-reconstruction

American Society of Plastic Surgeons—"Recovery after DIEP flap breast reconstruction": https://www.plasticsurgery.org/news/blog/recovery-after-diep-flap-breast-reconstruction

American Cancer Society—"What to Expect After Breast Reconstruction Surgery": https://www.cancer.org/cancer/breast-cancer/reconstruction-surgery/what-to-expect-after-breast-reconstruction-surgery.html

Dartmouth-Hitchcock Medical Center—"Instructions for Before and After Surgery": https://www.dartmouth-hitchcock.org/documents/breast_implant_reconstruction_201304120final.pdf

University of Michigan Health System—"DIEP/TRAM Flap Breast Reconstruction Post-Operative Instructions": http://www.med.umich.edu/1libr/Surgery/PlasticSurgery/BreastReconstruction/BreastRecon-DIEPTRAMpostop.pdf

Penn Medicine—"What to Expect After Breast Reconstruction: A Timeline" https://www.pennmedicine.org/cancer/about/focus-on-cancer/2019/october/what-to-expect-after-breast-reconstruction

Mayo Clinic—"Breast reconstruction with flap surgery": https://www.mayoclinic.org/tests-procedures/breast-reconstruction-flap/about/pac-20384937

Mayo Clinic—"Breast reconstruction with implants": https://www.mayoclinic.org/tests-procedures/breast-reconstruction-implants/about/pac-20384934

REFERENCES

1. Miller KD, Nogueira L, Mariotto AB, et al. Cancer treatment and survivorship statistics. *CA Cancer J Clin*. 2019;69(5):363–385.
2. Razdan SN, Cordeiro PG, Albornoz CR, et al. National breast reconstruction utilization in the setting of postmastectomy radiotherapy. *J Reconstr Microsurg*. 2017;33(5):312–317.
3. Ilonzo N, Tsang A, Tsantes S, Estabrook A, Thu Ma AM. Breast reconstruction after mastectomy: a ten-year analysis of trends and immediate postoperative outcomes. *Breast*. 2017;32:7–12.
4. Al-Ghazal SK, Sully L, Fallowfield L, Blamey RW. The psychological impact of immediate rather than delayed breast reconstruction. *Eur J Surg Oncol*. 2000;26(1):17–19.
5. Chao LF, Patel KM, Chen SC, et al. Monitoring patient-centered outcomes through the progression of breast reconstruction: a multicentered prospective longitudinal evaluation. *Breast Cancer Res Treat*. 2014;146(2):299–308.
6. Elder EE, Brandberg Y, Bjorklund T, et al. Quality of life and patient satisfaction in breast cancer patients after immediate breast reconstruction: a prospective study. *Breast*. 2005;14(3):201–208.
7. Girotto JA, Schreiber J, Nahabedian MY. Breast reconstruction in the elderly: preserving excellent quality of life. *Ann Plast Surg*. 2003;50(6):572–578.
8. Santosa KB, Qi J, Kim HM, Hamill JB, Wilkins EG, Pusic AL. Long-term patient-reported outcomes in postmastectomy breast reconstruction. *JAMA Surg*. 2018;153(10):891–899.
9. Pusic AL, Matros E, Fine N, et al. Patient-reported outcomes 1 year after immediate breast reconstruction: results of the mastectomy reconstruction outcomes consortium study. *J Clin Oncol*. 2017;35(22):2499–2506.
10. Teo I, Reece GP, Christie IC, et al. Body image and quality of life of breast cancer patients: influence of timing

and stage of breast reconstruction. *Psychooncology*. 2016; 25(9):1106–1112.
11. Poppler LH, Mundschenk MB, Linkugel A, Zubovic E, Dolen UC, Myckatyn TM. Tissue expander complications do not preclude a second successful implant-based breast reconstruction. *Plast Reconstr Surg*. 2019;143(1): 24–34.
12. American Society of Plastic Surgeons. *Plastic Surgery Statistics Report*. 2018.
13. Momeni A, Kanchwala S. Hybrid prepectoral breast reconstruction: a surgical approach that combines the benefits of autologous and implant-based reconstruction. *Plast Reconstr Surg*. 2018;142(5):1109–1115.
14. Tessler O, Guste J, Bartow MJ, et al. Stacked lateral thigh perforator flap as a novel option for autologous breast reconstruction. *Plast Reconstr Surg*. 2019;143(6): 1601–1604.
15. Netter FH, Machado CAG, Hansen JT, Benninger B, Brueckner JK, Netter FH. *Atlas of Human Anatomy*. 7th ed. 1 Vol. (various pagings). Philadelphia: Saunders Elsevier, 2014. Print.
16. Shiffman MA. *Breast Augmentation Principles and Practice*. Berlin: Springer; 2009. SpringerLink (Online Service). Available from: http://ezproxy.lib.usf.edu/login?url = http://dx.doi.org/10.1007/978-3-540-78948-2; https://login.ezproxy.net.ucf.edu/login?url = http://dx.doi.org/10.1007/978-3-540-78948-2; http://ezproxy.fiu.edu/login?url = http://dx.doi.org/10.1007/978-3-540-78948-2; http://link.springer.com/10.1007/978-3-540-78948-2.
17. Jarrell BE, Kavic SM. NMS surgery. Available from: <https://login.proxy.lib.fsu.edu/login?url = http://clerkship.lwwhealthlibrary.com/book.aspx?bookid = 1624; https://login.ezproxy.net.ucf.edu/login?url = http://clerkship.lwwhealthlibrary.com/book.aspx?bookid = 1624; http://ezproxy.fiu.edu/login?url = http://clerkship.lwwhealthlibrary.com/book.aspx?bookid = 1624>.
18. Hultborn A, Hulten L, Roos B, Rosencrantz M, Rosengren BAC. Effectiveness of axillary lymph node dissection in modified radical mastectomy with preservation of pectoral muscles. *Ann Surg*. 1974;179(3): 269–272.
19. Taghian NR, Miller CL, Jammallo LS, O'Toole J, Skolny MN. Lymphedema following breast cancer treatment and impact on quality of life: a review. *Crit Rev Oncol Hematol*. 2014;92(3):227–234.
20. Cooper A. *On the Anatomy of the Breast*. London: Longman, Orme, Green, Brown, and Longmans; 1840. vii, 193, 64 pp.
21. Zenn MR, Jones GE. *Reconstructive Surgery: Anatomy, Technique, and Clinical Applications*. St. Louis, MO: Quality Medical Pub; 2012. xxiv:911p.
22. Smith JW, Grabb WC, Thorne C. *Grabb and Smith's Plastic Surgery*. Philadelphia, PA: Wolters Kluwer Health/ Lippincott Williams & Wilkins; 2007.
23. Cordeiro PG, Pusic AL, Disa JJ, McCormick B, VanZee K. Irradiation after immediate tissue expander/implant breast reconstruction: outcomes, complications, aesthetic results, and satisfaction among 156 patients. *Plast Reconstr Surg*. 2004;113(3):877–881.
24. Baschnagel AM, Shah C, Wilkinson JB, Dekhne N, Arthur DW, Vicini FA. Failure rate and cosmesis of immediate tissue expander/implant breast reconstruction after postmastectomy irradiation. *Clin Breast Cancer*. 2012;12(6):428–432.
25. Fosnot J, Fischer JP, Smartt Jr. JM, Low DW. Kovach SJ, 3rd, Wu LC, et al. Does previous chest wall irradiation increase vascular complications in free autologous breast reconstruction? *Plast Reconstr Surg*. 2011;127(2): 496–504.
26. Rietjens M, De Lorenzi F, Andrea M, et al. Technique for minimizing donor-site morbidity after pedicled tram-flap breast reconstruction: outcomes by a single surgeon's experience. *Plast Reconstr Surg Global Open*. 2015; 3(8):e476.
27. Chang DW, Wang B, Robb GL, et al. Effect of obesity on flap and donor-site complications in free transverse rectus abdominis myocutaneous flap breast reconstruction. *Plast Reconstr Surg*. 2000;105(5):1640–1648.
28. Chang DW, Reece GP, Wang B, et al. Effect of smoking on complications in patients undergoing free TRAM flap breast reconstruction. *Plast Reconstr Surg*. 2000;105(7): 2374–2380.
29. Atisha DM, Tessiatore KM, Rushing CN, Dayicioglu D, Pusic A, Hwang S. A national snapshot of patient-reported outcomes comparing types of abdominal flaps for breast reconstruction. *Plast Reconstr Surg*. 2019; 143(3):667–677.
30. Seidenstuecker K, Legler U, Munder B, Andree C, Mahajan A, Witzel C. Myosonographic study of abdominal wall dynamics to assess donor site morbidity after microsurgical breast reconstruction with a DIEP or an ms-2 TRAM flap. *J Plast Reconstr Aesthet Surg*. 2016; 69(5):598–603.
31. Petit JY, Rietjens M, Ferreira MA, Montrucoli D, Lifrange E, Martinelli P. Abdominal sequelae after pedicled TRAM flap breast reconstruction. *Plast Reconstr Surg*. 1997; 99(3):723–729.
32. Fitoussi A, Le Taillandier M, Biffaud JC, Selinger R, Clough KB. [Functional evaluation of the abdominal wall after raising a rectus abdominis myocutaneous flap]. *Ann Chir Plast Esthet*. 1997;42(2):138–146.
33. Laitung JK, Peck F. Shoulder function following the loss of the latissimus dorsi muscle. *Br J Plast Surg*. 1985; 38(3):375–379.
34. Russell RC, Pribaz J, Zook EG, Leighton WD, Eriksson E, Smith CJ. Functional evaluation of latissimus dorsi donor site. *Plast Reconstr Surg*. 1986;78(3):336–344.
35. Fraulin FO, Louie G, Zorrilla L, Tilley W. Functional evaluation of the shoulder following latissimus dorsi muscle transfer. *Ann Plast Surg*. 1995;35(4):349–355.
36. Koh CE, Morrison WA. Functional impairment after latissimus dorsi flap. *ANZ J Surg*. 2009;79(1–2):42–47.
37. Umar M, Jahangir N, Hughes M, Malik Q, Kokan J, Waseem M. Incidence of shoulder functional morbidity

following ipsilateral mastectomy and latissimus dorsi flap reconstruction. *Acta Orthop Traumatol Turc*. 2019; 53:448–451.
38. Koh E, Watson DI, Dean NR. Quality of life and shoulder function after latissimus dorsi breast reconstruction. *J Plast Reconstr Aesthet Surg*. 2018;71(9):1317–1323.
39. Sowa Y, Morihara T, Kushida R, Sakaguchi K, Taguchi T, Numajiri T. Long-term prospective assessment of shoulder function after breast reconstruction involving a latissimus dorsi muscle flap transfer and postoperative radiotherapy. *Breast Cancer*. 2017;24(3):362–368.
40. Neumann CG. The expansion of an area of skin by progressive distention of a subcutaneous balloon; use of the method for securing skin for subtotal reconstruction of the ear. *Plast Reconstr Surg*. 1946;19(2):124–130. 1957.
41. Radovan C. Breast reconstruction after mastectomy using the temporary expander. *Plast Reconstr Surg*. 1982;69(2): 195–208.
42. Nigro LC, Blanchet NP. Animation deformity in postmastectomy implant-based reconstruction. *Plast Reconstr Surg Global Open*. 2017;5(7):e1407.
43. Dyrberg DL, Bille C, Gunnarsson GL, et al. Breast animation deformity. *Arch Plast Surg*. 2019;46(1):7–15.
44. Strasser EJ. Results of subglandular versus subpectoral augmentation over time: one surgeon's observations. *Aesthet Surg J*. 2006;26(1):45–50.
45. Bonomi S, Sala L, Cortinovis U. Prepectoral breast reconstruction. *Plast Reconstr Surg*. 2018;142(2): 232e–233ee.
46. Li S, Mu D, Liu C, et al. Complications following subpectoral versus prepectoral breast augmentation: a meta-analysis. *Aesthetic Plast Surg*. 2019;43(4):890–898.
47. Salibian AH, Harness JK, Mowlds DS. Staged suprapectoral expander/implant reconstruction without acellular dermal matrix following nipple-sparing mastectomy. *Plast Reconstr Surg*. 2017;139(1):30–39.
48. Artz JS, Dinner MI, Sampliner J. Breast reconstruction with a subcutaneous tissue expander followed with a polyurethane-covered silicone breast implant. *Ann Plast Surg*. 1988;20(6):517–521.
49. Oh C, Winocour SJ, Lemaine V. Latest trends in subpectoral breast reconstruction. *Semin Plast Surg*. 2019;33(4): 224–228.
50. Paydar KZ, Wirth GA, Mowlds DS. Prepectoral breast reconstruction with fenestrated acellular dermal matrix: a novel design. *Plast Reconstr Surg Global Open*. 2018; 6(4):e1712.
51. Tevlin R, Borrelli MR, Irizarry D, Nguyen D, Wan DC, Momeni A. Acellular dermal matrix reduces myofibroblast presence in the breast capsule. *Plast Reconstr Surg Global Open*. 2019;7(5):e2213.
52. Yang JY, Kim CW, Lee JW, Kim SK, Lee SA, Hwang E. Considerations for patient selection: prepectoral versus subpectoral implant-based breast reconstruction. *Arch Plast Surg*. 2019;46(6):550–557.
53. Storm-Dickerson T, Sigalove N. Prepectoral breast reconstruction: the breast surgeon's perspective. *Plast Reconstr Surg*. 2017;140:43S–48SS (6S Prepectoral Breast Reconstruction).
54. DelMauro MA, Chen K, Keller A. Reducing length of stay after microsurgical breast reconstruction with a standardized postoperative protocol. *J Reconstr Microsurg*. 2019; 35(8):557–567.
55. Rochlin DH, Leon DS, Yu C, Long C, Nazerali R, Lee GK. The power of patient norms: postoperative pathway associated with shorter hospital stay after free autologous breast reconstruction. *Ann Plast Surg*. 2019;82 (5S suppl 4):S320–S324.
56. Sebai ME, Siotos C, Payne RM, et al. Enhanced recovery after surgery pathway for microsurgical breast reconstruction: a systematic review and meta-analysis. *Plast Reconstr Surg*. 2019;143(3):655–666.
57. Bauermeister AJ, Zuriarrain A, Newman M, Earle SA, Medina 3rd MA. Impact of continuous two-team approach in autologous breast reconstruction. *J Reconstr Microsurg*. 2017;33(4):298–304.
58. Surgery UoMHSP. DIEP/TRAM flap breast reconstruction post-operative instructions. 2015. Available from: <http://www.med.umich.edu/1libr/Surgery/PlasticSurgery/BreastReconstruction/BreastRecon-DIEPTRAMpostop.pdf>.

FURTHER READING

Hamdi M, Weiler-Mithoff EM, Webster MH. Deep inferior epigastric perforator flap in breast reconstruction: experience with the first 50 flaps. *Plast Reconstr Surg*. 1999; 103(1):86–95.

Wormer BA, Valmadrid AC, Ganesh Kumar N, Al Kassis S, Rankin TM, Kaoutzanis C, et al. Reducing expansion visits in immediate implant-based breast reconstruction: a comparative study of prepectoral and subpectoral expander placement. *Plast Reconstr Surg*. 2019;144(2): 276–286.

CHAPTER 12

Rehabilitation of the Cancer Patient With Skeletal Metastasis

THERESA PAZIONIS, MD, MA, FRCSC • RACHEL THOMAS • MIRZA BAIG, BS

INTRODUCTION

Metastatic bone disease is a debilitating condition that arises in advanced stages of cancer. Tumors from different organ systems can metastasize to the bones, threatening skeletal support, muscular and nervous integrity, and movement.[1] A percentage of 60–80 patients with solid tumors will develop metastases.[2] The Oncology Services Comprehensive Electronic Records database contains data since 2004 from 52 academic and community oncology practices in the United States.[56] The incidence of bone metastasis at 1, 2, 5, and 10 years postdiagnosis for all tumor types is 4.8%, 5.6%, 6.9%, and 8.4%, respectively, with $N = 382{,}733$. Prostate cancer ($N = 22{,}801$) is the most likely tumor type to metastasize, achieving 18% incidence at 1 year and 29.2% at 10 years; however, breast cancer is the most common tumor pathology seen ($N = 137{,}720$) (3.4%—1 year, 4.2%—2 years, 6.0%—5 years, 8.1%—10 years). Gynecologic cancers by contrast exhibit relatively fewer bone metastasis ($N = 21{,}075$: 1.1%—1 year, 1.3%—2 years, 1.9%—5 years, 2.4%—10 years) and are more likely to present with visceral metastasis.[56]

Bone metastases frequently result in pathologic fractures that benefit from surgical intervention.[3] Early consultation with orthopedic oncology as a part of a multidisciplinary team is recommended. Although the majority of consultations received are nonsurgical in nature, early involvement of the orthopedics team allows for improved coordination of care and patient outcomes. The treatment goals of pathologic fracture management are generally to prevent tumors from metastasizing further, preserve movement, and reduce pain.[1] Several medical disciplines, including hematology and oncology, orthopedics, and physical medicine and rehabilitation (PM&R), must integrate care for the patient after skeletal metastasis. Patients with pathologic fractures due to metastatic bone disease can present the PM&R physician with unique challenges. PM&R treatment is vital to help patients recover from surgery, regain function to meet their personal medical goals, and make assessments regarding quality of life after cancer treatment. The purpose of this chapter is to provide background knowledge on the pathophysiology of metastatic bone disease, insight into orthopedic oncology procedures, and recommendations for optimal pain management and outcomes.

BACKGROUND

Pathophysiology

Skeletal metastases can be lytic (increased bone resorption), sclerotic (increased osteoblast activity), or mixed, based on the activity of osteoclasts and osteoblasts.[4] Most tumor-induced skeletal destruction is mediated by osteoclasts, spurred by malignant cells secreting osteoclast activators such as PGE, TGF-α/β, EGF, TNF, IL-1, and procathepsin D. Bone resorption and buildup are usually both accelerated in the affected bone, evidenced by increased osteoclast activity and resorption cavities even within sclerotic lesions.[5] Multiple myeloma, prostate, breast, lung, kidney, and thyroid tumors are the primary source of 80% of bone metastases.[1,6] The spine, pelvis, ribs, skull, and proximal femur are most likely to host skeletal metastases.[1] The most common symptom of acute BMD is a pain in the spine, pelvis, or extremities after the bone has been weakened by the tumor. Anemia also results from invasion of the spine, pelvis, ribs, skull, upper arm, and legs, since those regions of bone marrow produce a high level of RBCs. As the disease progresses and bone undergoes demineralization, pathologic fractures may result.[7]

Risk factors for metastasis have been identified in breast cancer patients. Age, menopausal status, BMI, histological type, grade, and tumor size have either unknown, conflicting relationships or no relationships to metastases.[8] While menopausal status may or may not be related, women undergoing

Breast Cancer and Gynecologic Cancer RehabilitationDOI: https://doi.org/10.1016/B978-0-323-72166-0.00012-8

chemotherapy for breast cancer develop low bone mineral density in response to the direct effect of chemotherapeutic drugs on bone cells, including osteoclasts, osteoblasts, and osteocytes. There is a decrease in circulating estrogen as a result of chemotherapy-induced ovarian dysfunction, resulting in a need to favor osteoblast activity during chemotherapy treatment.[9] Lymph node involvement may be a minor contributor to risk of metastases.[8] Genetic factors, such as intrinsic subtype, bone-specific metastasis-related genes (102-gene, 15-gene), and molecular changes, such as those related to the MAF protein, the prolactin receptor, bone sialoprotein, and BMP8, are also risk factors.[8]

Pharmaceuticals and Other Therapies

Commonly used treatments include bisphosphonates and the drug denosumab. Bisphosphonates are analogs of pyrophosphates and cause osteoclast apoptosis. Some studies show direct apoptotic effects on malignant tumor cells themselves. Bisphosphonates also exhibit antimyeloma and antitumor activity and increase overall survival for various malignancies.[10]

Denosumab is a human monoclonal antibody that inhibits RANK-L, preventing osteoclast development. The effect is to delay fractures in patients who already have bone metastases. Zoledronate is a popular drug with a similar effect, and denosumab is helpful when patients do not see results after taking zoledronate or have compromised renal function.[6] Other drugs include biologics, chemotherapeutic agents to halt development of rapidly dividing cells, and bone supportive medications.[6] Radiation therapy is widely used (see the "Pain Management" section).

ORTHOPEDIC ONCOLOGY PROCEDURES

Pathologic Fracture Management

As previously mentioned, the spine, pelvis, ribs, skull, and proximal femur are most likely to host skeletal metastases.[1] Mirel's and Harrington's criteria are the current standard evaluation tools to determine which patients are most likely to experience a pathologic fracture based on the lesion.[11] These criteria account for the type, site, and size of the metastatic lesion, as well as the patient's level of pain and its persistence.[12,13] Mirel's criteria[12] are the most commonly used and assign a score of 1–3 to the following tumor characteristics: site of lesion, nature of lesion, size of lesion, and pain (Table 12.1).

Mirel's score of 9 or greater confers a >30% risk of pathologic fracture, and prophylactic stabilization is recommended. Most lesions with a score of 7 or less are managed nonoperatively with possibility for radiotherapy, continued chemotherapeutics, or observation. A score of 8 confers only a 15% score of pathologic fracture, and multidisciplinary discussion should be undertaken and need for fixation should be decided on a case by case basis.

Patients experience a significant improvement in functional outcomes and a reduction in pain after surgically treated skeletal metastasis, according to a 2018 multicenter study examining PROMIS (Patient-Reported Outcomes Measurement Information System) scores.[3] Even patients with high-grade osteosarcomas (a rare primary tumor originating in the bone) benefit from surgical management of pathologic fracture. There is no additional risk of local recurrence for patients with this condition who undergo surgery, compared to patients who have not suffered a pathologic fracture and have no need for surgery.[14]

Intraoperative outcomes and postoperative return to mobility are improved in patients who receive prophylactic pathologic fracture surgery for metastases in the long bones.[11] Long bones require different surgical management than the other sites of skeletal metastases (i.e., vertebral sites). Surgical intervention can either focus on the entire bone or the affected segment of the bone. Focusing on the entire bone reduces the likelihood of later reoperation and also decreases the incidence of disease progression.[15]

TABLE 12.1
Mirel's Criteria

Score	Site of Lesion	Size of Lesion	Nature of Lesion	Pain
1	Upper limb	<1/3 of cortex	Blastic	Mild
2	Lower limb	1/3–2/3 of cortex	Mixed	Moderate
3	Trochanteric region	>2/3 of cortex	Lytic	Functional

Intramedullary nailing (IMN) is the preferred treatment for pathologic fracture of the long bones. The nail should be locked, and the diameter and length should be as large as possible. Ideally, the surgeon will be able to place the nail in the bone after reaming to ensure the correct size and fit before placing bone cement.[16] The load-sharing elements of intramedullary nails provide weight-bearing earlier than other methods of surgical management. Mobility postsurgery usually returns to the patient's presurgery status.[17] Evidence shows that prophylactic surgery with intramedullary nail (IMN) can reduce the risk of impending pathologic fracture. It is worth noting that reaming of the bone to insert the nail in IMN surgery does not increase metastatic dissection.[16] There are particular effects of intramedullary nailing on specific long bones. For example, the humerus may be shortened by this surgery, but this does not result in worse functional outcomes for the patient.[16] A recent study has shown that an intramedullary nail combined with an auxiliary plate and bone cement may contribute additional stability to the limb.[18]

The spine is a common site of bone metastasis. Metastasis often leads to extremely painful compression fractures, which usually occur on the anterior side of the vertebrae.[19] These fractures and the resulting collapse of these bones could cause paralysis or make the spinal cord more prone to metastatic compression, necessitating swift treatment as soon as the patient is identified as being at risk for fracture.[20] Patients with metastatic tumors to the spine experience significant pain reduction from surgical treatment via percutaneous vertebroplasty and kyphoplasty.[6,21] Polymethacrylate (PMMA) cement is injected into the defect during this procedure. Vertebroplasty can be accomplished by guiding a needle into the posterior vertebral body, while kyphoplasty uses balloon inflation to create a more amenable space for cement injection.[19] Prior to vertebroplasty, the surgeon must determine whether there is a risk for cancer to spread into the spinal cord.[2]

Limitations and Risks

Unfortunate outcomes can occur due to surgical and nonsurgical treatments. In some cases initial surgery to manage pathologic fracture fails. Patients can undergo a new fracture, or hardware can malfunction. Revision surgery in the long bones has been comparatively more successful with an endoprosthesis than with an intramedullary nail.[22] There is minimal follow-up time available in most patient populations to assess the long-term effects of percutaneous vertebroplasty and kyphoplasty. However, these procedures are minimally invasive, and their improved outcomes, compared to open surgery, have been demonstrated.[23,24] Radiation therapy can cause destruction of healthy tissue through tissue necrosis and fibrosis. The destruction of the microvasculature can also create a hypoxic environment, allowing free radical damage to progress.[2] The evidence from clinical trials on radiosurgery is inconclusive due to differing outcomes.[4] Pharmaceutical treatment to delay bone degradation, while effective, can have serious side effects. Bisphosphonates, for example, are nephrotoxic.[6] These drugs can also paradoxically increase the risk of fracture and hypercalcemia.[2]

Patients with cancer often also have compromised cardiopulmonary systems, and their postoperative outcomes can be risky due to fat or air embolisms.[17] Fat embolism syndrome is possible after intramedullary nailing procedures in particular.[15] The hypervascular nature of pathologic tissue in the bone being reamed for nail entry makes this syndrome more likely than in other procedures, as this process can open up paths into the circulatory system.[17] Evidence suggests that negative pressure reaming may reduce the chance of embolic syndromes postsurgery. Surgeons should consider using a reamer that irrigates and aspirates to lessen the risk.[17] PM&R physicians are highly qualified among clinicians to identify signs of stroke and embolic events and should be aware that postsurgery embolic events can occur in cancer patients due to their unique risks.

RECOMMENDATIONS FOR PHYSICAL MEDICINE AND REHABILITATION

Noninvasive Predictors of Pathologic Fracture

Since patients who undergo prophylactic treatment for pathologic fracture have better outcomes than those who undergo treatment after fracture, PM&R physicians should be prepared to identify impending pathologic fractures within their scope of practice to recommend orthopedic treatment.[11] Tumors that survive targeted treatment and/or continue to cause persistent pain indicate that patients require surgical intervention.[1] If patients are at risk for fracture and elect not to undergo surgery, it is imperative to obtain radiographic data when deweighting a limb to ensure that the redistributed weight will not compromise other areas of the skeleton.[25]

Technological tools for predicting pathologic fractures are improving tremendously. For patients receiving hormone treatment, the World Health Organization FRAX tool can be used. This tool predicts the 10-year fracture risk of patients by using data on bone mineral density, among other parameters, and can account for the osteoporotic changes brought on by hormone therapy by defining this treatment as a secondary osteoporosis parameter.[21] A study of men receiving prostate cancer androgen deprivation therapy treatment showed that this tool provides greater insight into fracture risk than bone mineral density alone.[26]

PathFX is an algorithm designed to provide insightful survival estimates for patients with pathologic fractures. The model requires inputs, including age, sex, performance status, red and white blood cell counts, site(s) of primary tumor, whether solitary or multiple metastases are present, whether organ metastases are present, and other optional inputs, including the physician's estimate of survival and whether lymph node metastases are present. The algorithm is validated using previously validated, large international data sets.[27–29] PathFX enables a multidisciplinary team of physicians to evaluate the survival estimates for patients at specific points in time and to use this information to make decisions with their families to meet the patient's personal goals. Those with longer survival estimates may opt for riskier surgeries, while those with shorter may decide upon palliative treatments with fewer side effects and less recovery time. Treating physicians, including orthopedic surgeons, oncologists, and PM&R doctors, can consult this tool to decide how to manage care as a multidisciplinary team while empowering the patient with the most accurate knowledge about their prognosis.

In a study of metastatic cancer to the spine originating from breast tumors, CT scans served as radiological predictors of impending vertebral pathologic fracture. Load-bearing capacity, axial rigidity, and bending rigidity determined from CT scans are appropriate radiographic criteria to assess the vertebral metastases.[30] A machine learning algorithm built with CT radiograph and clinical data has also demonstrated predictive capabilities for pathologic proximal femur fractures.[31] PM&R physicians, orthopedic surgeons, and oncologists should remain abreast of technological developments in the field as tools such as PathFX and algorithm-based prediction tools continue to develop.

In the clinical setting, PM&R physicians can implement tests to analyze patients' life expectancy and progression of metastasis. The results of short physical performance battery and fast gait speed tests can predict early mortality in survivors of cancer.[32] The 6-minute walk distance test, which observes the maximum distance a patient can move over a 30 m course in 6 minutes, was shown to be independently predictive of survival in patients with active metastatic cancer.[33] These tests may indicate decreasing function due to declining bone health, and subsequent reduction in survival estimates. Routine blood work should be implemented to check for hypercalcemia. Symptoms of hypercalcemia include dehydration, thirst, drowsiness, fatigue, anorexia, and constipation.[7,34] The consequences of uninhibited hypercalcemia include cardiac arrhythmias and renal failure.[7] While patients with mildly elevated calcium levels may not require immediate attention, levels above 3.5 mol/L constitute an oncologic emergency.[21]

Prevention of Pathologic Fracture Through Physical Medicine and Rehabilitation

Rehabilitation that begins upon cancer diagnosis has been termed "prehabilitation" in the literature. Prehabilitation has been shown to improve hospital stay, postoperative outcomes, and tolerance of cancer treatment.[35] However, evidence shows that targeted exercise therapy does not prophylactically prevent pathologic fracture. Patients benefit more from safety measures to reduce their fall risk.[2] Such efforts involve restricting forces with high resistance, high compression, or high rotational force/torque on the affected limb. The use of assistive devices to offload weight-bearing is recommended.[36] However, there is conflicting evidence on whether weight-bearing activity is more likely to result in pathologic fracture than nonweight-bearing activity.[21] Compensatory measures to prevent weight-bearing on the affected side, including or in addition to assistive devices, can be critical in preventing further injury. Increasing the tone and strength of supportive muscles can greatly reduce the pain a patient experiences from a compromised joint or vertebrae. Isometric contractions in particular are useful to stabilize and deweight an area of pain or clinical concern.[37] With regards to compensatory movements, clinicians should remember that overuse injuries are high in cancer survivors and educate patients about risks of repetitive compensation.[37]

Vertebral fractures present other challenges. Patients with vertebral metastases do not have a lower chance of pathologic fracture while wearing an immobilizing orthopedic corset.[38] Those who exhibit increasingly intense pain in the lower back are likely to have metastatic spinal cord compression (MSCC).[39] Patients with MSCC can also exhibit motor and sensory symptoms, along with bladder and bowel incontinence.[20,39]

This condition presents with pathologic fracture about 30%–40% of the time, which compounds the effects of MSCC. Pathologic fracture in the spine can also present with thoracic kyphosis accompanied by radicular pain and subsequent hypoventilation, and with abdominal pain leading to increased abdominal pressure that can impact food intake.[23] A higher number of vertebral metastases, higher growth rate of the primary tumor, more pain, larger tumors within the vertebral body, and involvement of the vertebral end plate and three columns have been associated with increased risk for pathological fracture. The presence of osteolytic lesions, more than 25% occupancy of the vertebral body, and involvement of the end plate and three columns are candidates for surgical stabilization.[40] Vertebral pathologic fracture is associated with reduced ambulatory function after decompression surgery for MSCC.[20] With knowledge of the risk factors and symptoms the PM&R physician can act swiftly once they suspect that a patient has spinal metastasis; quick recognition and treatment is critical to containing the problem. After surgery, 67%–100% of patients no longer have pain, with up to 70% having improved mobility.[23]

Changes in body composition are important in the context of pathologic fracture. Cancer patients can exhibit cachexia (overall weight loss, including the loss of muscle mass) and sarcopenia (loss of muscle mass and muscular atrophy).[36] The inclusion of nutritional experts to the multidisciplinary team of clinicians early on can help to delay or decrease cachexia and sarcopenia.[41] Patients suffering from metastatic bone disease in particular exhibit decreased muscle strength.[42] Monitoring the patient's degree of sarcopenia and concurrent decline in strength can be an important indicator for improper chemotherapeutic dosing and metastatic tumor progression.[43] Patients may become osteoporotic as a result of hormone treatments for cancers of the prostate, breast, and ovaries. To preserve bone mass, patients with bone metastases who are undergoing osteoporotic changes should perform functional loading activities for as long as they are able. This includes walking that results in a positive change for bone mass.[21]

Pain Management

Patients with bone metastases have a spectrum of goals during cancer treatment, and their wishes generally depend on their prognosis. Survival rates vary depending on the location of the primary tumor. In a recent study, 1-year survival after bone metastasis diagnosis was lowest in patients with lung cancer and highest in patients with breast cancer. At 5 years of follow-up, only patients with breast cancer had over 10% survival.[44] The poor prognosis for patients with bone metastases emphasizes the need for palliative care with the primary goal of pain reduction. Palliative treatments for advanced bone metastasis include radiation, chemotherapy and electrochemotherapy, embolization, radio-frequency ablation, and high-intensity focus ultrasound.[1]

Pain management is critical for patients with bone metastases. About 75% of patients with skeletal metastasis present with pain.[45] Surgical treatment for pathologic fracture generally relieves much of the severe pain associated with bone metastases and is the primary treatment for impending fracture or fractures that have already occurred.[45,46] For persistent or additional pending pathologic fractures after surgery, osteoprotegerin causes apoptosis of osteoclasts to reduce the risk of fractures and associated pain. Other options for residual pain, though not without their own side effects, include corticosteroids, opioids (though the analgesic effect decreases over time), NSAIDS, and ET-1, which antagonize the effect of nociceptive stimuli at receptors. Tricyclic antidepressants can also be used to change the perception of pain and any depressive symptoms that arise but carry their own side effects as well. Less effective options include bisphosphonates, such as zoledronate, that are effective in delaying disease progression but not as helpful for pain management.[47] Denosumab, like bisphosphonates, is less effective in pain management and more effective in preventing the physiological changes that lead to pain.[48]

Other courses for pain management include radiation therapy. Within 2 weeks of administration for metastases, patients report that pain declines dramatically. Both fractionated and nonfractionated courses of radiation are equally effective for pain reduction.[6] Radiation after surgery improves patient function and reduces the need for other surgeries to provide pain relief. The most common method of administration is local field radiation that relieves pain with minimal side effects in 50%–60% of cases and provides partial relief in 80%. In more severe cases hemibody irradiation is used for widespread metastatic disease. This can target larger fields of the upper body, midsection, or lower body, and supplements local field radiation. Injection of radiopharmaceuticals is also helpful for pain relief and easier to administer and to tolerate compared to hemibody radiation.[49] A short treatment schedule generally provides quick relief.[1]

Chemotherapeutic drugs have a wide variety of side effects, some of which are highly relevant in the PM&R scope of practice. Post chemotherapy, cancer patients are at a higher risk of balance impairment and falling.[50] Cancer patients also experience chronic fatigue due to treatment side effects and resulting general weakness that compounds their risk of falling.[51,52] This can discourage the patient from undergoing rehabilitation and therapy that is essential for a few reasons. The side effects of chemotherapy can be managed through a supervised therapeutic exercise program.[53] Aside from its benefits for chemotherapy, the importance of aerobic and resistance training in managing cancer recovery and relief from difficult treatments indicates that the patient's ability to move is integral to their fight against the disease.[2] For patients with comorbidities, aerobic exercise in particular has been noted to help with cardiac, vascular, and pulmonary diseases.[25] Patients with decreased bone density still benefit from rehabilitative weight-bearing activities, though engaging them in the exercises can be difficult due to pain.[36] Physical rehabilitation after pathologic fracture is a form of personal empowerment; patients with the freedom of movement have a new weapon in their arsenal to fight cancer.[2]

Functional pain has proven to be the most accurate predictor of pathologic fracture; pain associated with functional activity is considered a risk for pathologic fracture.[21,36] However, physical function and pain intensity are only moderately correlated. In cases where function and pain are not aligned, further examination may be necessary to assess disease progression.[54] Cancer patients may experience chemotherapy-induced neuropathies and nerve injury unrelated to function. As a result, they may experience musculoskeletal compromise with exaggerated pain or without any pain or sensation.[55] The Brief Pain Inventory tool is a reliable way to assess pain in patients with metastasis to the bone and is more useful than simple numerical pain measurements.[21] Breakthrough pain occurring during functional exercises, especially that associated with function, should be assessed by an orthopedist.[21] Neurological symptoms, as well as autonomic dysfunction, maybe the first indicators of new metastases.[36] Clinical judgment and patient monitoring are necessary to determine whether the patient needs to be reassessed by an oncologist and/or orthopedic surgeon.

CONCLUSION

Patients presenting with metastatic bone disease are managed effectively by a multidisciplinary team, including an orthopedic surgical oncologist. Management depends on overall patient functional status, current treatment regimen, tumor pathology, and risk of pathologic fracture. The majority of patients with metastatic bone disease are able to regain good to excellent functional status employing a multimodal approach to treatment.

REFERENCES

1. Mavrogenis AF, Angelini A, Vottis C, et al. Modern palliative treatments for metastatic bone disease. *Clin J Pain*. 2016;32(4):337–350. Available from: https://doi.org/10.1097/AJP.0000000000000255.
2. Cifu DX. *Braddom's Physical Medicine and Rehabilitation*, Elsevier, 2015.
3. Blank AT, Lerman DM, Shaw S, et al. PROMIS® scores in operative metastatic bone disease patients: a multicenter, prospective study. *J Surg Oncol*. 2018;118(3):532–535. Available from: https://doi.org/10.1002/jso.25159.
4. D'Oronzo S, Coleman R, Brown J, Silvestris F. Metastatic bone disease: pathogenesis and therapeutic options: update on bone metastasis management. *J Bone Oncol*. 2019;15:004. Available from: https://doi.org/10.1016/j.jbo.2018.10.004.
5. Coleman RE. Metastatic bone disease: clinical features, pathophysiology and treatment strategies. *Cancer Treat Rev*. 2001;27(3):165–176. Available from: https://doi.org/10.1053/ctrv.2000.0210.
6. D'Oronzo S, Coleman R, Brown J, Silvestris F. Metastatic bone disease: pathogenesis and therapeutic options: Update on bone metastasis management. *J Bone Oncol*. 2019;15:100205. Available from: https://doi.org/10.1016/j.jbo.2018.10.004. October 2018.
7. Coleman RE. Clinical features of metastatic bone disease and risk of skeletal morbidity. *Clin Cancer Res*. 2006;12(20):6243s–6249s. Available from: https://doi.org/10.1158/1078-0432.CCR-06-0931.
8. Pulido C, Vendrell I, Ferreira AR, et al. Bone metastasis risk factors in breast cancer. *Ecancermedicalscience*. 2017;11:715. Available from: https://doi.org/10.3332/ecancer.2017.715.
9. Mathis KM, Sturgeon KM, Winkels RM, Wiskemann J, De Souza MJ, Schmitz KH. Bone resorption and bone metastasis risk. *Med Hypotheses*. 2018;118:36–41. Available from: https://doi.org/10.1016/j.mehy.2018.06.013.
10. Macedo F, Ladeira K, Pinho F, et al. Bone metastases: an overview. *Oncol Rev*. 2017;11(1):321. Available from: https://doi.org/10.4081/oncol.2017.321.
11. Blank AT, Lerman DM, Patel NM, et al. Is prophylactic intervention more cost-effective than the treatment of pathologic fractures in metastatic bone disease? Clinical Orthopaedics and Related Research® A Publication of The Association of Bone and Joint Surgeons®. *Clin Orthop Relat Res*. 2015;474:1563–1570. Available from: https://doi.org/10.1007/s11999-016-4739-x.
12. Mirels H. Metastatic disease in long bones. A proposed scoring system for diagnosing impending pathologic fractures. *Clin Orthop Relat Res*. 1989;(249)256–264. Available from: http://www.ncbi.nlm.nih.gov/pubmed/2684463. Accessed 22.07.19.

13. Harrington KD. Orthopedic surgical management of skeletal complications of malignancy. *Cancer*. 1997;80(8 suppl):1614–1627. 10.1002/(sici)1097-0142(19971015) 80:8 + < 1614::aid-cncr12 > 3.3.co;2-0.
14. Ferguson PC, McLaughlin CE, Griffin AM, Bell RS, Deheshi BM, Wunder JS. Clinical and functional outcomes of patients with a pathologic fracture in high-grade osteosarcoma. *J Surg Oncol*. 2010;102(2):120–124. Available from: https://doi.org/10.1002/jso.21542.
15. Alvi HM, Damron TA. Prophylactic stabilization for bone metastases, myeloma, or lymphoma: do we need to protect the entire bone? *Clin Orthop Relat Res*. 2013;471(3):706–714. Available from: https://doi.org/10.1007/s11999-012-2656-1.
16. Anract P, Biau D, Boudou-Rouquette P. Metastatic fractures of long limb bones. *Orthop Traumatol Surg Res*. 2017;103(1):S41–S51. Available from: https://doi.org/10.1016/J.OTSR.2016.11.001.
17. Leddy LR. Rationale for reduced pressure reaming when stabilizing actual or impending pathological femoral fractures: a review of the literature. *Injury*. 2010;41:S48–S50. Available from: https://doi.org/10.1016/S0020-1383(10)70009-7.
18. Deng L, Yu L, Wei C, Wang B, Zhu S. [Intramedullary nail combined with auxiliary plate and bone cement in treatment of pathologic fracture of extremities caused by metastatic tumors]. *Zhongguo Xiu Fu Chong Jian Wai Ke Za Zhi*. 2017;31(12):1442–1446. Available from: https://doi.org/10.7507/1002-1892.201707047.
19. Patel A, Carter KR. *Percutaneous Vertebroplasty And Kyphoplasty*. StatPearls Publishing; 2019. Available from: http://www.ncbi.nlm.nih.gov/pubmed/30247838. Accessed 02.08.19.
20. Chaichana KL, Pendleton C, Wolinsky J-P, Gokaslan ZL, Sciubba DM. Vertebral compression fractures in patients presenting with metastatic epidural spinal cord compression. *Neurosurgery*. 2009;65(2):267–275. Available from: https://doi.org/10.1227/01.NEU.0000349919.31636.05.
21. Sheill G, Guinan EM, Peat N, Hussey J. Narrative review considerations for exercise prescription in patients with bone metastases: a comprehensive narrative review. *PM&R*. 2018;10(8):843–864. Available from: https://doi.org/10.1016/j.pmrj.2018.02.006.
22. Forsberg JA, Wedin R, Bauer H. Which implant is best after failed treatment for pathologic femur fractures? *Clin Orthop Relat Res*. 2013;471(3):735–740. Available from: https://doi.org/10.1007/s11999-012-2558-2.
23. Jurczyszyn A, Czepko R, Banach M, et al. Percutaneous vertebroplasty for pathological vertebral compression fractures secondary to multiple myeloma – medium-term and long-term assessment of pain relief and quality of life. *Adv Clin Exp Med*. 2015;24(4):651–656. Available from: https://doi.org/10.17219/acem/38556.
24. Itagaki MW, Talenfeld AD, Kwan SW, Brunner JWM, Mortell KE, Brunner MC. Percutaneous vertebroplasty and kyphoplasty for pathologic vertebral fractures in the medicare population: safer and less expensive than open surgery. *J Vasc Interv Radiol*. 2012;23(11):1423–1429. Available from: https://doi.org/10.1016/j.jvir.2012.08.010.
25. Cheville A. Rehabilitation of patients with advanced cancer. *Cancer*. 2001;92(S4):1039–1048. 10.1002/1097-0142(20010815)92:4 + < 1039::aid-cncr1417 > 3.0.co;2-l.
26. Saylor PJ, Kaufman DS, Michaelson MD, Lee RJ, Smith MR. Application of a fracture risk algorithm to men treated with androgen deprivation therapy for prostate cancer. *J Urol*. 2010;183(6):2200–2205. Available from: https://doi.org/10.1016/J.JURO.2010.02.022.
27. Piccioli A, Spinelli MS, Forsberg JA, et al. How do we estimate survival? External validation of a tool for survival estimation in patients with metastatic bone disease-decision analysis and comparison of three international patient populations. *BMC Cancer*. 2015;. Available from: https://doi.org/10.1186/s12885-015-1396-5.
28. Ogura K, Gokita T, Shinoda Y, et al. Can a multivariate model for survival estimation in skeletal metastases (PATHFx) be externally validated using Japanese patients? *Clin Orthop Relat Res*. 2017;475(9):2263–2270. Available from: https://doi.org/10.1007/s11999-017-5389-3.
29. Forsberg JA, Wedin R, Bauer HCF, et al. External validation of the Bayesian Estimated Tools for Survival (BETS) models in patients with surgically treated skeletal metastases. *BMC Cancer*. 2012;12(493). Available from: https://doi.org/10.1186/1471-2407-12-493.
30. Snyder BD, Cordio MA, Nazarian A, et al. Noninvasive prediction of fracture risk in patients with metastatic cancer to the spine. *Diagnosis*. 2009;. Available from: https://doi.org/10.1158/1078-0432.CCR-09-0420.
31. Oh E, Seo SW, Yoon YC, Kim DW, Kwon S, Yoon S. Prediction of pathologic femoral fractures in patients with lung cancer using machine learning algorithms: comparison of computed tomography-based radiological features with clinical features versus without clinical features. *J Orthop Surg*. 2017;25(2). Available from: https://doi.org/10.1177/2309499017716243. 23094990 1771624.
32. Brown JC, Harhay MO, Harhay MN. Physical function as a prognostic biomarker among cancer survivors. *Br J Cancer*. 2015;112(1):194–198. Available from: https://doi.org/10.1038/bjc.2014.568.
33. Jones LW, Hornsby WE, Goetzinger A, et al. Prognostic significance of functional capacity and exercise behavior in patients with metastatic non-small cell lung cancer. *Lung Cancer*. 2012;76(2):248–252. Available from: https://doi.org/10.1016/J.LUNGCAN.2011.10.009.
34. Willeumier JJ, van der Linden YM, van de Sande MAJ, Dijkstra PDS. Treatment of pathological fractures of the long bones. *EFORT Open Rev*. 2016;1(5):136–145. Available from: https://doi.org/10.1302/2058-5241.1. 000008.
35. Wittry S, Molinares D, Maltser S. *Handbook of Rehabilitation in Older Adults*. <https://books.google.com/books?hl = en&lr = &id = yMCKDwAAQBAJ&oi = fnd&pg = PA206&dq = rehabilitation + %2B + cancer + %2B + pathologic + fracture&ots = OS2SAVuYV9&sig =

p5hd81JegHjKPqAc6gCgy4dxB38#v = onepage&q = rehabilitation%2Bcancer%2Bpathologicfracture&f = false>; 2018 Accessed 02.08.19.

36. Maltser S, Cristian A, Silver JK, Morris GS, Stout NL. A focused review of safety considerations in cancer rehabilitation. *PM&R*. 2017;9:S415–S428. Available from: https://doi.org/10.1016/j.pmrj.2017.08.403.
37. Cheville AL, Smith SR, Basford JR. Rehabilitation medicine approaches to pain management. *Hematol Oncol Clin North Am*. 2018;32(3):469–482. Available from: https://doi.org/10.1016/J.HOC.2018.02.001.
38. Rief H, Förster R, Rieken S, et al. The influence of orthopedic corsets on the incidence of pathological fractures in patients with spinal bone metastases after radiotherapy. *BMC Cancer*. 2015;15(1):745. Available from: https://doi.org/10.1186/s12885-015-1797-5.
39. GAIN, Northern Ireland Cancer Network. *Guidelines for the Rehabilitation of Patients with Metastatic Spinal Cord Compression (MSCC) Assessment and Care Provision by Occupational Therapists and Physiotherapists in the Acute Sector*. <https://www.rqia.org.uk/RQIA/files/cb/cba33182-deab-46ae-acd1-d27279d9847c.pdf>; 2014 Accessed 02.08.19.
40. Hibberd CS, Quan GMY. Risk factors for pathological fracture and metastatic epidural spinal cord compression in patients with spinal metastases. *Orthopedics*. 2018;41(1):e38–e45. Available from: https://doi.org/10.3928/01477447-20171106-06.
41. Aapro M, Arends J, Bozzetti F, et al. Early recognition of malnutrition and cachexia in the cancer patient: a position paper of a European School of Oncology Task Force. *Ann Oncol*. 2014;25(8):1492–1499. Available from: https://doi.org/10.1093/annonc/mdu085.
42. Oldervoll LM, Loge JH, Lydersen S, et al. Physical exercise for cancer patients with advanced disease: a randomized controlled trial. *Oncologist*. 2011;16(11):1649–1657. Available from: https://doi.org/10.1634/theoncologist.2011-0133.
43. Prado CMM, Baracos VE, McCargar LJ, et al. Sarcopenia as a determinant of chemotherapy toxicity and time to tumor progression in metastatic breast cancer patients receiving capecitabine treatment. *Clin Cancer Res*. 2009;15(8):2920–2926. Available from: https://doi.org/10.1158/1078-0432.CCR-08-2242.
44. Svensson E, Christiansen CF, Ulrichsen SP, Rørth MR, Sørensen HT. Survival after bone metastasis by primary cancer type: a Danish population-based cohort study. *BMJ Open*. 2017;7(9):e016022. Available from: https://doi.org/10.1136/bmjopen-2017-016022.
45. Mandal CC, Siddiqui JA, Findlay DM, Soeharno H, Povegliano L, Choong PF. Multimodal treatment of bone metastasis—a surgical perspective. *Front Endocrinol*. 2018;9:518. Available from: https://doi.org/10.3389/fendo.2018.00518.
46. Lidar JBD, Dadia S, Lidar Z. Surgical management of metastatic bone disease. *J Bone Joint Surg Am*. 2009;91(6):1503–1516. Available from: https://doi.org/10.2106/jbjs.h.00175.
47. Ahmad I, Ahmed MM, Farhan Ahsraf M, et al. Pain management in metastatic bone disease: a literature review. *Cureus*. 2018;10(9):e3286. Available from: https://doi.org/10.7759/cureus.3286.
48. Porta-Sales J, Garzón-Rodríguez C, Llorens-Torromé S, Brunelli C, Pigni A, Caraceni A. Evidence on the analgesic role of bisphosphonates and denosumab in the treatment of pain due to bone metastases: a systematic review within the European Association for Palliative Care guidelines project. *Palliat Med*. 2017;31(1):5–25. Available from: https://doi.org/10.1177/0269216316639793.
49. Stea B, Hazard LJ, Gonzalez VJ, Hamilton R. The role of radiation therapy in the control of locoregional and metastatic cancer. *J Surg Oncol*. 2011;103(6):627–638. Available from: https://doi.org/10.1002/jso.21837.
50. Huang MH, Hile E, Croarkin E, et al. Academy of oncologic physical therapy EDGE task force. *Rehabil Oncol*. 2019;37(3):92–103. Available from: https://doi.org/10.1097/01.REO.0000000000000177.
51. Mitchell SA. Cancer-related fatigue: state of the science. *PM&R*. 2010;2(5):364–383. Available from: https://doi.org/10.1016/j.pmrj.2010.03.024.
52. Jason LA, Evans M, Brown M, Porter N. What is fatigue? Pathological and nonpathological fatigue. *PM&R*. 2010;2(5):327–331. Available from: https://doi.org/10.1016/j.pmrj.2010.03.028.
53. Wonders KY. The effect of supervised exercise training on symptoms of chemotherapy-induced peripheral neuropathy. *Int J Phys Med Rehabil*. 2014;02(04):1–5. Available from: https://doi.org/10.4172/2329-9096.1000210.
54. Janssen SJ, Pereira NRP, Thio QCBS, et al. Physical function and pain intensity in patients with metastatic bone disease. *J Surg Oncol*. 2019;. Available from: https://doi.org/10.1002/jso.25510. May:jso.25510.
55. Brown TJ, Sedhom R, Gupta A. Chemotherapy-induced peripheral neuropathy peripheral neuropathy. *JAMA Oncol*. 2019;5(5):750. Available from: https://doi.org/10.1001/jamaoncol.2018.6771.
56. Hernandez RK, Wade SW, Reich A, Pirolli M, Leide A, Lyman GH. Incidence of Bone Metastases in patients with solid tumors: analysis of oncology electronic medical records in the United States. *BMC Cancer*. 2018;18:44.

CHAPTER 13

Shoulder Dysfunction in Breast Cancer

DIANA MOLINARES, MD • ADRIAN CRISTIAN, MD, MHCM

INTRODUCTION

Shoulder dysfunction is a common complication seen in breast cancer survivors.[1] The incidence of ipsilateral shoulder pain, stiffness, swelling, and numbness is in over 80% of survivors.[2,3] The patients often present with difficulties with the movement of the affected upper extremity limiting their ability to carry objects, reach overhead, push or pull, as well as perform activities of daily living, such as grooming and self-feeding.[3] These functional deficits can affect breast cancer survivors' productivity and their ability to return to work.[4] Breast cancer survivors with decrease range of motion of the shoulder have 2.5 more likelihood to loose productivity compared to survivors who do not present shoulder dysfunction.[4] Women who have arm and shoulder morbidity after breast cancer treatment report higher levels of disability, which ultimately limits their ability to return to work.[5] This is especially the case of musicians, who even 5 years after treatment feel their identity and livelihood are threatened by the presence of shoulder pathology after breast cancer treatment.[5,6] Furthermore, more than a third of breast cancer survivors feel less capable and less confident to use their arm due to a shoulder problem, which[7] interferes with their ability to participate in recreational activities such as golf or tennis.[7]

ANATOMY AND BIOMECHANICS

The shoulder is the most mobile joint in the human body. It is composed of three bones and four articular surfaces: (1) the clavicle, which articulates with the sternum and the acromion to form the sternoclavicular and acromioclavicular joints, respectively; (2) the scapula, which articulates with the thorax to form the scapulothoracic joint; and (3) the proximal humerus, which articulates with the glenoid fossa to form the glenohumeral joint. Even though this is a "ball-and-socket" type of synovial joint, its stability comes from several different sources: static and dynamic restraints. The synovial capsule, labrum, and ligaments constitute the static restraints.[8] Static restraints are important at rest and at the end of range of motion.[8,9]

However, static structures alone are insufficient to stabilize the shoulder motion. Dynamic restraints play an important role during midrange of motion and are based on three general principles: concavity compression, muscle stiffness, and tendon compliance.[8] Concavity compression refers to compression of the humeral head into the glenoid fossa. This action is primarily accomplished by rotator cuff muscles (supraspinatus, infraspinatus, teres minor, and subscapularis), although, the deltoid and long head of the biceps also contribute. Most of the rotator cuff muscles are helpful in stabilizing the shoulder anteriorly during abduction, while the subscapularis muscles stabilize the shoulder posteriorly.[9]

Joint stability also depends on the interplay between the forces of the muscles, which is also known as torque.[8] The strength during shoulder adduction is the highest, which is two times the torque force of abduction. Extension, flexion, abduction, and internal and external rotations follow adduction from the strongest to the weakest.[9] These forces contribute to maintain the stability of the shoulder during active motion and during the influence of external forces. The last component of the dynamic restraints is the tendons. The tendon compliance allows them to store energy while they are being elongated and use it when they return to its original length, which contribute to keeping the head of the humerus in the right position.[8]

Breast cancer survivors have increased internal rotation of the scapula and reduced external rotation. The change in the alignment of these structures results in a smaller subacromial space and compression of

Breast Cancer and Gynecologic Cancer Rehabilitation DOI: https://doi.org/10.1016/B978-0-323-72166-0.00013-X

the rotator cuff structures. Scapula internal rotation also forces the head of the humerus joint into external rotation, which causes further impingement of the rotator cuff.[10]

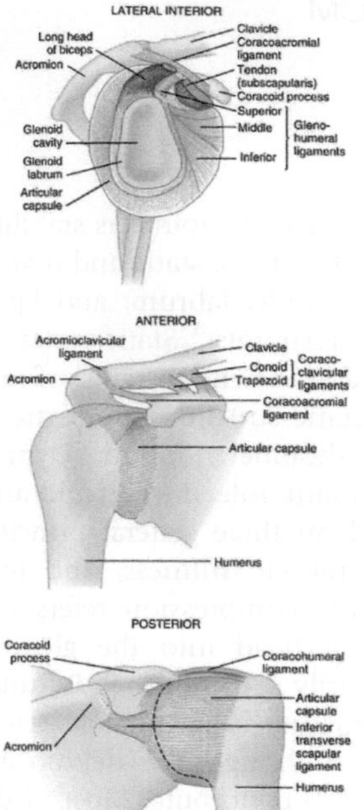

PATIENT ASSESSMENT

History and Self-Reported Function

As with other musculoskeletal complaints, a thorough evaluation and a detailed history are key elements when identifying the source of the dysfunction.[11] Symptom characteristics, onset, intensity, exacerbating/alleviating factors as well as associated functional limitations provide important clues about the source of the complaints. Preexisting shoulder pathology can often be exacerbated by breast cancer and its treatments; therefore it is important to understand the onset of the symptoms, history of trauma, occupation, and functional deficits present prior to the breast cancer diagnosis.[12]

The oncologic history, including staging and oncologic treatments, is indispensable when evaluating shoulder dysfunction. In cases of advanced breast cancer and worsening shoulder pain, metastatic disease to the proximal humerus or the scapula should be taken into consideration.[13] They frequently present with functional pain and/or pathologic fractures. Pain aggravated by movements and limitations in the range of motion can be observed during the physical examination.[14] However, with the increasing survival rate in breast cancer patients, most of the cases of shoulder dysfunction are consequences of the cancer treatment, rather than progression of the disease.[3,7] The extent of the cancer treatment is related to the risk of shoulder dysfunction. Patients who need conservative breast cancer surgery have less risk of developing shoulder dysfunction when compared to those who need more aggressive surgeries (i.e., mastectomy, lymph node dissection) or radiation therapy.[3,15]

Questionnaires to asses self-reported disability levels are commonly used to evaluate the impact of the symptoms in the functional level of the patients. The Disability of the Arm, Shoulder and Hand (DASH and Quick-DASH) is a validated tool that has been utilized to measure the self-reported upper extremity function in breast cancer patients.[7,16] One study found that up to 36% of breast cancer patients feel less capable of using their upper extremity and have moderate-to-severe difficulties participating in recreational activities that involve the use of the upper extremities, such as tennis or golf.[7] Although the results of the DASH could be influenced by the presence of lymphedema in the affected upper extremity, it is a tool that when used with a good history and examination can provide valuable information.

Physical Examination

Inspection

Unlike other patients, the breast cancer population frequently has clear evidence of asymmetries due to the presence of a mass, changes in the skin pigmentation due to radiation, or changes in the anatomy due to surgical interventions.[1,7] In these cases, knowing the muscles involved during the surgical procedure could help understand the changes in a patient's biomechanics. In addition, changes such as muscle atrophy can be the result of nerve injury, causing an imbalance of the forces of the shoulder muscles, critically important for its mobility and stability. Evaluation of the angle of the scapula for the presence of protrusion or winging could be another indication of injury of a peripheral nerve, such as the long thoracic nerve.[17]

Palpation

Palpation of the shoulder girdle is useful to identify points of tenderness, masses, deformities, or crepitus.[11] Deformities in the bony structure and crepitus are suggestive of possible fractures, while masses can be the result of enlarged lymph nodes, abscess, seroma, or presence of a tumor. Tendinopathy is often associated with tenderness along the trajectory of the tendon.[11] Furthermore, the presence of tender areas and palpable bands in the skeletal muscles, known as myofascial trigger points, is another cause of tenderness in this patient population.[18] During the palpation of the axillary area findings such as superficial tight cords are indicative of axillary web syndrome.[19] Although cording can be found in the chest or the arm, the axilla is the most common place. It is usually observed in patients that have undergone axillary node dissection.

Range of Motion

The large mobility of the shoulder is one of its most distinctive characteristics. Therefore it is not a surprise that the evaluation of the range of motion is a critical component of the physical examination. The shoulder is the most mobile joint in the body. It allows 150–180 degrees of forward flexion and 40–60 degrees of extension in the sagittal plane. In the coronal plane, abduction ranges between 150 and 180 degrees; and in the axial plane, external rotation ranges between 60 and 90 degrees, while internal rotation ranges between 50 and 70 degrees.[11] Breast cancer survivors have up to 60% reduction in flexion and abduction mobility 1 month after surgery, and 10% reduction at the 12-month mark.[20] A loss of 3–17 degrees of external rotation and 1–4 degrees of internal rotation have also been reported. Decreased mobility with passive motion is more indicative of pathologies such as adhesive capsulitis, degenerative changes of the glenohumeral joint, pectoralis tightness, or radiation fibrosis. On the contrary, preserved passive mobility with evidence of limitations during active range of motion is suggestive of rotator cuff dysfunction.[11,20–22]

Surgical interventions increase the risk of developing adhesive capsulitis.[22] Patients with this pathology present with multidirectional restrictions in the passive evaluation of the shoulder range motion. However, limitations are typically pronounced during external rotation.[23] Similarly, tightness of the pectoralis muscles can decrease the shoulder's range of motion in breast cancer survivors.[24] Anterior chest wall tightness in conjunction with scar tissue formation, radiation fibrosis, and patient acquisition of a protective posture causes malalignment of the shoulder structures.[3] These forces result in a forward depression of the shoulder girdle, which prompts a decrease in the size of the subacromial space and compression of the supraspinatus tendon and long head of the biceps tendon, subacromial bursa, and a portion of the glenohumeral joint capsule. This is known as the subacromial impingement syndrome and it is associated with rotator cuff dysfunction.

Rotator cuff disease is the leading cause of shoulder pain in the general population.[3] Shoulder malalignment is a major contributor to the development of rotator cuff pathology in the breast cancer population.[24] Dysfunction of the rotator cuff muscles presents with pain and weakness during shoulder active range of motion. In addition, patients report pain in the lateral and anterior aspect of the shoulder, which on occasion radiates to the ipsilateral elbow. The pain is usually exacerbated by overhead movements and is known to have an important impact in patient function.[3] Additional tests can be used for the evaluation of possible subacromial impingement syndrome and the integrity of the rotator cuff muscles. Neer and Hawkins-Kennedy are well-known impingement tests, while positive painful arc, drop arm, job tests, and pain with resisted internal and external rotation are suggestive of a rotator cuff pathology, likely involving the supraspinatus tendon.[11,25] For the evaluation of a possible subscapularis tear, the belly off test is the most sensitive test described by the literature.[25]

As the patient performs active range of motion of the shoulder, close attention needs to be given to the patient's general posture and bilateral scapula movements. The imbalance of the shoulder girdle muscles, pain and changes in the shoulder girdle alignment are likely to alter the motion of the scapula over the posterior chest wall.[3] Evaluation of the scapula alignment also includes the push-off wall test, which is useful to determine the presence of scapular winging caused by injury to the serratus anterior muscle or the long thoracic nerve (medial winging); or to the trapezius or cranial nerve XI (lateral winging).[3]

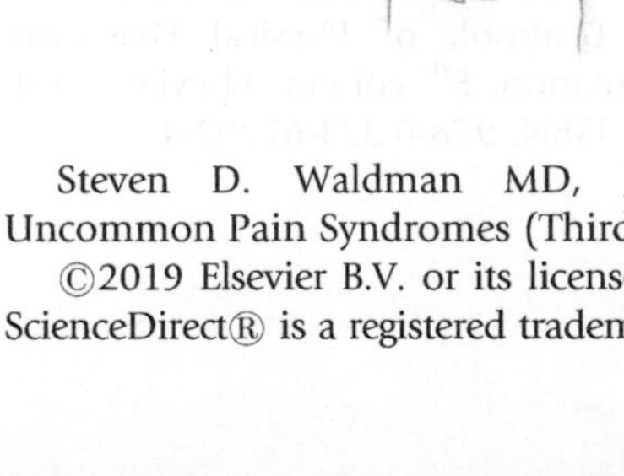

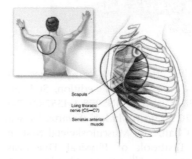

Winged scapula syndrome

Steven D. Waldman MD, JD, in Atlas of Uncommon Pain Syndromes (Third Edition), 2014

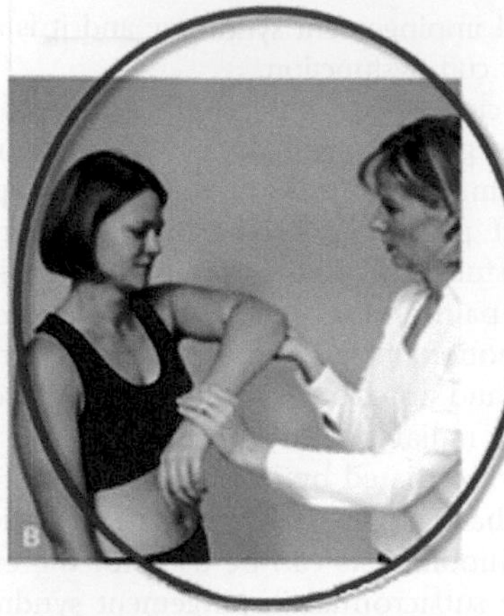

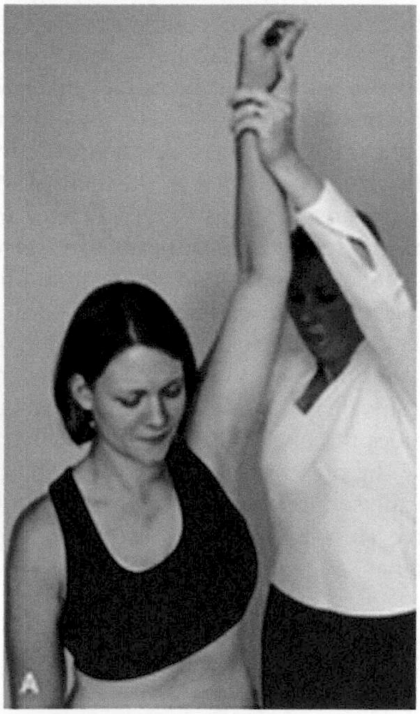

Kennedy-Hawkins: fig 5.87B from Magee DJ: Orthopedic Physical Assessment, 6th edition, St Louis, Saunders/Elsevier, 2014, p318, ISBN: 978-1-4557-0977-9.

Empty can: fig 20.36 from Mark H. Swartz, Darwin Chen and Jimmy Chan, The Musculoskeletal System; in: Swartz (ed): Textbook of Physical Diagnosis: History and Examination, 8th edition, Elsevier, 2021, ch20, pp429–472, ISBN: 978-0-323-67292-4.

Motor Exam

Bilateral evaluation of the shoulder girdle muscle strength is necessary for comparison. Isolation of the specific action(s) of each muscle is recommended to identify possible isolated muscle weakness due to nerve damage or injury to the muscle itself.[3] Weakness and decreased active range of motion are suggestive of tears of the muscle tendons.[25] In the breast cancer population, changes in the shoulder's biomechanics described previously put the supraspinatus muscle and its tendon at a higher risk of injury.[3,24,26,27] Similarly, examination of the anterior chest wall muscles should be included.[11] Pain in the anterior chest or anterior shoulder is suggestive of a pectoralis muscle pathology.[11]

Sensory

Sensory innervation of the shoulder is provided by the axillary, supraclavicular, and suprascapular nerves. The axillary nerve originates from the brachial plexus and provides sensation to the lateral, anterolateral, and posterolateral aspect of the shoulder. The supraclavicular nerve is originated out of branches of C3 and C4 nerve roots and provides sensation along the clavicle up to the superior aspect of the trapezius muscle region. Lastly, the suprascapular nerve, a branch of the upper trunk of the brachial plexus, carries the sensory inputs of the acromioclavicular joint and glenohumeral joint.

The intercostal nerves have an important role in the development of postmastectomy pain.[28] The intercostal brachial nerve, which is branch of the second intercostal nerve, provides sensory innervation to the upper thoracic dermatomes (T1 and T2), including the axilla, medial upper arm, and chest.[29] These sensory branches are often scarified during axillary dissections in the presence of positive lymph nodes. Chronic pain and postmastectomy pain syndrome are closely associated with injury to the intercostal brachial nerve. Furthermore axillary lymph node dissection is associated with pain, numbness, and stiffness, which negatively affect the quality of life of breast cancer survivors.[28] Perineural injections of the intercostal brachial nerve have shown benefits in the management of postmastectomy pain syndrome secondary to intercostal brachial neuralgia.[29] These findings confirm the role that injuries caused to this nerve have in the development of chronic pain syndrome in cancer survivors.[29]

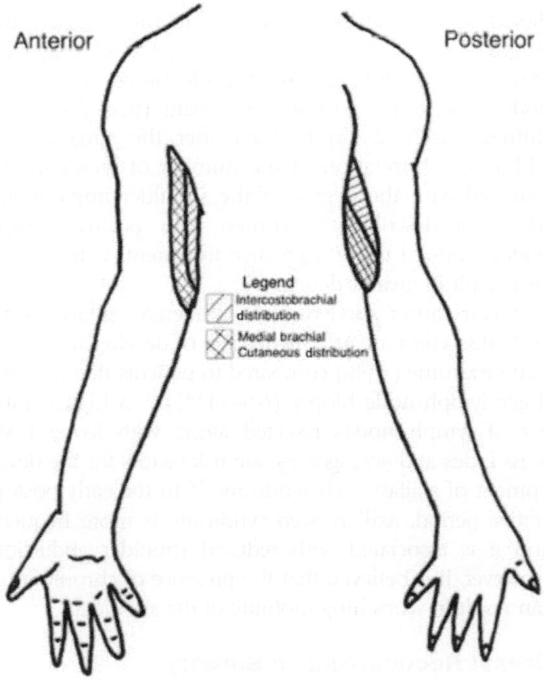

TUMOR-RELATED IMPAIRMENTS

Increasing efforts in breast cancer screening have resulted in earlier detection of the disease. Therefore impairments secondary to the tumors are less frequently seen. There is lack of studies that evaluate the direct effects of breast cancer mass to the function of the ipsilateral shoulder. However, it is believed that once diagnosed, there is a tendency for survivors to protect the affected side, limiting the level of activity that they are used to perform with the ipsilateral upper extremity. In a study performed by Flores and Dwyer, the shoulder range of motion of 33 women was tested after biopsy but before surgery.[30] Surprisingly, they found a significant reduction of the range of motion of the shoulder. Furthermore, African-American survivors were found to have greater reduction of shoulder flexion when compared to Whites.[30] More research needs to be conducted to understand the implication of breast cancer in shoulder function prior to the start of oncological treatments.

SURGICAL-RELATED IMPAIRMENTS

Functional limitations are believed to be at its peak in the first couple of months of surgery but have been reported even 6 years after surgery.[30–32] The most prevalent complaint is the difficulty to perform overhead activities, reported in 42%–56% of survivors[31,33,34] followed by pain, which is present in 22%–38% of the patients.[31] Flores and Dwyer measured the shoulder range of motions before and after breast cancer surgery.[30] In this study, all shoulder motions, except internal rotation, had a statistically significant reduced range of motion. However, abduction was found to be the most affected shoulder movement. Two weeks after surgery, the patients were able to achieve only 83 degrees of abduction, which is significantly below the 150–180 degrees that are considered normal.[11,25,30]

However, it is not only a matter of timing. The extent of the surgical intervention, conservative versus nonconservative surgery, and lymph node involvement plays a role in the risk of developing shoulder functional impairments.[3,7,19,35] A cross-sectional study performed in 150 breast cancer survivors reported greater pain and movement deviations in those patients that underwent mastectomy.[31]

Conserving Surgery

Breast-conserving surgery, including lumpectomy, partial mastectomy, or wide local excision, is associated with lower risk of postoperative shoulder dysfunction.[7,34,35] The average DASH score in postlumpectomy patients is 9.88 (0–100, where the higher the number the greater the disability)[7] and around 8% of the patients report shoulder stiffness.[35] However, the incidence of shoulder pain ranges between 8% and 31%, even 5 year after the surgery.[36] Breast cancer survivors tend to report lower levels of shoulder dysfunction (31% of survivors) compared to objective findings of 20 degrees or more of decreased range of motion (49% of survivors).[36] These findings suggest that patients may not notice smaller decreases in shoulder motion and/or develop compensatory strategies that allow them to continue to carry their prior level of activity.

Women who undergo breast-conserving surgery are not exempt from developing dysfunction of the shoulder girdle or shoulder pain. Shoulder impairments associated to breast-conserving surgery, although less frequent, can still have an impact in breast cancer survivors' function and quality of life. Therefore a thorough evaluation of the shoulder function by healthcare providers is highly recommended.

Mastectomy

Breast cancer survivors who undergo mastectomy are known to be at a higher risk of developing shoulder dysfunction, especially in the acute postoperative period.[3,7,10,20,26,27,31,32,34] The average DASH score in postmastectomy patients is 24.4 (> 20 is associated with major disability) 4 months after the surgery[7] and 12.9 at the year mark.[27] Similarly, 6 months postmastectomy, breast cancer survivors have a 20% prevalence of decreased shoulder range of motion, and 50% prevalence of difficulties with overhead activities, versus 10% and 47% 12 months after the surgery. Controversially, patients have higher levels of neck–shoulder pain at 12 months (40.6%) than at 6 months (38.5%) were observed.[37]

The perceived disability changes are associated with changes in the biomechanics of the shoulder function.[26,31] Patients who undergo mastectomy have greater upward rotation of the scapula.[27,31] This change could be a compensatory mechanism secondary to glenohumeral joint dysfunction, such as in cases of adhesive capsulitis.[31] Decrease in muscle activity observed in pectoralis major, upper trapezius, and rhomboid muscles are likely responsible for some of the biomechanical deviations.[33]

When evaluating shoulder range of motion, postmastectomy patients present limitations in all planes. However, abduction and flexion are affected the most.[20,35] Impaired flexion and abduction of more than 25 degrees has been reported in 24% and 38% of postmastectomy patients, respectively.[35] Limitations are greater in women with involvement of the nondominant side. Furthermore, patients who develop surgical seromas have reduced external rotation.[20] Tightness of the anterior chest wall muscles has been reported in 16% of breast cancer survivors who undergo mastectomy.[35]

Mastectomy is the strongest risk factor for the development of adhesive capsulitis.[22,38,39] Its incidence has been reported between 7.7% and 10.3% of the cases.[22,38] Moreover, patients who undergo reconstruction after mastectomy are at a bigger risk as well as those who receive adjuvant radiation therapy.[22] The onset of adhesive capsulitis is insidious. However, an onset as early as 4 months has been suggested.[38]

Lymph Node Dissection

Axillary lymph node dissection is another risk factor for the development of shoulder dysfunction.[15,20,31,40–43] Patients that undergo axillary lymph node dissection have a significant reduction in internal rotation strength with a mean loss of 2.2 kg.[40] Range of motion in all planes has also been described, with shoulder abduction and flexion being affected the most.[15] A reduction of 3.2 to 21 degrees of abduction and 5 to 6.3 degrees of flexion has been described at the 12-month mark.[15] Shoulder impairments associated with lymph node dissection are typically seen early in the postoperative period.[20] However, other studies suggest that patients that undergo sentinel lymph node biopsy or axillary node dissection report shoulder pain (9%–25%) and stiffness (14%–24%) 6 years after the surgery.[31] In addition, a correlation of the number of lymph nodes removed with the degree of the shoulder impairments has been described.[20] Women with positive lymph nodes required more aggressive treatment, which could also result in greater deficits.[35]

Breast cancer survivors who undergo axillary lymph node dissection are at a higher risk of developing axillary web syndrome (71%) compared to patients that undergo single lymph node biopsy (6%–41%).[19] A higher number of lymph nodes resected along with lower body mass index and younger age are risk factors for the development of axillary web syndrome.[19] In the early postoperative period, axillary web syndrome is more frequent, and it is associated with reduced shoulder abduction. However, it is believed that the presence of chronic cords can result in worsening mobility of the shoulder.[19]

Breast Reconstructive Surgery

As the flap options for breast reconstructive surgery increase, changes in shoulder biomechanics bring different challenges. Myung et al. evaluated the effects of implant insertion, latissimus dorsalis flap and transverse rectus abdominis musculocutaneous flap on the shoulder muscle strength.[44] Three months after the surgery there were no significant differences observed within groups. However, at the 6-month mark, the patients who underwent latissimus dorsalis flap had greater shoulder deficits.[44] These findings are similar to other studies that showed shoulder weakness 6 month after a latissimus dorsalis flap reconstruction, especially during abduction, internal rotation, and adduction.[45] Breast cancer survivors who undergo transverse rectus abdominis musculocutaneous flap show a faster recovery rate.[44]

Decrease in shoulder muscle strength translates into functional impairments that interfere with breast cancer survivor daily activities. Unilateral latissimus dorsi reconstruction is associated with functional impairment during the first 3 months after the surgery. Furthermore, bilateral extended autologous latissimus dorsi reconstruction has been associated with an increase in DASH scores of 25 points at 3 months and 18 points at 6 months (minimal clinically significant change = 12.7 points).[46] Although the tendency is to recover over time, due to the heterogenicity of the procedures and studies as well as potential confounding factors (i.e., access to therapy, lymph node involvement, age, body mass index), there is no consensus in the literature as per the long-term effects of latissimus dorsi reconstruction on shoulder function.[47]

The type of breast reconstruction after mastectomy has a significant impact on the shoulder associated morbidity. Survivors who undergo a reconstruction that involves the use of the latissimus dorsi have a higher risk of developing shoulder pathology. However, the use of expander–implants has also been associated with shoulder dysfunction. Around 23.8% of women who undergo expander–implants reconstruction develop shoulder impairments.[48] The implants inserted under the subpectoral space are thought to cause increased tension of the pectoralis muscle and tendon resulting in pectoralis tightness. During the procedure the muscle is also detached from the lower ribs and the sternum causing further injury to the muscle fibers. Pain associated to this intervention is exacerbated during the expansion period. As mentioned before, pain and pectoralis muscle tightness often result in changes in the biomechanics of the scapula and shoulder movement resulting in shoulder dysfunction. The use of expander–implants for breast cancer survivors has an odds ratio of 2.15 ($p + 0.010$) of developing shoulder dysfunction.[48] Most of the shoulder morbidity is secondary to decrease in the shoulder range of motion during abduction and flexion.

Table 3. Physical and Functional Effects Related to Breast Reconstruction

Reconstruction Method	Description	Potential Complications
Implant-based reconstruction	Placement of an implant behind the pectoralis major muscle; implants may be comprised of a saline solution or silicone gel or combination[76]	Decreased extensibility and strength of pectoral muscle[78]
Pedicled TRAM flap	Transfer of fat, abdominal skin, and one or both rectus abdominus muscles, which are tunnelled under the diaphragm[76]	Abdominal wall weakness with/without herniation[49] Loss of trunk extensor strength[79] Back pain/increases in back pain[80]
Free flap TRAM	Skin, fat, and a small portion of the lower rectus abdominus muscle is removed; microvascular surgery is performed to transplant the flap to the mastectomy site[76]	Pain: reconstructed breast, abdominal area, axilla, neck, and back[81]
DIEP flap TRAM	Preserves the anterior rectus sheath and integrity of abdominal muscle. Removes only the lower abdominal skin and fat along with deep inferior epigastric vessels, an artery, and a vein at the bottom of the rectus abdominis muscle[76]	Abdominal weakness: less weakness than pedicled or free flap TRAM[79]
Latissimus flap reconstruction	Often combined with a tissue expander or implant; the latismus muscle flap, with or without attached skin, is elevated off of the back and brought around to the front of the chest wall; the main thoracodorsal vessels remain attached to the body to ensure proper blood supply to the flap[76]	Shoulder pain[73] Impairment in shoulder flexion ROM[82] Impairment in shoulder strength and function[83] Difficulty with functional tasks (eg, reaching overhead) and athletic activities (eg, tennis, golf)[84]

DEIP, deep inferior epigastric artery perforation; ROM, range of motion; TRAM, transverse rectus abdominus muscle

Roundtable Meeting on a Prospective Model of Care for BreastCancer Rehabilitation, held February 24–25, 2011, at the American Cancer Society National Home Office, in Atlanta, Georgia.[49]

RADIATION IMPAIRMENTS

Neuromuscular dysfunction caused by the damage to the suprascapular, supraclavicular, and long thoracic nerves is part of the pathophysiology of radiation-related shoulder dysfunction. Additional fibrotic changes of shoulder tendons and ligaments result in loss of their elasticity and can result in reduction of the joint range of motion.[50] Myopathic changes are characterized by spasms that can compromise the blood supply causing further damage of the muscle and worsening of the shoulder dysfunction. Although these changes are challenging to notice during a physical examination, fibrosis, induration, and sclerosis of the skin are good reminders of the impact of radiation in the development of fibrosis of the shoulder components.[50–52]

Postmastectomy patients have a significant decrease in range of motion in all planes after receiving adjuvant radiation.[53–57] However, shoulder abduction is once again the most affected movement.[15,53,57] In a study performed in 30 women who underwent modified radical mastectomy and radiation therapy, subject ipsilateral shoulder had a 33-degree reduction in abduction when compared to the contralateral arm. Meanwhile, control patients (status post modified radical mastectomy without radiation) had only a loss of 6.9 degrees in abduction.[53]

Out of the breast cancer radiated survivors, those who received radiation to the axilla are at a significant higher risk of developing shoulder dysfunction than those who only received radiation to the chest.[15,34,57] Forty-nine percent of patients that undergo radiation that includes the axilla have decreased shoulder range of motion during abduction versus only 8% of patients whose radiation only includes the chest.[34] Patients also have decreased range of motion during flexion (39% chest/axillary radiation vs 4% chest-only radiation) and extension (45% chest/axillary radiation vs 14% chest-only radiation).[34]

Although morbidity related to radiation therapy could be present at any point after radiation is started, the impact of radiation in the function of the shoulder is more commonly seen as a late side effect. The presence of inflammatory infiltrates as well as changes in the deposit of proteins and collagen in nonmalignant tissue are important contributors to the shoulder morbidity associated with radiation.[50] These changes, often seen weeks or even years after radiation, are known as radiation fibrosis syndrome. Although changes in the tumor surrounding tissue start at the time of radiation, the clinical manifestations can present later on in life.[15,50,56,58]

Shoulder range of motion impairments are most commonly seen during the first few weeks after the surgery. During this postsurgical period, the efforts are focused on wound healing in preparation for adjuvant treatments. Wound healing is especially important for those women who need to undergo radiation treatment. However, shoulder range of motion and arm mobility also play important roles in their ability to undergo adjuvant radiation therapy.[59] Although different positions have been used to deliver radiation in breast cancer patients (supine vs prone vs crawl), in most cases overhead position of the arm is required. Limitations of the shoulder range of motion can cause pain during radiation treatments, or even prevent survivors from getting it.[59] There is not enough information in the literature that allows us to establish the incidence of these cases. However, treatments such as stretching of the pectoralis muscles and suprascapular nerve block have been found to have success on treating this condition.[59–61]

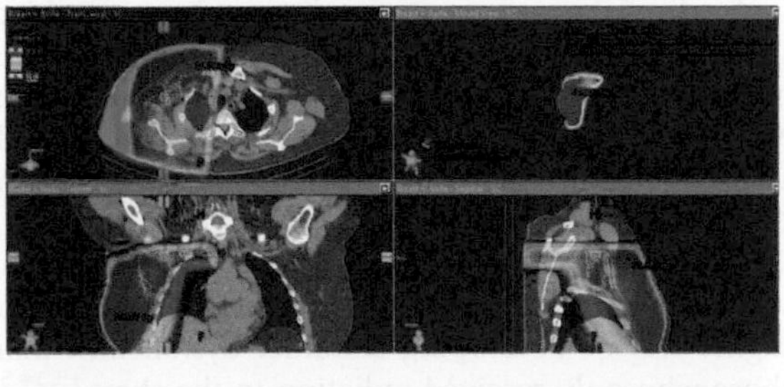

Radiation therapy plan treating breast and axilla. ARM node in green, level 1 axilla in cyan, level 2 axilla in blue, interpectoral space in yellow, level 3 axilla in white, level 4 axilla or lower supraclavicular fossa in red, breast PTV in pink. *ARM*, Axillary reverse mapping; *PTV*, planning target volume.

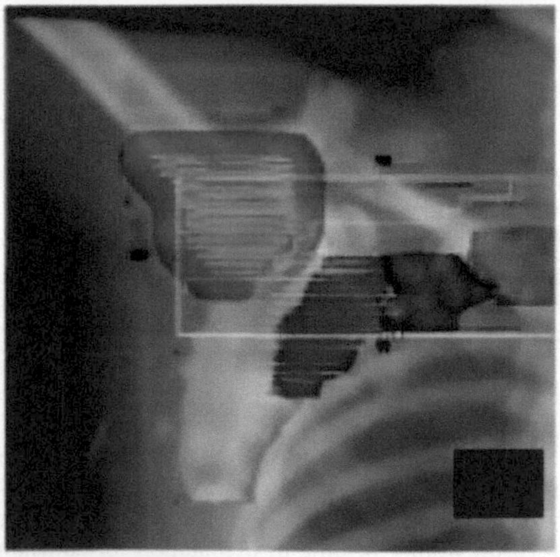

[62]

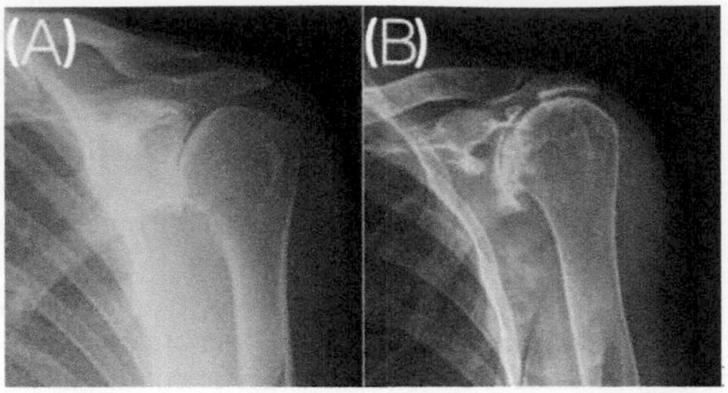

FIGURE 13.1 X-rays showing osteoarthritis of the shoulder joint in patients without a rotator cuff tear (A), and with a rotator cuff tear (B). Note the superior migration of the humeral head with acromion erosion in patients with rotator cuff arthritis.[63]

IMAGING

Radiography

Radiographs are a widely accessible and cost-effective tool that can provide valuable information of the shoulder bony structure. It is often the first imaging ordered in patients who present with shoulder pain. For breast cancer survivors, X-rays can help with the diagnosis of metastatic disease. Although smaller and noncortical metastases can be missed, radiographs are important in the evaluation of bone metastases, especially in symptomatic patients.[58]

In addition to the diagnosis of metastatic disease, X-rays can also be helpful in the detection of other shoulder pathologies, especially those involving degenerative changes. Osteoarthritic changes in the glenohumeral and acromioclavicular joint are characterized by sclerotic changes in the bony surface as well as loss of the articular space. Detection and follow-up of tendon calcification in cases of tendinitis can also be achieved with X-rays (Fig. 13.1).

Ultrasound

In the last couple of decades the popularity of musculoskeletal ultrasound (US) has increased. The large mobility of the shoulder joint makes US examination a great tool in the diagnosis of shoulder pathologies. During the US exam, dynamic movements of the joint can be evaluated live, which is helpful in the diagnosis of shoulder pathologies, such as impingement syndromes. In addition, partial and complete tendon tears, calcification or disruption of the fibrillar tendon pattern can be observed with this imaging.

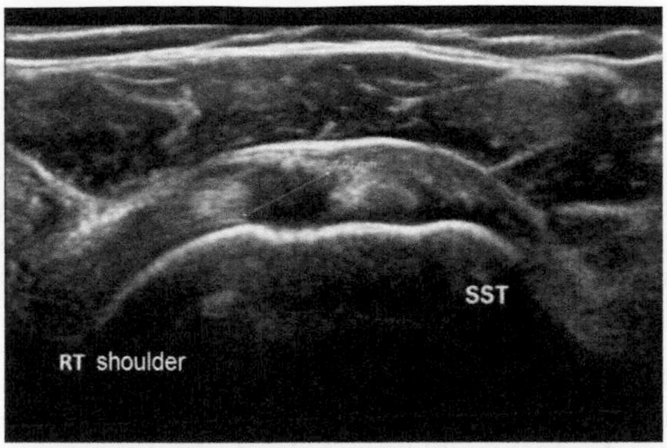

FIGURE 13.2 US LS of the right supraspinatus tendon showing a hypo-echoic area within involving its whole thickness denoting full thickness tear with a gap measuring 7 mm.[64]

US is also helpful in the detection of fluid and synovitis of the glenohumeral joint. Changes in the bone surface of the AC joint as well as the presence of osteophytes and effusions can be observed. In addition to the diagnostic advantages of the US in breast cancer survivors with shoulder impairments, US can be used to guide certain procedures, such as injection (Fig. 13.2).

MRI

Magnetic resonance in breast cancer survivors is useful in the assessment of malignant as well as noncancer-related shoulder pathologies. Evaluation of shoulder's soft tissue components provides valuable information for the diagnosis of pathologies such as rotator cuff injuries (tendonitis, tears, tendon calcification) and ligament disruption.

Nonetheless, MRI can provide information specific to pathologies secondary to breast cancer and its treatment. To start, MRI can detect the presence of metastasis in the bone marrow early in the process. T1-weighted and STIR sequences can provide this information without the use of contrast. It also can help evaluate the health of the shoulder muscles. A study performed in 57 women who underwent surgery with or without radiation found that both pectoralis muscles are decreased in size on the affected side.[33] In addition, MRI can reliably diagnose brachial plexopathy in symptomatic breast cancer survivors.[65] The diagnosis can be done in both patients who have symptoms secondary to cancer recurrence and whose symptoms are secondary to a nonmalignant causes, such as radiation plexopathy.[65,66] Furthermore, Diffusion-weighted MRIs can improve the visualization and therefore improve the detection of brachial plexus abnormalities in oncologic patients.[66]

In breast cancer survivors who present with clinical radiation fibrosis syndrome, MRI is able to detect soft tissue changes that correlate with the clinical degree of fibrosis.[67] Hoeller et al. was able to identify changes the axilla and the supraclavicular fossa characterized by an increase in signal intensity in T2-weighted sequence and STIR.[67] Other changes previously described include reduction of signal intensity of the fat in T1- and T2-weighted sequences and distortion of the neurovascular bundle.[67]

Positron Emission Tomography–Computed Tomography Scan

Breast cancer survivors typically undergo 18F-fluorodeoxyglucose (18F-FDG) positron emission tomography–computed tomography (PET/CT) to monitor the progression of the disease. However, after evidence of incidental uptake in the shoulder secondary to adhesive capsulitis, emphasis has been placed on the interpretations of these findings. There is a clear correlation between clinical findings and the level of 18F-FDG PET/CT uptake observed in the shoulder.[38] Breast cancer survivors with more severe symptoms of adhesive capsulitis have higher uptake in the shoulder, likely related to the level of inflammation. These findings can help physicians make an early diagnosis and therefore help them access appropriate treatment.

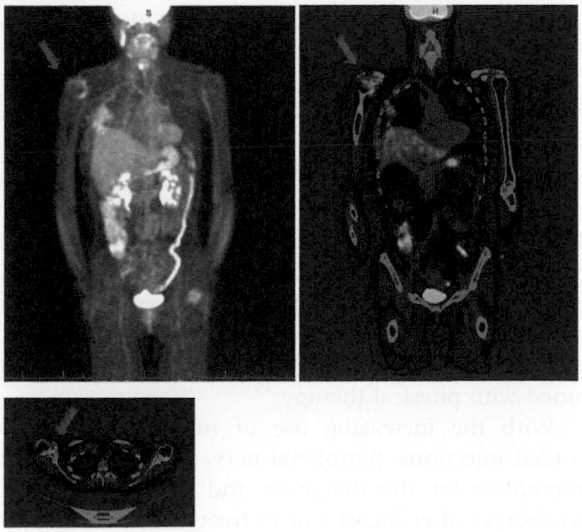

Increased uptake in the shoulder secondary to adhesive capsulitis.

SHOULDER REHABILITATION

Medications

Nonsteroidal antiinflammatory can provide significant benefits to breast cancer survivors who present shoulder dysfunction. The combination of NSAIDs and physical therapy has been proven to provide pain relief and functional gains in patients with rotator cuff pathology after breast cancer treatment.[68] Herrera and Stubblefield found a decrease of 4.57 points in the visual analog scale (from 8.28 to 3.71) in breast cancer survivors who had ipsilateral rotator cuff tendinopathy associated with lymphedema 4–6 weeks after starting treatment with NSAIDs and physical therapy.[68] NSAIDs have also been used for the treatment of axillary web syndrome; however, there is lack of literature that proves that the use of antiinflammatories change the course of the syndrome.[69,70]

Similarly, NSAIDs have been studied in cases of adhesive capsulitis. Despite the inflammatory nature of this pathology, there is no evidence (lack of control clinical trials) that supports the use of NSAID in patients with adhesive capsulitis, including those whose symptoms are secondary to breast cancer treatment. On the contrary, placebo-controlled clinical trials of the impact of steroidal antiinflammatory have shown short term improvement of the symptoms. However, no difference in the level of pain and range of motion is observed after steroids are stopped.

Recent studies with vitamin E and pentoxifylline have described some benefits in patients with radiation-induced fibrosis.[71] However, no significant benefits in the range of motion of the shoulder have been observed.[71]

Injections

Intraarticular steroid injections and physical therapy have shown to improve shoulder pain and range of motion of patients with adhesive capsulitis.[22] Similarly, subacromial steroid injections improve pain, mobility, and tolerance to therapy in breast cancer survivors.[39] Both impingement syndromes and rotator cuff tendinopathies can obtain pain relief as well as improvement in range of motion when combined with physical therapy.[39]

With the increasing use of musculoskeletal US-guided injections, peripheral nerve blocks propose an alternative for the diagnosis and treatment of pain syndromes after breast cancer treatment. As described in the anatomy section, the glenohumeral joint sensory input travels through the branches of the suprascapular nerve. Therefore blocking the suprascapular nerve can provide important benefits in the shoulder pain level of breast cancer patients, which can potentially translate in better mobility. Eighteen breast cancer survivors with postsurgical shoulder pain and movement limitations underwent US-guided suprascapular nerve blocks with evidence of statistically significant improvements in range of motion, pain severity, and disability (measured with the quick-DASH survey) 10 days after the procedure.[59]

Therapy

Therapy that promotes joint mobilization decreases the shoulder morbidity associated with breast cancer treatments.[18] Breast cancer survivors who start shoulder mobilization as early as postoperative day 1 have less reduction in shoulder range of motion. However, this may lead to a higher risk of seroma formation. To decrease this risk and promote mobility, a low-intensity program, with shoulder active mobilization, and wrist and elbow pumping, is recommended in the early postoperative period.[18] Both, exercising in groups or individually, are effective to achieve enhancements in shoulder mobility. However, when compared to HEP, supervised exercise programs seem to be more beneficial.[61,72,73] Patients that undergo physical therapy have less pain and better range of motion of the shoulder.[72] In addition, both Pilates and yoga-based exercises have shown to have benefits in mobility and shoulder pain in breast cancer survivors.

Despite the known effect of pectoralis tightness on shoulder range of motion, only one study evaluated the effect of a pectoralis stretching home exercise program, and no benefits were found.[73] Nevertheless, stretching in combination with a supervise resistance exercise program have significant improvements in flexion and abduction.[73] The combination of active, postural, progressively resistive, and proprioceptive neuromuscular exercises while in the acute hospitalization, followed by a home exercise program, improve shoulder mobility in the acute postoperative stay as well as 3 months after surgery.[73]

In addition, breast cancer survivors who present with late shoulder morbidity can benefit from therapy. Decreased mobility secondary to adhesive capsulitis, rotator cuff dysfunction, shoulder muscle weakness, axillary web syndrome, and radiation fibrosis can improve with a comprehensive treatment plan that includes a formal therapy program ideally followed by home exercises.

Similar to early mobilization after breast cancer surgery, preoperative exercise can positively impact the recovery of shoulder function. In a study performed with newly diagnosed breast cancer patients, survivors who underwent a preoperative education and exercise protocol, including range of motion and strengthening exercise, have a quicker recovery of the shoulder function.[32] Prehabilitation programs for breast cancer surgery have benefits in the preservation of shoulder range of motion and reduction of postoperative pain.[74] Preoperative grip strength, abduction, and shoulder flexion are good predictors of shoulder functional recovery. However, prehabilitation alone, without postoperative rehabilitation, has not shown to be enough.[74] Prehabilitation programs should focus on patients at higher risk of developing shoulder dysfunction, such as survivors who will undergo mastectomy, reconstructions, lymph node dissection, and adjuvant radiation treatment.

Other Treatments

Trigger point injections and deep tissue massage have shown benefits in breast cancer survivors with myopathic pain. In a study of 19 breast cancer survivors, US-guided trigger point injections of the subscapularis and/or pectoralis muscles were effective in decreasing shoulder pain caused by myofascial trigger points.[75] Moreover, myofascial release has shown benefits in shoulder pain and mobility of survivors that undergo breast-conserving surgery and radiation therapy. In addition, deep friction massage can potentially break fibrotic tissue caused by radiation therapy decreasing muscle spasms and associated pain [76]

CONCLUSION

Shoulder dysfunction is very common post breast cancer treatment with a significant adverse impact on the affected individual. Understanding the pertinent anatomy and the altered biomechanics of the joint due to the impact of the cancer treatment and preexisting conditions is important in determining the most appropriate treatment plan. Addressing shoulder impairments early in persons at risk for developing shoulder dysfunction is important to minimize functional loss.

REFERENCES

1. Lee CH, Chung SY, Kim WY, Yang SN. Effect of breast cancer surgery on chest tightness and upper limb dysfunction. *Medicine (Baltimore)*. 2019;98(19):e15524. Available from: https://doi.org/10.1097/MD.0000000000015524.
2. McCredie MR, Dite GS, Porter L, et al. Prevalence of self-reported arm morbidity following treatment for breast cancer in the Australian Breast Cancer Family Study. *Breast*. 2001;10(6):515–522. Available from: https://doi.org/10.1054/brst.2000.0291.
3. Ebaugh D, Spinelli B, Schmitz KH. Shoulder impairments and their association with symptomatic rotator cuff disease in breast cancer survivors. *Med Hypotheses*. 2011;77(4):481–487. Available from: https://doi.org/10.1016/j.mehy.2011.06.015.
4. Quinlan E, Thomas-MacLean R, Hack T, et al. The impact of breast cancer among Canadian women: disability and productivity. *Work*. 2009;34(3):285–296. Available from: https://doi.org/10.3233/WOR-2009-0926.
5. Thomas-Maclean RL, Hack T, Kwan W, Towers A, Miedema B, Tilley A. Arm morbidity and disability after breast cancer: new directions for care. *Oncol Nurs Forum*. 2008;35(1):65–71. Available from: https://doi.org/10.1188/08.ONF.65-71.
6. Schmalenberger S, Gessert CE, Giebenhain JE, Starr LD. Working after breast cancer treatment: lessons from musicians. *Med Probl Perform Art*. 2012;27(4):175–180.
7. Harrington S, Padua D, Battaglini C, et al. Comparison of shoulder flexibility, strength, and function between breast cancer survivors and healthy participants. *J Cancer Surviv.*. 2011;5(2):167–174. Available from: https://doi.org/10.1007/s11764-010-0168-0.
8. Hurov J. Anatomy and mechanics of the shoulder: review of current concepts. *J Hand Ther*. 2009;22(4):328–342. Available from: https://doi.org/10.1016/j.jht.2009.05.002. quiz 343.
9. Halder AM, Itoi E, An KN. Anatomy and biomechanics of the shoulder. *Orthop Clin North Am*. 2000;31(2):159–176.
10. Shamley D, Lascurain-Aguirrebeña I, Oskrochi R. Clinical anatomy of the shoulder after treatment for breast cancer. *Clin Anat*. 2014;27(3):467–477. Available from: https://doi.org/10.1002/ca.22267.
11. Bakhsh W, Nicandri G. Anatomy and physical examination of the shoulder. *Sports Med Arthrosc Rev*. 2018;26(3):e10–e22. Available from: https://doi.org/10.1097/JSA.0000000000000202.
12. Hose MK, Fontanesi J, Woytowitz M, Jarrin D, Quan A. Competency based clinical shoulder examination training improves physical exam, confidence, and knowledge in common shoulder conditions. *J Gen Intern Med*. 2017;32(11):1261–1265. Available from: https://doi.org/10.1007/s11606-017-4143-6.
13. Kim SY, Jung MW, Kim JM. The shoulder pain due to metastatic breast cancer – a case report. *Korean J Pain*. 2011;24(2):119–122. Available from: https://doi.org/10.3344/kjp.2011.24.2.119.
14. Kapur RA, McCann PA, Sarangi PP. Reverse geometry shoulder replacement for proximal humeral metastases. *Ann R Coll Surg Engl*. 2014;96(7):e32–e35. Available from: https://doi.org/10.1308/003588414X13946184903964.
15. Levangie PK, Drouin J. Magnitude of late effects of breast cancer treatments on shoulder function: a systematic review. *Breast Cancer Res Treat*. 2009;116(1):1–15. Available from: https://doi.org/10.1007/s10549-008-0246-4.

16. Dean LT, DeMichele A, LeBlanc M, et al. Black breast cancer survivors experience greater upper extremity disability. *Breast Cancer Res Treat.* 2015;154(1):117–125. Available from: https://doi.org/10.1007/s10549-015-3580-3.
17. Saied GM, Kamel RM, Dessouki NR. The effect of mastectomy and radiotherapy for breast carcinoma on soft tissues of the shoulder and its joint mobility among Egyptian patients. *Tanzan Health Res Bull.* 2007;9(2):121–125.
18. Groef A, de, van Kampen M, Dieltjens E, et al. Identification of myofascial trigger points in breast cancer survivors with upper limb pain: interrater reliability. *Pain Med.* 2018;19(8):1650–1656. Available from: https://doi.org/10.1093/pm/pnx299.
19. Koehler LA, Blaes AH, Haddad TC, Hunter DW, Hirsch AT, Ludewig PM. Movement, function, pain, and postoperative edema in axillary web syndrome. *Phys Ther.*. 2015;95(10):1345–1353. Available from: https://doi.org/10.2522/ptj.20140377.
20. Levy EW, Pfalzer LA, Danoff J, et al. Predictors of functional shoulder recovery at 1 and 12 months after breast cancer surgery. *Breast Cancer Res Treat.* 2012;134(1):315–324. Available from: https://doi.org/10.1007/s10549-012-2061-1.
21. Mitchell C, Adebajo A, Hay E, Carr A. Shoulder pain: diagnosis and management in primary care. *BMJ.* 2005;331(7525):1124–1128. Available from: https://doi.org/10.1136/bmj.331.7525.1124.
22. Yang S, Park DH, Ahn SH, et al. Prevalence and risk factors of adhesive capsulitis of the shoulder after breast cancer treatment. *Support Care Cancer.* 2017;25(4):1317–1322. Available from: https://doi.org/10.1007/s00520-016-3532-4.
23. Robinson CM, Seah KTM, Chee YH, Hindle P, Murray IR. Frozen shoulder. *J Bone Joint Surg Br.* 2012;94(1):1–9. Available from: https://doi.org/10.1302/0301-620x.94b1.27093.
24. Yang EJ, Park W-B, Seo KS, Kim S-W, Heo C-Y, Lim J-Y. Longitudinal change of treatment-related upper limb dysfunction and its impact on late dysfunction in breast cancer survivors: a prospective cohort study. *J Surg Oncol.* 2010;101(1):84–91. Available from: https://doi.org/10.1002/jso.21435.
25. O'Kane JW, Toresdahl BG. The evidenced-based shoulder evaluation. *Curr Sports Med Rep.* 2014;13(5):307–313. Available from: https://doi.org/10.1249/JSR.0000000000000090.
26. Shamley D, Srinaganathan R, Oskrochi R, Lascurain-Aguirrebeña I, Sugden E. Three-dimensional scapulothoracic motion following treatment for breast cancer. *Breast Cancer Res Treat.* 2009;118(2):315–322. Available from: https://doi.org/10.1007/s10549-008-0240-x.
27. Crosbie J, Kilbreath SL, Dylke E, et al. Effects of mastectomy on shoulder and spinal kinematics during bilateral upper-limb movement. *Phys Ther.* 2010;90(5):679–692. Available from: https://doi.org/10.2522/ptj.20090104.
28. Sclafani LM, Baron RH. Sentinel lymph node biopsy and axillary dissection: added morbidity of the arm, shoulder and chest wall after mastectomy and reconstruction. *Cancer J.*. 2008;14(4):216–222. Available from: https://doi.org/10.1097/PPO.0b013e31817fbe5e.
29. Wisotzky EM, Saini V, Kao C. Ultrasound-guided intercostobrachial nerve block for intercostobrachial neuralgia in breast cancer patients: a case series. *PMR.* 2016;8(3):273–277. Available from: https://doi.org/10.1016/j.pmrj.2015.10.003.
30. Flores AM, Dwyer K. Shoulder impairment before breast cancer surgery. *J Womens Health Phys Therap.* 2014;38(3):118–124. Available from: https://doi.org/10.1097/JWH.0000000000000020.
31. Shamley D, Lascurain-Aguirrebeña I, Oskrochi R, Srinaganathan R. Shoulder morbidity after treatment for breast cancer is bilateral and greater after mastectomy. *Acta Oncol.* 2012;51(8):1045–1053. Available from: https://doi.org/10.3109/0284186X.2012.695087.
32. Springer BA, Levy E, McGarvey C, et al. Pre-operative assessment enables early diagnosis and recovery of shoulder function in patients with breast cancer. *Breast Cancer Res Treat.* 2010;120(1):135–147. Available from: https://doi.org/10.1007/s10549-009-0710-9.
33. Shamley DR, Srinanaganathan R, Weatherall R, et al. Changes in shoulder muscle size and activity following treatment for breast cancer. *Breast Cancer Res Treat.* 2007;106(1):19–27. Available from: https://doi.org/10.1007/s10549-006-9466-7.
34. Sugden EM, Rezvani M, Harrison JM, Hughes LK. Shoulder movement after the treatment of early stage breast cancer. *Clin Oncol (R Coll Radiol).* 1998;10(3):173–181. Available from: https://doi.org/10.1016/s0936-6555(98)80063-0.
35. Nesvold I-L, Dahl AA, Løkkevik E, Marit Mengshoel A, Fosså SD. Arm and shoulder morbidity in breast cancer patients after breast-conserving therapy versus mastectomy. *Acta Oncol.* 2008;47(5):835–842. Available from: https://doi.org/10.1080/02841860801961257.
36. Tengrup I, Tennvall-Nittby L, Christiansson I, Laurin M. Arm morbidity after breast-conserving therapy for breast cancer. *Acta Oncol.* 2000;39(3):393–397. Available from: https://doi.org/10.1080/028418600750013177.
37. Kärki A, Simonen R, Mälkiä E, Selfe J. Impairments, activity limitations and participation restrictions 6 and 12 months after breast cancer operation. *J Rehabil Med.* 2005;37(3):180–188. Available from: https://doi.org/10.1080/16501970410024181.
38. Park JH, Lee YK, Kim DH, et al. Usefulness of 18F-fluorodeoxyglucose positron emission tomography-computed tomography in monitoring adhesive capsulitis after breast cancer treatment. *J Comput Assist Tomogr.* 2015;39(3):349–355. Available from: https://doi.org/10.1097/RCT.0000000000000222.
39. Stubblefield MD, Custodio CM. Upper-extremity pain disorders in breast cancer. *Arch Phys Med Rehabil.* 2006;87(3 suppl 1):S96–S99. Available from: https://doi.org/10.1016/j.apmr.2005.12.017. quiz S100-1.
40. Monleon S, Ferrer M, Tejero M, Pont A, Piqueras M, Belmonte R. Shoulder strength changes one year after axillary lymph node dissection or sentinel lymph node

biopsy in patients with breast cancer. *Arch Phys Med Rehabil*. 2016;97(6):953–963. Available from: https://doi.org/10.1016/j.apmr.2015.12.014.

41. Rietman JS, Dijkstra PU, Geertzen JHB, et al. Treatment-related upper limb morbidity 1 year after sentinel lymph node biopsy or axillary lymph node dissection for stage I or II breast cancer. *Ann Surg Oncol*. 2004;11(11):1018–1024. Available from: https://doi.org/10.1245/ASO.2004.03.512.
42. Verbelen H, Gebruers N, Eeckhout F-M, Verlinden K, Tjalma W. Shoulder and arm morbidity in sentinel node-negative breast cancer patients: a systematic review. *Breast Cancer Res Treat*. 2014;144(1):21–31. Available from: https://doi.org/10.1007/s10549-014-2846-5.
43. Kootstra JJ, Dijkstra PU, Rietman H, et al. A longitudinal study of shoulder and arm morbidity in breast cancer survivors 7 years after sentinel lymph node biopsy or axillary lymph node dissection. *Breast Cancer Res Treat*. 2013;139(1):125–134. Available from: https://doi.org/10.1007/s10549-013-2509-y.
44. Myung Y, Choi B, Kwon H, et al. Quantitative analysis of shoulder function and strength after breast reconstruction: A retrospective cohort study. *Medicine (Baltimore)*. 2018;97(24):e10979. Available from: https://doi.org/10.1097/MD.0000000000010979.
45. Forthomme B, Heymans O, Jacquemin D, et al. Shoulder function after latissimus dorsi transfer in breast reconstruction. *Clin Physiol Funct Imaging*. 2010;30(6):406–412. Available from: https://doi.org/10.1111/j.1475-097X.2010.00956.x.
46. Lohana P, Button J, Young D, Hart A, Weiler-Mithoff E. Functional recovery after bilateral extended autologous latissimus dorsi breast reconstruction: a prospective observational study. *J Plast Reconstr Aesthet Surg*. 2019;72(7):1060–1066. Available from: https://doi.org/10.1016/j.bjps.2019.01.013.
47. Steffenssen MCW, Kristiansen A-LH, Damsgaard TE. A systematic review and meta-analysis of functional shoulder impairment after latissimus dorsi breast reconstruction. *Ann Plast Surg*. 2019;82(1):116–127. Available from: https://doi.org/10.1097/SAP.0000000000001691.
48. Woo K-J, Lee K-T, Mun G-H, Pyon J-K, Bang SI. Effect of breast reconstruction modality on the development of postmastectomy shoulder morbidity. *J Plast Reconstr Aesthet Surg*. 2018;71(12):1761–1767. Available from: https://doi.org/10.1016/j.bjps.2018.07.033.
49. McNeely ML, Binkley JM, Pusic AL, Campbell KL, Gabram S, Soballe PW. A prospective model of care for breast cancer rehabilitation: postoperative and postreconstructive issues. *Cancer*. 2012;118(8 suppl):2226–2236. Available from: https://doi.org/10.1002/cncr.27468.
50. Hojan K, Milecki P. Opportunities for rehabilitation of patients with radiation fibrosis syndrome. *Rep Pract Oncol Radiother*. 2014;19(1):1–6. Available from: https://doi.org/10.1016/j.rpor.2013.07.007.
51. van Beek S, Jaeger K, de, Mijnheer B, van Vliet-Vroegindeweij C. Evaluation of a single-isocenter technique for axillary radiotherapy in breast cancer. *Med Dosim*. 2008;33(3):191–198. Available from: https://doi.org/10.1016/j.meddos.2007.06.003.
52. Farace P, Deidda MA, Amichetti M. Axillary irradiation omitting axillary dissection in breast cancer: is there a role for shoulder-sparing proton therapy? *Br J Radiol*. 2015;88(1054):20150274. Available from: https://doi.org/10.1259/bjr.20150274.
53. Blomqvist L, Stark B, Engler N, Malm M. Evaluation of arm and shoulder mobility and strength after modified radical mastectomy and radiotherapy. *Acta Oncol*. 2004;43(3):280–283. Available from: https://doi.org/10.1080/02841860410026170.
54. Caban ME, Freeman JL, Zhang DD, et al. The relationship between depressive symptoms and shoulder mobility among older women: assessment at one year after breast cancer diagnosis. *Clin Rehabil*. 2006;20(6):513–522. Available from: https://doi.org/10.1191/0269215506cr966oa.
55. Højris I, Andersen J, Overgaard M, Overgaard J. Late treatment-related morbidity in breast cancer patients randomized to postmastectomy radiotherapy and systemic treatment versus systemic treatment alone. *Acta Oncol*. 2000;39(3):355–372. Available from: https://doi.org/10.1080/028418600750013131.
56. Isaksson G, Feuk B. Morbidity from axillary treatment in breast cancer—a follow-up study in a district hospital. *Acta Oncol*. 2000;39(3):335–336. Available from: https://doi.org/10.1080/028418600750013104.
57. Johansson K, Ingvar C, Albertsson M, Ekdahl C. Arm lymphoedema, shoulder mobility and muscle strength after breast cancer treatment? A prospective 2-year study. *Adv Physiother*. 2001;3(2):55–66. Available from: https://doi.org/10.1080/14038190119371.
58. Heindel W, Gübitz R, Vieth V, Weckesser M, Schober O, Schäfers M. The diagnostic imaging of bone metastases. *Dtsch Arztebl Int*. 2014;111(44):741–747. Available from: https://doi.org/10.3238/arztebl.2014.0741.
59. Okur SC, Ozyemisci-Taskiran O, Pekindogan Y, Mert M, Caglar NS. Ultrasound-guided block of the suprascapular nerve in breast cancer survivors with limited shoulder motion – case series. *Pain Phys*. 2017;20(2):E233–E239.
60. Lee TS, Kilbreath SL, Refshauge KM, Pendlebury SC, Beith JM, Lee MJ. Pectoral stretching program for women undergoing radiotherapy for breast cancer. *Breast Cancer Res Treat*. 2007;102(3):313–321. Available from: https://doi.org/10.1007/s10549-006-9339-0.
61. Marazzi F, Masiello V, Marchesano D, et al. Shoulder girdle impairment in breast cancer survivors: the role of range of motion as predictive factor for dose distribution and clinical outcome. *Tumori*. 2019;105(4):319–330.
62. Offersen BV, Boersma LJ, Kirkove C, et al. ESTRO consensus guideline on target volume delineation for elective radiation therapy of early stage breast cancer, version 1.1. *Radiother Oncol.*. 2016;118(1):205–208. Available from: https://doi.org/10.1016/j.radonc.2015.12.027.
63. Pandya J, Johnson T, Low AK. Shoulder replacement for osteoarthritis: a review of surgical management. *Maturitas*. 2018;108:71–76. Available from: https://doi.org/10.1016/j.maturitas.2017.11.013.

64. Saraya S, El Bakry R. Ultrasound: can it replace MRI in the evaluation of the rotator cuff tears? *Egypt J Radiol Nucl Med.* 2016;47(1):193–201. Available from: https://doi.org/10.1016/j.ejrnm.2015.11.010.
65. Qayyum A, MacVicar AD, Padhani AR, Revell P, Husband JE. Symptomatic brachial plexopathy following treatment for breast cancer: utility of MR imaging with surface-coil techniques. *Radiology.* 2000;214(3):837–842. Available from: https://doi.org/10.1148/radiology.214.3.r00mr11837.
66. Andreou A, Sohaib A, Collins DJ, et al. Diffusion-weighted MR neurography for the assessment of brachial plexopathy in oncological practice. *Cancer Imaging.* 2015;15:6. Available from: https://doi.org/10.1186/s40644-015-0041-5.
67. Hoeller U, Bonacker M, Bajrovic A, Alberti W, Adam G. Radiation-induced plexopathy and fibrosis. Is magnetic resonance imaging the adequate diagnostic tool? *Strahlenther Onkol.*. 2004;180(10):650–654. Available from: https://doi.org/10.1007/s00066-004-1240-3.
68. Herrera JE, Stubblefield MD. Rotator cuff tendonitis in lymphedema: a retrospective case series. *Arch Phys Med Rehabil.* 2004;85(12):1939–1942. Available from: https://doi.org/10.1016/j.apmr.2004.06.065.
69. Moskovitz AH, Anderson BO, Yeung RS, Byrd DR, Lawton TJ, Moe RE. Axillary web syndrome after axillary dissection. *Am J Surg.* 2001;181(5):434–439. Available from: https://doi.org/10.1016/s0002-9610(01)00602-x.
70. Piper M, Guajardo I, Denkler K, Sbitany H. Axillary web syndrome: current understanding and new directions for treatment. *Ann Plast Surg.* 2016;76(suppl 3):S227–S231. Available from: https://doi.org/10.1097/SAP.0000000000000767.
71. Kaidar-Person O, Marks LB, Jones EL. Pentoxifylline and vitamin E for treatment or prevention of radiation-induced fibrosis in patients with breast cancer. *Breast J.* 2018;24(5):816–819. Available from: https://doi.org/10.1111/tbj.13044.
72. Beurskens CHG, van Uden CJT, Strobbe LJA, Oostendorp RAB, Wobbes T. The efficacy of physiotherapy upon shoulder function following axillary dissection in breast cancer, a randomized controlled study. *BMC Cancer.* 2007;7:166. Available from: https://doi.org/10.1186/1471-2407-7-166.
73. Kilbreath SL, Refshauge KM, Beith JM, et al. Upper limb progressive resistance training and stretching exercises following surgery for early breast cancer: a randomized controlled trial. *Breast Cancer Res Treat.* 2012;133(2):667–676. Available from: https://doi.org/10.1007/s10549-012-1964-1.
74. Yang A, Sokolof J, Gulati A. The effect of preoperative exercise on upper extremity recovery following breast cancer surgery: a systematic review. *Int J Rehabil Res.* 2018;41(3):189–196. Available from: https://doi.org/10.1097/MRR.0000000000000288.
75. Shin HJ, Shin JC, Kim WS, Chang WH, Lee SC. Application of ultrasound-guided trigger point injection for myofascial trigger points in the subscapularis and pectoralis muscles to post-mastectomy patients: a pilot study. *Yonsei Med J.* 2014;55(3):792–799. Available from: https://doi.org/10.3349/ymj.2014.55.3.792.
76. Warpenburg MJ. Deep friction massage in treatment of radiation-induced fibrosis: rehabilitative care for breast cancer survivors. *Integr Med (Encinitas).* 2014;13(5):32–36.

CHAPTER 14

Role of Interventional Pain Management in Breast Cancer

ASHISH KHANNA, MD

INTRODUCTION

Pain and decreased function in breast cancer are common and can be significant. One large study showed that 47% of women treated for breast cancer experienced pain and 58% reported sensory disturbances into the third year postoperatively, half rated this pain as moderate to severe.[1] Pain severe enough to limit function occurs in about 60% of cases.[2] As just one example of functional loss, consider arm morbidity after breast surgery and adjuvant treatments. As one might imagine, limitations in upper extremity range of motion have been linked to a reduction in ability to perform activities of daily living as well as a reduced health-related quality of life.[1,3] As such, pain and disability are among the most feared complications of breast cancer treatments.[4]

The evaluation of pain in this patient population requires an understanding of the pathophysiology and characteristics of breast cancer as a foundation. From there the patient-specific evaluation of the malignancy along with other comorbidities is used to clarify the cause(s) of the pain. Some pertinent questions are outlined in Table 14.2.

A careful history and physical examination will then focus on identifying pain generators. These can be divided into tumor- and treatment-related pain syndromes and then further divided into nociceptive and neuropathic pain syndromes. See Fig. 14.1 for common causes of pain in this population.

There are a few elements that require special attention during the physical exam of this unique population. For example, an inspection of the skin over irradiated areas and along the surgical incision should be done to evaluate for any signs of wound infection, adhesions, seromas, and neuromas. This should include the skin of the axilla for those who underwent nodal irradiation or lymphadenectomy. The muscles of the anterior and posterior chest wall should be palpated for asymmetry or myofascial pain. Observe for scapular winging. The shoulder should be moved through the full range of motion and inspected for any restrictions or weakness. Provocative maneuvers can be used to rule out rotator cuff or other musculoskeletal injuries to the shoulder girdle.[6]

POSTMASTECTOMY PAIN SYNDROME

Persistent breast pain following surgery is referred to as postmastectomy pain syndrome (PMPS). It is a collection of symptoms following any breast surgery, not just mastectomy, and can include lumpectomy, breast reconstruction, augmentation or reduction, and importantly is also inclusive of procedures done in the upper outer quadrant of the breast and axilla as well.[5] Though there are no universally accepted diagnostic criteria, it is agreed that pain must persist for more than 3 months postoperatively after all other causes of pain have been excluded. It typically presents with pain of neuropathic and/or musculoskeletal symptoms. Pain is commonly localized to the breast, chest wall, axilla, or ipsilateral shoulder or arm. This results in secondary limitations in functional range of motion and strength, including grip strength.[6] Risk factors for development of this type of pain are multifactorial and are presented in Table 14.1.[7]

RADIATION FIBROSIS SYNDROME

Under the umbrella of PMPS are several other syndromes that are seen in the breast cancer population that the clinician should be aware of. The first is radiation fibrosis syndrome, a collection of neuromuscular, musculoskeletal, and other complications resulting from radiation treatments. Nearly all patients will have some

Breast Cancer and Gynecologic Cancer Rehabilitation DOI: https://doi.org/10.1016/B978-0-323-72166-0.00014-1

TABLE 14.1
Risk Factors in Postmastectomy Pain Syndrome

Demographics	Younger age
	Lower socioeconomic status
Treatment and complication related	High degree of acute postoperative pain
	Extensiveness of axillary node dissection
	Intercostobrachial nerve injury
	Adjuvant chemotherapy or radiation
	Tumors location in upper outer quadrant
Psychosocial risk factors	Preoperative depression, anxiety, fatigue, sleep disturbance
	Maladaptive coping style (e.g., catastrophizing)

TABLE 14.2
Taking a Pain History

Severity	"How severe is your pain?"
Character	"How would you describe your pain?"
Location	"Where is your pain located? Can you point to it with one finger or is it diffuse?"
Radiation	"Does your pain travel or shoot anywhere?"
Timing	"When do you feel the pain the worst?"
Ameliorating/exacerbating factors	"What makes your pain better/worse?"
Impact	"How does this pain affect your daily life?"

symptoms in the acute period of radiation treatment. However, it is the late-term effects of radiation that manifest after years, even decades, that define this condition. Radiation fibrosis is a chronic, progressive, unpredictable, and nonreversible condition resulting from continued fibrotic changes to the radiated tissues. These tissues can be of any type—bone, muscle, skin, ligaments, viscera, or nerves. The proposed mechanism is a positive feedback loop resulting in proliferation of fibrin, into the microvasculature, which ultimately ends with progressive sclerosis of all tissues in the radiation field. Often times, symptoms will manifest when either neurovascular compromise and/or atrophy ultimately develop.[9] Sclerotic ligaments and tendons may shorten, resulting in loss of tissue elasticity and range of motion. Radiated musculature surrounding the shoulder, such as the rotator cuff, can become atrophied and lead to loss of function. Radiated chest wall musculature can begin to go into painful spasms, a result of ectopic firing of the injured motor nerves. This is seen particularly in the pectoralis major, serratus anterior, latissimus dorsi, and intercostal muscles.[7] The thoracodorsal, long thoracic, medial, and lateral pectoral nerves may also be in the radiation field and can lead to functional impairments.

Management of radiation fibrosis is largely symptomatic. Physical and occupational therapy can use manual techniques to mobilize fibrotic tissue. Stretching of the tissues causing shoulder dysfunction can improve range of motion and prevent further morbidity. There is some evidence that nerve stabilizers for neuropathic pain and opioid analgesics for nociceptive pain can be effective.[9] Botulinum toxin injections into painful spastic muscles, including those used for breast reconstruction, can also provide relief.[10] Though there is no known way to reverse radiation fibrosis, there is some evidence that its progress can be slowed using the combination of tocopherol and pentoxifylline. Tocopherol has vitamin E activity and is thought to be a free radical scavenger. Pentoxifylline limits fibroblast collagen proliferation and platelet aggregation among other properties. In combination, they serve to reduce oxidative stress and subcutaneous fibrosis. The optimal dose and duration has not been well defined, and there is evidence that high-dose tocopherol can increase all-cause mortality. In general, total dose vitamin E around 700–1000 IU/day and pentoxifylline 800 mg/day is recommended, with the author dividing it into twice-daily dosing. This combination is the only known treatment that could potentially slow the progression of radiation fibrosis.[11]

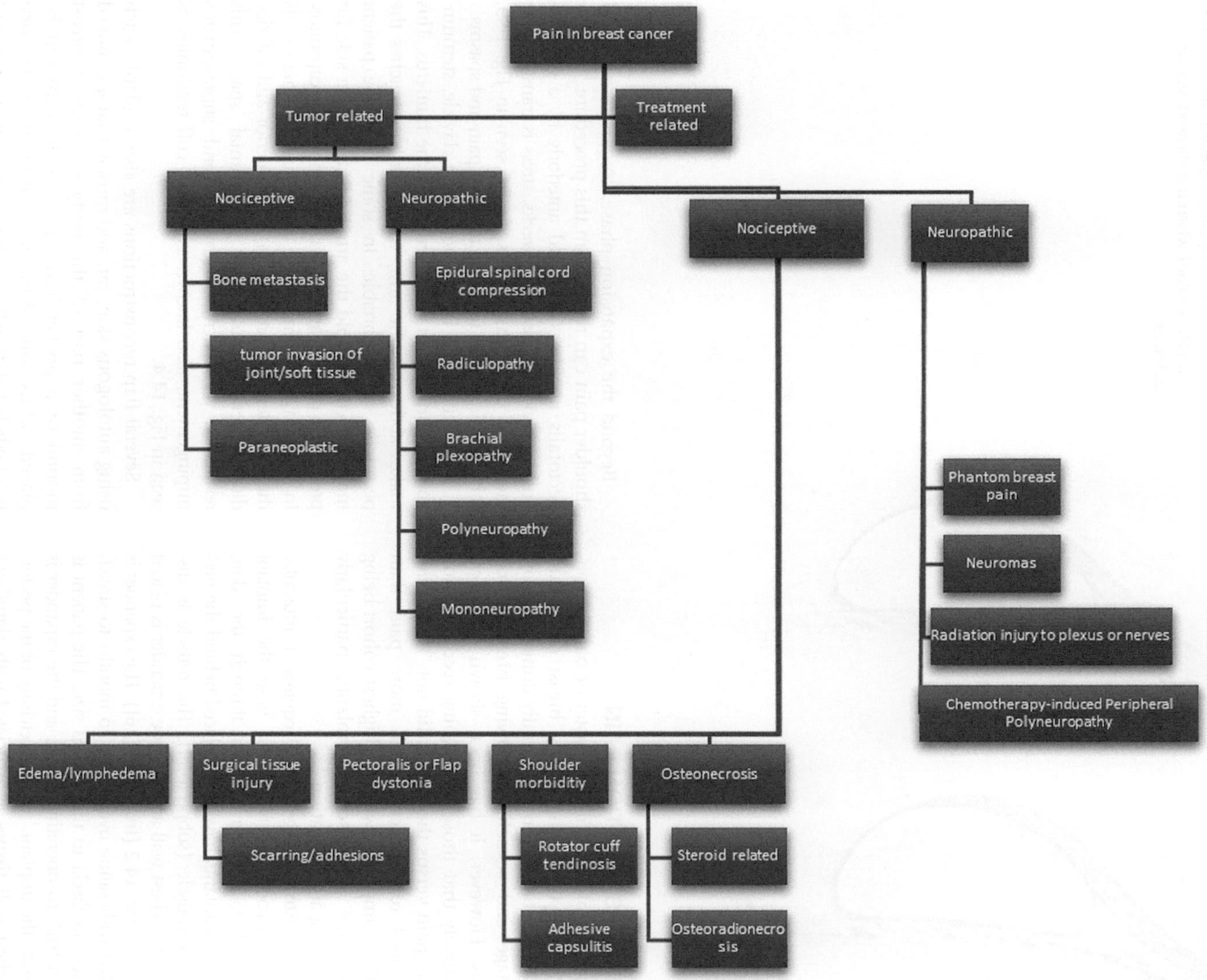

FIGURE 14.1 Pain generators in chronic breast pain.[8]

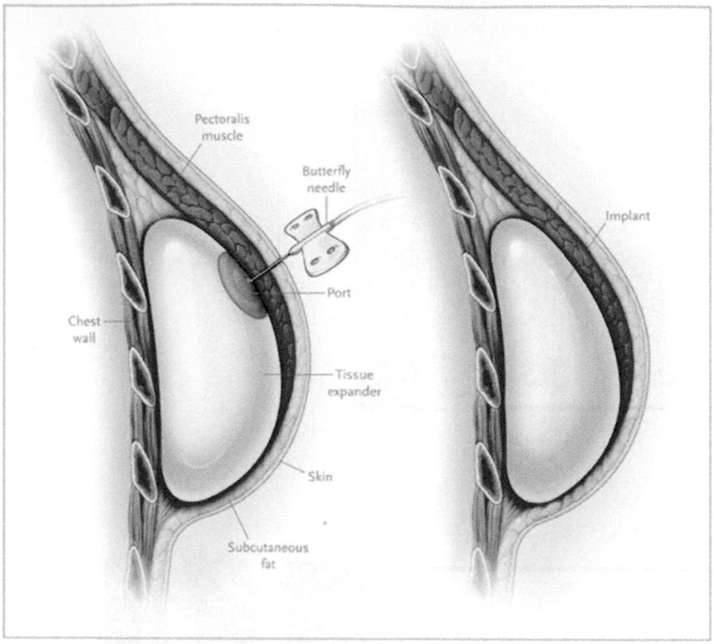

FIGURE 14.2 Tissue expanders are placed behind the pectoralis muscle and slowly expanded over time, stretching the pectoralis. It is then surgically replaced with the permanent implant when the desired size is achieved.

POSTRECONSTRUCTION PAIN

Another aspect of PMPS is the cluster of painful conditions seen in those undergoing breast reconstruction. Breast reconstruction is generally done to restore body image and sexuality following breast cancer treatments. However, it has been shown at 1 year postoperatively that those undergoing reconstruction have more pain versus those that did not. Those with implant-based reconstruction had more pain than those without implants, with the highest cohort being those that had submuscular implants, particularly those involving augmentation.[12]

Breast reconstruction generally requires a muscular "pocket" or myocutaneous flap to hold the implant in place and to prevent erosion through the skin. Traditionally, implants have been placed behind the pectoralis major muscle (subpectoral). The muscle is dissected from the chest wall and a tissue expander is placed beneath it. See Fig. 14.2 (from Ref. [16]). The expander is slowly filled with saline over weeks to months to stretch the muscle and fascia to the desired size. The patient is then taken back to operating room, and the expander is replaced with the implant.[13] This stretching of the pectoralis and chest wall tissues is associated with significant discomfort in the expansion phase. This pain can result in inadequate expansion as well as removal of the expanders, abandoning reconstruction.[14,15]

Beyond the expansion phase, long-term arm and shoulder pain can result from this procedure.[12] As the pectoralis muscle is stretched anteriorly by a continuously expanding vessel over weeks, stress is transferred to the points of attachment. As can be seen in Fig. 14.3, microscopic muscle tears can result in pain and spasms.

Thus tenderness is common at the clavicle, sternum, and, importantly, at the insertion of the humerus. This makes abducting the arm, which further stretches the pectoralis, uncomfortable. In some cases the patient may protectively hold the arm adducted at the side for prolonged periods and is at risk for adhesive capsulitis. In addition, stretching of the clavicular attachment pulls the shoulder into protraction. This anterior and inferior displacement narrows the subacromial space. This results in a subacromial bursitis and supraspinatus impingement, also known as rotator cuff tendonitis as seen in Fig. 14.4.

Several flap reconstructions are also available, each using autologous skin, fat, and muscle that are moved from another part of the body to create a breast mound or a pocket into which an implant can be placed. All use one of two surgical methods. The first is a pedicled flap, wherein the flap vasculature is kept intact and the tissue is "tunneled" underneath the skin to the chest wall. The second is a free flap, wherein the tissue is completely removed from the

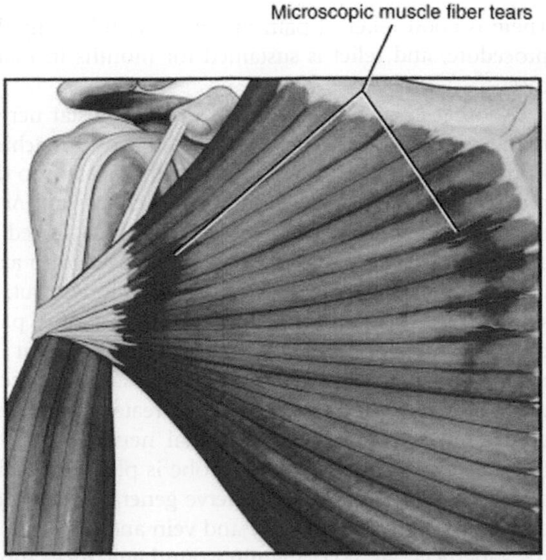

FIGURE 14.3 Stretching of the chest wall musculature results in microtears at the musculotendinous junction near the attachment points, resulting in pain and tenderness.

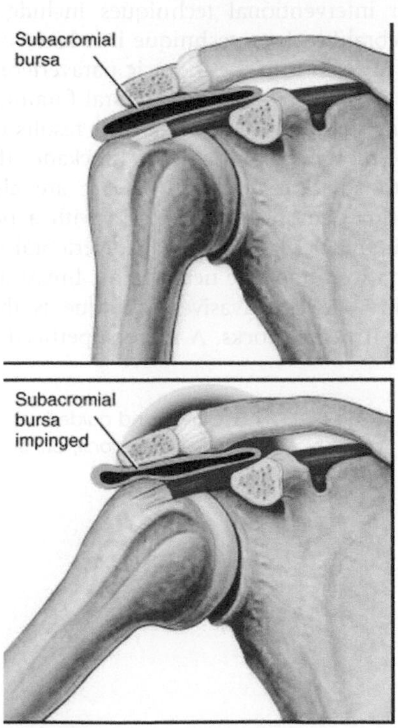

FIGURE 14.4 Subacromial bursitis and supraspinatus impingement as the result of a protracted shoulder, displacing the clavicle and acromion anteriorly and inferiorly. The result is a rotator cuff tendinopathy.

source and reattached to new vasculature in the chest wall using microsurgical techniques.[16]

Depending on the donor site and the amount of muscle removed, there can be functional implications. One of the most common pedicled myocutaneous flaps is the transverse rectus abdominis flap. Here, the rectus abdominis muscle, along with overlying soft tissue, is tunneled under the skin of the abdominal wall to the chest. This weakening of the truncal flexors results in a muscular imbalance with the extensors. Further, proprioceptive denervation may impact dynamic balance as truncal "righting" reflexes are impaired.[17] The latissimus dorsi flap similarly transposes a portion of that muscle from the mid-back around the body to the chest wall. Significant limitations in shoulder strength are likely to develop immediately postoperative, with varying degrees of recovery over time. This disruption of synergistic muscle patterns results in loss of shoulder function, which can sometimes persist for the long term.[18,19] Weakness is seen most prominently in shoulder extension, internal rotation, and adduction. These are movements in which the latissimus dorsi contributes and where compensation by surrounding muscles, such as the teres major, may be incomplete. In most cases, however, there is adequate compensation such that there is minimal functional impact with daily activities.[20]

INTERVENTIONAL PAIN TECHNIQUES

Breast pain has traditionally been treated with a combination of nociceptive pain medications, including NSAIDs and opiates, with or without neuropathic pain medications as appropriate, including gabapentinoids and antidepressants.[8] Other options include topical formulations of lidocaine, NSAIDs, and capsaicin as well as transcutaneous electrical nerve stimulation. However, a minority of patients may require a more invasive analgesic modality.

One postreconstruction issue is a focal dystonia of the muscles used for reconstruction. Hypoxia to serially expanded pectoral muscles as well as partial denervation to transposed flaps can result in continuous muscle fiber activity and spasms. This is termed neuromyotonia.[21] As with spasticity of other muscles, botulinum toxin injections are a treatment option that has shown success and can increase shoulder pain relief two-and-a-half fold. The dose to the pectoralis is usually 75–100 U, though up to 500 U has been shown to be safe.[22] The predicted spread is about 4.5 cm^2 so multiple injection sites within the muscle should be used.[23] Myocutaneous flaps, such as the latissimus dorsi flap, are also known to spasm and even demonstrate fasciculations. The toxin injections, by breaking these spasms and relaxing tonically contracted muscles, provide significant pain relief.[24] Ultrasound or EMG guidance is suggested for accuracy. Getting clearance from the plastic surgeon prior to doing any procedures on the flap is strongly recommended. For those that demonstrate success but desire a more long-term solution, referral back to the plastic surgeon for a neurectomy, a surgical removal of the nerve innervating the spastic flap, is a possibility.[25]

For those patients with severe pain along the incision with predominantly neuropathic symptoms, the postthoracotomy pain literature is instructive. Breast surgeries require violation of the chest wall tissues as do thoracotomies and, as such, a traumatic neuropathy resulting in severe allodynia and hyperalgesia surrounding the incisional area can be present. Though not entirely well understood, there is evidence that botulinum toxin has both nociceptive and neuropathic pain relief properties in addition to its antispasmotic properties.[26] Subcutaneous injections of 2–3 U of the toxin interspersed throughout the affected area about 1 cm^2 apart have shown promise in treating this condition.[27,28]

One regional anesthetic technique that shows promise in the management of breast pain is the ultrasound-guided serratus plane block. Here, blockade of the lateral cutaneous branches of the thoracic intercostal nerves T2–T12, but especially T2–T6, provides analgesia to the hemithorax. The patient is placed supine or in the lateral decubitus position. The ultrasound probe is placed at the midaxillary line, and a mixture of 10–20 mL of anesthetic and corticosteroid is injected between the muscle layers of the latissimus dorsi and the serratus anterior, as demonstrated in Figure 14.5. There is good relief of pain immediately following the procedure, and relief is sustained for months in many cases.[29–32]

Another cutaneous branch of the intercostal nerves is the intercostobrachial nerve, in this case branching from T1 and/or T2. It is responsible for sensation to the medial upper arm, axially, and lateral chest wall. As it traverses through the axilla, it is frequently sacrificed in axially node dissections and can be damaged with axillary radiation. Most often, it results in numbness but, in some cases, these injuries result in neuropathic pain called intercostobrachial neuralgia. Pain resistant to nerve-stabilizing medications and desensitization techniques have been successfully treated with an ultrasound-guided intercostobrachial nerve block. See Fig. 14.6. Here the ultrasound probe is placed over the posteromedial axilla with the nerve generally identified posterior to the axillary artery and vein and just deep to the superficial fascia. Using ultrasound guidance, about 3–5 mL of anesthetic and corticosteroid is used to hydrodissect the nerve while avoiding these vascular structures as well as the neighboring brachial plexus. Weeks to months of pain relief have been noted.[33–35]

Other interventional techniques include thoracic paravertebral blocks, a technique in which local anesthetic is injected into the thoracic paravertebral space, the area adjacent to the intervertebral foramina where the exiting spinal nerves emerge. This results in ipsilateral somatic and sympathetic blockade that may spread to adjacent levels.[36,37] There are also some case reports demonstrating success with a peripheral nerve stimulator placed in the paravertebral plexus as a solution to intractable neuropathic breast and chest wall pain.[38] A less invasive technique is the Pecs I and Pecs II nerve blocks. A more superficial block, it

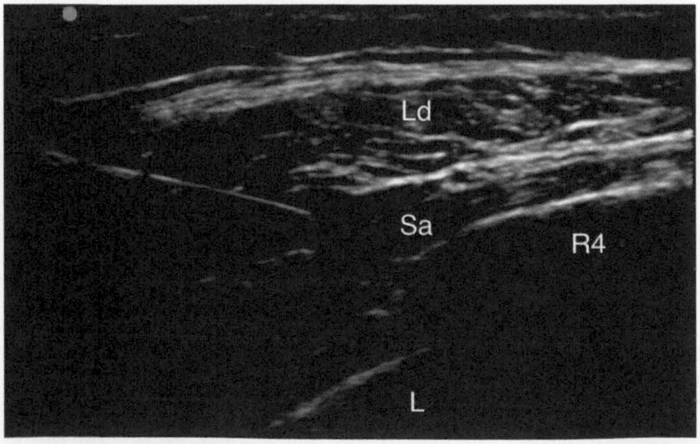

FIGURE 14.5 Ultrasound guided serratus plane block. *Ld: latissimus dorsi, Sa: serratus anterior, R4: 4th rib, L: lung.*

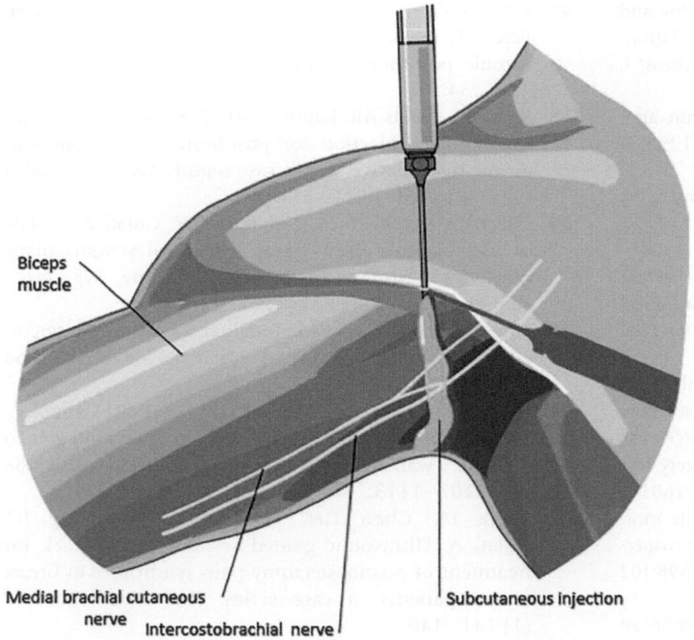

FIGURE 14.6 Medial brachial cutaneous and intercostobrachial nerve blocks. *From Waldman SD.* Atlas of Interventional Pain Management. *2nd ed. Philadelphia, PA: Saunders; 2004:p. 174. This is an Image from Elsevier/Sciencedirect.*

targets the lateral and median pectoral nerves at the interfacial plane between the pectoralis major and minor muscles. Both of these blocks have been shown to reduce postoperative pain following breast surgeries, though long-term success in the chronic breast pain population is variable.[39–42]

CONCLUSION

Pain and loss of function is routine following breast cancer surgeries. The perception that these issues will always resolve over time, or even worse, cannot be treated at all is unfortunately commonplace among members of the cancer care team. A multimodal approach involving conventional analgesics, interventional procedures, regional blocks plus holistic approaches should be considered in each case. A clinician attuned to taking a detailed cancer and pain history, performing a focused physical exam, and knowledgeable about treatment options can make a significant impact on the quality of life of patients affected by this most common cancer.

REFERENCES

1. Gartner R, Jensen MB, Nielsen J, Ewertz M, Kroman N, Kehlet H. Prevalence of and factors associated with persistent pain following breast cancer surgery. *JAMA.* 2009;302(18):1985–1992.
2. Cleeland CS, Gonin R, Hatfield AK, et al. Pain and its treatment in outpatients with metastatic cancer. *N Engl J Med.* 1994;330(9):592–596.
3. Campbell KL, Pusic AL, Zucker DS, et al. A prospective model of care for breast cancer rehabilitation: function. *Cancer.* 2012;118(8 suppl):2300–2311.
4. Azami-Aghdash S, Ghojazadeh M, Gareh Sheyklo S, et al. Breast cancer screening barriers from the womans perspective: a meta-synthesis. *Asian Pac J Cancer Prev.* 2015;16.
5. Macdonald L, Bruce J, Scott NW, Smith WCS, Chambers WA. Long-term follow-up of breast cancer survivors with post-mastectomy pain syndrome. *Br J Cancer.* 2005;92(2):225.
6. Stubblefield MD, Custodio CM. Upper-extremity pain disorders in breast cancer. *Arch Phys Med Rehabil.* 2006;87(3 suppl 1):S96–S99; quiz S100–101.
7. Wisotzky E, Hanrahan N, Lione TP, Maltser S. Deconstructing postmastectomy syndrome: implications for physiatric management. *Phys Med Rehabil Clin N Am.* 2017;28(1):153–169.
8. Saxena AK, Kumar S. Management strategies for pain in breast carcinoma patients: current opinions and future perspectives. *Pain Pract.* 2007;7(2):163–177.
9. Stubblefield MD. Radiation fibrosis syndrome: neuromuscular and musculoskeletal complications in cancer survivors. *P M R.* 2011;3(11):1041–1054.
10. Schwartz MS, Wren DR, Filshie J. Neuromyotonia in a muscle flap producing a convulsing breast: successful treatment with botulinum toxin. *Mov Disord.* 1998;13(1):188–190.

11. Kaidar-Person O, Marks LB, Jones EL. Pentoxifylline and vitamin E for treatment or prevention of radiation-induced fibrosis in patients with breast cancer. *Breast J.* 2018;24(5):816–819.
12. Wallace MS, Wallace AM, Lee J, Dobke MK. Pain after breast surgery: a survey of 282 women. *Pain.* 1996;66(2–3):195–205.
13. Radovan C. Breast reconstruction after mastectomy using the temporary expander. *Plast Reconstr Surg.* 1982;69(2):195–208.
14. Rimareix F, Masson J, Couturaud B, Revol M, Servant JM. Breast reconstruction by inflatable anatomical implant. Retrospective study of 65 cases. *Ann Chir Plast Esthet.* 1999;44.
15. Disa JJ, Ad-El DD, Cohen SM, Cordeiro PG, Hidalgo DA. The premature removal of tissue expanders in breast reconstruction. *Plast Reconstr Surg.* 1999;104(6):1662–1665.
16. Cordeiro PG. Breast reconstruction after surgery for breast cancer. *N Engl J Med.* 2008;359(15):1590–1601.
17. Edsander-Nord A, Jurell G, Wickman M. Donor-site morbidity after pedicled or free TRAM flap surgery: a prospective and objective study. *Plast Reconstr Surg.* 1998;102(5):1508–1516.
18. van Huizum MA, Hoornweg MJ, de Ruiter N, Oudenhoven E, Hage JJ, Veeger DJ. Effect of latissimus dorsi flap breast reconstruction on the strength profile of the upper extremity. *J Plast Surg Hand Surg.* 2016;50(4):202–207.
19. Giordano S, Kääriäinen M, Alavaikko J, Kaistila T, Kuokkanen H. Latissimus dorsi free flap harvesting may affect the shoulder joint in long run. *Scand J Surg.* 2011;100(3):202–207.
20. Lee K-T, Mun G-H. A systematic review of functional donor-site morbidity after latissimus dorsi muscle transfer. *Plast Reconstr Surg.* 2014;134(2):303–314.
21. Maddison P. Neuromyotonia. *Clin Neurophysiol.* 2006;117(10):2118–2127.
22. Winocour S, Murad MH, Bidgoli-Moghaddam M, et al. A systematic review of the use of botulinum toxin type A with subpectoral breast implants. *J Plast Reconstr Aesthet Surg.* 2014;67(1):34–41.
23. Marco E, Duarte E, Vila J, et al. Is botulinum toxin type A effective in the treatment of spastic shoulder pain in patients after stroke? A double-blind randomized clinical trial. *J Rehabil Med.* 2007;39(6):440–447.
24. Figus A, Mazzocchi M, Dessy LA, Curinga G, Scuderi N. Treatment of muscular contraction deformities with botulinum toxin type A after latissimus dorsi flap and sub-pectoral implant breast reconstruction. *J Plast Reconstr Aesthet Surg.* 2009;62(7):869–875.
25. Adkinson JM, Miller NF, Murphy Jr RX. Neurectomy for breast reconstruction-related spasms of the pectoralis major muscle. *J Plast Reconstr Aesthet Surg.* 2014;67(2):257–259.
26. Safarpour Y, Jabbari B. Botulinum toxin treatment of pain syndromes—an evidence based review. *Toxicon.* 2018;147:120–128.
27. Fabregat G, Asensio-Samper JM, Palmisani S, Villanueva-Perez VL, De Andres J. Subcutaneous botulinum toxin for chronic post-thoracotomy pain. *Pain Pract.* 2013;13(3):231–234.
28. Rashid S, Fields AR, Baumrucker SJ. Subcutaneous botulinum toxin injection for post-thoracotomy pain syndrome in palliative care: a case report. *Am J Hosp Palliat Care.* 2018;35(3):511–513.
29. Piracha MM, Thorp SL, Puttanniah V, Gulati A. "A tale of two planes": deep versus superficial serratus plane block for postmastectomy pain syndrome. *Reg Anesth Pain Med.* 2017;42(2):259–262.
30. Ohgoshi Y, Yokozuka M, Terajima K. [Serratus-intercostal plane block for breast surgery]. *Masui.* 2015;64(6):610–614.
31. Blanco R, Parras T, McDonnell JG, Prats-Galino A. Serratus plane block: a novel ultrasound-guided thoracic wall nerve block. *Anaesthesia.* 2013;68(11):1107–1113.
32. Zocca JA, Chen GH, Puttanniah VG, Hung JC, Gulati A. Ultrasound-guided serratus plane block for treatment of postmastectomy pain syndromes in breast cancer patients: a case series. *Pain Pract.* 2017;17(1):141–146.
33. Wisotzky EM, Saini V, Kao C. Ultrasound-guided intercostobrachial nerve block for intercostobrachial neuralgia in breast cancer patients: a case series. *PM R.* 2016;8(3):273–277.
34. Levy MH, Chwistek M, Mehta RS. Management of chronic pain in cancer survivors. *Cancer J.* 2008;14(6):401–409.
35. Loukas M, Hullett J, Louis Jr. RG, Holdman S, Holdman D. The gross anatomy of the extrathoracic course of the intercostobrachial nerve. *Clin Anat.* 2006;19(2):106–111.
36. Klein SM, Bergh A, Steele SM, Georgiade GS, Greengrass RA. Thoracic paravertebral block for breast surgery. *Anesth Analg.* 2000;90(6):1402–1405.
37. Karmakar MK. Thoracic paravertebral block. *Anesthesiology.* 2001;95(3):771–780.
38. Hegarty D, Goroszeniuk T. Peripheral nerve stimulation of the thoracic paravertebral plexus for chronic neuropathic pain. *Pain Physician.* 2011;14(3):295–300.
39. Blanco R, Fajardo M, Parras Maldonado T. Ultrasound description of Pecs II (modified Pecs I): a novel approach to breast surgery. *Rev Esp Anestesiol Reanim.* 2012;59(9):470–475.
40. Versyck B, van Geffen GJ, Van Houwe P. Prospective double blind randomized placebo-controlled clinical trial of the pectoral nerves (Pecs) block type II. *J Clin Anesth.* 2017;40:46–50.
41. Blanco R. The 'pecs block': a novel technique for providing analgesia after breast surgery. *Anaesthesia.* 2011;66(9):847–848.
42. KirvelÄ O, Antila H. Thoracic paravertebral block in chronic postoperative pain. *Reg Anesth Pain Med.* 1992;17(6):348–350.

CHAPTER 15

Aromatase Inhibitor Musculoskeletal Syndrome

MONICA GIBILISCO, DO • JONAS M. SOKOLOF, DO

INTRODUCTION

An aromatase inhibitor (AI) is a type of medication that stops the production of estrogen. This type of medication is the preferred treatment for hormone-receptor positive breast cancer in postmenopausal women. Since AIs cannot stop the ovaries from making estrogen, they are mostly used to treat postmenopausal women. The SOFT (Suppression of Ovarian Function Trial) study demonstrated that premenopausal women with hormone-receptor positive breast cancer could also be successfully treated with an AI if their ovarian function was suppressed. Ovarian suppression included either 5 years of triptorelin, surgical removal of the ovaries, or ovarian radiation.[1] AIs have been compared with tamoxifen, a selective estrogen receptor modulator. AIs and tamoxifen are both hormone therapies, but act in different ways. AIs lower the amount of estrogen in the body by stopping certain hormones from turning into estrogen, while tamoxifen blocks estrogen receptors on breast cancer cells. Hence, estrogen is still present in normal levels with tamoxifen use, while estrogen levels are low with the use of AIs. AIs are preferred for the use of hormone-receptor positive breast cancer in postmenopausal women over tamoxifen because studies have shown more benefits, reduced risk of cancer recurrence, and fewer side effects. Serious side effects of tamoxifen in postmenopausal women include endometrial cancer because tamoxifen acts as an antiestrogen in breast tissue but acts like estrogen in the uterus. This can stimulate the uterine lining to grow and increase the risk of endometrial cancer in postmenopausal women. AIs also have their side effects that can have an effect on a patient's quality of life and medication compliance. Their side effects include joint and muscle pain, osteoporosis, menopausal symptoms, hot flashes, vaginal dryness, and increased blood pressure. The arthralgia symptoms sometimes dominate patients' daily lives, and it is important to educate these patients on the necessity of exercise and rehabilitation.

ETIOLOGY AND PATHOGENESIS OF AROMATASE INHIBITOR MUSCULOSKELETAL SYNDROME

Estrogen Deprivation

The musculoskeletal side effects of AIs, including the arthralgia, myalgia, and stiffness, have been termed aromatase inhibitor musculoskeletal syndrome (AIMSS). The etiology of the syndrome is not well understood but is based off a few theories. Estrogen deprivation has been hypothesized as the major cause of AI arthralgia. It is unclear if the arthralgia is due to systemic or localized estrogen deficiency. Studies have shown that estrogen has chondroprotective effects by decreasing collagen degradation. Also, estrogen-based therapy has been associated with a reduced incidence of knee osteoarthritis and a reduced incidence of joint pain and swelling.[2] In an animal study, mice with surgically removed ovaries demonstrated accelerated cartilage turnover, which was presumed to be linked to their decreased amount of estrogen.[3] Since AIs stop the production of estrogen and estrogen decreases collagen and cartilage degradation, it can be inferred that this can be associated with the side effect of arthralgia.

Estrogen also has a natural antinociceptive property, meaning it blocks the detection of pain. This pathology is explained by opioid-containing neurons in the spinal cord which contain estrogen receptors.[4] Hence, patients taking AIs may also feel an increased sensation of pain which contributes to their arthralgia.

Lastly, there have been many studies in rheumatology that found that drops in estrogen causes cytokines to be released in high levels, which may accelerate bone loss. Research has demonstrated that synovial

Breast Cancer and Gynecologic Cancer Rehabilitation DOI: https://doi.org/10.1016/B978-0-323-72166-0.00015-3

cells express aromatase, and when aromatase induces the conversion of androstenedione to estradiol and estrone, IL-6 expression is decreased in the joint.[5] IL-6 is both a pro- and antiinflammatory cytokine, but it has been linked to being one of the main causes of increased bone loss in postmenopausal women.[6] Hence, when using an AI, a patient will have increased IL-6 expression, demonstrating another possible pathological explanation of AIMSS.

Tenosynovial Pathology

There have been several characteristic radiologic findings in patients with AIMSS. A key finding in some studies has been localized tenosynovial pathology to the hands and feet. In one study, 13 out of 28 patients with symptoms of AI arthralgia had evidence of tenosynovitis. In these patients, there was an absence of autoantibody development, which suggests more of a localized tenosynovitis instead of a systemic inflammatory process.[7] There were also less complaints of lower back and knee pain, which are more common for postmenopausal pain, which suggested that this pathology was most likely not due to osteoarthritis seen in menopause.

Another study showed 12 patients on AIs who reported severe morning stiffness and pain in their hands and wrists, causing impairment in closing and stretching both the hands and fingers. Trigger finger and carpal tunnel syndrome were the two most common reported clinical signs. Both ultrasound and MRI were used to demonstrate the radiologic findings. Ultrasound results showed fluid in the tendon sheath that enclosed the digital flexor tendons, and MRI results showed an enhancement and thickening of the tendon sheath. These MRI results were found in all 12 patients.[8]

A final study that suggested fluid retention within joints plays a key role in AI arthralgia showed that women, who were on AIs and also had chronic diuretic treatment for other medical conditions, were less likely to report muscle pains or stiffness.[9]

Autoimmunity

Some studies show absence of autoantibody development in AIMSS, while others show patients with elevated antinuclear antibodies and rheumatoid factor concentrations. One study selected 30 patients with AIMSS and 22 controls without the syndrome. Serum samples were collected at baseline and during treatment which tested for multiple inflammatory cytokines and lipid mediators. The study found there were no statistically significant changes during AI therapy between cases and controls for any of the inflammatory markers tested.[10] This study concluded that the syndrome is most likely not associated with a systemic inflammatory response, but a localized one.

Clinical Characteristics

AIMSS typically presents with symmetrical joint pain, stiffness, myalgia, and decreased grip strength. Almost all joints have been reported in research causing pain in AI arthralgia, but some studies have shown it most commonly targets the hands, knees, and back.[11] It has also been shown to present with carpal tunnel syndrome, trigger finger, and De Quervain's tendonitis.[8] The onset of symptoms varies; however, the median time has been shown to be 1.6 months. This ranges with some patients noticing symptoms a couple of weeks into treatment, while others did not start to feel symptoms until 10 months. Symptoms also tend to be their highest at about 6 months.[12]

Noncompliance

The pain and arthralgia that some of these patients face are so severe that these can lead to noncompliance of taking their AI. There have been several studies that demonstrate this. Among 437 patients using AIs, 47 prematurely discontinued their AI with an average of 29 months after initiation of therapy. Patients reported worsening joint pain, which they rated as a 4 or greater on the Brief Pain Inventory scale. A score of 0 meant no pain and a score of 10 meant the worse pain you can imagine. In this study, 11% of patients discontinued their therapy, with the number one cause being joint pain (57%).[13] The musculoskeletal pain in these breast cancer patients was so debilitating that they would rather not finish their treatments than experience it.

Diagnosis

Currently, no objective diagnostic criteria for AIMSS exists. This causes variation in the diagnosis of AIMSS, and in its incidence, since providers may be using different criteria to define it.

An MRI is a diagnostic test that can demonstrate changes in AIMSS. MRI studies in patients taking AIs have shown tenosynovial changes and increased intraarticular fluid.[14] Tenosynovial changes were defined as an increase in the amount of fluid in the tendon sheath or the thickening and enhancement of the tendon sheaths. Ultrasound can also show fluid in the tendon sheath. However, there does not have to be diagnostic test pathology to define AIMSS, since no definitive criteria exist.

Treatment

Medications

Medications can be used to try and treat the symptoms of AIMSS, but there is no true first line appropriate method identified as research is still in progress. Pain medications that can be used include acetaminophen, topical or oral nonsteroidal antiinflammatory drugs, and tramadol.

Glucosamine and chondroitin sulfate treatment showed moderate improvement in musculoskeletal symptoms after 24 weeks of treatment in patients with AI arthralgia.[15]

A trial of duloxetine showed clinically significant improvement in pain scores in patients on AIs.[16] Patients were treated with duloxetine for 8 weeks, and the results showed a 30% decrease in the average pain score over 8 weeks.

Calcitonin has been demonstrated to improve bone pain during AI treatment but did not have an effect on bone loss during the cancer treatment.[17]

Role of Rehabilitation Medicine

The physiatrist and members of the rehabilitation team, which commonly includes physical and occupational therapists, can be of great help to minimize the pain and improve the function of patients with AIMSS. The physiatrist has expertise in musculoskeletal medicine and can diagnose and treat the pain associated with this condition using medications and injections. They can also prescribe and monitor an effective treatment plan that includes physical and/or occupational therapy. Physical therapy can help these patients improve their physical abilities and regain strength, while occupational therapy can focus on improving activities of daily living.

Exercise

Exercise has been shown to improve a patient's musculoskeletal symptoms while taking an AI. One study demonstrated that 150 minutes per week of moderate intensity cardiovascular exercise and 2 days a week of resistance training provided a statistically significant improvement in the pain levels of patients with AI arthralgia.[18]

Another study investigated whether postmenopausal women on AI therapy differed from healthy postmenopausal women when they compared their responses to the same exact aerobic and resistance training programs. The results demonstrated that postmenopausal women on AI therapy and healthy postmenopausal women demonstrated similar improvements in body fat mass and estimated lower body strength. One difference was that healthy postmenopausal women demonstrated an increase in upper body strength after 6 months, while postmenopausal women on AI therapy demonstrated an improvement after 9 months of training. Overall, the study concluded that postmenopausal women on AI therapy have the ability to adapt to the same regimen of resistance and aerobic training as healthy postmenopausal women. This shows the importance of a combined exercise program for the treatment of AIMSS.[19]

Prophylaxis

In addition to arthralgias, women taking AIs are also at an increased risk for fractures. AI-associated bone loss is 2–4 × greater than bone loss in physiological postmenopausal bone loss in women.[20] Denosumab, intravenous and oral biphosphonates have been demonstrated to effectively prevent AI-associated bone loss in patients with breast cancer. The Adjuvant Denosumab in Breast Cancer Trial demonstrated the significant risk reduction of any clinical fracture in women taking denosumab in comparison to only calcium and vitamin D.[21] The Z-FAST trials (Zometa-Femara Adjuvant Synergy Trials) demonstrated that IV bisphosphonates also prevented AI-associated bone loss. This trial analyzed the efficacy of giving zoledronate to patients while starting AI therapy versus waiting to give zoledronate after a bone mineral density decrease to a *T*-score of <2.0. The delayed treatment resulted in a loss of bone mineral density at the lumbar spine and hip.[22] Oral bisphosphonates, such as risedronate, also demonstrated an increased bone mineral density by 2.2% in patients who started risedronate immediately versus a placebo for 2 years.[23] Women on AIs who develop osteoporosis are at an increased risk of bone fracture and musculoskeletal arthralgias. Recommendations have been made that patients on AIs should be offered biphosphonates and calcium to reduce the incidence of these symptoms.[24]

Risk Factors

There are no consistent predictors for the development of risk factors for AIMSS. Some studies have demonstrated an increased risk for arthralgias and musculoskeletal symptoms in women with a low BMI. Women who were overweight with a BMI of 25–30 were less likely to experience AI-related joint pain.[25]

Another risk factor that has demonstrated discordant information is the use of previous hormone replacement therapy such as tamoxifen. In one study, patients who were previously treated with tamoxifen were less likely to develop AI-related joint pain and stiffness, in comparison to those who had never received tamoxifen.[25] However, in another study, prior use of tamoxifen was related to discontinuation of AIs due to the aromatase-inhibitor-associated arthralgia.[26]

In another study in which patients were treated with a taxane, it was noted that those women were four times more likely to experience joint pain.[25]

A final risk factor that has also been researched has been the relationship between lengths of time since cessation of menstruation to onset of AI-associated arthralgia. Research has shown that the time since a woman's last menstrual period was inversely related to their report of AI-related arthralgia. This concept supports the theory that estrogen withdrawal plays a role in AIMSS since women have lower estrogen levels after menopause.[27]

CONCLUSION

In conclusion, AIMSS is very common in women taking an AI as part of their breast cancer treatment. Although the exact cause of AIMSS is not clearly known, there is speculation that estrogen has an important role in the proper function of joints and the reduction in estrogen as part of this treatment can contribute to the development of joint symptomatology in users. The early identification and initiation of treatment can help reduce pain, minimize loss of function, and maximize quality of life. Physiatrists can have a very important role in the assessment and treatment of this disabling condition.

REFERENCES

1. Francis PA, Regan MM, Fleming GF, et al. Adjuvant ovarian suppression in premenopausal breast cancer. *N Engl J Med.* 2015;(5)2436. <http://arktos.nyit.edu/login?url = http://search.ebscohost.com.arktos.nyit.edu/login.aspx?direct = true&db = edsgao&AN = edsgcl.403715857&site = eds-live&scope = site>.
2. Gaillard S, Stearns V. Aromatase inhibitor-associated bone and musculoskeletal effects: new evidence defining etiology and strategies for management. *Breast Cancer Res.* 2011;(2). Available from: https://doi.org/10.1186/bcr2818.
3. Din O, Dodwell D, Wakefield R, et al. Aromatase inhibitor induced arthralgia in early breast cancer: what do we know and how can we find out more? *Breast Cancer Res Treat.* 2010;120:525–538.
4. Dawson-Basoa M, Gintzler A. Gestational and ovarian sex steroid antinociception: synergy between spinal kappa and delta opioid systems. *Brain Res.* 1998;794:61–67.
5. Le Bail J, Liagre B, Vergne P, et al. Aromatase in synovial cells from postmenopausal women. *Steroids.* 2001;66:749–757.
6. Forsblad d'Elia H, Mattsson L, Ohlsson C, et al. Hormone replacement therapy in rheumatoid arthritis is associated with lower serum levels of soluble IL-6 receptor and higher insulin-like growth factor 1. *Arthritis Res Ther.* 2003;5:R202–R209.
7. Singer O, Cigler T, Moore AB, et al. Defining the aromatase inhibitor musculoskeletal syndrome: a prospective study. *Arthritis Care Res.* 2012;64(12):1910–1918. Available from: https://doi.org/10.1002/acr.21756.
8. Morales L, Pans S, Paridaens R, et al. Debilitating musculoskeletal pain and stiffness with letrozole and exemestane: associated tenosynovial changes on magnetic resonance imaging. *Breast Cancer Res Treat.* 2007;104:87–91.
9. Xepapadakis G, Ntasiou P, Koronarchis D, et al. New views on treatment of aromatase inhibitors induced arthralgia. *Breast.* 2010;19:249–250. Available from: https://doi.org/10.1016/j.breast.2010.03.031.
10. Henry NL, Pchejetski D, A'Hern R, et al. Inflammatory cytokines and aromatase inhibitor-associated musculoskeletal syndrome: a case-control study. *Br J Cancer.* 2010;103:291–296. Available from: https://doi.org/10.1038/sj.bjc.6605768.
11. Crew K, Greenlee H, Capodice J, et al. Prevalence of joint symptoms in postmenopausal women taking aromatase inhibitors for early stage breast cancer. *J Clin Oncol.* 2007;25:3877–3883.
12. Henry N, Giles J, Ang D, et al. Prospective characterization of musculoskeletal symptoms in early stage breast cancer patients treated with aromatase inhibitors. *Breast Cancer Res Treat.* 2008;111:365–372.
13. Chim K, Xie SX, Stricker CT, et al. Joint pain severity predicts premature discontinuation of aromatase inhibitors in breast cancer survivors. *BMC Cancer.* 2013;13(1):1–7. Available from: https://doi.org/10.1186/1471-2407-13-401.
14. Lintermans A, Laenen A, Van Calster B, et al. Prospective study to assess fluid accumulation and tenosynovial changes in the aromatase inhibitor-induced musculoskeletal syndrome: 2-year follow-up data. *Ann Oncol.* 2013;24(2):350–355. Available from: https://doi.org/10.1093/annonc/mds290.
15. Greenlee H, Crew KD, Shao T, et al. Phase II study of glucosamine with chondroitin on aromatase inhibitor-associated joint symptoms in women with breast cancer.

Support Care Cancer. 2013;21(4):1077–1087. Available from: https://doi.org/10.1007/s00520-012-1628-z.

16. Henry NL, Banerjee M, Wicha M, et al. Pilot study of duloxetine for treatment of aromatase inhibitor-associated musculoskeletal symptoms. *Cancer.* 2011;117:5469–5475.
17. Liu P, Yang D, Xie F, Zhour B, Liu M. Effect of calcitonin on anastrozole-induced bone pain during aromatase inhibitor therapy for breast cancer. *Genet Mol Res.* 2014;13(3):5285–5291.
18. Irwin ML, Cartmel B, Gross C, et al. Randomized exercise trial of aromatase inhibitor-induced arthralgia in breast cancer survivors. *J Clin Oncol.* 2015;33:1104–1111.
19. de Paulo TRS, Winters-Stone KM, Viezel J, et al. Comparing exercise responses to aerobic plus resistance training between postmenopausal breast cancer survivors undergoing aromatase inhibitor therapy and healthy women. *Disabil Rehabil.* 2019;41(18):2175–2182. Available from: https://doi.org/10.1080/09638288.2018.1460877.
20. Hadji P, Aapro MS, Body JJ, et al. Management of Aromatase Inhibitor-Associated Bone Loss (AIBL) in postmenopausal women with hormone sensitive breast cancer: joint position statement of the IOF, CABS, ECTS, IEG, ESCEO IMS, and SIOG. *J Bone Oncol.* 2017;7:1–12. Available from: https://doi.org/10.1016/j.jbo.2017.03.001. Published 2017 Mar 23.
21. Gnant M. Denosumab and fracture risk in women with breast cancer–Author's reply. *Lancet.* 2015;386(10008):2057–2058.
22. Coleman R, Bundred N, de Boer R, et al. Impact of zoledronic acid in postmenopausal women with early breast cancer receiving adjuvant letrozole: Z-FAST, ZO-FAST, and E-ZO-FAST. In: *Proceedings of the 32nd Annual San Antonio Breast Cancer Symposium.* San Antonio, TX [abstract 4082], December 9–13, 2009.
23. Van Poznak C, Hannon RA, Mackey JR. Prevention of aromatase inhibitor-induced bone loss using risedronate: the SABRE trial. *J Clin Oncol.* 2010;28:967–975.
24. Muslimani AA, et al. Aromatase inhibitor–related musculoskeletal symptoms: is preventing osteoporosis the key to eliminating these symptoms? *Clin Breast Cancer.* 2009;9(1):34–38.
25. Crew KD, Greenlee H, Capodice J, et al. *J Clin Oncol.* 2007;25(25):3877–3883.
26. Park L, Lee S, Bae S, et al. Aromatase inhibitor-associated musculoskeletal symptoms: incidence and associated factors. *J Korean Surg Soc.* 2013;85(5):205.
27. Mao JJ, Stricker C, Bruner D, et al. Patterns and risk factors associated with aromatase inhibitor-related arthralgia among breast cancer survivors. *Cancer.* 2009;115:3631–3639. Available from: https://doi.org/10.1002/cncr.24419.

CHAPTER 16

Systemic Therapy for Gynecologic Malignancies

JOHN P. DIAZ, MD, FACOG

INTRODUCTION

This chapter will review the use of chemotherapy in all gynecological cancers. The goal is to provide an overview of current therapeutic options. Chemotherapy is part of the multidisciplinary approach to the treatment of gynecologic malignancies. In recent years, traditional chemotherapy has been augmented with the growing knowledge of tumor genomics. The identification of molecular pathways, cell signaling, and tumorigenesis has the potential to revolutionize care as we move toward "personalized medicine."

Chemotherapy has evolved from single-agent therapy with alkylating agents and antimetabolites in the 1950s to the use of contemporary combination chemotherapy regimens that include the taxanes, platinums, anthracyclines, and other drugs.

OVARIAN CANCER

Epithelial cancers of ovarian, fallopian tubal, and peritoneal origin exhibit similar clinical characteristics and behavior. As a result, they are often combined together and define as epithelial ovarian cancer (EOC) in clinical trials and clinical practice. For this chapter, we will consider all histologies under the heading EOC. EOC is the most common cause of death among women with gynecologic malignancies and the fifth leading cause of cancer death in women in the United States. Approximately 75% of women have advanced-stage disease at the time of diagnosis.

Surgery remains the backbone of the treatment, either as the initial therapy or as a delayed primary procedure.[1] Systemic chemotherapy is central to the management of metastatic ovarian cancer. The established agents that continue to be used most frequently are carboplatin and paclitaxel. Following primary surgery, the conventional approach has been to use six cycles of standard carboplatin and paclitaxel at three weekly intervals, although alternatives are emerging. There are two options for the administration: intravenous (IV) chemotherapy alone or a combination of IV and intraperitoneal (IP) chemotherapy (IV/IP therapy). Primary cytoreductive surgery with the aim of optimal cytoreduction (i.e., no residual disease) remains the standard of care. In women who have had optimally resected disease, extended follow-up in four randomized trials has shown that IP chemotherapy with platinums and taxanes is highly effective in reducing the risk of recurrence and prolonging survival.[2–5] The adoption of IP chemotherapy has been mixed because of the perceived risk of toxicity and difficulties in managing IP catheters.

For those patients in whom IV therapy has been selected, the standard treatment is to administer carboplatin and paclitaxel every 3 weeks for a total of six cycles of therapy. An alternative regimen use dose-dense schedules with weekly IV paclitaxel in combination with three-week carboplatin. The initial experience came from the Japanese data, now with mature follow-up shows significant benefit to patients who received dose-dense schedules.[6] The downside of this schedule is that patients need more frequent attendances for treatment; however, the overall toxicity is lower.

Subsequently the European Trial MITO-7 demonstrated improved tolerability with the modified dose-dense regimen of a lower dose of weekly paclitaxel than in other dose-dense regimens over conventional dosing.[7] We typically suggest this regimen for medically frail patients. There is no clear consensus on the role of dose-dense versus conventionally dosed therapy. In general, trials have suggested similar or improved efficacy with dose-dense regimens relative to conventionally dosed therapy, though toxicities are typically higher. Two additional trials

Breast Cancer and Gynecologic Cancer Rehabilitation DOI: https://doi.org/10.1016/B978-0-323-72166-0.00016-5

evaluated the dose-dense regimen. ICON8 randomized almost 1600 patients to treatment with six cycles of either the standard every-3-week dosing regimen or with one of two different regimens, including once weekly carboplatin and dose-dense paclitaxel. This study failed to demonstrate a survival advantage of dose-dense over conventional schedule. Contrary to the Japanese trial, the patients who received the dose-dense regimen experienced greater toxicity.[8] In GOG 262, women with stage II–IV EOC who had either optimally or suboptimally cytoreduced disease were randomly assigned to conventionally dosed carboplatin and paclitaxel or to dose-dense therapy, carboplatin every 3 weeks plus weekly paclitaxel.[9] Bevacizumab administration was optional in both arms and was administered to 84% of patients. The majority of patients had stage III or IV disease. At a median follow-up of 28 months, there was no difference in survival between the dose-dense and the conventionally dosed treatment groups. While the study did not demonstrate and advantage to dose-dense over conventional treatment, a subset analysis suggested a treatment difference based on whether or not bevacizumab was administered. For those patients who were treated with chemotherapy only, dose-dense treatment prolonged progression-free survival (PFS) compared with conventional dosing. For those patients who were treated with chemotherapy and bevacizumab, PFS was similar among those treated with dose-dense versus conventionally dosed treatment.

Primary medical therapy, that is neoadjuvant chemotherapy (NACT), is now accepted as an alternative standard of care for patients who are deemed to be unlikely to obtain an optimal cytoreduction at the completion of their surgical effort or who are too frail to tolerate an aggressive surgical effort. Two important European trials, the European Organization for Research and Treatment of Cancer (EORTC) 55971 study and the UK-led CHORUS study, have shown that NACT followed by delayed primary surgery is not inferior to initial surgery in women with bulky supracolic omental disease and/or extensive liver metastases who are not suitable for optimal resection.[10,11] The medical management of first-line chemotherapy in the setting of ovarian cancer is complex and should be managed by oncologist with expertise and experience in this disease.

Recently, newer targeted agents that interfere with cell signaling pathways have become established. Bevacizumab and polyadenosine diphosphate-ribose polymerase (PARP) inhibitors have been incorporated in the upfront management of this disease.

Bevacizumab is a monoclonal antibody that targets the vascular endothelial growth factor (VEGF) receptor. The use of bevacizumab in frontline treatment was investigated by the Gynecological Oncology Group (GOG) 218 and the ICON 7 studies[12,13] and showed a significant improvement in PFS. This improvement was seen to be the most evident in women who had residual macroscopic disease. At this time, we reserve bevacizumab for those patients with high-risk factors who do not carry a BRCA mutation.

All newly diagnosed patients with ovarian cancer are recommended to undergo genetic testing. Women who are found to have a germ line or somatic breast cancer susceptibility gene (BRCA) may benefit from maintenance therapy with a PARP inhibitor following chemotherapy. This is based on multiple clinical trials showing that use of a PARP inhibitor as maintenance therapy affords a PFS advantage, even to women without a breast cancer susceptibility gene 1/2 (BRCA1/2) mutation.

In summary, advanced-stage EOC is initially treated with surgical cytoreduction followed by first-line chemotherapy. The choice among first-line treatments is made based upon the amount of disease remaining after surgery. Patients with <1 cm of disease in any one location are considered to have optimally cytoreduced. These patients should be treated with a platinum-plus-taxane combination. The individual regimen (dose-dense vs every 3 weeks) and route of administration (IV vs IV in combination with IP) may be individualized based on the patient. All patients should undergo genetic evaluation. For those patients who do not carry a BRCA mutation and are deemed to be high-risk, they may benefit from the addition of bevacizumab to their frontline treatment and continued as maintenance therapy. Those patients who carry a germ line or somatic BRCA mutation should be treated with a PARP Inhibitor as maintenance therapy at the completion of their upfront platinum-based chemotherapy.

RELAPSED DISEASE

In patients with relapsed disease, it is important to distinguish between platinum-sensitive and platinum-resistant disease. Platinum-resistant disease is normally defined as patients who develop recurrent disease within 6 months of completing their last dose of platinum. Platinum refractory disease is usually reserved for patients who develop resistance while receiving chemotherapy. Therefore platinum-sensitive disease refers to patients who develop recurrence beyond 6 months after completing their last dose of platinum.

The treatment-free interval following platinum chemotherapy predicts the response to second-line chemotherapy. Markman et al. and the French group GINECO23 have shown that beyond 12 months, the rate of response increases with rechallenge with carboplatin and paclitaxel. Nevertheless, a number of women have residual neuropathy, and this may influence the treatment options for recurrent disease. Carboplatin with gemcitabine is an acceptable alternative and two randomized controlled trials (CALYPSO and the Hellenic Cooperative Oncology Group) have shown that carboplatin and gemcitabine are not inferior to carboplatin and paclitaxel.[14,15] In older and less fit women, single-agent carboplatin remains a useful alternative with reasonable activity.

More recent drug developments have included adding tyrosine kinase inhibitors (TKIs) and VEGF receptor antagonists for treating relapsed disease, as in first-line therapy. The OCEANS study investigated the use of additional bevacizumab and found that it appears to show a significant benefit in this setting.[15] There is some debate as to whether it is better to use bevacizumab upfront or for relapse, and other debates have focused on retreating with bevacizumab when there has been prior exposure in first line.

Increasingly, patients are treated with multiple lines of therapy and other agents that may be used include liposomal doxorubicin, gemcitabine, topotecan, and dose-dense platinum schedules with taxanes or etoposide. Other new targeted agents remain under development and include folate receptor antagonists, antiangiogenesis agents, and other emerging TKIs.

PLATINUM RESISTANCE

>Rechallenge with platinum-based regimens has low response rates, many experts recognize this as an area for exploring new investigational agents or combinations. There are multiple agents with activity in platinum-resistant EOC, but there is not one universally preferred agent for use in the first-or subsequent-line treatment. A Cochrane systematic review of trials with platinum-resistant EOC concluded that topotecan, paclitaxel, and pegylated liposomal doxorubicin have similar efficacy, but different patterns of side effects.[3,16] A choice among these agents depends upon the clinician's experience, the side effect profile, and prior therapy. The use of bevacizumab in these patients in the Aurelia trial shows that improved PFS can be achieved, and some suggest reserving bevacizumab for this setting.[17]

BRCA MUTATION

The ability to identify germ line BRCA mutations in women has had a significant therapeutic impact over the last few years. The importance to recognize families with the BRCA mutation to facilitate family screening has been known. It is recommended that all patients with a newly diagnosed ovarian cancer undergo genetic counseling and subsequent testing. However, it was not recognized that this would have any impact on treatment. The development of the PARP inhibitors has led to interest as single-agent treat and in the maintenance setting. Several PARP inhibitors are available for the treatment of ovarian cancer, as maintenance therapy after first recurrence and initial diagnosis in BRCA wild type, germ line, somatic, and HRD patients.

UTERINE CANCER

Uterine or endometrial cancers are the most common gynecologic malignancy in developed countries and the second most common in developing countries. Among the different histologic types of adenocarcinomas, grade 1 and 2 endometrioid uterine cancers have a more favorable prognosis and typically present at an early stage. Other histologic types of uterine adenocarcinoma (e.g., serous, clear cell) are associated with a poorer prognosis. Women with advanced-stage or high-risk disease have a relatively poor prognosis following hysterectomy alone. As a result, adjuvant treatment is often recommended. The treatment may consist of radiation therapy, chemotherapy, or a combination of these two approaches.

Most recently, the use of carboplatin with paclitaxel has emerged as the standard of care, both for relapsed disease and in the adjuvant setting. This is based on the results of Gynecologic Oncology Group (GOG) 209.[18] This trial compared carboplatin plus paclitaxel with paclitaxel, doxorubicin, and cisplatin in 1300 women with chemotherapy-naïve advanced endometrial cancer, including women with stage III disease, and demonstrated that carboplatin and paclitaxel results in an equivalent overall response rate, similar PFS, and is less toxic.

Women with serous uterine carcinoma should have their tumor undergo HER2 immune-histochemistry (IHC) testing, with reflex to HER2 FISH for equivocal IHC, for possible treatment of advanced-stage or recurrent disease. Those patients whose tumor cares a HER2 profile may benefit from the addition of trastuzumab.[19] Similarly, recent studies have demonstrated a survival benefit to the addition of bevacizumab to carboplatin and paclitaxel in the management of advanced-stage and recurrent disease.[20]

An emerging area of interest is the role of immunotherapy in the management of recurrent endometrial cancer. Pembrolizumab is an immune checkpoint inhibitor that binds to and blocks programmed death (PD)-1. The phase Ib KEYNOTE-028 trial demonstrated a durable antitumor response in patients with PD ligand 1 (PD-L1)–positive tumors. The FDA approved pembrolizumab for uterine cancers with unresectable or metastatic, microsatellite instability-high (MSI-H), or deficient mismatch repair (dMMR) solid tumors that have progressed following prior treatment and have no satisfactory alternative treatment options.[21] The combination of pembrolizumab and lenvatinib, a multiple kinase inhibitor, has been approved for the management of treatment of patients with advanced endometrial cancer who have disease progression following prior systemic therapy. The indication applies to patients who are not candidates for curative surgery or radiation and who have disease that is not MSI-H or dMMR.[22]

Numerous important molecular pathways are disrupted in endometrial cancer, in particular the mechanistic target of rapamycin, phosphatase and tensin homolog, and the phosphoinositide 3-kinase. Emerging treatment developments are targeting these pathways, and further trials are ongoing on the use medications in endometrial cancer.

CERVICAL CANCER

Chemotherapy in cervical cancer has been used most frequently concomitantly with radiation for primary treatment. Following the National Cancer Institute consensus statement in 2000, the use of weekly cisplatin in combination with pelvic radiation was recommended, and it has now become the gold standard of care.[23] For those patients who present with metastatic disease or at the time of recurrence, systemic chemotherapy provides a role for palliative chemotherapy.

The GOG has conducted a number of studies over the past 20 years, including GOG 169, 179, 204, and 240, which have helped to determine the optimal regimens for recurrent disease. These trials have demonstrated that cisplatin with paclitaxel was superior to cisplatin alone. Cisplatin and topotecan appeared to show a benefit but when cisplatin and paclitaxel, cisplatin and topotecan, and a nonplatinum schedule of topotecan with paclitaxel were compared, no advantage over the newer regimens was shown and cisplatin/paclitaxel has reemerged as the preferred standard treatment.[24]

Bevacizumab has been investigated to determine if it improves outcomes compared to chemotherapy alone. GOG 240 study, in which bevacizumab was added to these agents, has shown a significant improvement in both progression-free and overall survival.[25] As a result, bevacizumab was approved for the treatment of metastatic and recurrent cervical cancer. In the second-line setting a choice among active agents must be tailored to the individual patient, with consideration to prior therapies received, residual toxicity, and performance status. In these patients, MMR/MSI testing or PD-L1 testing should be performed. Pembrolizumab has been a preferred regimen for second-line option for treating PD-L1–positive or MSI-H/dMMR cervical tumors.[26]

VAGINAL AND VULVAR CANCER

Vulvar and vaginal cancers are similar to cervical cancer and are squamous and often HPV-associated. As such, the treatment of cervical cancer is also used for vulvar and vaginal cancers.

UTERINE SARCOMAS

Uterine sarcomas include leiomyosarcomas (LMSs), endometrial stromal sarcomas, and undifferenced uterine sarcomas. Carcinosarcomas should be managed as high-risk endometrial cancers and will not be included here. LMSs are aggressive tumors. Active drugs for LMS include doxorubicin, either alone or combined with ifosfamide, and, more recently, docetaxel and gemcitabine combinations have emerged. The benefits of adjuvant chemotherapy are unclear. However, due to their aggressive nature, oncologists often treat these tumors with systemic chemotherapy. Low-grade endometrial stromal sarcomas are generally more indolent and respond to hormonal manipulation but may also respond to combinations of carboplatin and paclitaxel or platinum, doxorubicin, and ifosfamide.

CONCLUSION

Gynecological cancers require a multidisciplinary approach. Chemotherapy may be used as an adjuvant therapy or for the management of locally advanced or recurrent tumors. Traditional chemotherapy drugs have probably reached a plateau for development and tailored therapy with personalized medicine is emerging. Tumor tissue with identification of the molecular pathways will be the way forward, together with greater use of recognizing the importance of genetic differences as already shown for ovarian cancer and BRCA mutations.

REFERENCES

1. Kyrgiou M, et al. Survival benefits with diverse chemotherapy regimens for ovarian cancer: meta-analysis of multiple treatments. *J Natl Cancer Inst.* 2006;98:1655.
2. Markman M, et al. Phase III trial of standard-dose intravenous cisplatin plus paclitaxel versus moderately high-dose carboplatin followed by intravenous paclitaxel and intraperitoneal cisplatin. *J Clin Oncol.* 2001;19:1001–1007.
3. Alberts DS, et al. Intraperitoneal cisplatin plus intravenous cyclophosphamide versus intravenous cisplatin plus intravenous cyclophosphamide for stage III ovarian cancer. *N Engl J Med.* 1996;335:1950–1955.
4. Armstrong DK, et al. Intraperitoneal cisplatin and paclitaxel in ovarian cancer. *N Engl J Med.* 2006;354:34–43.
5. Tewari D, et al. Long-term survival advantage and prognostic factors associated with intraperitoneal chemotherapy treatment in advanced ovarian cancer: a gynecologic oncology group study. *J Clin Oncol.* 2015;33:1460–1466.
6. Katsumata N, et al. Long-term results of dose-dense paclitaxel and carboplatin versus conventional paclitaxel and carboplatin for treatment of advanced epithelial ovarian, fallopian tube, or primary peritoneal cancer (JGOG 3016): a randomised, controlled, open-label trial. *Lancet Oncol.* 2013;14:1020–1026.
7. Pignata S, et al. Carboplatin plus paclitaxel once a week versus every 3 weeks in patients with advanced ovarian cancer (MITO-7): a randomised, multicentre, open-label, phase 3 trial. *Lancet Oncol.* 2014;15:396.
8. Clamp AR, et al. Weekly dose-dense chemotherapy in first-line epithelial ovarian, fallopian tube, or primary peritoneal carcinoma treatment (ICON8): primary progression free survival analysis results from a GCIG phase 3 randomised controlled trial. *Lancet.* 2019;394(10214):2084.
9. Chan JK, et al. Weekly vs. every-3-week paclitaxel and carboplatin for ovarian cancer. *N Engl J Med.* 2016;374:738.
10. Vergote I, et al. Primary surgery or neoadjuvant chemotherapy followed by interval debulking surgery in advanced ovarian cancer. *Eur J Cancer.* 2011;47(suppl 3):S88–S92.
11. Kehoe S, et al. Chemotherapy or upfront surgery for newly diagnosed advanced ovarian cancer: results from the MRC CHORUS trial. *J Clin Oncol.* 2013;31(suppl):5500.
12. Burger RA, et al. Incorporation of bevacizumab in the primary treatment of ovarian cancer. *N Engl J Med.* 2011;365:2473.
13. Oza AM, et al. Standard chemotherapy with or without bevacizumab for women with newly diagnosed ovarian cancer (ICON7): overall survival results of a phase 3 randomised trial. *Lancet Oncol.* 2015;16:928.
14. Pujade-Lauraine E, et al. Pegylated liposomal doxorubicin and carboplatin compared with paclitaxel and carboplatin for patients with platinum-sensitive ovarian cancer in late relapse. *J Clin Oncol.* 2010;28:3323–3329.
15. Aghajanian C, et al. OCEANS: a randomized, double-blind, placebo-controlled phase III trial of chemotherapy with or without bevacizumab in patients with platinum sensitive recurrent epithelial ovarian, primary peritoneal, or fallopian tube cancer. *J Clin Oncol.* 2012;30:2039–2045.
16. Peng LH, et al. Topotecan for ovarian cancer. *Cochrane Database Syst Rev.* 2008;2:CD005589.
17. Pujade-Lauraine E, et al. Bevacizumab combined with chemotherapy for platinum-resistant recurrent ovarian cancer: the AURELIA open-label randomized phase III trial. *J Clin Oncol.* 2014;32:1302.
18. Miller D, et al. Randomized phase III noninferiority trial of first line chemotherapy for metastatic or recurrent endometrial carcinoma: a Gynecologic Oncology Group study. *Gynecol Oncol.* 2012;125S:771.
19. Fader AN, et al. Randomized phase II trial of carboplatin-paclitaxel versus carboplatin-paclitaxel-trastuzumab in uterine serous carcinomas that 4 overexpress human epidermal growth factor receptor 2/neu. *J Clin Oncol.* 2018;36:2044–2051.
20. Rose PG, et al. Paclitaxel, carboplatin, and bevacizumab in advanced and recurrent endometrial carcinoma. *Int J Gynecol Cancer.* 2017;27:452–458.
21. Le DT, et al. PD-1 blockade in tumors with mismatch-repair deficiency. *N Engl J Med.* 2015;372:2509–2520.
22. Makker V, et al. Lenvatinib plus pembrolizumab in patients with advanced endometrial cancer: an interim analysis of a multicentre, open-label, single-arm, phase 2 trial. *Lancet Oncol.* 2019;20:711–718.
23. Institute NC. *Clinical Announcement: Concurrent Chemoradiation for Cervical Cancer.* Washington, DC: United States Department of Public Health; 1999.
24. Moore DH, et al. Prognostic factors for response to cisplatin-based chemotherapy in advanced cervical carcinoma: a Gynecologic Oncology Group Study. *Gynecol Oncol.* 2010;116:44.
25. Tewari KS, et al. Improved survival with bevacizumab in advanced cervical cancer. *N Engl J Med.* 2014;370:734.
26. Frenel JS, et al. Safety and efficacy of pembrolizumab in advanced, programmed death ligand 1-positive cervical cancer: results from the phase Ib KEYNOTE-028 trial. *J Clin Oncol.* 2017;35:4035–4041.

CHAPTER 17

Principles of Radiation Therapy in Gynecologic Cancer

ALLIE GARCIA-SERRA, MD

GENERAL OVERVIEW OF RADIATION THERAPY

Ionizing radiation has been used for decades to kill cancer cells. The field of radiation oncology was once known as therapeutic radiology. Megavoltage X-rays are used to penetrate tissues that create double-stranded DNA breaks thereby killing cancer cells. Radiation affects both cancer cells and healthy cells. However, the cancer cells due to mutations do not have the capacity to repair double stranded DNA breaks and therefore die while the healthy cells are able to repair the cellular damage. If the healthy cells are unable to recover from the effect of radiation, then a long term side effect ensues. The goal of radiation oncology is to maximize the therapeutic ratio. The therapeutic ratio is defined as maximum tumor cell killing while respecting normal tissue tolerance levels, that is, minimizing late tissue toxicity or late effects.[1] Sometimes, this is achieved by increasing the total tumor dose while decreasing the dose to the surrounding normal tissues. An example of this would be proton therapy that will be described more later. Another example of being able to increase tumor cell kill without damaging the normal surrounding tissue would be the use of radiosensitizing chemotherapy in addition to radiation therapy. Both of these examples enhance the tumoricidal effect while potentially preserving normal surrounding healthy tissue.

Radiation causes side effects that can be globally classified into two groups: acute side effects and late side effects. Acute side effects are those that come on during the treatment and usually subside within 3 months post treatment. These effects resolve and usually the patient's function returns to that of baseline. However, radiation can also cause late effects that can happen months to years after the radiation treatment has been delivered. The side effects caused by radiation are strictly determined by the anatomical region being treated. For example, in gynecologic malignancies typically, it is the female pelvis that is being treated with radiation plus or minus the inclusion of lymph nodes within the para-aortic (abdominal) region. For the most part, acute pelvic side effects include bladder changes (frequency, urgency, dysuria, nocturia, and worsening overflow incontinence) as well as rectal changes, including diarrhea, mucus in stools, and hemorrhoidal tissue flare. Most of the side effects are managed conservatively with the use of medications such as Pyridium for dysuria and Imodium for diarrhea. These symptoms will resolve several weeks after the treatment is completed. Late effects due to radiation therapy include changes to the vagina, such as vaginal stenosis, strictures or adhesions, dyspareunia (painful intercourse), vaginal dryness, as well as pelvic floor dysfunction, lymphedema, and ovarian dysfunction.

There are different ways to deliver radiation therapy. The majority of the radiation therapy is performed utilizing external beam radiation therapy as opposed to internal techniques with the utilization of brachytherapy. Typically, external beam is delivered using linear accelerators where X-rays are made by accelerating electrons in a vacuum through a tube which then hit a metal target and turn into photons, or high energy X-rays. This creates the X-ray beam that will be delivered a specific anatomical area in the patient. The majority of radiation oncology facilities use photon energy to treat cancer cells. A minority of facilities are now using proton beam. Protons are positively charged particles that are created in a cyclotron and then diverted into a treatment machine. Proton therapy has the advantage of having no exit dose as opposed to photon energy that has entrance and exit dose. Therefore proton therapy has the added benefit of potentially protecting nearby critical structures in a situation where the area being treated is located in close proximity to a critical structure, for example, spinal cord. Not everybody is a candidate for proton therapy. Proton

Breast Cancer and Gynecologic Cancer Rehabilitation DOI: https://doi.org/10.1016/B978-0-323-72166-0.00017-7

therapy is also not widely available due to it being cost-prohibitive.

Most of the external beam radiation is delivered utilizing photon energy. Very sophisticated ways of delivering this photon energy are on the market. Modern-day equipment is capable of delivering the radiation beam to within millimeter accuracy. Image-guided radiation therapy uses computed tomography (CT) images to confirm the position of the patient and treatment field to improve the accuracy of treatment. There is also a linear accelerator that is mounted adjacent to an magnetic resonance imaging (MRI) magnet that allows for MRI-guided radiation therapy. This is especially useful when the target is moving or if there is a critical structure within the area being treated that can be identified most accurately with MRI due to better soft tissue delineation. Most facilities use CT-based linear accelerators where CT images are obtained prior to treatment. There are also very accurate and precise treatment delivery systems to treat small tumors to exceptionally high doses. Examples include Gamma Knife for treatment of brain tumors (stereotactic radiosurgery) and CyberKnife for treatment of brain tumors and tumors within the body (stereotactic body radiotherapy).

Another way of delivering a concentrated dose of radiation therapy is with the utilization of brachytherapy. "Brachy" in Greek means close therefore brachytherapy means "close therapy."[2] Modern-day equipment uses a small but powerful radioactive seed the size of a rice grain, typically Iridium-192. The source is radioactive and undergoes radioactive decay properties. The source is transmitted into a series of applicators that are located inside the patient to deliver a concentrated dose of radiation to a small area. The value of brachytherapy is that it delivers a high dose to a small area that allows us to protect the normal surrounding tissue, thereby enhancing the therapeutic ratio. There are two broad categories of brachytherapy. An intracavitary treatment uses an applicator that is placed within a cavity, such as an applicator that is placed inside the vagina. An example of intracavitary brachytherapy is a vaginal cylinder for the postoperative treatment of endometrial cancer or cervical cancer. A vaginal cylinder is placed inside the vagina in the clinic after which the radioactive seed is transmitted through the inside of the vaginal cylinder that is hollow and thereby treats the top of the vagina to a certain dose. The radioactive seed stays inside the patient as long as necessary to deliver a specific dose (usually less than 10 minutes). This treatment is easy to perform and has very limited morbidity due to its ability to deliver a concentrated dose to within 5 mm of the applicator. A second example of an intracavitary brachytherapy applicator is tandem and ovoid or ring applicator that is used for primary treatment of unresectable cervical cancer. The tandem is a metal applicator that is placed inside the uterus and the ovoids or ring are placed inside the vagina. The units are fastened together and held in position with vaginal packing for definitive treatment of cervical cancer. Typically, these applicators are placed in the operating room with general anesthesia or conscious sedation since the procedure can be uncomfortable especially if the cervix needs to be dilated to accommodate the applicator inside the uterus. Another type of brachytherapy treatment is using interstitial brachytherapy applicators. These are a series of thin long needles that are placed either into the vagina or the paracervical/parametrial tissues to treat either locally advanced vaginal cancer or cervical cancer, respectively. Brachytherapy is an important component of definitive treatment of cervical cancer. Patients who do not receive brachytherapy as a part of their treatment have inferior survival rates.[3] Another example of an interstitial brachytherapy application is the use of radioactive seeds implanted into the prostate for treatment of prostate cancer.

The first step in radiation treatment planning is a targeted CAT scan of the area being treated that is performed in the radiation department. This is called a CT simulation. This scan is utilized to define the target(s) to be treated and the normal tissues to be avoided. Often, the pretreatment diagnostic MRI or positron emission tomography (PET) scan is fused to the planning CT to confidently delineate the area of gross tumor. The treatment plan is then generated with the aid of the dosimetrists and medical physicists. After the plan is approved and quality assurance has taken place by the medical physicists, the patient begins her daily treatment. This includes a series of daily, Monday through Friday, treatments that may take 15–20 minutes daily for up to several weeks. In general, when the pelvis is treated for a gynecologic malignancy, the treatment duration is approximately 5–6 weeks of daily external beam radiation therapy. A brachytherapy treatment may follow the initial pelvic field to boost the dose to the area of concern. The treatment delivery system is painless. The patient lays on the treatment table. The gantry which is the head of the treatment machine that contains the X-ray beam will rotate around the patient to deliver the radiation from multiple angles to treat the designated area in a conformal manner. The radiation only affects the area being treated. Therefore if the patient is having side effects outside of the pelvis, likely the symptoms are due to another cause (e.g., chemotherapy or other comorbid conditions.) The patient is not radioactive during the external beam treatment. The radiation stays within the linear accelerator. The equipment never touches the patient and the patient can resume her daily activities on most occasions. Very frequently the patient will also receive concurrent radiosensitizing chemotherapy. It is known that chemotherapy can enhance the response to radiation therapy, and therefore in certain cases radiosensitizing chemotherapy is used in conjunction with the pelvic radiotherapy to enhance overall survival such as the case with definitive treatment of cervical carcinoma with radiation.[4] In this example the patient will receive chemotherapy once a week through a peripheral vein or a port-a-cath. The infusion takes several hours to perform. The patient will also need to receive her pelvic radiation that day as well. It is common for patients to feel fatigued amongst other side effects during the course of treatment especially since these treatment days can be long.

Typically, a full bladder and an empty rectum are preferred for pelvic treatment of a gynecologic malignancy. There can be significant organ motion due to bladder filling such as is the case in cervical carcinoma. The cervix can move up to 2 cm in superior to inferior direction due to bladder filling.[5] The cervix tumor will also shrink during the treatment, and therefore the treatment plan may need to be adjusted along the way to make sure that the tumor is still being adequately covered within the radiation fields. Prior to each treatment, a quick CT-scan image is obtained on the treatment table in order to ascertain that the radiation is being delivered to the correct area. This on-table, pretreatment CT-scan image is fused with the planning CT-scan image to confirm an exact match. Sometimes, minor modifications have to be made in up to six degrees of freedom. At times, the patient is given feedback to increase bladder filling or conversely decrease rectal filling in order to obtain a better match in position of the internal organs. Obtaining pretreatment imaging is called image-guided radiation therapy that is now being routinely used. This allows us to decrease the amount of radiation exposure to the normal surrounding tissue (bladder, rectum, and bowel). Since we use three-dimensional treatment planning (treatments are based on a pretreatment CT scan image), dose approximations to the normal surrounding organs are known and kept to accepted standards. This helps decrease the chance of causing a severe permanent tissue complication (i.e., small bowel obstruction, perforation, and fistula). The treatment planning process is the most important component of the overall treatment followed by meticulous treatment delivery by trained radiation therapist. The medical physicist is the right hand of the radiation oncologist. The medical physicist verifies the treatment parameters and confirms that the treatment is being delivered as planned. Another important job of the physicist is to make sure that the machines are calibrated correctly. This avoids situations of over or under dosing of patients. The pretreatment daily CT scans that are called cone beam CTs are checked by the physician daily. This allows the physician to confirm that there has been accurate treatment delivery as well as it gives us the ability to assess for tumor response. If there has been significant tumor shrinkage during the treatment, sometimes the patient is replanned (undergoes a new CT simulation) and the treatment is adjusted to its new tumor volume (adaptive replanning.)

The radiation oncologist sees the patient in initial consultation and determines if radiation is appropriate for the patient. If so, the most important question is determining if the patient is curable. In most cases there is significant multidisciplinary interaction between the radiation oncologist, gynecologic oncologist and/or medical oncologist. Rehabilitative physician, ancillary staff, including social workers, nurse navigators, and dietitians, are also important components of the oncology team. When patients receive chemotherapy during the radiation, optimal timing of the two treatments is crucial. If the patient has undergone surgery, the timing and start of adjuvant (postoperative) radiation therapy are critical. Typically, the time frame is 6–8 weeks postoperative if the patient is well healed. In certain cases where there is the possibility of a rapid recurrence such as in head and neck carcinomas, timely initiation of adjuvant treatment is paramount. If there is a long delay between surgery and initiation of treatment, there is the possibility of tumor recurrence. While the patient is undergoing daily treatments, the radiation oncologist sees the patient once-per-week to manage any treatment-related side effects. Once the patient has completed treatment, the patient is seen in follow-up to assess for signs or symptoms of tumor recurrence and for any possible late effects due to radiation therapy. Usually, patients will continue to be seen for ongoing surveillance over the next 5 years.

Most recurrences tend to occur within the first several years of treatment. In gynecologic cancers, initially there is a peak recurrence time of approximately 8 months followed by later recurrence up to 2–3 years posttreatment.[6] Recurrences can be seen even later than this. If there is prompt detection of early recurrence, then there may be a localized treatment that can be offered for salvage such as surgery or a focused stereotactic radiation technique. In more advanced cases a pelvic exenteration that removes all the internal pelvic organs, including the bladder and rectum, may be an option if there is no evidence of metastatic disease. Patients who have human papilloma Virus (HPV)-related disease remain at risk for additional malignancies within the lower genital tract. Therefore a careful history, clinical exam, and complementary diagnostic imaging remain an important part of the overall surveillance.

Managing late radiation effects is an important part of follow-up. Late effects of radiation to the pelvis can include changes to the bladder, rectum, vagina, bowel, skin, and connective tissues, including bone and nerves. These complications tend to occur the first few years posttreatment. Large, locally advanced tumors tend to cause the most side effects due to the volume of radiated tissues. For example, treatment of a large cervical tumor invading the bladder may cause a fistula after the tumor regresses. Radiation cystitis may also occur. This is a small ulceration of the bladder mucosa due to too much radiation to a particular part of the bladder. This is managed with bladder irrigation and catheterization. Occasionally, fulguration is needed to stop the bleeding. Radiation proctitis can be managed with steroid suppositories or argon plasma coagulation. Radiation enteropathy, including obstruction perforation or fistula, is a severe complication of the bowel that occurs when dose is greater than 60 Gy are delivered to the bowel loops.[6] Occasionally, surgical intervention is needed. Duodenal injury may present with bleeding ulceration or stricture formation. Long-term changes to the skin may include fibrosis, telangiectasia, and either hyper or hypopigmentation. In cases where there is a late radiation complication that is not amenable to conservative treatment, hyperbaric oxygen treatments may be useful to help successfully treat radiated tissues. Hyperbaric oxygen helps deliver oxygen to damaged tissues and thereby reverse the late radiation effect.

There are specific late effects due to radiation therapy to the pelvis that may be amenable to rehabilitation. These are discussed in this section.

Vaginal Side Effects

Physical changes to the vagina may include vaginal stenosis, strictures, adhesions, and synechiae. These can make the vagina narrower and shorter. Vaginal synechiae are webs of fibrotic scar tissue that can form after radiation to the vagina. The formation of vaginal synechiae is dose dependent. Synechiae may require disruption using either digital manipulation or manipulation with a dilator. In extreme cases, surgical disruption in the operating room with general anesthesia may be necessary as this can be painful for the patient. In addition, disruption of the scar tissue can cause significant bleeding. Vaginal dilators can be used to treat and prevent vaginal narrowing and scar tissue formation, although the data is inconclusive. A Cochrane Database review by Miles and Johnson concluded that there was no reliable evidence to show that routine dilator use improved late effects of radiation to the vagina.[7] Women who are compliant with dilator use have less late toxicity such as vaginal shortening and stenosis as well as dyspareunia (painful intercourse). We counsel the patient to use the vaginal dilator 10 minutes a day three times per week and to remain sexually active if possible. Discomfort and bleeding is expected and is normal. The dilator should be used long term. If the patient already has significant narrowing, there are graduated vaginal dilator kits that can be used in order to gradually reexpand the vagina.

A common complaint postradiation therapy is dyspareunia. Painful sexual intercourse is related to physical changes of the vagina such as synechiae and vaginal canal shortening due to surgery. It can also be caused by vaginal dryness. There are two components to vaginal moisture. The cervix produces moisture to the top of the vagina and the Bartholin's glands, that sit at either side of the entrance to the vagina, produce the rest of the lubrication. Many of these patients have undergone a hysterectomy where the cervix is removed. In addition, Bartholin's glands are extremely sensitive to low radiation doses and lose function after low doses. As a result of radiation therapy, vaginal dryness occurs. In addition, patients who had either their ovaries surgically removed or had the ovaries treated with radiation therapy can also have vaginal dryness due to loss of estrogen production. Supplementation with personal lubricants is extremely important to ease the sexual dysfunction. Occasionally, vaginal estrogen creams can be used with good result. Typically, this is contraindicated in the case of endometrial cancer, since endometrial cancer is estrogen sensitive. Always have the patient consult with her gynecologic oncologist prior to initiation of hormonal creams or other hormonal supplements. Vaginal shortening, due to surgery and/or radiation, can affect the depth of penetration and therefore sexual satisfaction. Unfortunately, there is no way to alter the length of the vaginal canal. Working with a trained vaginal rehabilitation therapist is also useful.

Psychosocial changes also occur. Anxiety over sexual intercourse occurs in both the patient and her partner in most cases. The partner typically worries about hurting the patient, especially if there is postcoital bleeding. Bleeding causes anxiety in the patient as this is the most frequent presenting symptom of both cervical and endometrial cancer. Sexuality counseling is an important component of rehabilitation. Jensen et al published in the *International Journal of Radiation Oncology Biology and Physics* a longitudinal study of self-reported sexual function and vaginal changes after radiation following treatment for cervical cancer.[8] One hundred and eighteen patients were assessed using a validated self-assessment questionnaire. A percentage of 85 of patients had low or no sexual interest, 35% had moderate-to-severe lack of lubrication, 55% had mild-to-severe dyspareunia, and 30% were dissatisfied with their sexual life. A reduced vaginal dimension was reported in 50% of the patients and 45% were never or only occasionally able to complete sexual intercourse. A greater emphasis needs to be placed on vaginal rehabilitation. A patient is encouraged to work together with their partner as a team in order to restore sexual intimacy.

Ovarian Dysfunction

Extremely low doses of radiation will cause ovarian dysfunction. Doses in the order of 200 cGy will cause severe irreparable and permanent loss of endocrine function of the ovary.[9] This leads to early menopause. Menopausal symptoms include hot flashes, emotional lability, weight gain, decreased libido, and vaginal dryness or atrophy. Estrogen replacement may be considered in certain cases, although it is not usually recommended for endometrial cancers specifically adenocarcinoma that is an especially estrogen-sensitive tumor. For patients who are premenopausal who become menopausal due to treatment but still have a uterus may be candidates for both estrogen and progesterone replacement; low doses up to age 49 may be acceptable. Long-term hormonal supplementation is not indicated. Always consult with the gynecologic oncologist to determine the safety of hormone replacement.

Ovarian transposition also known as oophoropexy is a surgical approach to try to limit the radiation dose to the ovaries. The gynecologic surgeons move the ovaries out of the radiation field in an attempt to preserve ovarian function. The ovaries are typically ligated to the peritoneum as high and lateral as possible. This procedure can be performed laparoscopically with minimal morbidity.[10] Despite moving the ovaries out of the field of radiation, retention of ovarian hormonal function may not occur for multiple reasons. Vascular changes to the ovaries may cause ovarian infarction (i.e., loss of blood supply) and therefore loss of function. Occasionally, the ovaries migrate down into the lower abdomen due to gravity.

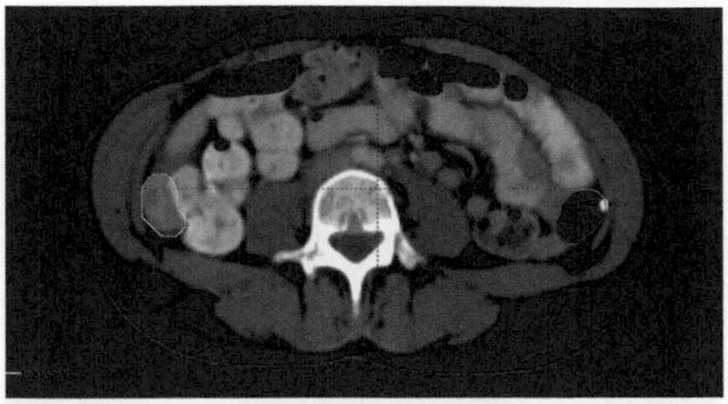

FIGURE 17.1 (Left) Axial CT slice used for radiation treatment planning. Left ovary in yellow and right ovary in pink transposed to the abdomen. Hyperdense metal surgical clip seen on right ovary.

For example, a 34-year-old patient was diagnosed with cervical cancer. She underwent a radical hysterectomy and lymph node sampling as well as and ovarian transposition. Her ovaries were secured into her upper lateral abdomen (see Figs. 17.1 and 17.2). A dose–volume histogram allows us to see how much dose is to be delivered to a certain volume of a specific organ. In the dose–volume histogram displayed next, the mean doses to the ovaries were less than 200 cGy (right ovary 139 cGy and left ovary 194 cGy) (see Fig. 17.3).

Mean radiation doses to the ovaries were kept within acceptable range. However, the patient became menopausal 3 months after completion of treatment. This was biochemically proven with markedly elevated follicle-stimulating hormone (FSH) levels confirming menopausal status. She is now 3 years post treatment and is using vaginal estrogen cream supplementation and remains sexually active.

Pelvic Floor Dysfunction

Pelvic floor dysfunction or disorders include pelvic organ prolapse, urinary incontinence, anal incontinence, and sexual dysfunction. The etiology of pelvic floor disorders is often multifactorial. For example, patients may be obese (known risk factor for endometrial cancer) and/or diabetic or other comorbid conditions with baseline urinary incontinence or organ prolapse. Also, she may undergo multiple lines of treatment such as surgery, radiation, and

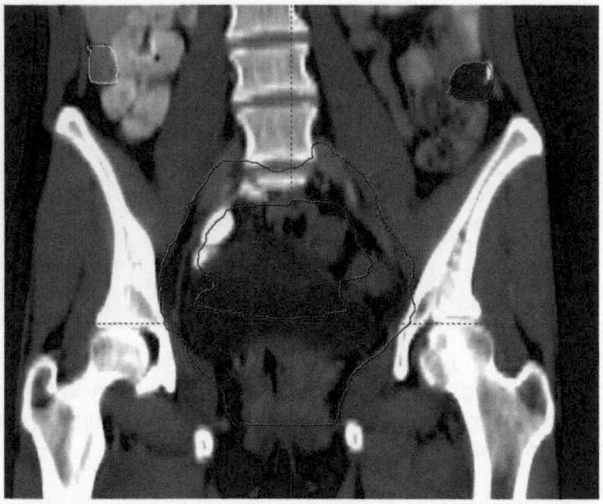

FIGURE 17.2 (Right) Coronal CT slice showing ovaries in yellow and pink and radiation isodose line of 45 Gy in red.

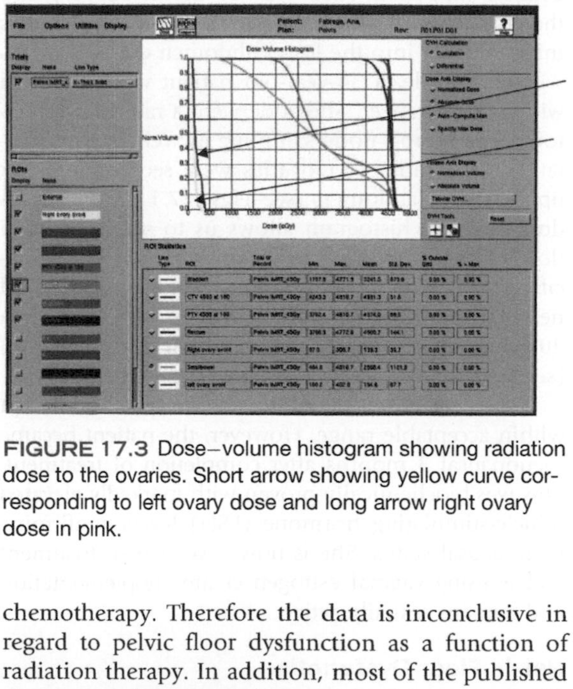

FIGURE 17.3 Dose–volume histogram showing radiation dose to the ovaries. Short arrow showing yellow curve corresponding to left ovary dose and long arrow right ovary dose in pink.

chemotherapy. Therefore the data is inconclusive in regard to pelvic floor dysfunction as a function of radiation therapy. In addition, most of the published data comes from mailed questionnaires to a specific patient population (i.e., retrospective data.) For these reasons, it is difficult to discern the exact radiation-related rate of complication.

Segal et al. performed a retrospective cohort study of endometrial cancer survivors.[11] A questionnaire was sent out to the patients in regard to urinary function and other pelvic floor disorders. A percentage of 41 of 149 endometrial cancer survivors received radiation therapy. The rates of urinary incontinence in women who received vaginal brachytherapy or whole pelvic radiation therapy were not significantly different, approximately 50%. Fecal incontinence rates also were similar in both groups. On multivariate analysis, significant risk factors for urinary incontinence were age and body mass index (BMI). Treatment with radiation was not associated with urinary incontinence or fecal incontinence. Radiation therapy was, however, related to sexual dysfunction. In patients with cervical cancer, it was recently documented that patients undergoing more radical surgery for cervix cancer had higher rates of urinary dysfunction, including both urinary retention and incontinence.[12] Since patients with cervical cancer often undergo both surgery and radiation therapy, it is difficult to discriminate the added risk of radiation therapy to pelvic floor dysfunction in these patients.

There are useful validated questionnaires for measuring pelvic floor disorders as follows: urinary incontinence severity: the Sandvik Incontinence Severity; anal incontinence: the Wexner Fecal Incontinence Scale; sexual function: the Pelvic Organ Prolapse/ Urinary Incontinence Sexual Questionnaire (PISQ-12).[13] Rutledge et al. used these validated questionnaires in order to determine risk of pelvic floor disorders and sexual dysfunction in patients who were treated for gynecologic malignancies. This was a cohort study where 108 control patients and 260 survivor questionnaires were completed. There was a statistically increased risk of worse moderate-to-severe urinary incontinence, fecal incontinence and less sexual desire, and less ability to climax in survivors.

Muscles can undergo either atrophy or fibrosis due to radiation therapy. Physical therapy can be of help in either case. (Fig. 17.4) is an example of a young female who underwent postoperative radiation therapy to the pelvis for the diagnosis of cervical cancer. The large arrow is showing the obturator internus muscle contained within the high-dose radiation field (green isodose line displays prescription dose). It is necessary to treat this area due to the possible spread to the obturator lymph nodes that drain the uterus. This in turn can cause destabilization of the hip joint and difficulty with external rotation of the ipsilateral leg. The short arrow demonstrates the location of the piriformis muscle also within the high-dose radiation field. The piriformis muscle originates at the internal surface of the sacrum that is also necessary to cover due to potential spread to the presacral lymph nodes. This muscle also helps with stabilization and rotation of the hip joint (Fig. 17.4).

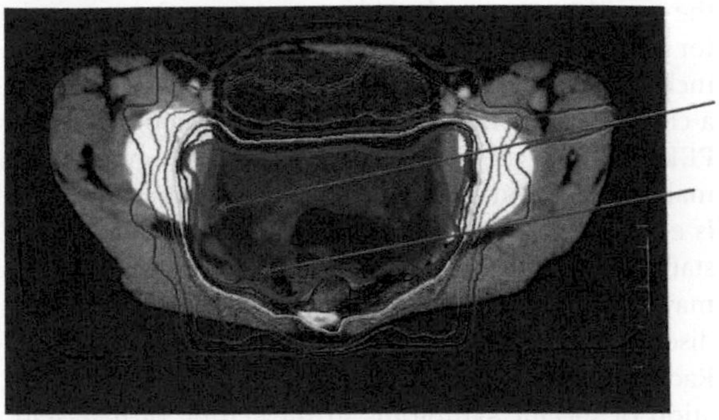

FIGURE 17.4 Axial Ct slice displaying radiation field, including obturator internus muscle (*long arrow*) and piriformis muscle (*short arrow*).

In regards to urinary incontinence, this is a multifactorial event. Most patients who present with baseline urinary incontinence and receive radiation therapy experience worsening of the urinary incontinence. The etiology of this is unclear. It is postulated that perhaps there is some fibrosis of the pelvic floor muscles leading to incontinence. Nerve damage is less likely as nerves are more "radiation tolerant." Pelvic floor strengthening exercises, including Kegel exercises, may be of benefit. Urinary retention can occur as a consequence of surgery. This is typically mitigated by "timed voiding." Fecal incontinence is not typically seen as a radiation-related side effect in the treatment of gynecologic disorders. Normally, fecal incontinence can be seen as a result of high-dose radiation therapy for primary treatment of anal canal squamous cell carcinomas or low rectal tumors probably due to muscular changes in the sphincter region. Usually, the fecal incontinence in this setting is self-limiting and temporary. High-fiber diet and again Kegel exercises may benefit these patients. The role of nerve stimulators remains undetermined although likely to help fecal incontinence.[14]

Lymphedema

Lymphedema causes pain, impaired mobility and can increase the risk of infection and thromboembolic events. The impaired mobility may limit physical activities, limit social activities as well as sleep. There is a retrospective questionnaire-based Swedish study published in 2013 that noted 36% of cancer survivors reported lower extremity lymphedema yet few patients actually sought professional help for this problem.[15] Lymphedema develops as a result of impaired lymphatic flow either due to surgical disruption of the lymphatics, including lymph node dissection or radiation therapy, or usually a combination of the two. Risk factors for lymphedema include the following: increased BMI, lymphadenectomy, number of removed lymph nodes, removal of circumflex iliac lymph nodes, and adjuvant treatment, including both radiation and chemotherapy.[16] Due to the morbidity of lymphadenectomy, there has been a consensus movement in gynecologic oncology toward sentinel lymph node mapping specifically for staging of endometrial cancer and vulvar cancer.

Sentinel lymph node techniques started in the 1980s mostly with melanoma and subsequently breast cancer staging. Sentinel lymph node techniques allow for examination of the lymph node with the highest propensity of being involved and only proceeding with completion lymph node dissection if that sentinel lymph node is found to be positive at the time of surgery on frozen section. Sentinel lymph node mapping techniques are associated with less risk of lymphedema due to removal of less number of lymph nodes as well as less manipulation of the lymphatic flow. There are some patients in whom the sentinel lymph node mapping fails and thereby the sentinel lymph node cannot be detected. Patients with clinically positive lymph nodes and high BMI may have a baseline of obstructed lymphatics, and therefore the sentinel lymph node fails. Therefore the sentinel lymph node technique is not valid for all patients. There is a comprehensive review article on sentinel lymph node mapping and staging in endometrial cancer referenced here.[17]

Patients who require postoperative (adjuvant) radiation therapy after initial surgery for endometrial cancer, cervical cancer, or even vulvar cancer remain at risk for the development of lymphedema. Most lymphedema results are retrospective and questionnaire-based but can range between 20% and 40%. Over the last 20 years, data has shown that vaginal cuff brachytherapy is equally successful in decreasing the chances of a vaginal recurrence as compared to pelvic radiotherapy in certain lower risk endometrial cancers.[18] This translates into less patients receiving pelvic radiation thereby decreasing the rates of lower limb lymphedema. It has been published that vaginal cuff brachytherapy does not increase the chances of developing permanent lymphedema.[19]

The gold-standard in management of lymphedema is complete decongestive therapy that includes the use of manual lymph drainage, compression therapy, exercise, and skin care. Meticulous compliance with the rehabilitation program is necessary for optimal success.

Bone

Pelvic insufficiency fractures are a known side effect of radiation therapy to the bone. Common areas of insufficiency fractures include the sacral ala or pubic bone. These fractures commonly occur when large fields of radiation are used such as treatment of vulvar cancer where the inguinal lymph nodes need to be treated either therapeutic or prophylactically. Insufficiency fractures to the pelvis occur at doses greater than 40–45 Gy. Additional risk factors include low body mass index, postmenopausal status as well as osteoporosis or osteopenia. Cigarette smoking may also be related. Usually, these fractures occur from 3 to 24 months after radiation therapy.[20] At MD Anderson it was noted that there was a 10% rate of insufficiency fractures after radiation therapy to the pelvis. Approximately 45% were symptomatic. Rest and analgesics are the recommended treatment. Insufficiency fractures rarely require surgical intervention. Bone-density studies and bone-strengthening pharmacologic agents should be considered. Of note, on follow-up PET imaging sacral insufficiency fractures present themselves as areas of increased FDG uptake that can be confused for metastases. Usually, bone marrow edema related to prior radiation therapy is also seen on MRI that can help determine the etiology of the FDG-avid lesion (Figs. 17.5–17.9).

CANCER SURVEILLANCE

Long-term follow-up in cancer patients is of utmost importance not only for early detection of recurrent disease but also for management of long-term toxicity related to curative treatment. In gynecologic malignancies the majority of the recurrences occur within the first 3 years. There is a peak incidence of recurrence of approximately 8 months.[6] Continued follow-up with the oncology team should occur every 3–6 months for up to 5 years posttreatment. Cancer surveillance includes both a detailed history and physical but also a clinical exam and on occasion radiographic imaging. PET scans are extremely sensitive in most gynecologic malignancies and help detect early recurrences. If there is early detection of recurrent disease that is not metastatic, localized treatment (either radiation or surgery) may result in long-term cures. For distant metastatic disease, salvage chemotherapy is typically utilized. Radiation therapy may still be recommended for palliation of specific symptoms in the setting of metastatic

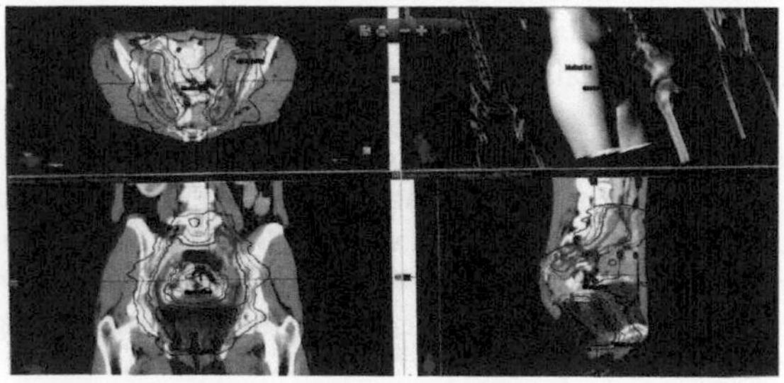

FIGURE 17.5 Axial, coronal, and sagittal CT images displaying the radiation isodose lines, blue color represents the 45 Gy line and the pink line represents the 50 Gy line. Upper sacrum lies within the 45 Gy isodose line best seen on the Sagittal view.

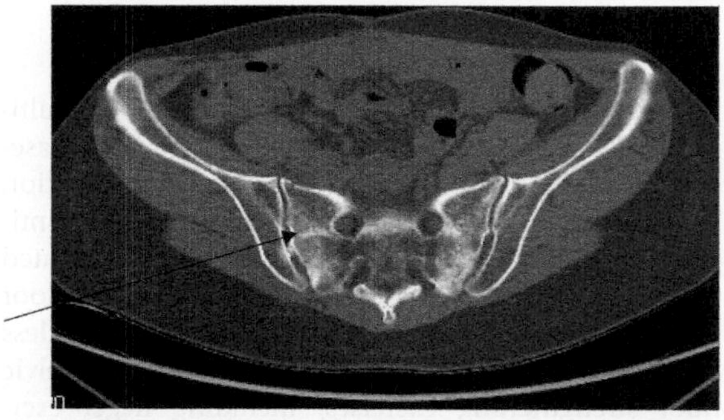

FIGURE 17.6 Axial scan images displaying "bone window" view showing sacral insufficiency fracture on the right sacral ala.

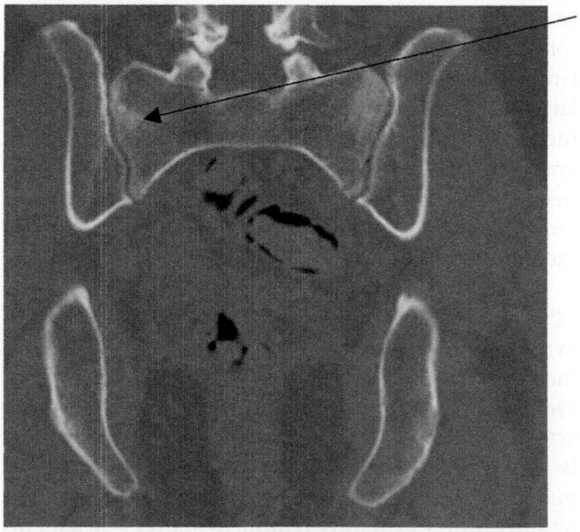

FIGURE 17.7 Coronal CT scan images displaying "bone window" view showing sacral insufficiency fracture on the right sacral ala.

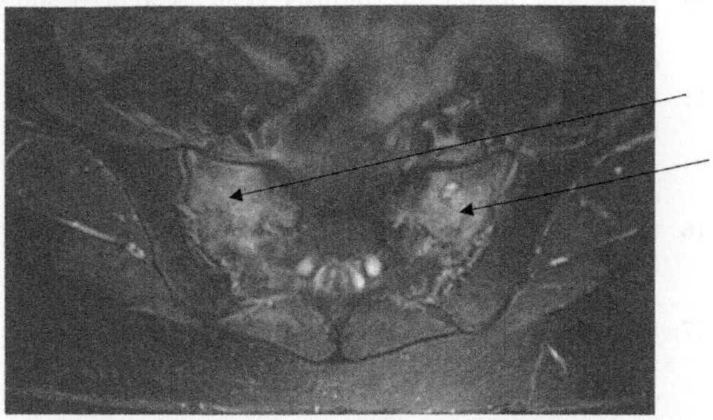

FIGURE 17.8 Axial view T2 fat-suppressed MRI of the pelvis showing bone marrow radiation-related changes within the bilateral sacral ala (displayed as white/hypodense changes in the bone). Images taken 8 months postcompletion of external beam radiation to the pelvis.

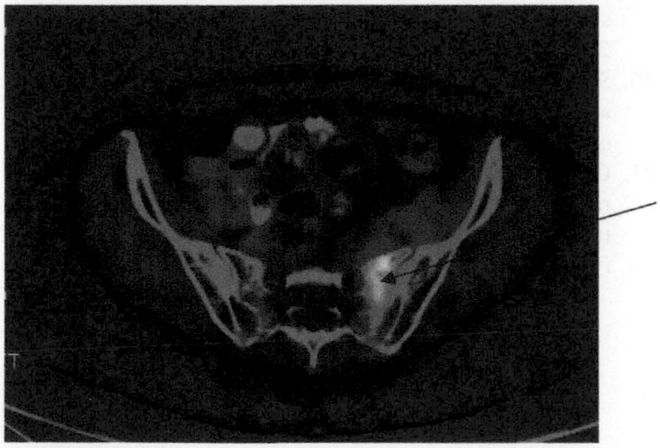

FIGURE 17.9 Axial PET/CT showing FDG-avid region at the left sacrum consistent with a left sacral insufficiency fracture on a separate patient one and half years after completion of radiation treatment.

disease. Radiation therapy is useful for palliating pain or bleeding, for example.

Patients who have tested positive for HPV (human papillomavirus) within the genital tract and have had one malignancy within the genital tract remain at increased risk for a secondary malignancy due to the HPV virus. For example, a patient with HPV-related cervical cancer remains at risk for HPV-related vaginal or anal carcinoma. Routine age-appropriate cancer screening, including mammograms and colonoscopy, is also important. Any patient who has had radiation to the pelvis and presents with rectal bleeding should be sent for a colonoscopy for further workup or if the patient has hematuria, a cystoscopy should be performed. These patients remain at risk for secondary malignancies due to radiation therapy. Usually, there is a latency period of approximately 15 years. Therefore in older patients (age 70 or 80), this is not much of a concern. However, in younger patients age 20 or 30, this can be a true risk. In Portec-1 trial where endometrial cancer patients were randomized to either pelvic radiation or observation, the patients who received pelvic radiation had a higher chance of secondary malignancy at a median follow-up of 15 years (22% vs 16% in the observation group).[21]

Lifestyle modifications, including weight loss, smoking cessation as well as adherence to a regular exercise program, are also especially important in cancer survival. Obesity is a risk factor for endometrial cancer as well as recurrence of endometrial cancer due to increased levels of circulating estrogen. It is well known that peripheral adipose tissue specifically that within the abdominal region produces circulating estrogen. Since a significant proportion of endometrial cancer patients are overweight, these cancer survivors should be counseled on the importance of maintaining a healthy weight. Smoking cessation is paramount. Smokers who undergo radiation therapy can have inferior outcomes due to tissue hypoxia. In addition, smoking can increase not only posttreatment complications such as tissue necrosis and delays with wound healing but also the risk of secondary malignancies. There is no benefit to smoking. Exercise is linked with superior survival outcomes, such as in the case of breast cancer. Genetic counseling is also important to determine if the patient is at risk for an additional malignancy due to a germ line genetic mutation such as Lynch syndrome, BRCA 1 or 2. Genetic testing is also important for determining the risk of additional family members being diagnosed with a malignancy.

REFERENCES

1. Chargari C, Magne N, Guy JB, et al. Optimize and refine therapeutic index in radiation therapy: overview of a century. *Cancer Treat Rev*. 2016;45:58–67.
2. Halperin EC, Perez CA, Brady LW, eds. *Principles and Practice of Radiation Oncology*. 6th ed. Philadelphia, PA: Lippincott Williams & Wilkins; 2013.
3. Karlsson J, Dreifaldt AC, Mordhorst LB, et al. Differences in outcome for cervical cancer patients treated with or without brachytherapy. *Brachytherapy*. 2017;16:133–140.
4. Green J, Kirwan J, Tierney J, et al. Concomitant chemotherapy and radiation therapy for cancer of the uterine cervix. *Cochran Database Syst Rev*. 2005;3:CD002225.
5. Beadle BM, Jhingran A, Salehpour M, et al. Cervix regression and motion during the course of external beam

chemoradiation for cervical cancer. *Int J Radiat Oncol Biol Phys*. 2009;73:235–241.
6. Eifel P, Klopp A. *Gynecologic Radiation Oncology: A Practical Guide*. 1st ed. Philadelphia, PA: Wolters Kluwer; 2017 [chapters 9 and 10].
7. Miles T, Johnson N. Vaginal dilator therapy for women receiving pelvic radiotherapy. *Cochrane Database Syst Rev*. 2014;(9)CD007291.
8. Jensen PT, Groenvold M, Klee MC, et al. Longitudinal study of sexual function and vaginal changes after radiotherapy for cervical cancer. *Int J Radiat Oncol Biol Phys*. 2003;56:937–949.
9. Wallace WH, Thomson AB, Kelsey TW. The radiosensitivity of the human oocyte. *Hum Reprod*. 2003;18:117–121.
10. Moawad Nash S, Santamaria E, Rhoton-Vlasak A, et al. Laparoscopic ovarian transposition before pelvic cancer treatment: ovarian function and fertility preservation. *J Minim Invasive Gynecol*. 2017;24:28–35.
11. Segal S, John G, Sammel M, et al. Urinary incontinence and other pelvic floor disorders after radiation therapy and endometrial cancer survivors. *Maturitas*. 2017;105: 83–88.
12. Derks M, van der Velden J, Frijstein MM, et al. Long-term pelvic floor function and quality of life after radical surgery for cervical cancer: a multicenter comparison between different techniques for radical hysterectomy with pelvic lymphadenectomy. *Int J Gynecol Cancer*. 2016;26:1538–1543.
13. Rutledge TL, Heckman SR, Qualls C, et al. Pelvic floor disorders and sexual function in gynecologic cancer survivors: a cohort study. *Am J Obstet Gynecol*. 2010;203: 514.e1–514.e7.
14. Thaha MA, Abukar AA, Thin NN, et al. Sacral nerve stimulation for faecal incontinence and constipation in adults. *Cochrane Database Syst Rev*. 2015;8:CD004464.
15. Dunberger G, Lindquist H, Waldenström AC, et al. Lower limb lymphedema in gynecological cancer survivors—effect on daily life functioning. *Support Care Cancer*. 2013;11:3063–3070.
16. Biglia N, Zanfagnin V, Daniele A, et al. Lower body lymphedema in patients with gynecologic cancer. *Anticancer Res*. 2017;37:4005–4015.
17. Holloway R, Abu-Rustum N, Backes F, et al. Sentinel lymph node mapping and staging and endometrial cancer: a society of gynecologic oncology literature review with consensus recommendations. *Gynecol Oncol*. 2017;146:405–415.
18. Nout RA, Smit VT, Putter H, et al. Vaginal brachytherapy versus pelvic external beam radiotherapy for patients with endometrial cancer of high-intermediate risk (PORTEC-2): an open-label, non-inferiority, randomised trial. *Lancet*. 2010;375:816–823.
19. Quick A, Seamon L, Abdel-Rasoul M, et al. Sexual function after intracavitary vaginal brachytherapy for early-stage endometrial carcinoma. *Int J Gynecol Cancer*. 2012;22:703–708.
20. Schmeler KM, Jhingran A, Iyer RB, et al. Pelvic fractures after radiotherapy for cervical cancer: implications for survivors. *Cancer*. 2010;116:625–630.
21. Creutzberg CL, Nout RA, Lybeert ML, et al. Fifteen-year radiotherapy outcomes of the randomized PORTEC-1 trial for endometrial carcinoma. *Int J Radiat Oncol Biol Phys*. 2011;81:631–638.

CHAPTER 18

Surgical Gynecologic Oncology

NICHOLAS C. LAMBROU, MD • ANGEL AMADEO, BS

INTRODUCTION

Gynecologic oncology was defined as a subspecialty of obstetrics and gynecology in 1969. Gynecologic oncologists undergo fellowship training after residency to gain additional surgical expertise, including gastrointestinal, urologic, and complex abdominal and pelvic surgery. Gynecologic oncology requires a multidisciplinary approach to treatment, including surgery, chemotherapy, and radiation therapy. This chapter focuses on the surgical aspects of gynecologic oncology. Topics will include endometrial, cervical, ovarian, and vulvar carcinoma. Vaginal cancer is primarily treated with radiation therapy or with radical upper vaginal surgery, which is similar to the treatment of cervix cancer.

ANATOMY

In performing gynecologic surgery, understanding the three-dimensional pelvic anatomy is critical. The true pelvis is a bowl-shaped structure formed from the sacrum, pubis, ilium, ischium, the ligaments that interconnect these bones and the muscles that line their inner surface (Fig. 18.1). The true pelvis is considered to start at the level of the plane passing through the promontory of the sacrum, the arcuate line on the ilium, the iliopectineal line, and the posterior surface of the pubic crest. This plane or "inlet" lies at an angle of between 35 and 50 degrees up from the horizontal and above this the bony structures are sometimes referred to as the false pelvis.

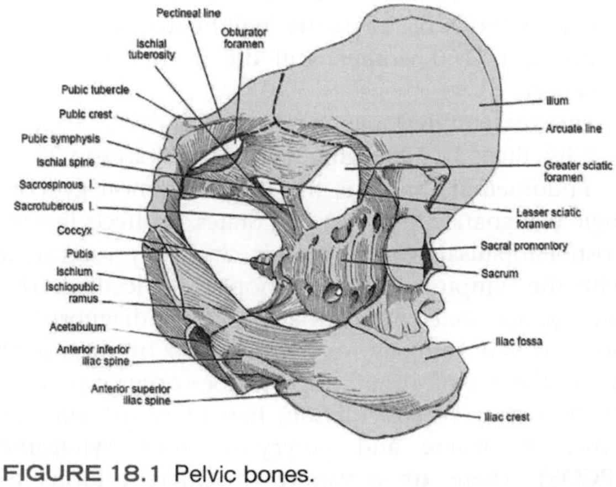

FIGURE 18.1 Pelvic bones.

Muscles arising within the pelvis form two groups. Piriformis and obturator internus, although forming part of the walls of the pelvis, are considered as primarily muscles of the lower limb. Levator ani and coccygeus form the pelvic diaphragm and delineate the lower limit of the true pelvis. The fasciae investing the muscles are continuous with visceral pelvic fascia above, perineal fascia below, and obturator fascia laterally (Fig. 18.2).

The true pelvis contains the internal iliac arteries and veins and the lymphatics, which drain the majority of the pelvic viscera. The common and external iliac vessels and the lymphatics, which drain the lower limb, lie along the pelvic brim and in the lower retroperitoneum and are described together with the vessels of the true pelvis.

At the pelvic brim the common iliac vessels will bifurcate into the internal and external iliac vessels (Fig. 18.3). The ureter will then cross over the iliac vessels from the lateral side to the medial. In surgery due to gynecologic cancer, this level is important as a defining location for pelvic and para-aortic lymph node dissections. The ovaries derive their blood supply directly from a branch of the aorta located within the infundibulopelvic ligament. The external iliac artery, after bifurcation at the level of sacral promontory, will travel along the iliopsoas muscle to provide blood to the lower limbs. From the anterior aspect of the external iliac artery, the inferior epigastric artery will branch off and travel along the anterior abdominal wall.

The internal iliac artery is the major blood supply to the pelvic organs. The anterior division of the internal iliac artery will supply blood to the bladder via the superior vesical artery and to the uterus via the uterine artery. The uterine artery will be the only vessel to cross the

Breast Cancer and Gynecologic Cancer Rehabilitation DOI: https://doi.org/10.1016/B978-0-323-72166-0.00018-9

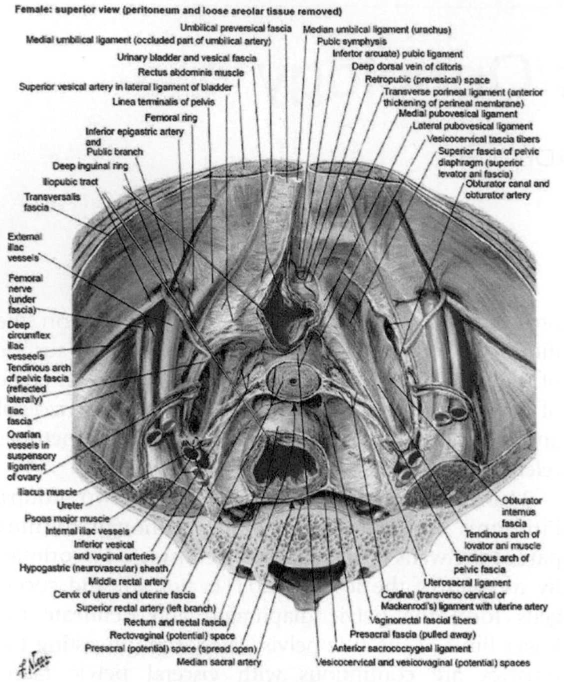

FIGURE 18.2 Pelvic basin.

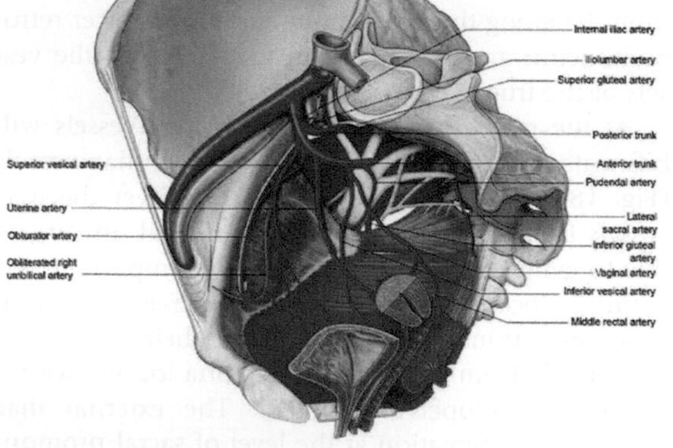

FIGURE 18.3 Pelvic vessels.

ureter horizontally (this is commonly referred to as "water under the bridge" where the ureter travels below the uterine artery as the artery crosses medially). The location of the ureter in relationship to the pelvic vessels is critical to understand surgically and a common area of concern to avoid iatrogenic injury.

The inferior hypogastric nerve plexus will innervate both the uterus and the urinary bladder, which is a combination of the inferior hypogastric nerve and the pelvic splanchnic nerve.

ENDOMETRIAL CARCINOMA

Introduction and Epidemiology

The endometrium is the inner lining of the uterus. During a woman's menstrual cycle, this part of the uterus will undergo changes due to hormones, estrogen and progesterone. When high levels of estrogen are produced, the endometrium thickens in order to provide implantation for embryo during pregnancy. When a woman's egg is not fertilized, estrogen levels drop, while progesterone levels increase, causing the endometrial lining to shed turning the lining into menstrual flow.[1,2] The endometrium is also the initial mutation point for most uterine cancers. Cancers begin to form in the body when the DNA of a cell is mutated.[3] Normal cells in the body have the ability to replicate as needed in the body, die when old and damaged, listen to signals to stop when come to close to other cells, and stay restricted to the specified area in the body. When a cell's genes become mutated and form into cancer cells, the cells will begin to replicate out of control forming a tumor over time, ignore signaling from other cells and invade nearby tissue, and cells will deviate from their specified area and spread throughout the body forming new tumors (metastasize). When the cells of the endometrium begin to mutate and become cancerous, the patient is said to have endometrial cancer.

The American Cancer Society's estimates for cancer of the uterus in the United States for 2019 are[4] as follows:

- About 61,880 new cases of cancer in the uterine corpus (body of the uterus) will be diagnosed.[4]
- About 12,160 women will die from endometrial cancer.
- Five-year survival rate for Stage I is 95%, Stage II 75%, Stage III 52%, and Stage IV decreases to 25%.

Endometrial cancer is the most common gynecologic malignancy in the United States. It affects mostly postmenopausal women and is classically associated with the symptom of postmenopausal bleeding. The average age that endometrial cancer is diagnosed is 60. It is very unlikely for a woman to be diagnosed under the age of 45 although it does occur especially in the setting of anovulation, hereditary risk such as Lynch syndrome and polycystic ovary syndrome (PCOS). There are a variety of different forms of endometrial cancer, but the most common is an endometrioid tumor. This tumor is typically caught early and associated with a very favorable prognosis. Risk factors include hypertension, anovulation, nulliparity, diabetes mellitus, and obesity.

Another important form of endometrial cancer is serous carcinoma. This form of endometrial cancer is less common and behaves more similar to ovarian carcinoma, with none of the risk factors associated with endometrioid type. Serous carcinoma is grouped in a category of endometrial cancer called high-risk endometrial cancer and most often requires adjuvant chemotherapy and/or radiation therapy after initial surgical staging.[5] Serous carcinomas are more associated with distinctive molecular alteration, while endometrioid tumors are more clearly associated with estrogen imbalance. Genetics may play a role in both of these diagnoses and evaluation for hereditary syndromes is important in every diagnosis of endometrial carcinoma.

Diagnosis and Staging

Endometrial cancer is most commonly diagnosed due to the presence of symptoms.[6] The most common symptom pertaining to endometrial cancer is postmenopausal bleeding as this occurs in 90% of cases.[7] Other less common symptoms associated with endometrial cancer are nonbloody vaginal discharge, pelvic pain, the presence of a mass, and unexpected weight loss. Once a patient presents symptoms such as postmenopausal bleeding, a gynecologist will perform a series of test to obtain the diagnosis, including a transvaginal ultrasound followed by a tissue diagnosis with either and office endometrial biopsy or operative dilatation and curettage. Endometrial biopsy is the most common test in determining endometrial cancer and can be done in the doctor's office. In an endometrial biopsy a physician will insert a thin flexible tube into the vaginal canal and through the cervix in order to reach the uterus, then using suction the tube will extract a small sample of tissue from the endometrial lining. In some cases, either endometrial biopsy cannot be attained or the results can be inconclusive. If an office biopsy is unsuccessful or not performed, the patient may need to undergo an outpatient procedure called a dilation and curettage. This procedure can be done either with sedation or general anesthesia; the physician will begin by dilating the cervix, then the doctor will scrap endometrial tissue that will be sent to pathology to determine the presence of cancer cells. When endometrial carcinoma is confirmed, the patient will be referred to a gynecologic oncologist for a consultation to plan surgical staging and treatment.

The stage of a cancer is determined using two main systems: the FIGO (International Federation of Gynecology and Obstetrics) system and the American Joint Committee on Cancer TNM staging system. Both of these systems use three main factors to stage[8]:

- The extent (size) of the tumor (*T*): How far has the cancer has grown into the uterus? Has the cancer reached nearby structures or organs?
- The spread to nearby lymph nodes (N): Has the cancer spread to the para-aortic lymph nodes? These are the lymph nodes in the pelvis or around the aorta (the main artery that runs from the heart down the back of the abdomen and pelvis).
- The spread (metastasis) to distant sites (M): Has the cancer spread to distant lymph nodes or distant organs in other parts of the body?

Numbers or letters following T, N, and M provide more detail about each of these factors. Higher numbers mean the cancer is more progressed. Once a person's T, N, and M categories have been determined, this information is combined in a process called stage grouping to assign an overall stage.

The staging system in Table 18.1 uses the pathological stage. The stage is found by examining tissue removed during an operation. In cases where surgery is not possible right away, the cancer will be given a clinical stage instead. A clinical stage is determined using results from a physical exam, biopsy, and imaging test done prior to surgery.

Surgery

The uterus is composed of the uterine corpus and the uterine cervix. The uterine cervix can be described as a supporting structure that allows separation of the vagina and the endometrial cavity and serves to maintain support during pregnancy.[9] The uterus itself is composed of three main layers: endometrium, myometrium, and serosa. The endometrium is the lining of the uterine cavity, which contains a superficial layer consisting of glandular epithelium and stroma. The myometrium is the thickest tissue of the uterus, which is composed of smooth muscle fibers. The final composition of the uterus is the serosa, which is composed of visceral peritoneum. Superior to the uterus hangs the ovaries and fallopian tubes.

The blood supply to the pelvis comes initially from the aorta, which descends down into the abdominal aorta. The ovarian artery forms directly from the aorta and branches off inferiorly to the renal artery. In the pelvis the ovarian artery will then descend to the infundibulopelvic ligament, which supplies the ovary. Following the bifurcation of the ovarian artery, the abdominal aorta

TABLE 18.1
Most recent American Joint Committee on Cancer system That Went Into Effect January 2018.

Stage	Stage Grouping	FIGO Stage	Stage Description[a]
I	T1 N0 M0	I	The cancer is growing inside the uterus. It may also be growing into the glands of the cervix, but not into the supporting connective tissue of the cervix (T1). It has not spread to nearby lymph nodes (N0) or to distant sites (M0).
IA	T1a N0 M0	IA	The cancer is in the endometrium (inner lining of the uterus) and may have grown less than halfway through the underlying muscle layer of the uterus (the myometrium) (T1a). It has not spread to nearby lymph nodes (N0) or to distant sites (M0).
IB	T1b N0 M0	IB	The cancer has grown from the endometrium into the myometrium. It has grown more than halfway through the myometrium but has not spread beyond the body of the uterus (T1b). It has not spread to nearby lymph nodes (N0) or to distant sites (M0).
II	T2 N0 M0	II	The cancer has spread from the body of the uterus and is growing into the supporting connective tissue of the cervix (called the cervical stroma). But it has not spread outside the uterus (T2). It has not spread to nearby lymph nodes (N0) or to distant sites (M0).
III	T3 N0 M0	III	The cancer has spread outside the uterus but has not spread to the inner lining of the rectum or urinary bladder (T3). It has not spread to nearby lymph nodes (N0) or to distant sites (M0).
IIIA	T3a N0 M0	IIIA	The cancer has spread to the outer surface of the uterus (called the serosa) and/or to the fallopian tubes or ovaries (the adnexa) (T3a). It has not spread to nearby lymph nodes (N0) or to distant sites (M0).
IIIB	T3b N0 M0	IIIB	The cancer has spread to the vagina or to the tissues around the uterus (the parametrium) (T3b). It has not spread to nearby lymph nodes (N0) or to distant sites (M0).
IIIC1	T1–T3 N1, N1mi, or N1a M0	IIIC1	The cancer is growing in the body of the uterus. It may have spread to some nearby tissues but is not growing into the inside of the bladder or rectum (T1–T3). It has also spread to pelvic lymph nodes (N1, N1mi, or N1a), but not to lymph nodes around the aorta or distant sites (M0).
IIIC2	T1–T3 N2, N2mi, or N2a M0	IIIC2	The cancer is growing in the body of the uterus. It may have spread to some nearby tissues but is not growing into the inside of the bladder or rectum (T1–T3). It has also spread to lymph nodes around the aorta (para-aortic lymph nodes) (N2, N2mi, or N2a), but not to distant sites (M0).
IVA	T4 Any N M0		The cancer has spread to the inner lining of the rectum or urinary bladder (called the mucosa) (T4). It may or may not have spread to nearby lymph nodes (any N) but has not spread to distant sites (M0).
IVB	Any T Any N M1	IVB	The cancer has spread to inguinal (groin) lymph nodes, the upper abdomen, the omentum, or to organs away from the uterus, such as the lungs, liver, or bones (M1). The cancer can be any size (any T) and it might or might not have spread to other lymph nodes (any N).

[a]Additional categories that are not described or listed above are as follows:

- TX: Main tumor cannot be assessed due to lack of information.
- T0: No evidence of primary tumor.
- NX: Regional lymph nodes cannot be assessed due to lack of information.[8]

will continue and bifurcate again into the common iliac arteries. The common iliac then divides into the external and internal iliac, which provide branches that supply blood to the pelvic organs. The internal iliac artery branches off into anterior and posterior divisions with the anterior division supplying the pelvic organs. The uterine artery travels through the cardinal ligament and is the primary blood supply to the uterus Fig. 18.4.

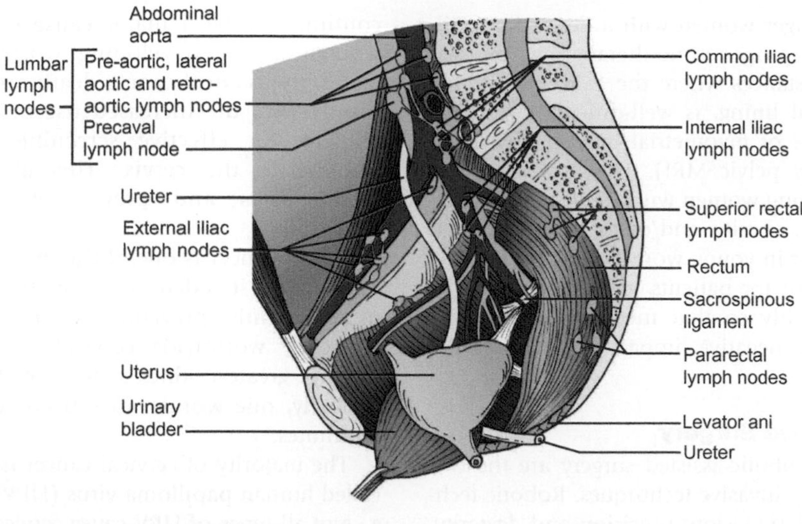

FIGURE 18.4 Blood supply to the reproductive organs.

Standard treatment for endometrial cancer includes a total hysterectomy, bilateral salpingo-oophorectomy (BSO), and surgical staging. A total hysterectomy includes removal of the uterus and the cervix. A BSO procedure will consist of the physician removing both ovaries and fallopian tubes.

The staging includes a surgical assessment of the lymph nodes (either sentinel or lymphadenectomy) and pelvic washings. To obtain pelvic washings the surgeon will fill the pelvic cavity with saline, then using suction the fluid is collected and sent to pathology for testing of cancer cells.[10] Although this does not change the surgical staging, pelvic washings may be used to provide adjuvant therapy recommendations.

Lymphadenectomy

Pelvic and para-aortic lymphadenectomy is a procedure that is used in intermediate-risk and high-risk endometrial cancers.[11,12] Lymphadenectomy is a procedure in which the surgeon will remove the lymph nodes that primarily drain the pelvic organs. With endometrial carcinoma the iliac basins are the regional lymph nodes most commonly involved. Factors that are associated with para-aortic lymph node dissemination are advanced stage, high histological grade, deep myometrial involvement, cervical involvement, lympho-vascular space involvement, and pelvic lymph node metastasis.[12,13] Risks associated with lymph node staging include iatrogenic injury to the vessels, nerves, or ureter during the dissection. Postoperative risks include a higher risk of deep vein thrombosis, lower extremity lymphedema, and musculoskeletal neuropathy. Fortunately with the use of minimally invasive surgery these risks are minimal.

Sentinel Lymph Node Staging

Sentinel lymph nodes are defined as the first lymph nodes in lymphatic drainage from a particular organ. With the widespread adoption of minimally invasive robotic surgery in endometrial cancer, sentinel lymph node staging has become a new standard of care.[14] Multiple sentinel lymph node mapping techniques include the use of dyes such as methylene blue, isosulfan blue, patent blue, and indocyanine green.[15] The injection of these dyes is performed intraoperatively directly into the cervix. The surgeon will then visualize the lymph nodes that turn the color of the dye, which allows for identification of the sentinel lymph node. The benefit of sentinel lymph node staging is to minimize the number and amount of lymph nodes removed to obtain accurate surgical staging. In addition, sentinel lymph nodes are processed differently by the pathologist than a routine lymph node sampling. Sentinel lymph nodes are examined under closer detail called micro-staging and this may allow for the identification of tiny cancer cells that may have otherwise gone undetected.

Fertility preservation

Although endometrial cancer is most often associated with postmenopausal women, it may also be diagnosed in younger women with a desire for fertility. In this setting, progesterone therapy may be used in specific circumstances where the cancer is limited to the endometrial lining, is well-differentiated, and shows no evidence of myometrial invasion by imaging (confirmed by pelvic MRI). This scenario most often occurs in young women with associated risk factors such as PCOS, obesity, and/or diabetes, although this may also occur in young women with no risk factors. It is important for patients in this setting to be counseled thoroughly so that medical management does not have a negative impact on her overall prognosis.

Minimally Invasive Surgery

Laparoscopy and robotic-assisted surgery are the two forms of minimally invasive techniques. Robotic technology introduced 3D vision, precision and dexterity, which has become widely adopted among gynecologic oncologists.[16,17] Robotic and laparoscopic surgery provides the benefits of enhanced surgical visualization due to the abdominal insufflation and improved clinical outcomes associated with smaller incisions. Patients are routinely able to go home the same or the following day from surgery. From a technical standpoint, during surgery, the patient is securely positioned into a Trendelenburg position which allows gravity to displace the intestines towards the upper abdomen and permits clear visualization of the pelvis during surgery. Prior to placing the patient into the Trendelenburg position, the physician will insert the primary trocar into a 12-mm incision at the umbilicus, avoiding the retroperitoneal vessels and the intestinal tract.[18] CO_2 insufflation is then performed followed by the insertion of the other laparoscopic or robotic trocars. It is important that the uterus is removed intact and is most often accomplished by vaginal extraction after all of the surrounding vessels and attachments have been isolated. When the uterus is too large to be removed vaginally, a separate Pfannenstiel incision may be used for removal of the specimen. Multiple studies have shown the advantages of minimally invasive procedures, including a lower risk of postoperative complications and enhanced postoperative recovery in comparison to traditional open surgery.[19]

Cervical Carcinoma

Introduction and Epidemiology

Cervical cancer was once one of the most common causes of cancer death for American women and continues to be a major cause of death of young women in the developing world. In the United States, the cervical cancer death rate dropped significantly with the increased use of the Pap test that allowed for effective screening of precancerous changes in the cervix. This allowed for earlier interventions and prevention of cancer from developing.

Cervix cancer is one of the most preventable types of cancers if it is detected early, treated correctly, and more recently prevented with HPV vaccinations. However, worldwide cervical cancer remains one of the greatest threats to the lives of women. Globally, one woman dies from cervix cancer every 2 minutes.

The majority of cervical cancer is caused by a virus called human papilloma virus (HPV):

- Not all types of HPV cause cervical cancer. Some of them cause genital warts, but other types may not cause any infections.
- The diagnosis of cervical cancer is established through a biopsy of the cervix. This may be a result of an abnormal Pap test or of a lesion visualized at the time of a speculum examination. In the setting of an abnormal Pap test, a colposcopy is performed where an examination of the cervix is performed with the use of a colposcope. A colposcope is an instrument that provides a magnification of the cervix to more closely identify the areas of abnormality. When an abnormality is seen, a biopsy is performed using a punch biopsy and/or endocervical curettage. The *punch biopsy* involves using a sharp tool to pinch off small samples of cervical tissue. *Endocervical curettage uses a* curet or a thin brush to scrape a tissue sample from the inside of the cervix. In settings where further biopsy tissue is indicated or needed to establish a diagnosis, a *LEEP* (loop electroexcisional procedure) or cone biopsy may be recommended. A LEEP uses a thin, low-voltage electrified wire to obtain a small tissue sample. Generally, this is done under local anesthesia in the office or an outpatient operating room. A *cone biopsy* (conization) is similar to a LEEP and is performed with a scalpel, excision of a portion of the cervix. This may be both diagnostic and therapeutic in select cases. This is most often performed in an outpatient surgical setting.

Cervical cancer tends to occur in midlife and is most frequently diagnosed in women between the ages of 35 and 44. It rarely develops in women younger than 20. Many older women do not realize that the risk of developing cervical cancer is still present as they age. More than 15% of cases of cervical cancer are found in women over 65. However, these cancers rarely occur in women who have been getting regular tests to screen for cervical cancer before they were 65.

In the United States, Hispanic women are most likely to get cervical cancer, followed by African-Americans, Asians and Pacific Islanders, and Whites. American-Indians and Alaskan natives have the lowest risk of cervical cancer in this country.

Initial stages of cervical cancer show no signs or symptoms. Signs and side effects of further developed cervical cancer include

- vaginal bleeding after intercourse
- abnormal vaginal discharge with foul odor
- pelvic pain during intercourse

Staging

Cervical cancer spreads by direct extension into the parametrium, vagina, uterus, and adjacent organs such as the bladder and rectum. It also spreads through the lymphatics to the pelvic lymph nodes (obturator, external and internal iliac) and the para-aortic region. In advanced or recurrent disease, cervix cancer may also metastasize through hematogenous spread to the liver, lung, and distant organs.

Until recently, cervical cancer staging was limited to the physical examination and limited additional studies when applicable. Tumor size and lymph node involvement remain important prognostic factors for women with cervical cancer and in 2018 the International Federation of Gynecology and Obstetrics (FIGO) published an updated cervical cancer staging system. Among the changes the list of tests and procedures that may be used to assign stage was expanded to include imaging and pathologic findings where available, tumor size criteria for some stages were revised, and lymph node metastases were included in staging.[20]

International Federation of Gynecology and Obstetrics (FIGO) Staging of Cancer of the Cervix Uteri (2018)

Stage	Description
I	The carcinoma is strictly confined to the cervix (extension to the uterine corpus should be disregarded)
IA	Invasive carcinoma that can be diagnosed only by microscopy, with maximum depth of invasion <5 mm
IA1	Measured stromal invasion <3 mm in depth
IA2	Measured stromal invasion ≥ 3 and <5 mm in depth
IB	Invasive carcinoma with measured deepest invasion ≥ 5 mm (greater than Stage IA), lesion limited to the cervix uteri
IB1	Invasive carcinoma ≥ 5 mm depth of stromal invasion and <2 cm in greatest dimension
IB2	Invasive carcinoma ≥ 2 and <4 cm in greatest dimension
IB3	Invasive carcinoma ≥ 4 cm in greatest dimension
II	The carcinoma invades beyond the uterus but has not extended onto the lower third of the vagina or to the pelvic wall
IIA	Involvement limited to the upper two-thirds of the vagina without parametrial involvement
IIA1	Invasive carcinoma <4 cm in greatest dimension
IIA2	Invasive carcinoma ≥ 4 cm in greatest dimension
IIB	With parametrial involvement but not up to the pelvic wall
III	The carcinoma involves the lower third of the vagina and/or extends to the pelvic wall and/or causes hydronephrosis or nonfunctioning kidney and/or involves pelvic and/or para-aortic lymph nodes
IIIA	The carcinoma involves the lower third of the vagina, with no extension to the pelvic wall
IIIB	Extension to the pelvic wall and/or hydronephrosis or nonfunctioning kidney (unless known to be due to another cause)
IIIC	Involvement of pelvic and/or para-aortic lymph nodes, irrespective of tumor size and extent (with r and p notations)
IIIC1	Pelvic lymph node metastasis only
IIIC2	Para-aortic lymph node metastasis
IV	The carcinoma has extended beyond the true pelvis or has involved (biopsy proven) the mucosa of the bladder or rectum. (A bullous edema, as such, does not permit a case to be allotted to Stage IV)
IVA	Spread to adjacent pelvic organs
IVB	Spread to distant organs

Surgery—Radical Hysterectomy

Radical hysterectomy with pelvic lymphadenectomy is considered the gold standard surgical treatment for patients with cervical cancer clinically confined to the cervix and upper vagina (FIGO Stages IB–IIA), with an overall survival ranging from 50% to 90%, depending on the presence of pathologic risk factors.[21–23]

In general, radical hysterectomy is defined by the additional surgical complexity taken to remove the tissue adjacent to the cervix (parametrium) and upper vagina (Fig. 18.1). One of the greatest surgical challenges in performing this operation is in the creation of a safe surgical distance from the ureters (they must be dissected free from the pelvic brim down to their insertion into the bladder), the bladder, and the rectum. In order to perform a radical hysterectomy, the surgeon must open the avascular surgical planes that are located in the retroperitoneum (Fig. 18.2). Potential intraoperative and postoperative complications include injury to the surrounding organs. Vesico-vaginal, uretero-vaginal, and rectovaginal fistulas are among the most serious surgical risks in addition to pelvic hemorrhage. Uretero-vaginal and vesico-vaginal fistulas occur in approximately 2%–4% of patients and postoperative ureteral obstruction occurs less than 1% of the time.[24]

Ovarian Preservation

When describing types of hysterectomy, it is important to note that it does not imply the removal of the ovaries. In fact, since cervix cancer often affects young women, the standard of care is to preserve the ovaries when indicated. Often an ovarian transposition is performed at the time of hysterectomy to move the ovaries to a position above the pelvic brim in order to be outside of the area of radiation if needed. This is performed to protect the ovaries from radiation and allow continued hormonal production. Unfortunately, it is only successful in preventing ovarian failure less than 50% of the time.[25]

Stage IA, Cervix Cancer and Fertility

The cervix may be preserved in select cases of early stage microinvasive cervix cancer (Stage IA). This is achieved by performing a cervical conization in which a portion of the cervix is removed. In all other cases the cervix must be removed for oncologic treatment.

Stage IA2

Since there is a small risk of lymph node metastases in these cases,[26–28] pelvic lymphadenectomy is recommended in addition to modified radical hysterectomy.[29]

In low-risk cases, simple hysterectomy or trachelectomy, with either pelvic lymphadenectomy or sentinel lymph node assessment, may be adequate surgical treatment.[30,31]

When the patient desires fertility, she may be counseled on other surgical options, including a radical trachelectomy.[32] In young women desiring fertility sparing, a radical trachelectomy may be performed for Stage IA2–IB1 tumors measuring less than or equal to 2 cm in largest diameter.[33] The cervix along with the parametrium is removed followed by anastomosis of the uterus with the vaginal end. Trachelectomy may be performed by open abdominal, vaginal, or by minimally invasive routes. The abdominal route is generally preferred. Even in the most experienced hands, a radical trachelectomy is a very challenging surgical procedure and patients should be individualized and counseled carefully regarding this option and risks.

Stages IB1, IB2, and IIA1

Performing a radical hysterectomy creates permanent and irreversible sterilization and patients must be counseled on this. Ovarian preservation and oocyte retrieval should be discussed with patients interested in in vitro fertilization and surrogate pregnancy options.[34]

Surgical treatment is an acceptable treatment modality for the treatment of Stage IB1, IB2, and IIA1 lesions. It would usually consist of a radical hysterectomy with pelvic lymphadenectomy. The routes of surgery may be open or minimally invasive, that is, laparoscopic or robotic.

Despite many retrospective studies supporting the safety and efficacy of minimally invasive surgical approaches to radical hysterectomy,[35–38] recent data have suggested a worsened prognosis when performed by a laparoscopic or robotic route.[39,40] Although minimally invasive surgery offers many clinical benefits to the patient, including shortened recovery, less blood loss, and a quicker return to daily activities, these recent data have challenged the oncologic outcomes of these procedures. Many gynecologic oncologists have since returned to the recommendation of open radical hysterectomy for Stage IB–IIA cervical carcinoma.

Once final pathology is available, the patient is considered as low risk with the following criteria: largest tumor diameter less than 2 cm, cervical stromal invasion less than 50%, no lympho-vascular space invasion, clear margins, and negative lymph nodes. Radiation will be recommended in the setting where there are risk factors identified after radical hysterectomy.

Complications and side effects associated with surgery and/or pelvic radiation

Short- and long-term side effects of radical hysterectomy include neurologic affects to the bladder, which may lead to urinary retention. In addition, sexual function may be greatly impacted due to a shortened vagina.[41–43] When radiation is added after radical hysterectomy, the risk of vaginal stenosis increases greatly. Patients are educated on the use of vaginal dilators to help prevent vaginal stenosis, but this is not generally very effective.

One of the risks associated with radical pelvic surgery is injury to the autonomic nerves (i.e., hypogastric nerve, splanchnic nerve, and pelvic plexus). Side effects include impairment of urination, defecation, and sexual function. This may be associated with a deterioration of the postoperative quality of life (QOL).[44,45] A nerve-sparing approach to radical hysterectomy is advised when possible although outcomes are not consistent.

Long-term side effects associated with radiation include gastrointestinal side effects such as radiation enteritis.[46–48]

Total Pelvic Exenteration

Aside from radical hysterectomy, perhaps the single most defining surgical procedure for the practicing gynecologic oncologist is pelvic exenteration. The availability of modern antibiotics, surgical intensive care units, and improvements in surgical reconstruction have decreased morbidity in patients undergoing pelvic exenteration and may help to improve overall survival in these patients.[49] Total pelvic exenteration is indicated for persistent or recurrent disease located in the pelvis with no distant metastases.[50] Pelvic exenteration involves the en bloc removal of pelvic organs due to a central recurrence of cancer located within a radiated field. This radical procedure involves the removal of all pelvic organs, including the bladder, uterus, cervix, vagina, rectosigmoid colon, and sometimes the vulva. The resection is followed by a reconstructive phase to address the urinary system, bowel function, and pelvic defect created by the large en bloc resection. Total pelvic exenteration can be further classified into anterior/posterior and infra-levator versus supra-levator.[51] The supra-levator exenteration includes removal of the uterus, cervix, upper vagina, and bladder (anterior) and or rectosigmoid colon (posterior). Infra-levator exenteration is required for disease that has extended to the lower vagina, vulva or perineum, including the anus and urethra. A large defect is created with the infra-levator procedure and requires reconstruction usually with myocutaneous flap reconstruction.[52,53] The benefit of the supra-levator exenteration includes preservation of the pelvic floor muscles. Urinary diversions both continent and incontinent are options to address the removal of the bladder.[54,55] A permanent colostomy is often required due to the removal of the rectosigmoid colon especially in patients who have had pelvic radiation, but a low rectal or colo-anal anastomosis may be used in carefully selected patients.[56,57]

Ovarian, Fallopian Tube, and Primary Peritoneal Carcinoma

The majority of cancers that develop from the ovary, fallopian tubes, and peritoneum are serous carcinomas that present and behave in a similar fashion. In addition, their management is the same. For simplicity, we will refer to ovarian carcinoma including fallopian tube and primary peritoneal diagnoses. Ovarian cancer is associated with the highest mortality of all gynecologic cancers in the western world.[58] The reason for this is that the majority of patients are diagnosed with advanced stage or when the disease has spread beyond the ovaries and onto peritoneal surfaces. Ascites is also often present (Fig. 18.1). In addition, there are no currently effective screening tools available to diagnosis ovarian cancer either in its premalignant state or at an early stage.

However, recent advances both in surgery and in adjuvant chemotherapy and biologic therapy have extended both the overall survival and progression-free survival of patients with this diagnosis. More than ever before, refinements in surgical techniques and how we care for women after surgery are improving outcomes for all stage of ovarian cancer. In a recent publication, of 11,541 women in the study with ovarian cancer, 3582 (31%) survived for more than 10 years following diagnosis.[59]

In addition, recent advances in genetic screening and in the understanding of how many diagnoses of ovarian cancer likely originated in the fallopian tubes have allowed for earlier surgical interventions to prevent this disease from occurring in high-risk populations.[60–62] It has become widely acceptable to electively remove the fallopian tubes at the time of hysterectomy for benign disease as a strategy to prevent ovarian/fallopian tube cancer.[63–66]

Depending upon the stage and extent of disease at presentation, the most effective treatment for ovarian cancer involves a combination of surgery and chemotherapy. The cornerstone of ovarian cancer treatment includes a maximum effort to remove or "debulk" as much disease as possible followed by six cycles of chemotherapy with carboplatin and paclitaxel. This surgical procedure is called cytoreductive surgery with an effort to reduce the burden of disease to nothing that is visible or minimally visible to the naked eye.

One of the key concepts of treating patients with ovarian cancer is the idea of recurrences. The vast majority of women with advanced ovarian cancer will respond to treatment, including surgery and chemotherapy. However, the majority will also recur. The window of time between the completion of initial therapy and the time to recurrence is the best prognostic indicator to a woman's overall survival from this diagnosis. For example, patients that recur within 6 months of the completion of treatment have a worse prognosis than those that recur after 6 months.

When a woman experiences her first recurrence from ovarian cancer, it often responds to therapy with a complete response. However, the time to second recurrence is usually less than with the first. It is common for a patient with ovarian cancer to experience many recurrences throughout her lifetime, each one treated differently, either with surgery, chemotherapy, biologic therapy, targeted radiation, or more recently with immunotherapy. Each of these treatments has its own specific side effects, all of which may be cumulative during a woman's lifetime.

Epidemiology

The American Cancer Society's estimates for ovarian cancer in the United States for 2019 are as follows:

- About 22,530 women will receive a new diagnosis of ovarian cancer.
- About 13,980 women will die from ovarian cancer.
- Ovarian cancer ranks fifth in cancer deaths among women, accounting for more deaths than any other cancer of the female reproductive system. A woman's risk of getting ovarian cancer during her lifetime is about 1 in 78. Her lifetime chance of dying from ovarian cancer is about 1 in 108. (These statistics do not count low malignant potential ovarian tumors.)

This cancer mainly develops in older women. About half of the women who are diagnosed with ovarian cancer are 63 years or older. It is more common in white women than African-American women. The rate at which women are diagnosed with ovarian cancer has been slowly falling over the past 20 years.[67]

Diagnosis and Staging

The two systems used for staging ovarian cancer the FIGO (International Federation of Gynecology and Obstetrics) system and the AJCC (American Joint Committee on Cancer) TNM staging system are basically the same. The table below represents the most recent AJCC system effective January 2018. It is the staging system for ovarian, fallopian tube, and primary peritoneal cancers.[68]

AJCC Stage	Stage Grouping	FIGO Stage	Stage Description[a]
I	T1 N0 M0	I	The cancer is only in the ovary (or ovaries) or fallopian tube(s) (T1). It has not spread to nearby lymph nodes (N0) or to distant sites (M0).
IA	T1a N0 M0	IA	The cancer is in one ovary, and the tumor is confined to the inside of the ovary; or the cancer is in one fallopian tube and is only inside the fallopian tube. There is no cancer on the outer surfaces of the ovary or fallopian tube. No cancer cells are found in the fluid (ascites) or washings from the abdomen and pelvis (T1a). It has not spread to nearby lymph nodes (N0) or to distant sites (M0).
IB	T1b N0 M0	IB	The cancer is in both ovaries or fallopian tubes but not on their outer surfaces. No cancer cells are found in the fluid (ascites) or washings from the abdomen and pelvis (T1b). It has not spread to nearby lymph nodes (N0) or to distant sites (M0).
IC	T1c N0 M0	IC	The cancer is in one or both ovaries or fallopian tubes and any of the following are present: • The tissue (capsule) surrounding the tumor broke during surgery, which could allow cancer cells to leak into the abdomen and pelvis (called *surgical spill*). This is Stage *IC1*.

			• Cancer is on the outer surface of at least one of the ovaries or fallopian tubes or the capsule (tissue surrounding the tumor) has ruptured (burst) before surgery (which could allow cancer cells to spill into the abdomen and pelvis). This is Stage *IC2*. • Cancer cells are found in the fluid (ascites) or washings from the abdomen and pelvis. This is Stage *IC3*. It has not spread to nearby lymph nodes (N0) or to distant sites (M0).
II	T2 N0 M0	II	The cancer is in one or both ovaries or fallopian tubes and has spread to other organs (such as the uterus, bladder, the sigmoid colon, or the rectum) within the pelvis or there is primary peritoneal cancer (T2). It has not spread to nearby lymph nodes (N0) or to distant sites (M0).
IIA	T2a N0 M0	IIA	The cancer has spread to or has invaded (grown into) the uterus or the fallopian tubes, or the ovaries (T2a). It has not spread to nearby lymph nodes (N0) or to distant sites (M0).
IIB	T2b N0 M0	IIB	The cancer is on the outer surface of or has grown into other nearby pelvic organs such as the bladder, the sigmoid colon, or the rectum (T2b). It has not spread to nearby lymph nodes (N0) or to distant sites (M0).
IIIA1	T1 or T2 N1 M0	IIIA1	The cancer is in one or both ovaries or fallopian tubes, or there is primary peritoneal cancer (T1) and it may have spread or grown into nearby organs in the pelvis (T2). It has spread to the retroperitoneal (pelvic and/or para-aortic) lymph nodes only. It has not spread to distant sites (M0).
IIIA2	T3a N0 or N1 M0	IIIA2	The cancer is in one or both ovaries or fallopian tubes, or there is primary peritoneal cancer and it has spread or grown into organs outside the pelvis. During surgery, no cancer is visible in the abdomen (outside of the pelvis) to the naked eye, but tiny deposits of cancer are found in the lining of the abdomen when it is examined in the lab (T3a). The cancer might or might not have spread to retroperitoneal lymph nodes (N0 or N1), but it has not spread to distant sites (M0).
IIIB	T3bN0 or N1 M0	IIIB	There is cancer in one or both ovaries or fallopian tubes, or there is primary peritoneal cancer and it has spread or grown into organs outside the pelvis. The deposits of cancer are large enough for the surgeon to see but are no bigger than 2 cm (about 3/4 in.) across (T3b). It may or may not have spread to the retroperitoneal lymph nodes (N0 or N1), but it has not spread to the inside of the liver or spleen or to distant sites (M0).
IIIC	T3c N0 or N1 M0	IIIC	The cancer is in one or both ovaries or fallopian tubes, or there is primary peritoneal cancer and it has spread or grown into organs outside the pelvis. The deposits of cancer are larger than 2 cm (about 3/4 in.) across and may be on the outside (the capsule) of the liver or spleen (T3c). It may or may not have spread to the retroperitoneal lymph nodes (N0 or N1), but it has not spread to the inside of the liver or spleen or to distant sites (M0).
IVA	Any T Any N M1a	IVA	Cancer cells are found in the fluid around the lungs (called a malignant pleural effusion) with no other areas of cancer spread such as the

			liver, spleen, intestine, or lymph nodes outside the abdomen (M1a).
IVB	Any T Any N M1b	IVB	The cancer has spread to the inside of the spleen or liver, to lymph nodes other than the retroperitoneal lymph nodes, and/or to other organs or tissues outside the peritoneal cavity such as the lungs and bones (M1b).

[a]The following additional categories are not described in the table:

- *TX*: Main tumor cannot be assessed due to lack of information.
- *T0*: No evidence of a primary tumor.
- *NX*: Regional lymph nodes cannot be assessed due to lack of information.

Surgery for Epithelial Ovarian Cancer. For epithelial ovarian cancer, surgery has two main goals: staging and debulking. These procedures are usually performed by a gynecologic oncologist who is fellowship trained in this specific type of surgery.

Staging Epithelial Ovarian Cancer

The first goal of ovarian cancer surgery is to *stage* the cancer—to see how far the cancer has spread from the ovary. Usually, this includes a hysterectomy, along with both ovaries and fallopian tubes (BSO). In addition, the omentum is also removed (an *omentectomy*). If there is no apparent spread to the omentum, then performing a lymph node sampling of the pelvic and para-aortic lymph nodes is advised to determine accurate surgical staging.[69–71] If there is fluid in the pelvis or abdominal cavity, it will be sent for cytology. If not, then washings are obtained by instilling sterile saline into the abdominal cavity and retrieving it for cytology evaluation. In addition, a series of random peritoneal biopsies are obtained from the pelvis, abdomen, and diaphragmatic peritoneum to assess for microscopic disease. Staging is very important because ovarian cancers at different stages are treated differently. If the staging is not done correctly, the patient is at risk to being over or under treated.

Surgery—Debulking and Cytoreduction

The other important goal of ovarian cancer surgery is to remove as much of the tumor as possible—this is called *debulking*. Debulking is very important when ovarian cancer has already spread throughout the abdomen at the time of surgery.[72] The aim of debulking surgery is to leave behind no visible cancer or no tumors larger than 1 cm (less than 1/2 in.).[73,74] This is called *optimally debulked. Patients whose tumors have been optimally debulked have a better outlook* (prognosis) *than those left with larger tumors after surgery* (*called suboptimally debulked*).[75–78]

In some cases, other organs might be affected by debulking. Gynecologic oncologists are fellowship trained to perform both gastrointestinal and urinary surgery when these organs are affected by a gynecologic malignancy. Ovarian cancer is the most common of the gynecologic cancers to affect multiple organs within the abdomen.

The rectosigmoid colon is positioned in the pelvis between the tubes and ovaries and behind the uterus. When ovarian cancer begins to spread locally, it is common to extend to the sigmoid colon. In some cases, this is only superficial and a surgical plane can be developed between the two organs. However, when the tumor has fused between the ovary and the colon and has invaded the colon serosa and/or mucosa, then performing a sigmoid resection at the time of ovarian debulking is indicated.[79–81] When planned in advance and depending upon the extent of disease, an ostomy may be avoided. In other cases where disease is too extensive (mostly in the recurrent setting) or there are other risk factors, a colostomy may be required either temporarily or permanent.[82,83]

Malignant small bowel obstruction is a risk associated with ovarian cancer. In these cases a part of the small intestine may need to be removed. Just like with the colon, the small intestine can either be reconnected (which is most common) or an ileostomy might be made. This is usually temporary; however, when the disease has progressed such as in recurrent carcinomatosis, this may be permanent.[84–86] Furthermore, when extensive carcinomatosis is involved, surgical options are limited. Percutaneous gastrostomy for palliative relief and other palliative options are indicated in this setting.

Chemotherapy

Intravenous chemotherapy is an integral part of the effective management of ovarian cancer. It may be given after surgery (adjuvant) or prior to surgery (neoadjuvant). Taxol and carboplatin are the established first-line therapies for ovarian cancer. When counseling a patient at diagnosis, patients are usually informed that chemotherapy has over a 75% chance of creating a complete clinical response. This is defined as normalization of CA 125 and/or no radiographic evidence of disease. The time interval from completion of chemotherapy until first recurrence is an important prognostic factor and may be unpredictable. A patient with a recurrence occurring after 6 months from completion of chemotherapy is considered "platinum-sensitive" and is often retreated with a platinum regimen usually in combination with another chemotherapy. A patient with recurrence within 6 months of completion of treatment is considered "platinum resistant." These patients have a worse prognosis and rarely respond to chemotherapy. A patient with progression of cancer during initial adjuvant chemotherapy is considered "platinum refractory." This carries the most ominous prognosis with a short overall survival.[87–89]

Most patients with ovarian cancer diagnosed at Stage III or IV (the majority) will have a complete response to initial surgery and chemotherapy. Over their lifetime, it is common to encounter multiple recurrences over a variety of time periods, using various choices of chemotherapy, surgical intervention, biologic therapy, and occasionally targeted radiation therapy to treat each reoccurrence.

Surgery for Ovarian Germ Cell Tumors and Ovarian Stromal Tumors

For germ cell tumors and stromal tumors, the main goal of surgery is to remove the cancer.

Most ovarian germ cell tumors are treated with a hysterectomy and BSO. If the cancer is in only one ovary and you still want to be able to have children, only the ovary containing the cancer and the fallopian tube on the same side are removed (leaving behind the other ovary and fallopian tube and the uterus).

Ovarian stromal tumors are often confined to just one ovary, so surgery may just remove that ovary. If the cancer has spread, more tissue may need to be removed. This could mean a hysterectomy and BSO and even debulking surgery.

Sometimes, after childbearing is finished, surgery to remove the other ovary, the other fallopian tube, and the uterus may be recommended, for both germ cell and stromal ovarian tumors.

Vulvar Intraepithelial Neoplasia, Paget's Disease of Vulva and Vulvar Carcinoma

Vulvar Intraepithelial Neoplasia

Vulvar intraepithelial neoplasia includes three categories of dysplasia (VIN I, II, III). Whether or not this represents a continuum is unclear. Similar to cervical intraepithelial neoplasia, these lesions appear to be HPV-related and initial evaluation includes colposcopy of the vulva with biopsy to confirm diagnosis. Wide local excision is most commonly recommended with 5 mm margins.

Although usually curative with wide local excision, there is a 3%–7% risk of progression to cancer after treatment and therefore continued surveillance is advised.

Paget's Disease of Vulva

Paget's disease of the vulva presents as red lesions of the vulva often associated with pruritis and discomfort or pain. The mean age at presentation is 65 years and most often in postmenopausal white women. Biopsy is important to establish the diagnosis as this can often be misdiagnosed as eczema or dermatitis. Paget's disease is classified as a carcinoma in situ and carries a 10% risk of underlying or associated carcinoma. Treatment includes wide local excision of the vulva or radical vulvectomy when an invasive component is present. Other topical therapies, including topical steroids and immunotherapy, are also integrated into the treatment of Paget's disease.

Vulvar Carcinoma

Invasive vulvar carcinoma accounts for 5%–8% of all female genital malignancies. The American Cancer Society's estimates for vulvar cancer in the United States for 2019 are about 6070 cancers of the vulva will be diagnosed and about 1280 women will die of this cancer.

Almost all women with invasive vulvar cancers will have the following symptoms:

- an area on the vulva that looks different from normal and could be lighter or darker than the normal skin around it or look red or pink
- a bump or lump, which could be red, pink, or white and could have a wart-like or raw surface or feel rough or thick
- thickening of the skin of the vulva
- itching
- pain or burning
- bleeding or discharge not related to the normal menstrual period
- an open sore (especially if it lasts for a month or more)

After a woman is diagnosed with vulvar cancer, it will be staged to determine the best course of treatment.

Vulvar cancer stages range from Stage I to IV. As a rule, the lower the number, the less the cancer has spread. A higher number, such as Stage IV, means cancer has spread more. Prognosis is closely linked to the stages of disease.

Types of Vulvectomy

Surgical vulvectomy includes four basic types of surgery.[90] In this type of operation, all or part of the vulva is removed.

- A *wide local excision* is an option for treating VIN or other vulvar lesion with a removal of skin and minimal underlying tissue.
- In a *simple vulvectomy* the entire vulva is removed (the inner and outer labia; sometimes the clitoris too) as well as tissue just under the skin. This is not commonly performed. More commonly, a *simple partial vulvectomy* is performed, removing the affected lesion and surrounding margin (similar to a wide local excision).
- A *partial or modified radical vulvectomy* removes part of the vulva, including the deep tissue, and may include the addition of a unilateral or bilateral inguinal lymphadenectomy to evaluate the regional lymph nodes.
- In a *complete radical vulvectomy* the entire vulva and deep tissues, including the clitoris, are removed.

Radical vulvectomy with unilateral or bilateral inguinal lymph node dissection.

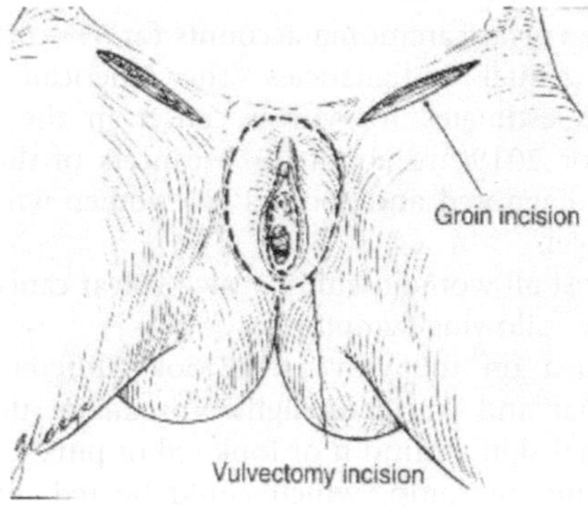

Inguinal Lymph Node Dissection

Surgery to remove lymph nodes in the groin is called an inguinal lymph node dissection. Usually, only lymph nodes on the same side as the cancer are removed. If the cancer is in or near the middle, then both sides may have to be done.

The groin incision is made from the iliac crest along the inguinal ligament and carried deep, down through membranes that cover the femoral nerves, veins, and arteries. This exposes most of the inguinal lymph nodes, which are then removed as a solid piece. A major vein, the saphenous vein, may or may not be closed off by the surgeon. Some surgeons will try to save it in an effort to reduce leg swelling (lymphedema) after surgery, but some doctors will not try to save the vein since the problem with swelling is mainly caused by the lymph node removal.

After the surgery a drain is placed into the incision and the wound is closed. The drain may remain for weeks after surgery and is removed once there is minimal lymphatic or serous drainage.

Sentinel Lymph Node Biopsy

This procedure can help some women avoid having a full inguinal node dissection. It is used to find and remove the lymph nodes that drain the area where the cancer is and is evolving as a standard of care. These lymph nodes are known as sentinel lymph nodes because cancer would be expected to spread to them first.

To find the sentinel lymph node(s) a small amount of radioactive material and/or blue dye is injected into the tumor site on the day before surgery. The groin is scanned to identify the side (left or right) that picks up the radioactive material. This is the side where the lymph nodes will be removed. During the surgery to remove the cancer, blue dye will be injected again into the tumor site. This allows the surgeon to find the sentinel node by its blue color and then remove it. Sometimes two or more lymph nodes turn blue and are removed.

If a lymph node near a vulvar cancer is abnormally large, it is more likely to contain cancer and a sentinel lymph node biopsy is usually not done. Instead, a fine needle aspiration biopsy or surgical biopsy of that lymph node is done to check for cancer cells.

Complications and Side Effects of Vulvar Surgery

Removal of wide areas of vulvar skin often leads to problems with wound healing, wound infections, or failure of the skin graft to take. The more tissue removed, the greater the risk of wound complications. Good hygiene and careful wound care are important as well as specific preoperative counseling. Wound care may take weeks or months and patients should anticipate a prolonged recovery from radical vulvar surgery.

Complications of vulvar and groin node surgery include wound seromas, wound infections, wound openings, pain with sitting, and permanent disfigurement. Sexual dysfunction may be permanent depending upon the degree of radicality and vulvar tissue removed.

Lymphedema is risk associated with removal of groin lymph nodes. This may be temporary or chronic and often requires lymphedema therapy for management.

The urine stream may change depending upon the amount of tissue removed near or adjacent to the urethra.

After vulvar surgery, women often feel discomfort if they wear tight slacks or jeans because the "padding" around the urethral opening and vaginal entrance is gone. The area around the vagina also looks very different.

Sexual impact of vulvectomy cannot be underestimated. Despite reconstructive techniques, there are permanent changes to the vulva, which may include the clitoris. Women often fear their partners will feel turned off by the scarring and loss of the outer genitals.

It may be difficult for women who have had a vulvectomy to reach orgasm.

With scarring of the introitus, vaginal dilators can sometimes help stretch the opening. When scarring is severe, the surgeon can sometimes use skin grafts to widen the entrance. Sometimes, a special type of physical therapy called pelvic floor therapy may help.

Pelvic Exenteration

Pelvic exenteration is an extensive operation that when used to treat vulvar cancer includes vulvectomy and often removal of the pelvic lymph nodes as well as one or more of the following structures: the lower colon, rectum, bladder, uterus, cervix, and vagina. How much has to be removed depends on how far the cancer has spread into nearby organs. This is very complex surgery that can lead to many different kinds of complications.

If the bladder is removed, a new way to store and pass urine is needed. Usually, a short piece of intestine is used to function as a new bladder. This may be connected to the abdominal wall so that urine can be drained when the woman places a catheter into a small opening (urostomy) or urine may drain continuously into a small plastic bag that sticks to the belly over the opening.

If the rectum and part of the colon are removed, a colostomy, either permanent or temporary, may be needed.

Vulvar Reconstruction

Sometimes these procedures remove a large area of skin from the vulva, requiring skin grafts from other parts of the body to cover the wound. But, most of the time the surgical wounds can be closed without grafts and still provide a very satisfactory appearance. If a skin graft is needed, the gynecologic oncologist may do it. Otherwise, it may be done by a plastic/reconstructive surgeon after the vulvectomy.

Reconstructive surgery is available for women who have had more extensive surgery. A reconstructive surgeon can take a piece of skin and underlying fatty tissue and sew it into the area where the cancer was removed. Several sites in the body can be used, but it is complicated by the fact that the blood supply to the transplanted tissue needs to be kept intact. This is where a skillful surgeon is needed because the tissue must be moved without damaging the blood supply. If you are having flap reconstruction, ask the surgeon to explain how it will be done, because there is no set way of doing it.

CONCLUSION

Gynecologic surgery is an integral part of the management of endometrial, cervical, ovarian, and vulvar cancers in both the staging and debulking of the cancer. Commonly performed surgeries include total hysterectomy, BSO, lymphadenectomy, vulvectomy, and pelvic exenteration. An understanding of pertinent anatomy involved by the cancer, stage of cancer, and type of surgery performed is essential for clinicians involved in the rehabilitation of persons with gynecologic cancer.

REFERENCES

1. Murali R, Davidson B, Fadare O, et al. High-grade endometrial carcinomas: morphologic and immunohistochemical features, diagnostic challenges and recommendations. *Int J Gynecol Pathol.* 2019;38(suppl 1):S40–S63.
2. National Cancer Institute. Endometrial Cancer Treatment (PDQ®)—Health Professional Version. January 19, 2018.
3. National Comprehensive Cancer Network. Uterine Cancer Guidelines For Patients. October 2018.
4. American Cancer Society. *Facts & Figures 2019*. Atlanta, GA: American Cancer Society; 2019.
5. Zhang L, Kwan SY, Wong KK, Solaman PT, Lu KH, Mok SC. Pathogenesis and Clinical Management of Uterine Serous Carcinoma. *Cancers (Basel)*. 2020;12(3). pii: E686. https://doi:10.3390/cancers12030686
6. Endometrial Cancer Early Detection. *Diagnosis, and Staging*. American Cancer Society; 2019, Published March

27. Available from: https://www.cancer.org/content/dam/CRC/PDF/Public/8611.00.pdf. Accessed 19.09.19.
7. Endometrial cancer. Mayo Clinic. <https://www.mayoclinic.org/diseases-conditions/endometrial-cancer/symptoms-causes/syc-20352461>; July 25, 2019. Accessed 09.09.19.
8. Endometrial Cancer Stages. American Cancer Society. <https://www.cancer.org/cancer/endometrial-cancer/detection-diagnosis-staging/staging.html>; March 27, 2019. Accessed 21.09.19.
9. Barber MD, Park AJ. Surgical pelvic female anatomyWaltham, MA In: Rose BD, ed. *UpToDate*. 2013.
10. Rodriguez EF, Monaco SE, Khalbuss W, Marshall Austin R, Pantanowitz L. Abdominopelvic washings: a comprehensive review. *CytoJournal*. 2013;10:7.
11. Fowler JM, Backes FJ. Pelvic and Paraaortic Lymphadenectomoy in Gynecologic Cancers. November 2018.
12. Mariani A, Dowdy S, Podratz K. The role of pelvic and para-aortic lymph node dissection in the surgical treatment of endometrial cancer: a view from the USA. *Obstet Gynaecol*. 2009;11:199–204.
13. AlHilli MM, Mariani A. *Int J Clin Oncol*. 2013;18:193. Available from: https://doi.org/10.1007/s10147-013-0528-7.
14. Stewart KI, Eska JS, Harrison RF, Suidan R, Abraham A, Chisholm GB, et al. Implementation of a sentinel lymph node mapping algorithm for endometrial cancer: surgical outcomes and hospital charges. *Int J Gynecol Cancer*. 2020;30(3):352–357. Available from: https://doi.org/10.1136/ijgc-2019-000941.
15. Kim S, Ryu KJ, Min KJ, Lee S, Jung US, Hong JH, Song JY, Lee JK, Lee NW. Learning curve for sentinel lymph node mapping in gynecologic malignancies. **sentinel lymph node**. mapping in gynecologic malignancies. *J Surg Oncol* 2020;121(4):599–604. https://doi.org/10.1002/jso.25853.
16. Gehrig PA, Cantrell LA, Shafer A, Abaid LN, Mendivil A, Boggess JF. *What is the optimal minimally invasive surgical procedure for endometrial cancer staging in the obese and morbidly obese woman?* 1st ed. *Gynecologic Oncology*. 111. Chapel Hill, NC: Elsevier; 2008:41–45.
17. Hurd W.W. Gynecologic Laparoscopy Treatment & Management; September 2018.
18. Silva E, Silva A, de Carvalho JPM, et al. Introduction of robotic surgery for endometrial cancer into a Brazilian cancer service: a randomized trial evaluating perioperative clinical outcomes and costs. *Clin (Sao Paulo)*. 2018;73(suppl 1):e522s.
19. Frumovitz M, Escobar P, Ramirez PT. Minimally invasive surgical approaches for patients with endometrial cancer. *Clin Obstet Gynecol*. 2011;54(2):226–234.
20. Bhatla N, Aoki D, Sharma DN, Rengaswamy S. Cancer of the cervix uteri. *Int J Gynecol Obstet*. 2018;143(suppl 2):22–36.
21. Clark JG. A more radical method of performing hysterectomy for cancer of the uterus. *Bull Johns Hopkins Hospital*. 1895.
22. Wertheim E. The extended abdominal operation for carcinoma uteri. *Am J Obstet Gynecol*. 1912;LXVI (2).
23. Meigs JV. The Wertheim operation for carcinoma of the cervix. *Am. J. Obst & Gynec*. 1945;49:542–543.
24. Ralph G, Tamussino K, Lichgenegger W. Urological complications after radical hysterectomy with or without radiotherapy for cervical cancer. *Arch Gynecol Obstet*. 1990;248:61–65.
25. Yin L, Lu S, Zhu J, Zhang W, Ke G. Ovarian transposition before radiotherapy in cervical cancer patients: functional outcome and the adequate dose constraint. *Radiat Oncol*. 2019;14(1):100. Available from: https://doi.org/10.1186/s13014-019-1312-2.
26. van Meurs H, Visser O, Buist MR, et al. Frequency of pelvic lymph node metastases and parametrial involvement in stage IA2 cervical cancer: a population-based study and literature review. *Int J Gynecol Cancer*. 2009;19:21–26.
27. Costa S, Marra E, Martinelli GN, et al. Outcome of conservatively treated microinvasive squamous cell carcinoma of the uterine cervix during a 10-year follow-up. *Int J Gynecol Cancer*. 2009;19:33–38.
28. Bouchard-Fortier G, Reade CJ, Covens A. Non-radical surgery for small early-stage cervical cancer. Is it time? *Gynecol Oncol*. 2014;132:624–627.
29. Bhatla N, Aoki D, Sharma DN, Rengaswamy S. Cancer of the cervix uteri. *Int J Gynecol Obstet*. 2018;143(suppl 2):22–36.
30. Coutant C, Cordier AG, Guillo E, Ballester M, Rouzier R, Daraï E. Clues pointing to simple hysterectomy to treat early-stage cervical cancer. *Oncol Rep*. 2009;22:927–934.
31. Frumovitz M, Sun CC, Schmeler KM, et al. Parametrial involvement in radical hysterectomy specimens for women with early-stage cervical cancer. *Obstet Gynecol*. 2009;114:93–99.
32. Shepherd JH, Spencer C, Herod J, Ind TE. Radical vaginal trachelectomy as a fertility-sparing procedure in women with early-stage cervical cancer- cumulative pregnancy rate in a series of 123 women. *BJOG*. 2006;113:719–724.
33. Abu-Rustum NR, Sonoda Y, Black D, et al. Fertility-sparing radical abdominal trachelectomy for cervical carcinoma: technique and review of the literature. *Gynecol Oncol*. 2006;103:807–813.
34. Matsuo K, Machida H, Shoupe D, et al. Ovarian conservation and overall survival in young women with early-stage cervical cancer. *Obstet Gynecol*. 2017;129(1):139–151.
35. Malzoni M, Tinelli R, Cosentino F, Perone C, Vicario V. Feasibility, morbidity, and safety of total laparoscopic radical hysterectomy with lymphadenectomy: our experience. *J Minim Invasive Gynecol*. 2007;14(5):584–590.
36. Salicrú S, Gil-Moreno A, Montero A, Roure M, Pérez-Benavente A, Xercavins J. Laparoscopic radical hysterectomy with pelvic lymphadenectomy in early invasive cervical cancer. *J Minim Invasive Gynecol*. 2011;18(5):555–568.
37. Gil-Moreno A, Puig O, Pérez-Benavente MA, et al. Total laparoscopic radical hysterectomy (type II-III) with

pelvic lymphadenectomy in early invasive cervical cancer. *J Minim Invasive Gynecol.* 2005;12(2):113–120.
38. Shazly SA, Murad MH, Dowdy SC, Gostout BS, Famuyide AO. Robotic radical hysterectomy in early stage cervical cancer: a systematic review and meta-analysis. *Gynecol Oncol.* 2015;138(2):457–471.
39. Ramirez PT, Frumovitz M, Pareja R, et al. Minimally invasive versus abdominal radical hysterectomy for cervical cancer. *N Engl J Med.* 2018;379(20):1895–1904.
40. Melamed A, Margul DJ, Chen L, et al. Survival after minimally invasive radical hysterectomy for early-stage cervical cancer. *N Engl J Med.* 2018;379(20):1905–1914.
41. Sun H, Cao D, Shen K, et al. Piver type II vs. type III hysterectomy in the treatment of early-stage cervical cancer: midterm follow-up results of a randomized controlled trial. *Front Oncol.* 2018;8:568. Available from: https://doi.org/10.3389/fonc.2018.00568.
42. Plotti F, Nelaj E, Sansone M, et al. Sexual function after modified radical hysterectomy (Piver II/Type B) vs. classic radical hysterectomy (Piver III/Type C2) for early stage cervical cancer. A prospective study. *J Sex Med.* 2012;9(3):909–917.
43. Jongpipan J, Charoenkwan K. Sexual function after radical hysterectomy for early-stage cervical cancer. *J Sex Med.* 2007;4(6):1659–1665.
44. Fujii S, Takakura K, Matsumura N, et al. Anatomic identification and functional outcomes of the nerve sparing Okabayashi radical hysterectomy. *Gynecol Oncol.* 2007;107:4–13.
45. Roh JW, Lee DO, Suh DH, et al. Efficacy and oncologic safety of nerve- sparing radical hysterectomy for cervical cancer: A randomized controlled trial. *J Gynecol Oncol.* 2015;26:90–99.
46. Smyrniotis V, Kostopanagiotou G, Gamaletsos E, et al. A safe method of gut resection in women with complicated post-radiation enteritis after cervix cancer. *Eur J Gynaecol Oncol.* 2003;24(2):195–197.
47. Chen SW, Liang JA, Yang SN, et al. Radiation injury to intestine following hysterectomy and adjuvant radiotherapy for cervical cancer. *Gynecol Oncol.* 2004;95(1):208–214.
48. Yang J, Ding C, Zhang T, et al. Clinical features, outcome and risk factors in cervical cancer patients after surgery for chronic radiation enteropathy. *Radiat Oncol.* 2015;10:128.
49. Averette HE, Lichtenger M, Sevin BU, et al. Pelvic exenteration: a 15 year experience in a general metropolitan hospital. *Am J Obstet Gynecol.* 1984;150:179–184.
50. Berek JS, Howe C, Lagasse LD, Hacker NF. Pelvic exenteration for recurrent gynecologic malignancy: survival and morbidity analysis of the 45-year experience at UCLA. *Gynecol Oncol.* 2005;99(1):153–159.
51. Magrina JF, Stanhope CR, Weaver AL. Pelvic exenterations: supralevator, infralevator, and with vulvectomy. *Gynecol Oncol.* 1997;64:130–135.
52. Berger JL, Westin SN, Fellman B, et al. Modified vertical rectus abdominis myocutaneous flap vaginal reconstruction: an analysis of surgical outcomes. *Gynecol Oncol.* 2012;125(1):252–255.
53. Soper JT, Secord AA, Havrilesky LJ, Berchuck A, Clarke-Pearson DL. Comparison of gracilis and rectus abdominis myocutaneous flap neovaginal reconstruction performed during radical pelvic surgery: flap-specific morbidity. *Int J Gynecol Cancer.* 2007;17(1):298–303.
54. Salom EM, Mendez LE, Schey D, et al. Continent ileocolonic urinary reservoir (Miami pouch): the University of Miami experience over 15 years. *Am J Obstet Gynecol.* 2004;190(4):994–1003.
55. Urh A, Soliman PT, Schmeler KM, et al. Postoperative outcomes after continent versus incontinent urinary diversion at the time of pelvic exenteration for gynecologic malignancies. *Gynecol Oncol.* 2013;129(3):580–585.
56. Benn T, Brooks RA, Zhang Q, et al. Pelvic exenteration in gynecologic oncology: a single institution study over 20 years. *Gynecol Oncol.* 2011;122(1):14–18.
57. Lambrou NL, Pearson JM, Averette HE. Pelvic exenteration of gynecologic malignancy: indications, and technical and reconstructive considerations. *Surg Oncol Clin N Am.* 2005;14(2):289–300.
58. Momenimovahed Z, Tiznobaik A, Taheri S, Salehiniya H. Ovarian cancer in the world: epidemiology and risk factors. *Int J Womens Health.* 2019;11:287–299.
59. Cress RD, Chen YS, Morris CR, Petersen M, Leiserowitz GS. Characteristics of long-term survivors of epithelial ovarian cancer. *Obstet Gynecol.* 2015;126(3):491–497.
60. Salvador S, Gilks B, Köbel M, Huntsman D, Rosen B, Miller D. The fallopian tube: primary site of most pelvic high-grade serous carcinomas. *Int J Gynecol Cancer.* 2009;19:58–64.
61. Crum CP, Drapkin R, Miron A, et al. The distal fallopian tube: a new model for pelvic serous carcinogenesis. *Curr Opin Obstet Gynecol.* 2007;19(1):3–9.
62. Crum CP, Drapkin R, Kindelberger D, Medeiros F, Miron A, Lee Y. Lessons from BRCA: the tubal fimbria emerges as an origin for pelvic serous cancer. *Clin Med Res.* 2007;5(1):35–44.
63. Pölcher M, Hauptmann S, Fotopoulou C, et al. Should fallopian tubes be removed during hysterectomy procedures? – A statement by AGO ovar. *Geburtshilfe Frauenheilkd.* 2015;75(4):339–341. Available from: https://doi.org/10.1055/s-0035-1545958.
64. Van Lieshout LAM, Pijlman B, Vos MC, et al. Opportunistic salpingectomy in women undergoing hysterectomy: Results from the HYSTUB randomised controlled trial. *Maturitas.* 2018;107:1–6.
65. Kim M, Kim YH, Kim YB, et al. Bilateral salpingectomy to reduce the risk of ovarian/fallopian/peritoneal cancer in women at average risk: a position statement of the Korean Society of Obstetrics and Gynecology (KSOG). *Obstet Gynecol Sci.* 2018;61(5):542–552.
66. Paul PG, Mannur S, Shintre H, Paul G, Gulati G, Mehta S. Thirteen years of experience with opportunistic bilateral salpingectomy during TLH in low-risk

premenopausal women. *J Obstet Gynaecol India*. 2018;68 (4):314–319.
67. Howlader N, Noone AM, Krapcho M, et al., eds. *American Cancer Society. Cancer Facts & Figures 2019*. Atlanta, GA: American Cancer Society; 2019, Lifetime Risk (Percent) of Being Diagnosed with Cancer by Site and Race/Ethnicity; Males, 18 SEER Areas, 2012–2014 SEER Cancer Statistics Review, 1975–2014, National Cancer Institute. Bethesda, MD. Available from: https://seer.cancer.gov/csr/1975_2014/. based on November 2016 SEER data submission, posted to the SEER web site, April 2017.
68. Prat J, FIGO Committee on Gynecologic Oncology. *Staging classification for cancer of the ovary, fallopian tube, and peritoneum. American Joint Committee on Cancer. Ovary, Fallopian Tube, and Primary Peritoneal Carcinoma. AJCC Cancer Staging Manual*. 8th ed. New York: Springer; 2017:681–690. Int J Gynecol Obstet. 2014;124(1):1–5.
69. Cannistra SA, Gershenson DM, Recht A. Ch 76 – Ovarian cancer, fallopian tube carcinoma, and peritoneal carcinoma. In: DeVita VT, Hellman S, Rosenberg SA, eds. *Cancer: Principles and Practice of Oncology*. 10th ed. Philadelphia, PA: Lippincott Williams & Wilkins; 2015.
70. Morgan M, Boyd J, Drapkin R, Seiden MV. Ch 89 – Cancers arising in the ovary. In: Abeloff MD, Armitage JO, Lichter AS, Niederhuber JE, Kastan MB, McKenna WG, eds. *Clinical Oncology*. 5th ed. Philadelphia, PA: Elsevier; 2014:1592.
71. Young RC, Decker DG, Wharton JT, et al. Staging laparotomy in early ovarian cancer. *JAMA*. 1983;250:3072.
72. Hoskins WJ. Epithelial ovarian carcinoma: principles of primary surgery. *Gynecol Oncol*. 1994;55:S91.
73. Hoskins WJ, McGuire WP, Brady MF, et al. The effect of diameter of largest residual disease on survival after primary cytoreductive surgery in patients with suboptimal residual epithelial ovarian carcinoma. *Am J Obstet Gynecol*. 1994;170:974.
74. McCreath WA, Chi DS. Surgical cytoreduction in ovarian cancer. *Oncol (Huntingt)*. 2004;18:645.
75. Schorge JO, McCann C, Del Carmen MG. Surgical debulking of ovarian cancer: what difference does it make? *Rev Obstet Gynecol*. 2010;3(3):111–117.
76. Bristow RE, Tomacruz RS, Armstrong DK, et al. Survival effect of maximal cytoreductive surgery for advanced ovarian carcinoma during the platinum era: a meta-analysis. *J Clin Oncol*. 2002;20:1248.
77. Eisenkop SM, Friedman RL, Wang HJ. Complete cytoreductive surgery is feasible and maximizes survival in patients with advanced epithelial ovarian cancer: a prospective study. *Gynecol Oncol*. 1998;69:103.
78. Allen DG, Heintz AP, Touw FW. A meta-analysis of residual disease and survival in stage III and IV carcinoma of the ovary. *Eur J Gynaecol Oncol*. 1995;16: 349.
79. Scarabelli C, Gallo A, Franceschi S, et al. Primary cytoreductive surgery with rectosigmoid colon resection for patients with advanced epithelial ovarian carcinoma. *Cancer*. 2000;88:389.
80. O'Hanlan KA, Kargas S, Schreiber M, et al. Ovarian carcinoma metastases to gastrointestinal tract appear to spread like colon carcinoma: implications for surgical resection. *Gynecol Oncol*. 1995;59:200.
81. Weber AM, Kennedy AW. The role of bowel resection in the primary surgical debulking of carcinoma of the ovary. *J Am Coll Surg*. 1994;179:465.
82. Tseng JH, Suidan RS, Zivanovic O, et al. Diverting ileostomy during primary debulking surgery for ovarian cancer: associated factors and postoperative outcomes. *Gynecol Oncol*. 2016;142(2):217–224.
83. Tamussino KF, Lim PC, Webb MJ, et al. Gastrointestinal surgery in patients with ovarian cancer. *Gynecol Oncol*. 2001;80:79.
84. Glasgow MA, Shields K, Vogel RI, Teoh D, Argenta PA. Postoperative readmissions following ileostomy formation among patients with a gynecologic malignancy. *Gynecol Oncol*. 2014;134(3):561–565. Available from: https://doi.org/10.1016/j.ygyno.2014.06.005.
85. Martinez Castro P, Vargas L, Mancheño A, et al. Malignant bowel obstruction in relapsed ovarian cancer with peritoneal carcinomatosis: an occlusive state. *Int J Gynecol Cancer*. 2017;27(7):1367–1372.
86. Lee YC, Jivraj N, O'Brien C, et al. Malignant bowel obstruction in advanced gynecologic cancers: an updated review from a multidisciplinary perspective. *Obstet Gynecol Int*. 2018;2018:1867238.
87. Kobayashi-Kato, M, et al. Platinum-free interval affects efficacy of following treatment for platinum-refractory or -resistant ovarian cancer. *Cancer Chemother Pharmacol*. 2019;84(1):33–39.
88. Oronsky B, et al. A brief review of the management of platinum-resistant-platinum-refractory ovarian cancer. *Med Oncol*. 2017;34(6):103. Available from: https://doi.org/10.1007/s12032-017-0960-z.
89. Parikh R, Kurosky SK, Udall M, et al. Treatment patterns and health outcomes in platinum-refractory or platinum-resistant ovarian cancer: a retrospective medical record review. *Int J Gynecol Cancer*. 2018;28 (4):738–748.
90. Dellinger TH, Hakim AA, Lee SJ, et al. Surgical management of vulvar cancer. *J Natl Compr Cancer Netw*. 2017;15(1):121–128.

CHAPTER 19

Pelvic Floor Dysfunction in Gynecologic Cancer

LOUISE V. GLEASON, MSPT, PRPC

INTRODUCTION

This chapter will introduce the clinician to the role of pelvic floor therapy for rehabilitation of gynecological (GYN) cancer survivors. This population is unlike others with pelvic floor dysfunction because of overlapping local and systemic side effects of their cancer treatment. Many women do not seek evaluation of their pelvic floor symptoms for a variety of personal reasons or due to a lack of awareness on the part of the patient and their health-care providers.[1] It is imperative that the rehabilitation specialists caring for these patients are well versed on the management of pelvic floor dysfunction. The goal of this chapter is to review the body systems affected by GYN cancer and investigate evidence-based rehabilitation interventions to treat them.

GYN cancers represent approximately 6% of the 1.8 million new cancer diagnoses that will be made in the United States in 2019. Uterine cancers are the most common, of all the cancers affecting the female reproductive system, followed by ovarian, cervical, and vulvar cancers. According to the National Cancer Institute annual report to the nation, the estimate of new cases for GYN-related cancers in 2019 is 109,000 with an overall survivorship of nearly 70%.[2] Acute management of GYN cancers includes surgery, chemotherapy, radiation, hormonal, and targeted therapies, which can be used alone or jointly. These treatments are known to have long-term effects that significantly impact physical activity levels and quality of life.[3] There is a growing body of research that identifies the impact GYN cancer treatments have on the pelvic floor, including bladder, bowel, and sexual function.[4] The need for survivorship rehabilitation services in this population will certainly continue to increase as the general population ages.

GYN cancer survivors constitute a unique population, different from other women who have had pelvic injuries or age-related hormonal changes. Neron et al. compared pelvic floor dysfunction between GYN cancer survivors 1 year after hysterectomy, healthy controls in the general population, and controls with a history of benign hysterectomy. They found that the GYN cancer survivors had more pelvic floor dysfunction and greater severity of symptoms affecting quality of life than the other two groups.[5] Ramaseshan et al. performed a systematic review to describe the prevalence of pelvic floor disorders among GYN cancer survivors and concluded that pelvic floor dysfunctions, including urinary and fecal incontinence, urinary retention, dyspareunia, vaginal dryness, prolapse, and sexual dysfunction, are up to three times more prevalent in GYN cancer survivors than controls.[6] In a study of 152 women with suspected GYN malignancy who were scheduled for surgical intervention, Bretschneider et al. looked at the prevalence of pelvic floor disorders and found that this population had a high rate of pelvic floor symptoms even before surgical or adjuvant treatments.[7]

The specific nature of GYN cancer treatment affects the pelvic structures acutely and leaves long-term systemic side effects. Surgical scars and radiation damage last for many years after the initial recovery phase. Chemotherapy-related cytotoxicity could cause pancytopenia and immunocompromise that may limit or restrict patient participation in activities such as exercise or sexual intercourse. Cognitive side effects, "chemo brain," cardiac function, and cancer-related fatigue (CRF) as a result of chemotherapy regimens are significant considerations during rehabilitation. Hormonal changes can affect bone mineral density and risk of osteoporosis. Cancer survivors can be impacted by decreased activity levels years after active treatment, and studies show that there is a need for intervention in this population.[3] Research supports that ongoing support and education throughout a survivorship program have the greatest potential for

Breast Cancer and Gynecologic Cancer Rehabilitation DOI: https://doi.org/10.1016/B978-0-323-72166-0.00019-0

successful outcomes. Rehabilitation for each survivor is about restoring the quality of life that was disrupted by her cancer.

Pelvic floor rehabilitation must address multiple different body systems. The pathophysiology and tissue damage within each of the following systems will be examined separately: musculoskeletal, urinary, anorectal, and sexual. A brief review of the healthy physiology will help the clinician understand evaluation techniques that are readily available in the rehabilitation clinic as well as diagnostic imaging and testing performed outside the rehab setting. Due to these complex system interactions, management of the pelvic floor requires the integration of multiple clinical specialties as part of the comprehensive survivorship team. Valid and reliable quality of life questionnaires and assessment tools are available to assess and measure outcomes of pelvic floor therapy. These can be helpful to communicate within the multidisciplinary survivorship team.

Evidence-based treatment options are available for the general rehabilitation practitioner as well as the pelvic floor specialist. Treatment options available to all rehabilitation clinicians will focus on patient education, behavioral modifications, self-care, exercise, and ongoing support. More specialized biofeedback, electrical stimulation, manual therapy, and dilator training will also be reviewed. In following the *International Classification of Functioning, Disability and Health* we will look at how to write treatment goals that address the functional limitations and activity level of the whole person and ultimately can lead to greater participation in society and decreased handicap or disability.[8]

PELVIC FLOOR EVALUATION: ASSESSING SYSTEMS

Evaluation of the pelvic floor will be broken down into each of the following four systems: musculoskeletal, bladder, bowel, and sexual function.

The main functions of the pelvic floor are postural stabilization, support of the pelvic organs, sphincter control, and sexual function. It also helps control intraabdominal pressure, which is important in generating a strong Valsalva maneuver, during vomiting or coughing to clear the airway (Fig. 19.1). When pelvic floor pathology or pain exists, these basic functions are affected. The initial evaluation is an opportunity to assess all aspects of pelvic health in each of these domains.

The pelvic floor rehabilitation intake visit should begin with history taking and assessment of the patient's signs and symptoms, pain, vital signs, posture, and

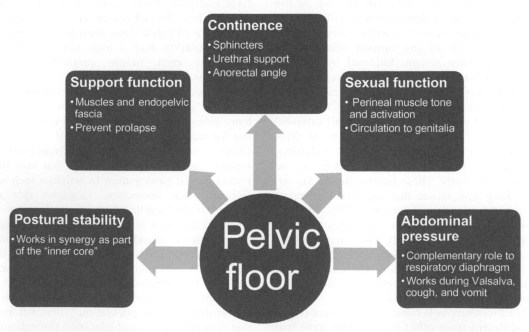

• Prevent prolapse

• Works in synergy as part of the "inner core"

• Complementary role to respiratory diaphragm
• Works during Valsalva, cough, and vomit

FIGURE 19.1 Pelvic floor function.

balance. A thorough screen of the abdominal wall, spine, sacroiliac joint (SIJ), hip, and lower extremities should be performed and can identify contributing musculoskeletal factors originating outside the pelvis. Sensation and reflex testing of the lumbar and sacral dermatomes and myotomes should be performed. Each of the following sections will review normal function of the pelvic floor, bladder, bowel, and sexual organs as well as how cancer treatments may cause impairments.

The treating therapist must be able to clearly articulate what they are doing next and why, in order to avoid any misunderstandings or appearances of sexual misconduct. Patients must be cognitively intact. She must be able to understand the instructions and able to give permission in order to be appropriate for modalities to the pelvic floor. It should always be made clear that the woman has a choice in her treatment and a chaperone should be available.

Pelvic Floor Musculoskeletal System

Anatomy and Physiology

The pelvic floor can be divided grossly into three muscular layers. The superficial layer consists of the ischiocavernosus, bulbocavernosus, transverse perineal, and external anal sphincter (EAS) muscles. The middle layer consists of the sphincter urethrae and the sphincter pubovaginalis as well as the internal transverse perineal muscles. The deepest layer, known as the levator ani, consists of the puborectalis, ischiococcygeus, and coccygeus muscles. The anterior muscle attachment is at the pubic symphysis and the fibers run along the arcus tendineus levator ani (ATLA) laterally to the ischial spine and posteriorly to the coccyx and sacrum. The piriformis and obturator internus are also important muscles of the deeper anatomy. The obturator internus muscle borders the levator ani and the endopelvic fascia along the ATLA (Fig. 19.2).

During voluntary contraction the pelvic floor muscles lift superiorly and the sphincters tighten. During relaxation the general motion is descent and opening. The pelvic floor muscles are composed of approximately 70% slow twitch fibers and 30% fast twitch fibers. The percentage of fast twitch fibers is higher as you move anteriorly.[9] Innervation of the pelvic floor muscles is by the branches of the pudendal nerve (S2, S3, S4) and the nerves to the levator ani and coccygeus (S3, S4). Normal sacral reflexes include the bulbocavernosus–clitoral reflex, anal wink, and cough reflexes.

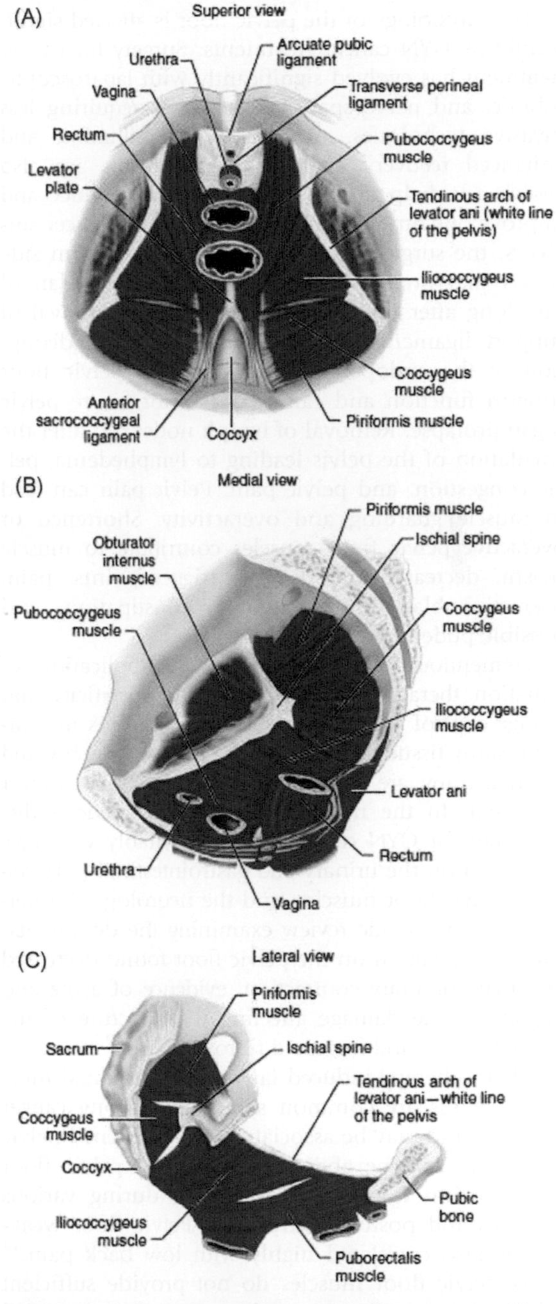

FIGURE 19.2 Anatomy of the pelvic floor muscles. Three views: (A) Superior, (B) Medial, (C) Lateral views. *From Fielding JR, Llave A. Chapter 5: Magnetic resonance imaging of the female pelvis: technique, anatomy, and pitfalls. In: Fielding JR, Brown D, Thurmond AS, eds.* Gynecologic Imaging: Expert Radiology Series. *Saunders: Elsevier; 2011:71–102; Figs. 5–20.*

The physiology of the pelvic floor is affected significantly by GYN cancer treatments. Surgery for cancer treatment has evolved significantly with laparoscopic, robotic, and nerve sparing procedures requiring less invasive techniques. Accelerated rehabilitation and enhanced recovery after surgery protocols are also evolving to help improve the patient experience and improve outcomes.[10] Most importantly for cancer survivors, the surgical interventions have long-term side effects that impact a physical therapy (PT) plan of care long after the initial healing phase. Removal of support ligaments during hysterectomy and disruption of the endopelvic fascia decreases pelvic floor support function and can be a risk for future pelvic organ prolapse. Removal of lymph nodes can alter the circulation of the pelvis leading to lymphedema, pelvic congestion, and pelvic pain. Pelvic pain can lead to muscle guarding and overactivity. Shortened or overactive pelvic floor muscles contribute to muscle spasm, decreased blood flow, trigger points, pain, overactive bladder, dyspareunia, constipation, and possible pudendal neuralgia.[11]

Tremendous advancement in the application of radiation therapies has led to greater specificity and dosage control with considerable implications in sparing healthy tissue. External beam radiation therapy and brachytherapy are commonly used with GYN cancer treatment. In the narrow space of the pelvic girdle, treatment for GYN cancer almost inevitably will have an impact on the urinary and gastrointestinal (GI) systems, pelvic floor muscles, and the neurological innervation. A systematic review examining the detrimental effects of radiation on the pelvic floor found decreased maximal voluntary contraction, evidence of acute and ongoing tissue damage affecting the structure of the pelvic muscles and increased fibrotic tissue.[12]

Chemotherapy-induced fatigue and proximal muscle weakness are common symptoms among cancer survivors and may be associated with weakened pelvic floor muscles. The abdominal wall and pelvic floor cocontraction is a normal response during various exercises and postural activities.[13] Pelvic floor weakness is also correlated highly with low back pain.[14] Weak pelvic floor muscles do not provide sufficient sphincter contraction strength or organ support and are associated with urinary and fecal incontinence, sexual dysfunction, and pelvic organ prolapse.

Assessing Muscle Function of the Pelvic Floor

The most simple pelvic floor muscle assessment is observation, which can reveal one of the following outcomes: (1) the patient is able to contract with visible lift, (2) is not able to generate visible lift, or (3) strains to produce a downward descent of the perineum. External observation does not provide accurate information related to the deeper structures. As an initial screening tool, however, it provides useful information about the client's ability to generate perineal lift and identify the appropriate muscles without producing a Valsalva maneuver or using excessive accessory muscle overflow. A simple external muscle test, palpating medial to the ischial tuberosities through clothing with the patient in hook lying position, can provide the treating therapist with similar information. External palpation provides an added benefit of greater patient privacy and may be useful when internal work is contraindicated (Fig. 19.3A–D). The validity and reliability of external palpation has not been studied for research purposes,[15] but it may still be a useful screening tool in the clinic, at the bedside in acute care, or in other outpatient therapy settings that do not specialize in pelvic rehabilitation.

Practitioners who are trained in pelvic floor therapy may choose an internal muscle assessment. Manual muscle testing is the most convenient method to use in the rehabilitation clinic. Vaginal palpation is a low-cost tool and can discriminate between pelvic floor circumferential squeeze and lift, though the discrimination is poor[15] (Fig. 19.4). Note, however, that vaginal palpation is not appropriate less than 6 weeks postoperative or postpartum, in the presence of suspected or confirmed infection, severe vaginal atrophy, active cancer, active bleeding, or whenever the patient does not or is not able to give permission. Rectal palpation may also be a useful alternative approach for palpating the pelvic floor muscles and may be necessary to assess the anal sphincters. Kegel described vaginal palpation as a method to assess the ability to perform a correct or incorrect pelvic floor contraction, and he developed the "perineometer" to measure vaginal squeeze pressure and thereby quantify strength.[16,17]

The Modified Oxford scale and Laycock PERFECT scale are two strength grading systems that are commonly used in pelvic floor rehabilitation. The Modified Oxford scale uses a six-point rating system from 0 to 5 with (+/−) for added specificity. A score of 0 means there is no palpable contraction. A score of 5 represents a strong contraction with palpable lift. The Laycock PERFECT scale is a reliable and validated tool for assessing pelvic floor muscle strength, which begins with the "P" for power using the Modified Oxford scale but additionally describes "E" endurance, "R" repetitions, and "F" fast twitch muscle properties as well. The Laycock PERFECT scale additionally

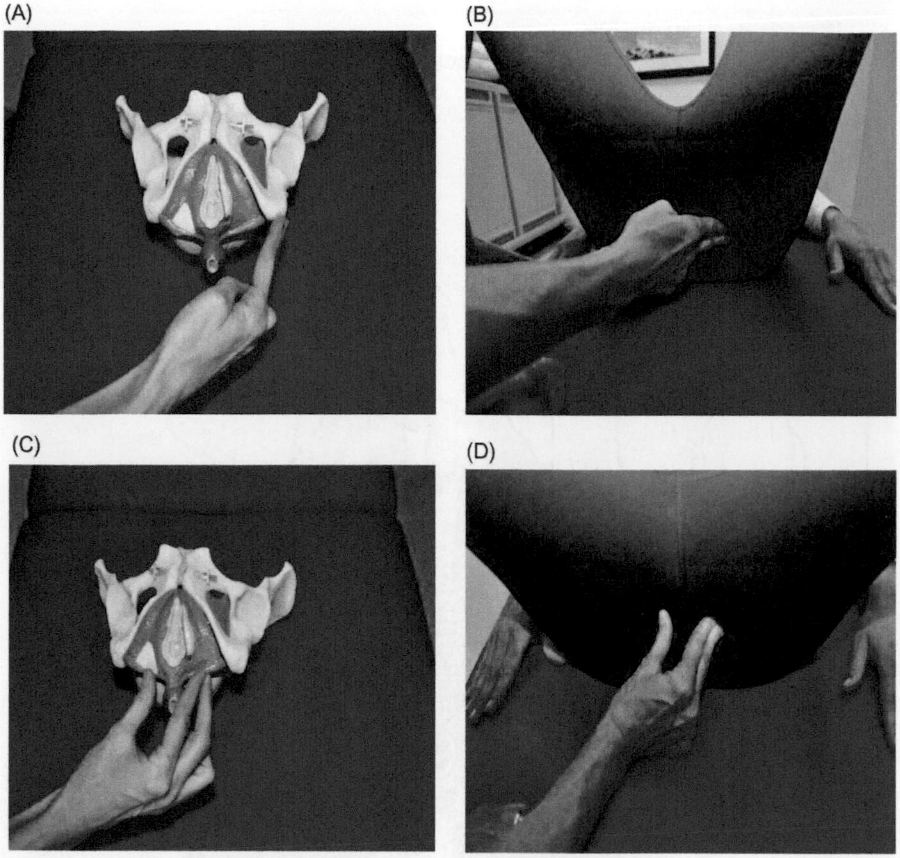

FIGURE 19.3. External palpation: (A and B) the ischial tuberosities serve as a landmark. (C and D) The therapist palpates the perineum medial to the ischial tuberosities during a pelvic floor contraction to assess, if the patient can lift the perineum correctly or produces an erroneous outward push.

provides a basis to recommend parameters for subsequent exercise prescription, which will be discussed later in the chapter.[18]

The initial digital exam will also provide assessment of muscle symmetry, individual muscle strength, range of motion and tone, and tissue integrity. Cough test and Valsalva should be performed to assess laxity and prolapse during the initial assessments. Findings may vary in supine, sitting, and standing.

Electromyography (EMG) is a useful tool to examine the electrical potentials of the pelvic floor muscles during rest, reflexive activities, and voluntary contractions. Fine needle or concentric needle EMG can be used percutaneously to target local areas within a muscle and provide very specific information. However, this is not routinely performed in the PT setting. A doctor may also order EMG studies of the pudendal nerve motor latency.

Surface EMG (sEMG) with vaginal, rectal, or external electrodes can be an excellent method of pelvic floor evaluation in the rehabilitation setting and can be used for muscle reeducation through biofeedback. Manual assessment and sEMG together can differentiate overactive or paradoxical contraction from a shortened or contracted pelvic floor, which may be electrically more silent and may not be clearly discernable from manual palpation alone. External sEMG is not muscle specific and therefore cannot measure the action potentials from a single muscle, but it is useful to assess overall behavior and activation patterns. Dual channel sEMG is useful in differentiating pelvic floor from accessory muscles such as the rectus abdominus or gluteal muscles. Impedance from subcutaneous tissues and variation in electrode placement make it difficult to describe normative data. sEMG can, nevertheless, be an excellent tool to assess the behavior

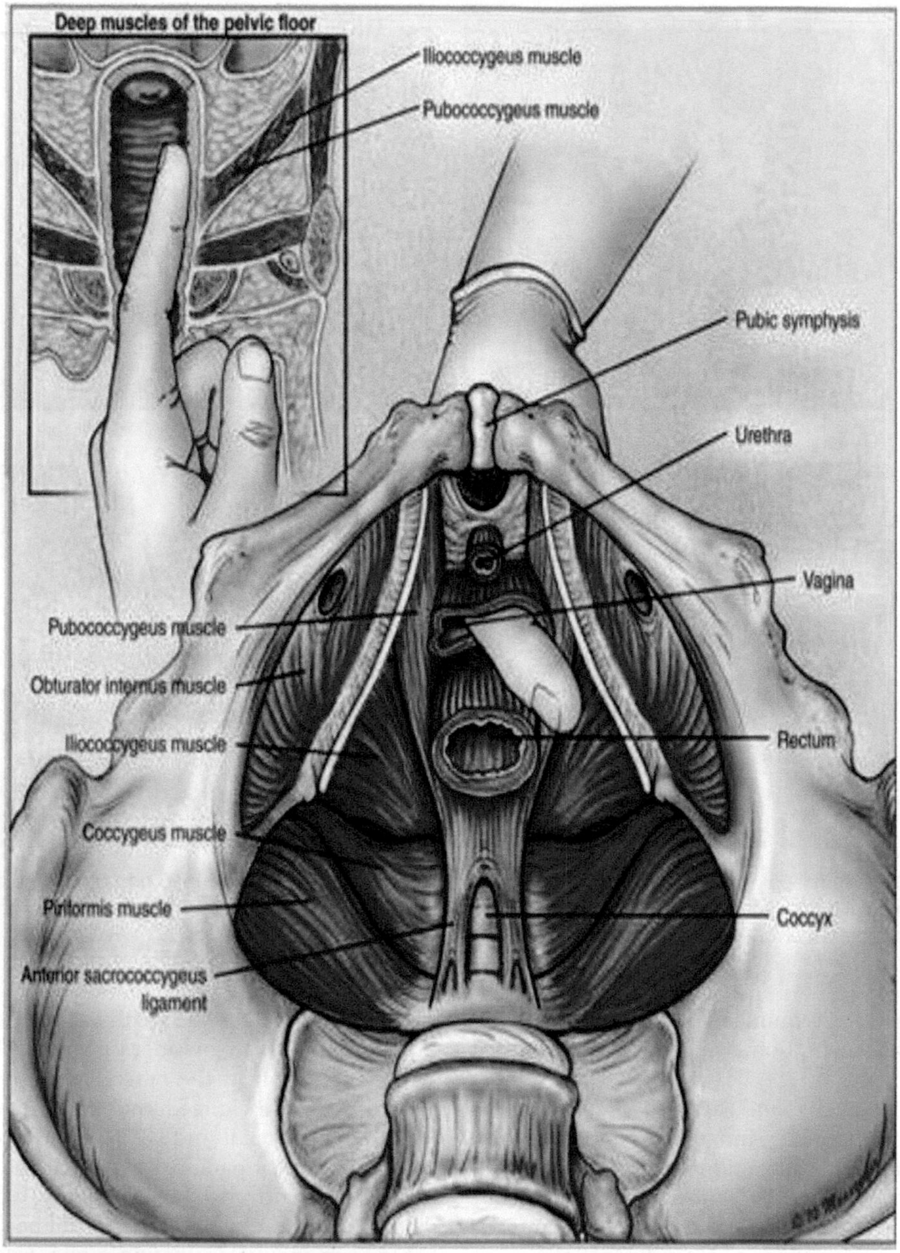

FIGURE 19.4 Digital manual assessment of the pelvic floor: the therapist can identify circumferential squeeze and perineal lift using an internal assessment, as well as areas of muscle weakness or asymmetry. *Reprinted from Sarton J. Assessment of the pelvic floor muscles in women with sexual pain.* J Sex Med. *2010;7(11):4, with permission from Elsevier.*

of the muscle relative to fatigue, coordination, and general return to resting levels after activity.[15]

Pressure manometry can also be used for quantifying the amount of pressure generated within the vagina or rectum and many machines provide dual lead assessments for combined sEMG and manometry. Pressure measurements are not able to discriminate between forces produced intraabdominally or generated by the pelvic floor and therefore they are best used in conjunction with other observation.

The inward drawing action on the sensor lead wire can help determine if the correct muscle action is occurring.[15]

Ultrasonography is becoming more easily accessible and some facilities may have this technology available to rehabilitation practitioners. Visualization of correct movement and timing of the pelvic floor muscles can provide the patient and the therapist with real-time perspective on the actions of the pelvic floor muscles. Physicians may order ultrasound or dynamic MRI to identify the anatomy of impaired pelvic structures, which can impact the rehabilitation plan of care.

Bladder/Urinary System

Anatomy and Physiology

The healthy adult bladder receives urine via the ureters from the kidneys. As the bladder fills the muscular wall of the bladder, detrusor muscle is relaxed and gently accommodates a typical volume of up to 500 mL of urine, while the smooth muscle of the urethra remains closed. Autonomic sympathetic signals via the superior hypogastric plexus and hypogastric nerves and parasympathetic signals carried by the pelvic splanchnic nerves pass through the inferior hypogastric plexus to control the micturition reflex and urination. The somatic pelvic floor muscles, which are primarily innervated by the pudendal nerve and nerves to the levator ani, must contract with increased abdominal pressure to prevent accidental leaking. Autonomically controlled smooth muscle of the vesicle neck and circular and longitudinal muscle fibers of the internal urethral sphincter also help to control urinary continence through tonic activity at rest (Fig. 19.5). The supportive connective tissue acts like a sling behind the urethra to support the urethra as intraabdominal pressures rise. In addition, coaptation of the vaginal lumen also helps to keep the urethra closed at rest.[19]

During micturition the pelvic floor muscles must relax to allow for opening of the external urethral sphincters along with contraction of the detrusor muscle for optimal bladder emptying. Typical post-voiding residual values range from 0 to 75 mL of urine in the bladder. Normal bladder voiding frequency is approximately every 3–4 hours and 0–1 times at night for most adults based on 48–64 oz of fluid intake every 24 hours.

Cancer treatment may cause both bladder storage and voiding dysfunction. Donovan et al. found that bladder storage and incontinence symptoms were more prevalent in the cancer survivor group than in noncancer control groups.[4] Bladder irritation can occur as a result of infection, surgery, radiation, diet, and anxiety and leads to overactive bladder, urinary frequency and urgency, nocturia, and urge incontinence. Surgical damage to the bladder innervation can lead to autonomic dysfunction of the micturition reflexes, decreased somatic control, neurogenic bladder, or internal sphincter deficiencies. Chemotherapy is associated with peripheral neuropathy, which may have sensory, motor, and autonomic components. For successful control of the bladder and bowel, a patient must have sensory awareness of bladder and rectal filling as well as proprioceptive awareness of the pelvic floor. Radiation fibrosis can significantly limit the elasticity of the bladder, vagina, and rectum and alters the ability to produce proper lubrication or protective secretions. The urethral and vaginal tissues are estrogen sensitive and can be affected by radiation and chemotherapy-induced mucositis.

Medical assessment of the patient with urinary incontinence should include a thorough history, physical examination by the physician, urine test to rule out infection, and assessment of postvoid residual volumes. Urodynamic testing may be ordered to examine bladder function. Stress incontinence, volume at first urge, postresidual volumes, and retention of urine can be detected with this procedure. Ultrasound and other imaging techniques can identify obstruction, postvoid volume, and abnormalities that may affect rehabilitation prognosis. Although pelvic floor therapy cannot treat all of these urological conditions, the physical therapist may have an important role in differential diagnosis by fully evaluating and treating the pelvic floor muscles.

Assessing Bladder Function

At the time of the evaluation the therapist should be able to identify predominant bladder storage problems such as stress, urge, or mixed incontinence. The International Continence Society defines incontinence as "involuntary loss of urine that is social or hygienic problem and is objectively demonstrable."[20] Urinary stress incontinence due to muscle weakness or damage is a common side effect after GYN cancer treatments and patients may benefit from pelvic floor rehabilitation for weak, uncoordinated muscles or to build endurance. The evaluation can identify the level of effort or intensity that is required to cause stress incontinence and therefore set strength training goals for functional rehabilitation. Urge incontinence may also result from the treatments affecting the

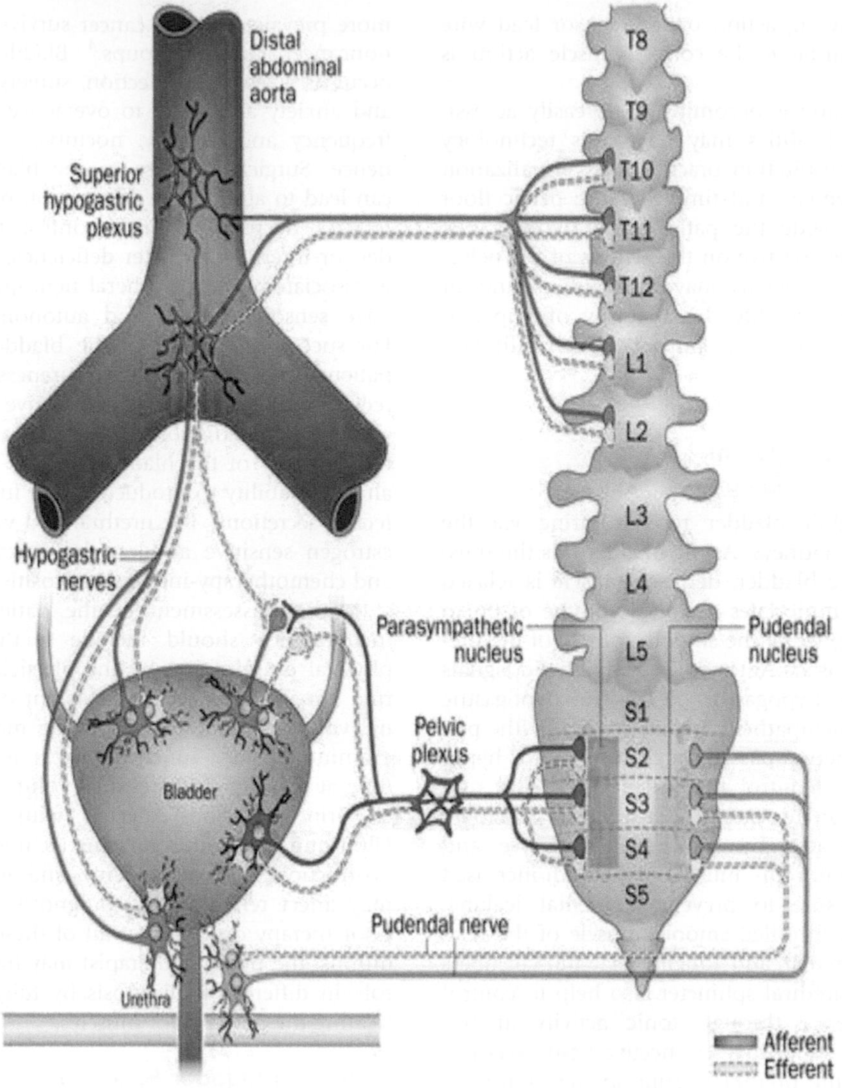

FIGURE 19.5 Innervation of the bladder and pelvic floor: micturition is controlled by sympathetic, parasympathetic, and somatic controls, which can be vulnerable to the effects of cancer therapy. *Reprinted from Wit EMK, Horenblas S. Urological complications after treatment of cervical cancer.* Nat Rev Urol. *2014, with permission from Springer Nature.*

neurological controls of the bladder and urethra. Overflow incontinence and functional incontinence may be present as a result of changes in mobility and fatigue that prevent the patient from getting to the bathroom in a consistent and timely manner.

Conversely, a patient may have voiding dysfunction such as urinary retention or difficulty voiding. Voiding dysfunction may be the result of overactive pelvic floor muscles. Mechanical or neurological changes after cancer therapy may cause increased resistance, urethral obstruction, neurogenic bladder, decreased detrusor muscle contraction, or poor coordination of the bladder and sphincter during micturition.

Objective measures and subjective reports are important to begin assessing the level of impairment and setting patient-specific functional goals. A careful interview and symptom review is crucial as well as careful analysis of the patient's fluid intake and voiding behaviors. Quality of life questionnaires, such as the Pelvic Floor Distress Inventory (PFDI-20), Pelvic Floor Impact Questionnaire,[21] and Sandvik Scale,[22] are valid and reliable baseline measurements to compare pre- and posttherapy progress. Bladder diaries are useful to help quantify the frequency of leaks initially and as follow-up to reinforce awareness and compliance to healthy toileting practices. Three-day diaries are considered valid and reliable. Formal pad tests where each pad is weighed may be used for research but are less desirable for patient assessment. Instead, observations about the number and saturation of pads can be easily documented on the bladder diaries (Fig. 19.6). There are various smartphone apps that can facilitate keeping a bladder log.

Bladder diary				Name:			Date:	
Hour	Intake		Output		Leaks		Notes	Pad change
	Amount	Beverage	Urine/stool	Amount	Stress	Urge		
6:00 a.m.								
7:00 a.m.								
8:00 a.m.								
9:00 a.m.								
10:00 a.m.								
11:00 a.m.								
12:00 p.m.								
1:00 p.m.								
2:00 p.m.								
3:00 p.m.								
4:00 p.m.								
5:00 p.m.								
6:00 p.m.								
7:00 p.m.								
8:00 p.m.								
9:00 p.m.								
10:00 p.m.								
11:00 p.m.								
12:00 a.m.								
1:00 a.m.								
2:00 a.m.								
3:00 a.m.								
4:00 a.m.								
5:00 a.m.								

FIGURE 19.6 A simple bladder diary can be a useful tool to assess bladder habits.

Anorectal/Bowel Function

Anatomy and Physiology

Understanding how a healthy GI system functions is imperative before assessing patients who have undergone GYN cancer treatment. Digestion begins with consuming food and liquids by mouth. An appropriate appetite and regular meal times help maintain a consistent rhythm of digestion and elimination. Food entering the stomach triggers the gastrocolic reflex, which stimulates intestinal peristalsis. Stool is moved through the small intestines and colon into the rectum. Stretching of receptors in the rectal wall triggers the intrinsic defecation reflex and causes relaxation of the internal anal sphincter (IAS). Another reflex called the parasympathetic defecation reflex is activated by stretch of the rectal walls and causes increased peristaltic activity, which helps lead to defecation. If the woman is not able to defecate, increased sympathetic output and tonic contraction of the EAS and puborectalis, which hold the anorectal angle at approximately 80–100 degrees, can suppress peristalsis. The IAS closes and defecation is deferred. Over time deferring fecal urge may lead to constipation. Liquid stool, however, can pass the anorectal angle more easily, which can cause soiling.

Adjuvant chemotherapy and radiation as well as surgical resection of tissue can affect the function of the intestines; decrease rectal compliance; reduce or increase rectal sensitivity; and lead to fecal incontinence, constipation, and other problems with the bowel. The normal gastrocolic reflex, peristaltic activity, and intestinal mucosa may be impacted, which can lead to accelerated or impaired motility. GI toxicity is a common side effect, which can lead to chronic diarrhea. Narcotic pain management and decreased mobilization are known causes of decreased bowel motility and constipation. Neuropathy, decreased sampling reflex, reduced rectal sensation, pain, guarding, and fear may also lead to paradoxical pelvic floor contractions, outlet obstructive constipation, fecal smearing, and soiling, all of which have a devastating effect on quality of life.

Patients referred for fecal incontinence may have imaging in the form of colonoscopy, dynamic MRI defecography with or without contrast mimicking stool in the colon, or ultrasound. Other diagnostic testing that may be ordered include rectal sensation testing, balloon expulsion testing, or EMG studies of the anal sphincter or pudendal nerve.[23] The physician, as part of comprehensive survivorship support, may order additional motility studies, allergy sensitivity tests, and nutritional evaluations.

Assessing Bowel Function

Questionnaires and pen-and-paper tools such as the Bristol Stool Chart, Longo ODS, Wexner, and PFDI-20 are useful to quantify subjective reports and objectively measure bowel symptom severity.[24,25] Diaries and food logs can be helpful for patients to self-assess their habits and identify triggers that can lead to clustered bowel movements, urgency, and diarrhea.

As with urinary dysfunction, a thorough assessment of the pelvic floor muscles is necessary to evaluate bowel dysfunction. If possible, a rectal assessment allows better access to the EAS and IAS resting and squeeze pressure. Biofeedback and anorectal manometry can be used to assess muscle electrical activity and physical pressure within the anal canal, respectively. These assessments can be done on the exam table for ease of the therapist, but a functional assessment of the patient sitting on a commode may be more appropriate. Muscle strength should be assessed with special attention to muscle endurance. Reflexive mechanisms for fecal continence require sustained EAS control for 45—60 seconds in order to override the recto-anal inhibitory reflex and facilitate closure of the IAS when it is inappropriate to respond to fecal urgency. A thorough assessment for rectal wall prolapse and sensation is also important during the rehabilitation evaluation.

Genitalia and Sexual Health

Anatomy and Physiology

Fertility and reproductive medicine are not within the scope of the pelvic floor PT; however, sexual health can and should certainly be addressed. Objective assessment is extremely difficult, since female sexual function is a complex blend of physiological, physical, emotional, and psychological factors. Early research conducted by Masters and Johnson in the 1960s and 1970s characterized sexual response as a linear phasic system for women and men alike, which included excitement, plateau, orgasm, and resolution. Under this model, sexual desire was considered to emerge from an inherent internal drive. Clinical assessment tools were developed by the scientific and medical community to assess and define each phase of the sexual response. The initial phase includes central and peripheral changes to the autonomic nervous system, nonspecific increased sympathetic cardiovascular and respiratory responses, and increased pelvic muscle tone.[26] Increased blood flow to the genitals and genital vasocongestion causes engorgement of the vulva, clitoris, and vagina as well as and genital lubrication and increased tactile sensitivity. Healthy orgasm is the result of sympathetic signals that trigger climax, which is accompanied by rhythmic muscle contraction and a sensation of pleasure or euphoria. Resolution is the return to homeostasis and reabsorption of engorged fluid.

More recent studies have looked at the sexual response of women and moved toward newer models, such as the Incentive Motivation Model, in which desire and arousal are reciprocally reinforcing. Basson proposed a more circular model and included a greater role of subjective context–dependent stimulation and cognitive feedback.[27,28] Research by Chivers and Brotto suggested reconceptualizing sexual desire as a motivational state evoked by sexual stimuli and responsive to contextual factors, which significantly influence how and when desire is assessed.[29]

Desire and arousal are two aspects of sexual behavior that are significantly impacted by the cancer treatment journey. Changes in personal relationships with a partner, body image, and CRF could be very significant. The relationship between physiological arousal and sexual desire is complex and not directly sequential as initially proposed by the early research. Modern models of the female sexual response cycle also address issues of gender identity and orientation, which can add additional layers of complexity to sexual rehabilitation. A referral to a psychologist specializing in sexual health is often recommended for GYN cancer survivors.

Radiation produces long-term side effects, including atrophy of vaginal mucosa, obliteration of muscle and vasculature, atrophy, fibrosis, telangiectasia, mucosal pallor, adhesions, decreased elasticity, fragility of vaginal tissues, dyspareunia, and postcoital bleeding. Studies estimate that the frequency of radiation-induced vaginal stenosis after radiation therapy for uterine, cervical, and vaginal cancers to be between 1.25% and 88%, with the highest probability occurring after cervical cancer treatments.[30] Vaginal atrophy and vaginal dryness are common menopausal symptoms. Women who have already gone through menopause may have vaginal atrophy prior to their cancer treatments and be at a greater risk for vaginal stenosis.[30] These changes often continue to evolve over the 10 years following radiation therapy; therefore ongoing patient monitoring and education is critical.[31]

Assessing Sexual Function

All rehabilitation therapists should screen their clients for sexual dysfunction by asking them if they have concerns about their sexual health. The interview should include open-ended questions related to prior sexual history, sexual identity, and goals for future sexual activity. Past experiences, abuse, current relationships, and motivations for sex are as important as the physical condition of the vagina in assessing a woman's sexual health. Neither self-reported frequency nor self-reported desire of sexual relations is an accurate measure of a woman's physical sexual responses.[29,32] Sexual function questionnaires such as the female sexual distress scale and female sexual function index (FSFI) are more objective measures and should be used in conjunction with the interview process.[33,34]

During external assessment of the pelvic floor, physical therapists should check the integrity and mobility of the tissues of the perineum, vulva, vaginal vestibule, vaginal walls as well as the anus, thighs, and lower abdomen for fibrotic changes, swelling, irritation, sensation, and adhesions through gentle palpation. A Q-tip test can be performed for gentle pressure in all areas of the external vulva or vaginal vestibule to assess localized vestibulodynia. The fascial layers of the pelvic floor connect with the hip adductors, abdominal wall, and deep hip rotators. These can be impacted by fibrotic changes from radiation and limited mobility of the hip and back joints. Muscle assessment particularly of the superficial muscles by palpation is important. Sensation and sacral reflexes should be checked as well.

During the initial vaginal evaluation, assessing the patient's tolerance of vaginal palpation as well as her openness to internal vaginal treatments will help the therapist set realistic goals for her plan of care. The presence of vaginal stenosis, narrowing of the urogenital hiatus, vaginal length, tissue mobility, and adhesions are significant in determining future treatment options such as vaginal dilation or manual techniques. Some patients need additional time to accept the physical changes to their body and may be more appropriate for external work or supportive education.

REHABILITATION: TREATING PELVIC FLOOR DYSFUNCTION

They are listed grossly from most general to most specialized: education, exercise, biofeedback, electrical stimulation, manual therapy, and vaginal dilators.

In the next section, we will look at the most common pelvic floor treatment interventions, and some of the research that supports their use. They are listed grossly from most general to most specialized.

Education

Patient education is a primary component of pelvic floor rehabilitation for all GYN oncology patients. With cancer survivorship rates improving overall, there is a significant need to educate patients about the long-term effects following cancer treatment and how these can impact pelvic floor function. Motivation to participate and belief in the effectiveness of pelvic floor rehabilitation are dependent on the successful communication between therapist and patient. Research shows that the amount of education provided needs to be tailored to each patient and must avoid causing excessive fear, frustration, or anxiety.[35] Some patients are ready to learn how to cope with the "new normal" and can handle reeducation for bowel and bladder and sexual health. Other patients need more time to cope with these changes and a more supportive approach. Involving family and caregivers may be useful for some, but other patients are not prepared to share the details of their intimate pelvic dysfunctions with family and friends for a variety of social and cultural reasons. Patients who have cognitive limitations or learning impairments must have instructions that are designed to their specific needs. Smartphone apps, links to online resources, videos, and podcasts can supplement a traditional paper handout and provide various different learning tools for your patients.

Behavioral Modifications

Many pelvic floor symptoms related to urogenital and bowel function respond dramatically to behavioral modifications. Daily routine, fluid, diet, voiding, and toileting habits can significantly improve urinary urgency and frequency and bowel irregularity. Behavioral modifications have been shown to improve the quality of life in patients with stress and urgency incontinence,[36] and especially those that are accompanied by clinical or group support programs to reinforce initial teaching over the treatment period.[37] Quality of life questionnaires and bladder diaries can begin the process of identifying behaviors that lead to lower urinary tract symptoms. Patients may perceive their frequency to be elevated or insufficient when it is in fact within normal limits or the opposite. Any changes arising after cancer therapy may be perceived as problematic, and simple education can be useful to assuage those concerns. Risk factors for urinary incontinence may include elevated BMI, caffeine intake, carbonated beverages, and constipation.[38]

Controlling urinary urgency and frequency are two steps in bladder training and can help manage overactive bladder. The onset of urinary urgency is a complex, reflexively mediated, neurological process. The treating therapist can teach the patient strategies for urge suppression. These include breathing and relaxation, pelvic floor contractions, and mental distraction techniques. Once the patient has tools to help control urgency, a bladder training program to increase voiding intervals can begin. Bladder training to regulate overactive bladder typically involves increasing the interval between voids by some prescribed amount each week, typically 5–20 minutes, until reaching a set goal or returning within normal limits. A 3-hour interval will allow for watching a movie or concert uninterrupted or traveling by car for a road trip. In a case where sensory awareness to bladder filling is impaired, however, patients may need a timed voiding schedule every 3–4 hours to avoid overflow or sudden onset of urgency.

Bowel function can also be affected by timing and control of defecation. Establishing a healthy bowel routine to manage constipation requires proper stimulation of the autonomic nervous system driving digestion, opportunity to find a bathroom, and the ability to respond to urge by relaxing the pelvic floor and avoiding paradoxical contractions. Regular physical activity, diet, and water intake are also highly important for good bowel management.

Poor pelvic floor support function can cause positional obstruction and patients can be taught strategies for perineal splinting, double voiding, toileting posture, or Crede maneuver to help facilitate better bladder and bowel emptying. Ergonomic education and postural awareness also help patients adapt their environment in proactive ways to facilitate their best function and recovery. These components of a comprehensive treatment plan are most effective when based on specific patient's quality of life goals.

Diet and Fluid Intake

Comprehensive cancer rehabilitation today includes consultation with a registered dietician or nutritionist experienced with oncology survivorship. This interdisciplinary approach has great potential to help patients with pelvic floor dysfunction as the bladder and bowel are directly impacted by diet. Weight management, fatigue, muscle recovery, and hydration all have significant roles in the recovery of this patient population. Excessive fluid intake will naturally lead to frequent urination. Teaching patients to time their consumption and voiding intervals throughout the day can be very helpful, but there is little consensus on how much is enough water to drink. The National Academies of Sciences, Engineering, and Medicine has determined that an adequate total daily fluid intake for women is about 11.5 cups (2.7 L) of fluids a day, including fluids from water, other beverages, and food. About 20% of daily fluid intake usually comes from food and the rest from drinks.[39] This equates with nine cups per day; however, this adequate intake does not represent a minimum threshold for individual hydration. As a treating clinician it is important to educate your patients on signs of dehydration. Patients with urinary symptoms often manipulate their intake well above and below this amount and may be unaware of how much they actually consume. In addition, patients benefit from education regarding bladder irritants and diuretics to avoid such as caffeine, carbonated beverages, acidic drinks, and artificial sweeteners. Patients may also experience dry mouth and should be educated on products to help moisturize their mouths and lips, avoiding products such as mouthwashes that contain alcohol.

GI toxicity and mucositis are common side effects after chemotherapy and radiation with devastating effects on bowel control. Patients with bowel control issues are in great need of nutritional counseling services with a registered dietician or nutritionist. Controlling the consistency and frequency of stool is very important in managing the anorectal outlet function. Learning to manage portion sizes; identifying food irritants; and balancing fluid, fiber, and other nutrients can help regulate the stools and minimize mass movements and dumping syndromes. Appetite and food tolerances can be seriously altered during cancer treatment. The loss and return of taste and pleasure with eating may have a significant impact on the patient's social role within her family, as mealtime is a critical time for personal interaction.

Self-Care

Hygiene products and self-care techniques are an important part of maintaining vulvar and perineal health. Urinary and fecal control pads are different than feminine hygiene products and offer more absorbency ranges and styles. Perineal skin care products, moisturizers and barrier creams can protect the skin from breakdown, but most people are unaware of these products and may have misconceptions about their use.

Research has shown that vaginal and sexual health rehabilitation can improve the quality of life among GYN cancer survivors and should be part of comprehensive survivorship care with education being a significant component of every program.[31,41,42] Baseline vaginal dryness and decreased lubrication during sexual arousal are symptoms that commonly occur in postmenopausal women. After GYN cancer treatment this dryness can be even more problematic and proper self-care should be reviewed with patients. Topical hormone creams, tablets, or rings can be inserted vaginally and provide replacement hormones to help keep the area moist and reduce vaginal atrophy. Hormonal treatments, however, may be not advised for cancer survivors or patients may choose to avoid them. Hyaluronic acid vaginal creams[40] and vaginal moisturizers, such as Replens, are typically used to keep the tissues of the vagina and vulvar area moist during daily life.[41] Many women are unaware of these products to keep the tissues healthy and reduce irritation, itching, and odor. Vaginal moisturizers used at a frequency sufficient to control symptoms after cancer therapy, three to five times per week, were found to improve vaginal and vulvar symptoms as well as improved scores on the FSFI for sexual response.[42] Lubricants are more specifically for decreasing friction during sexual relations and help reduce dyspareunia. These are usually water or silicon based. Psychotherapists who specialize in sexual rehabilitation can compliment pelvic floor PT by addressing the psychosocial aspects of sexual relationships.

Exercise

Strength, Endurance, and Power

Among GYN cancer survivors, pelvic floor exercises have been shown to improve pelvic floor dysfunction and quality of life.[43] Pelvic floor muscle exercises have been known to improve urinary incontinence, bowel incontinence, constipation, support dysfunction, and pelvic organ prolapse. Studies have revealed that pelvic floor muscle training improves the sexual function of women with urinary incontinence and women with a diagnosis of sexual dysfunction by increasing pelvic floor muscle strength.[44–46] In addition, the research shows that pelvic floor muscle rehabilitation is more likely to succeed with a supervised program than with self-administered exercises.[47]

In the literature there is very little agreement on what the best pelvic floor strengthening protocols should look like.[47] Treatment protocols are highly variable and outcome measures differ between various

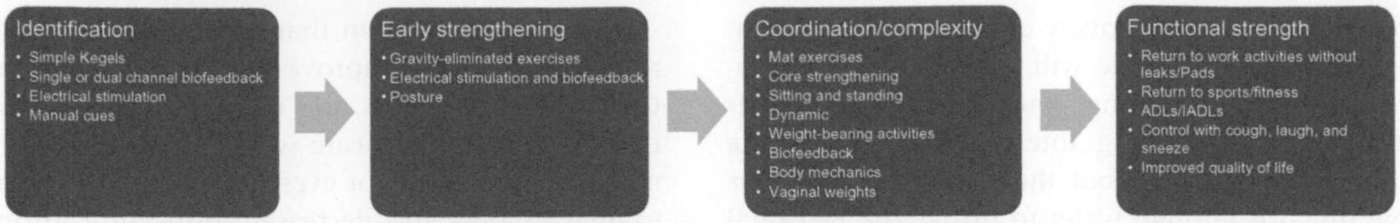

FIGURE 19.7 Progression of pelvic floor strengthening exercises. (A) Identification, (B) Early Strengthening, (C) Coordination/complexity, (D) Functional strength.

studies. There is some basic consensus, however, that pelvic floor muscle training should follow principles of muscle physiology and include elements of overload, specificity, and reversibility.[48] Muscle training should include exercises to address endurance, power, coordination, velocity, and flexibility. The treating therapist has considerable leeway in crafting a program that suits the specific needs of the GYN cancer patients.

Proper identification of the correct muscle action is the first step in muscle reeducation (Fig. 19.7A). Diaphragmatic breathing is an excellent tool to help quiet the autonomic nervous system and relax the patient so that she can feel and observe the pelvic floor motion. Research indicates that pelvic floor muscle isolation is not necessary for pelvic floor muscle strengthening to occur.[13] It is important, however, that the patient is able to accurately contract the pelvic floor in order for strengthening to take place and that rest intervals are appropriate. Vaginal dilators or manual digital insertion can also provide additional proprioceptive feedback for improved muscle awareness during strengthening. In cases of severely decreased awareness, the therapist can teach exercises that utilize overflow from other muscle groups such as hip abduction and adduction to help facilitate the pelvic floor.

Once the muscles are identified, exercise progression can begin. Initial strengthening exercises are based on the evaluation findings. The PERFECT scale was designed to lead directly from the evaluation process into exercise prescription.[18] Supine or side lying exercises such as Kegels or simple bridges limit resistance against gravity and are particularly useful during early rehabilitation phases (Figs. 19.7B and 19.8A and B). Pelvic floor exercises must address slow and fast twitch muscular fibers as well as coordination. Elevator Kegels are an example of a graded coordination exercise. The patient visualizes their pelvic floor beginning on the ground floor, relaxed, and then incrementally elevating to the second and third floor with the concentric contraction and then descending as the pelvic floor eccentrically lowers back to the ground floor.

Patients should progress to less supported or gravity-resisted positions such as quadruped exercises or seated hip abduction and adduction with the ball and band, which incorporate the obturator internus and other hip rotators as well as the adductors (Figs. 19.7C and 19.8C and D). Exercise advancement and progressive overloading should proceed to even more difficult standing activities such as lunges or squats and finally begin to mimic functional movement patterns during dynamic standing (Fig. 19.8E). Eventually, higher impact exercises such as jumping or jogging in place may provide additional eccentric loading of the muscles prior to contraction and evoke balance and postural reflexes (Fig. 19.7D). The transition from local exercise to global movement can help to restore spontaneous movement patterns and reinforce more complex motor plans. Vaginal weights or cones can be used to increase resistance or provide proprioceptive feedback for higher level activities and greater endurance. For survivors whose goals are to become very physically active and return to sports competition or personal fitness, core strengthening and progression into sport-specific rehabilitation should also be encouraged.

Muscle overloading is important for strength gains, but caution should be used to avoid excessive fatigue during survivorship rehab. This is especially true in respect to pelvic floor weakness. Excessive fatigue can often exacerbate symptoms of urinary leaking. Improper technique as a result of fatigue often leads to excessive isometric contraction of accessory muscle groups and patient complaints of soreness, spasm, or cramping.

Core Stabilization and Postural Control Strategies

Research has demonstrated how important a role the pelvic floor has for pelvic girdle stabilization prior to postural activities and load transfer through the spine and pelvis. Most pelvic floor muscle action is tonic and reflexively controlled. For optimal support of the pelvic joints and organs, including the bladder neck, there must exist sufficient passive form closure, active

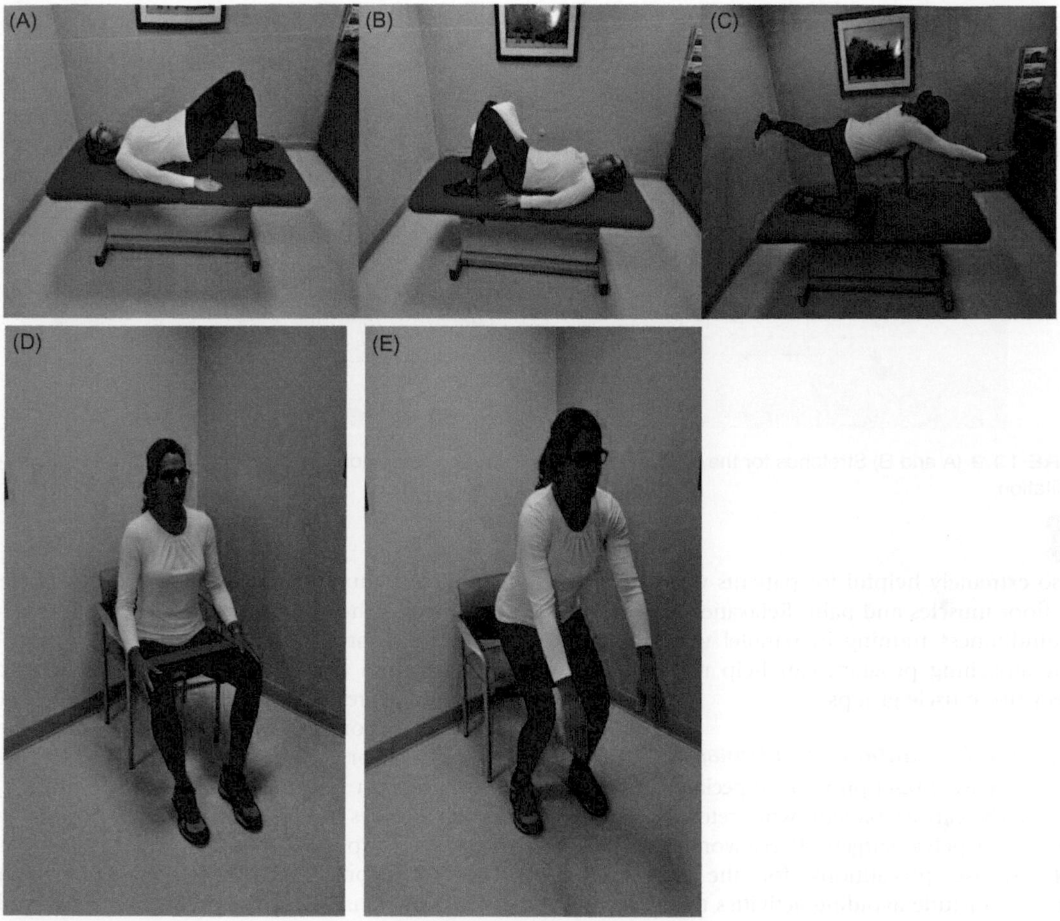

FIGURE 19.8 Pelvic floor exercise progression from hook lying to dynamic standing: (A) gravity-assisted bridges, (B) gravity neutral hip adduction, (C) quadruped bird dog, (D) seated hip abduction, (E) dynamic sit to stand.

force closure, and optimal motor control.[11] If pelvic floor muscle recruitment is delayed as a result of pain or side effects of oncology treatment, then there will be insufficient support during load transfers through the pelvis. This may lead to SIJ pain, back pain, strain on the pelvic floor, organ prolapse, or incontinence.[14,49]

Proximal weakness is a major factor in GYN cancer rehabilitation. Core stabilization exercises are especially relevant for this population. Supine bridges, supine marching, and quadruped exercises, for example, provide support to the pelvic organs on the bony pelvis and are a natural way to transition from simple pelvic floor contractions into more purposeful activities. Exercise in the forms of Yoga and Pilates is also very helpful for improving patient awareness of the pelvic floor. Returning to group classes offers additional social benefits as well. Compliance with pelvic floor home exercise programs has been shown to degrade after supervised interventions cease; however, integrating pelvic floor activation with regular activities of daily living, behavioral modifications, and pleasurable fitness activities may help to improve ongoing adherence to pelvic floor exercise programs.[50,51]

Stretching and Down Training

Increased muscle tone, guarding, and overactivity may be addressed with stretching and relaxation exercises for the muscles of the hips, pelvis, low back, and abdomen. These include stretching the hip adductors, hip external rotators, hip extensors, and groin (Fig. 19.9A and B). Techniques to help facilitate downregulation of the sympathetic nervous system

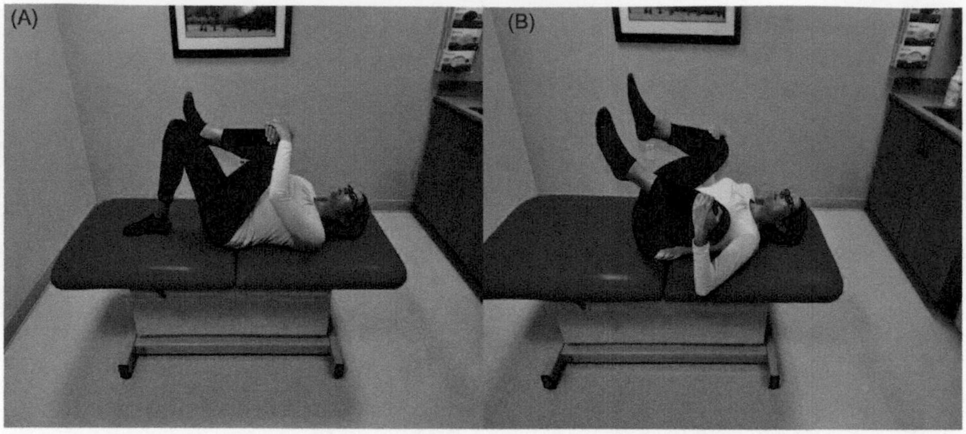

FIGURE 19.9 (A and B) Stretches for the hip rotators, gluteal muscles, and adductors are important for pelvic floor rehabilitation.

are also extremely helpful for patients with overactive pelvic floor muscles and pain. Relaxation, meditation, and mindfulness training in parallel with a patient-specific stretching program can help restore balance to overactive muscle groups.

Pelvic Floor Precautions and Prolapse

Correct exercise prescription is especially important for the GYN cancer patient who returns to fitness activities after pelvic surgery. Every woman should be taught exercise precautions for the pelvic floor. Precautions include avoiding activities that excessively strain the pelvic floor muscles or stretch the connective tissues of the pelvic floor and reduce "stiffness" of the supportive tissues. While not everyone will have symptoms of pelvic floor descent or pelvic organ prolapse, it is important for oncology patients to return to exercise gradually and be aware of exercise modifications that can protect their recovering pelvic floor. Proper breathing techniques also help to decrease intraabdominal pressure and reduce straining of the pelvic floor, which is seen during Valsalva maneuvers. Additional support in the form of a pessary (disposable or prescription) may be prescribed by a physician and can help address laxity by providing extrinsic support. Pessaries may not be appropriate for patients who have compromised vaginal tissue integrity post-radiation treatment or significant vaginal atrophy as they may lead to vaginal breakdown.

Biofeedback

Patients with weaker and less coordinated pelvic floor muscles as well as those with overactivity may benefit from neuromuscular reeducation using biofeedback to augment their exercises. Biofeedback provides the patient with an audio or visual representation of the muscle action they are trying to achieve. This can be helpful to reinforce correct muscle action and sequencing for patients with poor proprioceptive awareness or decreased muscle identification. Feedback can be presented through audio tones, visual displays on a computer screen or an analog device, or simple observation.

sEMG is commonly used in pelvic floor rehabilitation. The signal is measured in microvolt/milliamp, but the display can be a range of lights, a graphic display, or a video clip such as the opening and closing of a flower to help motivate the patient. The choice of electrode type and placement depends on the patient and the goals for therapy that day. Internal vaginal or rectal electrodes offer the ability to position the electrode within the vagina or anal sphincters and may also allow the delivery of electrical stimulation during the same treatment session. Internal sensors are usually contraindicated in patients who are less than 6 weeks postoperative and have any active or suspected infection, severe vaginal atrophy, vaginal or rectal bleeding, active cancer or tumor at the site, during pregnancy, or after denervation of the area. Vaginal stenosis or prolapse may make placement of the vaginal electrode difficult or painful. It is important to perform a careful digital assessment in advance of placing any rectal or vaginal electrodes.

External electrodes offer greater patient mobility and allow for treatment in standing positions and dynamic movements. Dual channel sEMG can provide feedback for improved muscle identification or coordination. For example, the accessory lead may help the patient identify the contracting muscles and eliminate erroneous contractions of the gluteus maximus or abdominal wall. sEMG biofeedback alone cannot differentiate between a correct muscle contraction and the incorrect electrical activity caused by Valsalva or excessive gluteal contractions; therefore the therapist must play an active role in ongoing observation of patient performance with these devices. Some systems may also be equipped with pressure manometry, which can measure the circumferential squeeze pressure within the vagina or anus.

Other types of biofeedback may include pelvic floor exercise trainers, observation with a mirror, palpation of the perineum, or inserting a dilator or finger into the vagina to palpate for movement. Studies have shown that biofeedback can be helpful in augmenting exercises for pelvic floor rehabilitation.[52,53] As with pelvic floor exercises, the therapist must assess that the patient is performing the contractions correctly by observing the proper perineal lift.

Strengthening With Biofeedback

As with exercise prescription alone, the therapist should assess the patient's initial resting tone, strength, power, endurance, and coordination before initiating pelvic floor exercises in order to set appropriate parameters and goals. For example, a very weak patient, who demonstrates 1/5 muscle strength for 3 seconds endurance, a total of three repetitions, and cannot perform fast twitches correctly due to breath holding and Valsalva, may benefit from fewer repetitions with more rest periods, for example, 1 set × 5 repetitions of 3 seconds work with 10–15 seconds rest and an emphasis on technique. A stronger patient with an evaluation of 3/5 strength; 10 repetitions with 6 seconds endurance, and 8 fast twitches in 10 seconds may be more independent with biofeedback and would benefit from 2 to 3 sets × 10 repetitions × 10 seconds work, 10 seconds rest; progressing to shorter rest intervals.

Coordination and Sequencing

Pelvic floor dysfunctions such as urinary and fecal incontinence as well as lumbopelvic instability can be caused by poor pelvic floor sequencing as discussed earlier. Biofeedback can demonstrate the order of muscle activation during particular movement patterns. The "knack," or protective contraction of the pelvic floor prior to coughing, is a good example of how the sequencing of pelvic floor contraction prior to the onset of intraabdominal pressure can improve urethral support and reduce stress urinary incontinence. Similarly, engagement of the pelvic floor and transverse abdominus prior to sit-to-stand transfers helps improve force closure through the pelvis and may reduce shear through a painful SIJ and decrease intraabdominal pressure during the transfer. Exercises that promote graded coordination of the pelvic floor include biofeedback with a pyramid or step up pattern as well as using goal lines for intermediate level and lighter contractions. Elevator Kegels work well with sEMG biofeedback as the patients can visualize the effects of their efforts clearly with the visual display. Paradoxical contraction of the pelvic floor can be addressed with biofeedback. In some patients with outlet dysfunction constipation, a poorly timed pelvic floor contraction can inhibit successful rectal emptying. Improved coordination may help reduce incomplete evacuation.

Down Training With Biofeedback

Overactive pelvic floor muscles are often associated with pain and dysfunction. Muscle guarding as a result of existing pain, poor posture, or apprehension about pain with intercourse can also lead to increased electrical potential on sEMG. Biofeedback is an effective tool to help patients identify muscle overactivity and implement effective relaxation strategies. In the clinical setting, external electrodes are convenient to use as they afford greater mobility and can be used with dilator training, various positioning, and during exercises. Long rest intervals between contractions (10–20 seconds) and coordination exercises (e.g., down elevator Kegels) afford the patient time to recognize and practice effective muscle relaxation techniques. Biofeedback during sets of exercises measures the ability of the patient to return to resting tone between contractions and thereby demonstrate a measure of how the patient tolerates her exercise program.

Electrical Stimulation

Pelvic floor electrical stimulation (PFES) has been shown to be a useful treatment for muscle reeducation and strengthening as well as bladder inhibition.[54] Stimulation of the pelvic floor muscles may also provide local sensory awareness of the pelvic floor so that patients can better identify the muscles for effective strengthening or relaxation. Studies have shown that PFES can improve subjective symptoms of urinary urgency and frequency in patients with overactive bladder as measured on quality of life questionnaires.[54] Stimulation of afferent neurons carrying signals to the S2 and S3 nerve roots may indirectly inhibit detrusor muscle activity via the parasympathetic hypogastric nerves.

Unfortunately, most of the evidence supporting the use of electrical modalities with the pelvic floor has been tested outside of the GYN cancer population. Transcutaneous electrical nerve stimulation has been shown to be safe and effective in relieving pain among cancer patients, and a review of low-frequency neuromuscular electrical stimulation (NMES) among adult cancer survivors suggests that NMES is safe and helps improve quality of life.[55] There is preliminary evidence that PFES with exercise and/or biofeedback is beneficial in treating for patients after prostate cancer.[56] Recently Li et al. found that low-frequency electrical stimulation with cervical cancer patients after hysterectomy helped reduce urinary retention in the acute phase and suggested accelerated recovery of pelvic floor muscle strength.[57] There is a significant need to build on this data with randomized control trials (RCTs) in the GYN cancer population.

External perineal, vaginal, or rectal electrodes can be used with electrical stimulation. The contraindications for PFES use in the general population include pacemaker, unstable arrhythmia, unstable seizure disorder, complete denervation, and pregnancy. Other contraindications that should be carefully considered with GYN cancer survivors are the integrity of the skin and vaginal mucosa, especially after radiation. The same contraindications for use on rectal or vaginal probes used for biofeedback apply to electrical stimulation.

Percutaneous posterior tibial nerve stimulation, implantable sacral nerve root stimulators,[58,59] or high-intensity focused electromagnetic technology[60,61] are additional FDA-approved electrical modalities for treating the pelvic floor that are neither well tested among GYN cancer survivors nor typically available in the rehab setting.

Manual Therapy

Manual therapy is commonly used to treat pelvic floor dysfunctions. Tissue mobility goals may be to improve tolerance of GYN assessment with a speculum or return to sexual intimacy without pain. Periurethral muscle tightness and spasm can contribute to urine retention and voiding dysfunction and may respond favorably to manual release. Abdominal or colon massage may be helpful stimulating the bowel.[62] The patient or patient's partner can be educated on manual pelvic floor techniques as part of the home program, and a self-guided manual program can be very useful in sexual rehabilitation.[63]

Therapists with pelvic floor training can perform perineal massage and internal vaginal or rectal work. A variety of manual techniques have been reported in the literature for stretching and mobilizing the vaginal tissue and pelvic floor specifically for pain-related sexual dysfunction. These include trigger point massage, myofascial release, connective and scar tissue release, strain–counterstrain, and visceral manipulation.[45] Gentle exploration with one or two fingers by the therapist can help stretch vaginal wall and pelvic floor muscles. Instrument-assisted manual therapy utilizing a wand or small dilator can facilitate reaching areas of the pelvic floor that may be difficult to reach. Postradiation changes such as severe vaginal stenosis, atrophy, skin breakdown, or bleeding may be contraindications for internal manual work. Good communication between the treating therapist and the medical team is very important.

Vaginal Dilators

Progressively sized dilators, usually made of plastic or silicone, are introduced sequentially into the vagina to increase circumferential stretch of the vaginal walls and connective tissue. Gentle exploration, manual therapy, progressive dilation, and penetrative intercourse two to three times a week are generally recommended to help prevent complications and keep the vaginal canal from sticking together. There is a lack of RCTs that demonstrates that dilator use is beneficial, though it is widely believed that it can help prevent complications of vaginal adhesions after radiotherapy.[64,65] Research is conflicted on the merits and risks of vaginal dilation after radiation. Initiating therapy with vaginal dilators too soon after radiation can cause additional tissue damage.[64] Contraindications for vaginal dilator use would include broken or inflamed tissue, infection, active bleeding, and presence of local tumor, pain, or absence of patient consent.

Directions on dilator use should include verbal and visual education tools, specific goal setting, opportunities to practice, and encouragement. A proper warm-up, stretching, and frame of mind are very important prior to introducing an instrument into the vagina. The patient should begin with good hand hygiene and a quiet, private environment where they can position themselves comfortably to begin treatment. The dilator should be washed and well lubricated before it is gently introduced for therapy. Treatment may include static gentle stretching by

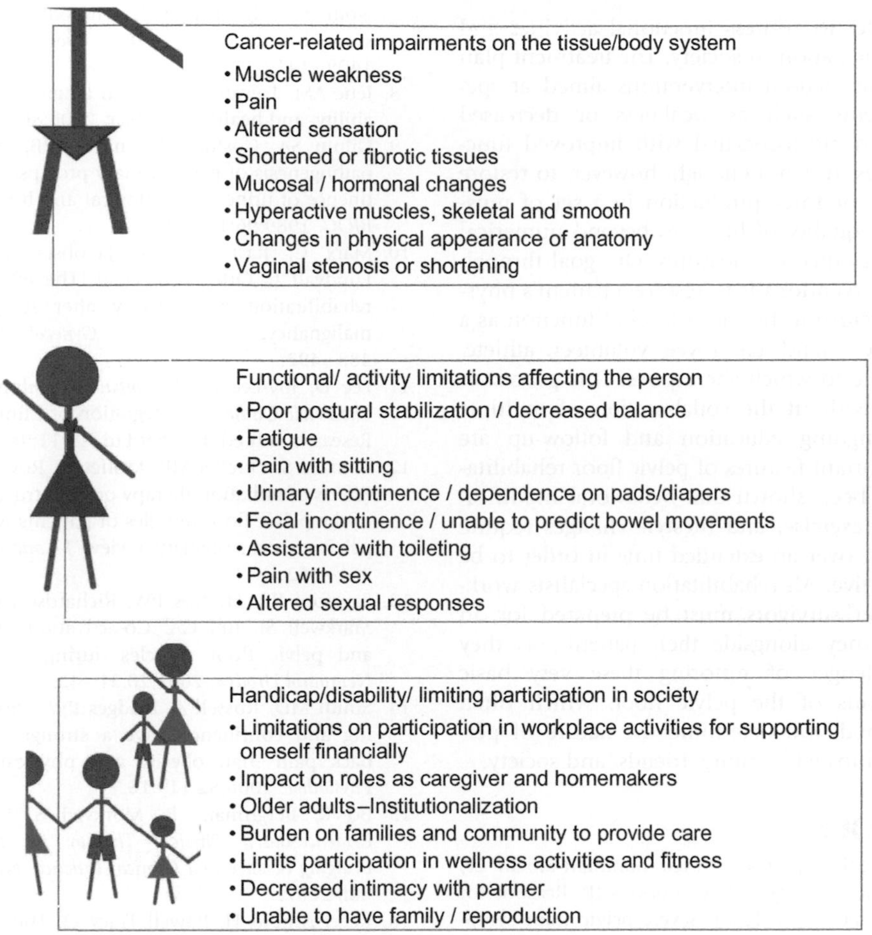
Cancer-related impairments on the tissue/body system
• Muscle weakness
• Pain
• Altered sensation
• Shortened or fibrotic tissues
• Mucosal / hormonal changes
• Hyperactive muscles, skeletal and smooth
• Changes in physical appearance of anatomy
• Vaginal stenosis or shortening
Functional/ activity limitations affecting the person
• Poor postural stabilization / decreased balance
• Fatigue
• Pain with sitting
• Urinary incontinence / dependence on pads/diapers
• Fecal incontinence / unable to predict bowel movements
• Assistance with toileting
• Pain with sex
• Altered sexual responses
Handicap/disability/ limiting participation in society
• Limitations on participation in workplace activities for supporting oneself financially
• Impact on roles as caregiver and homemakers
• Older adults–Institutionalization
• Burden on families and community to provide care
• Limits participation in wellness activities and fitness
• Decreased intimacy with partner
• Unable to have family / reproduction

FIGURE 19.10 Pelvic floor dysfunction and disability.

moving the dilator against the tight tissues, Kegel contractions against the dilator, or inserting and removing the dilator or combinations. Patient compliance with vaginal dilator use is greatly influenced by the support of their health-care providers.[66]

COMMUNICATING THERAPY GOALS

The craft of documenting measurable and objective therapy goals is based on the therapist's ability to blend multiple factors. He or she must determine the patient's wishes and needs as well as the realistic potential for each case, then identify the correct impairment, choose the appropriate intervention, and estimate the correct time frame for the anticipated outcome, while satisfying the requirements of reimbursement.

Fig. 19.10 summarizes the levels of impairments, dysfunction and disability, with some examples that relate to the pelvic floor (Fig. 19.10). Fig. 19.10 can be helpful in crafting the language of goal writing. An example could be: the patient will improve pelvic floor muscle strength (impairment) in order to reduce stress incontinence and return to work without needing to wear pads (function) in 6 weeks (time frame).

SUMMARY

As the population of cancer survivors increases, pelvic floor therapy interventions will be required by more and more women and should be readily available as part of a comprehensive cancer rehabilitation program. Therapeutic interventions can be used to affect changes at the level of the tissue, muscles, and body systems in order to address functional activities and ultimately participation in society. The treatment plan should describe focused interventions aimed at specific impairments such as weakness or decreased mobility, which are associated with improved functional outcomes. It is not enough, however, to restore tissue mobility or force production in a set of muscles. Improved quality of life goes beyond numerical data on patient outcome measures. Our goal through therapeutic interventions is to restore a patient's physical ability to return to her prior level of function as a mother, spouse, friend, employee, volunteer, athlete, or whatever role to which she aspires. This process is not complete without the collaboration of multiple disciplines. Ongoing education and follow-up are extremely important features of pelvic floor rehabilitation, as it has been shown that behavioral modifications for diet, exercise, and lifestyle changes require clinical support over an extended time in order to be optimally effective. All rehabilitation specialists working with cancer survivors must be prepared for an emotional journey alongside their patients, as they face the challenges of restoring these very basic human functions of the pelvic floor, which often define adulthood and determine the nature of personal relationships with family, friends, and society.

REFERENCES

1. Hazewinkel MH, Sprangers MAG, Taminiau-Bloem EF, van der Velden J, Burger MPM, Roovers JP. Reasons for not seeking medical help for severe pelvic floor symptoms: a qualitative study in survivors of gynaecological cancer. *BJOG*. 2010;117:39–46.
2. Howlader N, Noone A, Krapcho M, Miller D, Brest A, Yu M, et al. *SEER Cancer Statistics Review, 1975–2016*. Bethesda, MD: National Cancer Institute; 2019.
3. Lin K-Y, Edbrooke L, Granger C, Denehy L, Frawley H. The impact of gynaecological cancer treatment on physical activity levels: a systematic review of observational studies. *Braz J Phys Ther*. 2019;23(2):79–92.
4. Donovan KA, Boyington AR, Judson PL, Wyman JF. Bladder and bowel symptoms in cervical and endometrial cancer survivors. *Psychooncology*. 2014;23:672–678.
5. Neron M, Bastide S, Tayrac RD, Masia F, Ferrer C, Labaki M, et al. Impact of gynecologic cancer on pelvic floor disorder symptoms and quality of life: an observational study. *Sci Rep*. 2019;9:2250.
6. Ramaseshan AS, Felton J, Roque D, Rao G, Shipper AG, Sanses TVD. Pelvic floor disorders in women with gynecologic malignancies: a systematic review. *Int Urogynecol J*. 2018;29:459–476.
7. Bretschneider CE, Doll KM, Bensen JT, Gehrig PA, Wu JM, Geller EJ. Prevalence of pelvic floor disorders in women with suspected gynecological malignancy: a survey-based study. *Int Urogynecol J*. 2016;27: 1409–1414.
8. Jette AM. Toward a common language for function, disability, and health. *Phys Ther*. 2006;86:726–734.
9. Gilpin SA, Gosling JA, Smith ARB, Warrell DW. The pathogenesis of genitourinary prolapse and stress incontinence of urine. A histological and histochemical study. *BJOG*. 1989;96:15–23.
10. Marx C, Rasmussen T, Jakobsen DH, Ottosen C, Lundvall L, Ottesen B, et al. The effect of accelerated rehabilitation on recovery after surgery for ovarian malignancy. *Acta Obstet Gynecol Scand*. 2006;85: 488–492.
11. Lee D, Joy-Lee L. *The Impaired lumbopelvic-hip complex. The Pelvic Girdle*, An Integration of Clinical Expertise and Research. 4th ed. Elsevier Ltd.; 2011:91–128.
12. Bernard S, Ouellet MP, Moffet H, Roy JS, Dumoulin C. Effects of radiation therapy on the structure and function of the pelvic floor muscles of patients with cancer in the pelvic area: a systematic review. *J Cancer Surviv*. 2016;10: 351–362.
13. Sapsford RR, Hodges PW, Richardson CA, Cooper DH, Markwell SJ, Jull GA. Co-activation of the abdominal and pelvic floor muscles during voluntary exercises. *Neurourol Urodyn*. 2001;20:31–42.
14. Smith MD, Russell A, Hodges PW. Disorders of breathing and continence have a stronger association with back pain than obesity and physical activity. *Aust J Physiother*. 2006;52:11–16.
15. Bo K, Berghmans B, Morkved S, Van Kampen M. *Evidence-Based Physical Therapy for the Pelvic Floor, Bridging Science and Clinical Practice*. New York: Elsevier Ltd; 2007.
16. Kegel Arnold H, Powell Tracy O. The physiologic treatment of urinary stress incontinence. *J Urol*. 1950;63: 808–813.
17. Kegel AH. Progressive resistance exercise in the functional restoration of the perineal muscles. *Am J Obstet Gynecol*. 1948;56:238–248.
18. Laycock J, Jerwood D. Pelvic floor muscle assessment: the PERFECT scheme. *Physiotherapy*. 2001;87:631–642.
19. Ashton-Miller J, DeLancey JOL. Functional anatomy of the female pelvic floor. In: Bo K, Berghmans B, Morkved S, Van Kampen M, eds. *Evidence Based Physical Therapy for the Pelvic Floor Bridging Science and Clinical Practice*. New York: Elsevier; 2007:19–33.
20. D'Ancona C, Haylen B, Oelke M, Abranches-Monteiro L, Arnold E, Goldman H, et al. The International Continence Society (ICS) report on the terminology for adult male lower urinary tract and pelvic floor symptoms and dysfunction. *Neurourol Urodyn*. 2019;38: 433–477.
21. Wren P, Janz N, Brubaker L, Fitzgerald M, Weber AM, LaPorte FB, et al. Reliability of health-related quality-of-life measures 1 year after surgical procedures for pelvic floor disorders. *Am J Obstet Gynecol*. 2005;192:780–788.

22. Sandvik H, Seim A, Vanvik A, Hunskaar S. A severity index for epidemiological surveys of female urinary incontinence: comparison with 48-hour pad-weighing tests. *Neurourol Urodyn*. 2000;19:137–145.
23. Bharucha AE. Management of fecal incontinence. *Gastroenterol Hepatol*. 2008;4:807–817.
24. Rockwood TH. Incontinence severity and QOL scales for fecal incontinence. *Gastroenterology*. 2004;126: S106–S113.
25. Coffin B, Caussé C. Constipation Assessment Scales in adults: a literature review including the new Bowel Function Index. *Expert Rev Gastroenterol Hepatol*. 2011;5: 601–613.
26. Zuckerman M. Physiological measures of sexual arousal in the human. *Psychol Bull*. 1971;75:297–329.
27. Basson R. The female sexual response: a different model. *J Sex Marital Ther*. 2000;26:51–65.
28. Basson R. A model of women's sexual arousal. *J Sex Marital Ther*. 2002;28:1–10.
29. Chivers ML, Brotto LA. Controversies of women's sexual arousal and desire. *Eur Psychol*. 2017;22:5–26.
30. Morris L, Do V, Chard J, Brand AH. Radiation-induced vaginal stenosis: current perspectives. *Int J Womens Health*. 2017;9:273–279.
31. Katz A. Interventions for sexuality after pelvic radiation therapy and gynecological cancer. *Cancer J*. 2009;15: 45–47.
32. Bakker RM, Kenter GG, Creutberg CL, Stiggelbout AM, Derks M, Mingelen W, et al. Sexual distress and associated factors among cervical cancer survivors: a cross-sectional multicenter observational study. *Psychooncology*. 2016;26.
33. Wiegel M, Meston C, Rosen R. The female sexual function index (FSFI): cross-validation and development of clinical cutoff scores. *J Sex Marital Ther*. 2005;31:1–20.
34. Giraldi A, Rellini A, Pfaus J, Bitzer J, Laan E, Jannini E, et al. Questionnaires for assessment of female sexual dysfunction: a review and proposal for a standardized screener. *J Sex Med*. 2011;8:2681–2706.
35. Boulton M, Adams E, Horne A, Durrant L, Rose P, Watson E. A qualitative study of cancer survivors' responses to information on the long-term and late effects of pelvic radiotherapy 1–11 years post treatment. *Eur J Cancer Care*. 2015;24:734–747.
36. Goode PS, Burgio KL, Johnson TM, Clay OJ, Roth DL, Markland AD, et al. Behavioral therapy with or without biofeedback and pelvic floor electrical stimulation for persistent postprostatectomy incontinence: a randomized controlled trial. *JAMA*. 2011;305:151–159.
37. Goode PS, Burgio KL, Locher JL, Roth DL, Umlauf MG, Richter HE, et al. Effect of behavioral training with or without pelvic floor electrical stimulation on stress incontinence in women: a randomized controlled trial. *JAMA*. 2003;290:345–352.
38. Chiarelli P. Lifestyle interventions for pelvic floor dysfunction. In: Bo K, Berghams B, Morkved S, Van Kampen M, eds. *Evidence-Based Physical Therapy for the Pelvic Floor*. New York: Churchill Livingstone, Elsevier; 2007:147–154.
39. Medicine IO. *Dietary Reference Intakes for Water, Potassium, Sodium, Chloride, and Sulfate*. Washington, DC: The National Academies Press; 2005.
40. Jokar A, Davari T, Asadi N, Ahmadi F, Foruhari S. Comparison of the hyaluronic acid vaginal cream and conjugated estrogen used in treatment of vaginal atrophy of menopause women: a randomized controlled clinical trial. *Int J Community Based Nurs Midwifery*. 2016;4: 69–78.
41. Edwards D, Panay N. Treating vulvovaginal atrophy/genitourinary syndrome of menopause: how important is vaginal lubricant and moisturizer composition? *Climacteric*. 2016;19:151–161.
42. Carter J, Stabile C, Seidel B, Baser R, Goldfarb S, Goldfrank D. Vaginal and sexual health treatment strategies within a female sexual medicine program for cancer patients and survivors. *J Cancer Surviv*. 2016;11.
43. Yang EJ, Lim J-Y, Rah UW, Kim YB. Effect of a pelvic floor muscle training program on gynecologic cancer survivors with pelvic floor dysfunction: a randomized controlled trial. *Gynecol Oncol*. 2012;125:705–711.
44. Ghaderi F, Bastani P, Hajebrahimi S, Jafarabadi MA, Berghmans B. Pelvic floor rehabilitation in the treatment of women with dyspareunia: a randomized controlled clinical trial. *Int Urogynecol J*. 2019;30:1849–1855.
45. Rosenbaum T, Annette Owens Md P. The role of pelvic floor physical therapy in the treatment of pelvic and genital pain-related sexual dysfunction (CME). *J Sex Med*. 2008;5:513–523.
46. Piassarolli VP, Hardy E, Andrade NF, Ferreira Nde O, Osis MJ. Pelvic floor muscle training in female sexual dysfunctions. *Rev Bras Ginecol Obstet*. 2010;32:234–240.
47. Dumoulin C, Glazener C, Jenkinson D. Determining the optimal pelvic floor muscle training regimen for women with stress urinary incontinence. *Neurourol Urodyn*. 2011; 30:746–753.
48. Marques A, Stothers L, Macnab A. The status of pelvic floor muscle training for women. *Can Urol Assoc J*. 2010; 4:419–424.
49. Hodges PW, Sapsford R, Pengel LHM. Postural and respiratory functions of the pelvic floor muscles. *Neurourol Urodyn*. 2007;26:362–371.
50. Borello-France D, Burgio KL, Goode PS, Ye W, Weidner AC, Lukacz ES, et al. Adherence to behavioral interventions for stress incontinence: rates, barriers, and predictors. *Phys Ther*. 2013;93:757–773.
51. Venegas M, Carrasco B, Casas-Cordero R. Factors influencing long-term adherence to pelvic floor exercises in women with urinary incontinence. *Neurourol Urodyn*. 2018;37:1120–1127.
52. Newman D. Pelvic floor muscle rehabilitation using biofeedback. *Urol Nurs*. 2014;34:193–202.
53. Dannecker C, Wolf V, Raab R, Hepp H, Anthuber C. EMG-biofeedback assisted pelvic floor muscle training is an effective therapy of stress urinary or mixed

incontinence: a 7-year experience with 390 patients. *Arch Gynecol Obstet.* 2005;273:93.
54. Wang AC, Wang Y-Y, Chen M-C. Single-blind, randomized trial of pelvic floor muscle training, biofeedback-assisted pelvic floor muscle training, and electrical stimulation in the management of overactive bladder. *Urology.* 2004;63:61–66.
55. O'Connor D, Caulfield B, Lennon O. The efficacy and prescription of neuromuscular electrical stimulation (NMES) in adult cancer survivors: a systematic review and meta-analysis. *Support Care Cancer.* 2018;26:3985–4000.
56. Kannan P, Winser SJ, Fung B, Cheing G. Effectiveness of pelvic floor muscle training alone and in combination with biofeedback, electrical stimulation, or both compared to control for urinary incontinence in men following prostatectomy: systematic review and meta-analysis. *Phys Ther.* 2018;98:932–945.
57. Li H, Zhou C-K, Song J, Zhang W-Y, Wang S-M, Gu Y-L, et al. Curative efficacy of low frequency electrical stimulation in preventing urinary retention after cervical cancer operation. *World J Surg Oncol.* 2019;17:141.
58. Scaldazza CV, Morosetti C, Giampieretti R, Lorenzetti R, Baroni M. Percutaneous tibial nerve stimulation versus electrical stimulation with pelvic floor muscle training for overactive bladder syndrome in women: results of a randomized controlled study. *Int Braz J Urol.* 2017;43:121–126.
59. Tutolo M, Ammirati E, Van der Aa F. What is new in neuromodulation for overactive bladder? *Eur Urol Focus.* 2018;4:49–53.
60. Samuels JB, Pezzella A, Berenholz J, Alinsod R. Safety and efficacy of a non-invasive high-intensity focused electromagnetic field (HIFEM) device for treatment of urinary incontinence and enhancement of quality of life. *Lasers Surg Med.* 2019;51:760–766.
61. Hlavinka TC, Turčan P, Bader A. The use of HIFEM technology in the treatment of pelvic floor muscles as a cause of female sexual dysfunction: a multi-center pilot study. *J Womens Health Care.* 2019;08.
62. McClurg D, Lowe-Strong A. Does abdominal massage relieve constipation? *Nurs Times.* 2011;107:20–22.
63. Gallo-Silver L. The sexual rehabilitation of persons with cancer. *Cancer Pract.* 2000;8:10–15.
64. Miles T, Johnson N. Vaginal dilator therapy for women receiving pelvic radiotherapy. *Cochrane Database Syst Rev.* 2014;9:CD007291.
65. Kachnic LA, Bruner DW, Qureshi MM, Russo GA. Perceptions and practices regarding women's vaginal health following radiation therapy: a survey of radiation oncologists practicing in the United States. *Pract Radiat Oncol.* 2017;7:356–363.
66. Lee Y. Patients' perception and adherence to vaginal dilator therapy: a systematic review and synthesis employing symbolic interactionism. *Patient Prefer Adherence.* 2018;12:551–560.

CHAPTER 20

Cancer-Related Cognitive Impairment: Diagnosis, Pathogenesis, and Management

AILEEN M. MORENO, LCSW • RICHARD A. HAMILTON, PHD • M. BEATRIZ CURRIER, MD

INTRODUCTION

Pertinent Definitions and Terms

Individuals living with cancer often experience a multitude of adverse effects that can negatively impact quality of life. One of the most prevalent and disabling sequelae is cancer-related cognitive impairment (CRCI), defined as the pattern of cognitive deficits reflecting the CNS toxic effects of cancer and its treatment. CRCI is most commonly categorized by a pattern of cognitive deficits in verbal memory, sustained attention, executive function, and processing speed.[1] It is important to note that visual memory was not assessed in most studies of CRCI. It is highly unlikely that the toxic effects of cancer treatment would only affect focal brain regions or be unilateral. Multiple bilateral areas of cerebral dysfunction are more likely. Other cognitive domains can also be affected such as visual memory, verbal fluency, and upper extremity fine motor dexterity.[2]

This pattern of cognitive impairments is often referred to as "chemo brain." This colloquial term was originally coined based upon the previously accepted understanding that chemotherapy treatments were the primary culprit for these types of cognitive changes. However, neuroscience research in this area reveals the neurotoxic effects of systemic chemotherapy are only one possible etiology for this debilitating syndrome. While an exact pathophysiology is still unknown, it is now widely thought that other factors such as systematic inflammation associated with cancer and its treatment (surgery, chemotherapy, radiotherapy), hormonal therapies, premorbid and/or comorbid depression/anxiety, chronic sleep disturbance, external stressors (e.g., marital/family problems, financial/ health insurance issues), alcohol/ substance abuse, and genetic predisposition to cognitive impairment may also contribute to the development of CRCI. In fact, many of these factors often overlap, making it challenging to distinguish the likely cause of cognitive changes in patients with cancer. The term "chemo brain" is now most commonly referred to in the medical literature as CRCI or cancer-related cognitive impairment.

Prevalence and Course of Cognitive Impairment in Patients With Breast and Gynecological Cancers

Multiple longitudinal prospective studies, comparing pre- and posttreatment cognitive function predominantly in breast cancer survivors, have been conducted to identify the prevalence and course of CRCI. These large, multicenter studies have used neuropsychological testing across multiple time points up to 6–24 months after the cancer diagnosis. These studies have found a CRCI prevalence rate ranging from 12% to 82% across the cancer treatment trajectory.[3–26] A review by Janelsins et al. highlights studies of CRCI that found prevalence rates of 30% among breast cancer patients pretreatment, 75% of patients during treatment, and 35% of patients posttreatment.[27] In the largest multicenter, longitudinal prospective

Breast Cancer and Gynecologic Cancer Rehabilitation DOI: https://doi.org/10.1016/B978-0-323-72166-0.00020-7

controlled study of 581 breast cancer survivors and 364 controls matched for age, education, and menopausal status, Janelsins et al. assessed cognitive function at three time points, including prechemotherapy, postchemotherapy, and 6 months after chemotherapy.[3] Janelsins et al. found a significantly higher rate of cognitive decline postchemotherapy compared to prechemotherapy among the breast cancer survivors and matched controls (45% and 10%, respectively, $P < .001$). Six months after completing chemotherapy, a statistically significant rate of cognitive decline persisted in the breast cancer survivors compared to the controls (37% and 14%, respectively, $P < .001$). Notably, pretreatment baseline cognitive reserve, as measured by the Wide Range Achievement Test, significantly correlated with cognitive decline rates in this sample.

In a longitudinal age-matched controlled study utilizing neuropsychological testing in 132 breast cancer patients after surgery but prior to adjuvant therapy (chemotherapy or radiotherapy), investigators found a significantly higher rate of cognitive deficits among 22% of breast cancer patients as compared to only 4% of age-matched healthy controls.[28] This finding of postsurgery pretreatment cognitive decline in breast cancer patients (prior to receiving adjuvant therapy) propelled the hypothesis that the biology of the proinflammatory tumor microenvironment may contribute to the pathogenesis of CRCI, independent of the neurotoxicity of chemotherapy.[28] However, other factors such as the effects of anesthesia, pain medication, and postsurgery emotional sequelae should be considered in future research.

Specifically, several studies have found that 20%–30% of patients with breast cancer have lower than expected cognitive performance pretreatment, based on age and education.[28–30] In addition, a review done by Ahles et al. indicates that cross-sectional studies of breast cancer survivors have found that 17%–75% experienced cognitive deficits in domains, including attention, concentration, working memory, and executive function, from 6 months to 20 years after chemotherapy exposure.[29,31,32] Furthermore, according to Van Arsdale et al., studies evaluating cognitive dysfunction in women with ovarian cancer have shown that 17%–80% have been reported to have cognitive deficits with symptoms, including decreased memory, attention, and executive function lasting 5–10 years following treatment.[33] To date, the literature suggests that presentation and course of CRCI among breast and gynecological cancer patients are highly variable. This syndrome may manifest with subtle or dramatic cognitive deficits, and its course may be transient or permanent and stable or progressive. A possible contributing factor to the variable presentation of CRCI is the fact that not all the studies cited utilized the same neuropsychological tests. In addition, the testing that was done was more of a neuropsychological screening than a comprehensive battery. It is possible that a more comprehensive test battery would demonstrate other areas of cognitive dysfunction. However, time and cost constraints of a comprehensive neuropsychological test battery may limit its utility in clinical settings.

Much more research is needed to better understand the debilitating sequelae of CRCI. Most studies have been conducted with breast cancer patients under the age of 60.[29] More studies evaluating the incidence of CRCI among patients with gynecological cancers (i.e., endometrial, ovarian, cervical, and vulvar) are needed. That said, the assessment approach for CRCI would likely be the same across cancer types; and its treatment is primarily tied to the specific cognitive deficits found on neuropsychological testing.

Impact of Cognitive Impairment on Quality of Life and Function in Breast and Gynecological Cancers

The highly variable and unpredictable course of CRCI can make its impact more challenging to manage and difficult to treat. For patients experiencing CRCI, returning to school and/or work can be quite daunting due to its negative impact on an individual's daily functioning. Sometimes, patients may find themselves needing to temporarily interrupt their academic studies, extend a medical leave of absence from work, change jobs/careers, or even apply for disability, all of which can have financial implications on the heels of an already financially burdensome time. Furthermore, CRCI's reach often extends its interference into other areas, including familial and societal roles as well as emotional consequences. Patients often describe becoming more withdrawn due to feelings of self-consciousness over cognitive difficulties that can sometimes lead to depression. Their self-confidence and self-esteem can be rattled and they often make statements such as "I can't made decisions" or "I can no longer multitask." They often feel guilty over their perceived burden placed on loved ones. Some other common descriptions given by patients include (1) "Going back to work has been very difficult because I'm not as sharp or quick on my feet as I was before and I'm afraid my co-workers will think I'm not capable anymore"; (2) "I always had the best memory, everyone knew me for it, and now I can't even remember simple things like movies I've seen or things I've read"; (3) "I often have trouble finding words I want to say, I can picture it in my mind and can describe it, but I can't think of the actual word, so I now avoid having conversations whenever possible because I'm embarrassed when it happens"; or (4) "I went back to graduate school a few months before my diagnosis and going back now after finishing chemo I'm finding it really hard to listen to lectures while keeping up with taking good notes." Patients also frequently report discontinuing pleasurable activities or hobbies due to their CRCI symptoms. See Table 20.1 for more examples of CRCI symptom presentation.

Given the advancing age of the average gynecological cancer patient population, these women may present with other comorbid medical conditions that may contribute to or exacerbate any presenting cognitive difficulties, in addition to expected aging cognitive decline. Hence, a thorough assessment, including past and current medical history, is critical.

STRUCTURAL AND FUNCTIONAL NEUROANATOMICAL CORRELATES OF CANCER-RELATED COGNITIVE IMPAIRMENT

Normal cognitive function can be characterized into six cognitive domains with specific functions that are mediated by different regions of the brain.[34] Present research indicates that CRCI may impact up to four of these cognitive domains, including sustained attention, executive function, processing speed, and learning/working memory. The areas most impacted by chemotherapy include brain hub regions such as the prefrontal cortex and hippocampus that are critical for executive functioning and memory. Moreover, brain network connectivity is also impacted by chemotherapy that may interfere with sustained attention and processing speed. See Table 20.1 for a list of cognitive domains and their respective functions, including examples of related CRCI symptom presentation.[34]

To date, the greatest body of research on CRCI includes structural and functional neuroimaging studies of breast cancer patients who have received chemotherapy.[35–40] See Table 20.2 for neuroanatomical correlates of CRCI in breast cancer patients treated with chemotherapy. McDonald et al. conducted prospective longitudinal controlled voxel-based morphometry measurements of structural MRIs among 48 breast cancer patients with chemotherapy compared to age-matched breast cancer patients without chemotherapy and age-matched controls across three time points; baseline, 1 month postchemotherapy, and 12 months postchemotherapy.[37,38] These studies showed reduced gray matter volume in the frontal lobe, medial temporal lobe, and cerebellum that correlated with neuropsychological testing deficits.[37,38] A cross-sectional structural MRI study of 339 breast cancer patients with and without chemotherapy was compared with healthy controls at 1 and 3 years after treatment.[39] This study found a reduction in neocortical gray matter persisted at year 1 and normalized by year 3 after chemotherapy. In two cross-sectional diffusion tensor imaging studies among breast cancer patients who received chemotherapy, reduced white matter integrity correlated with worsening attention and verbal memory.[35,40]

A review by Simó et al. reports that prospective structural neuroimaging (MRI) studies have shown that there is a widespread decrease in white matter volume prior to treatment with chemotherapy and with functional MRI an increased level of activation of the frontoparietal attentional network of cancer patients compared to controls.[41] However, Simó et al. also report that once patients were exposed to chemotherapy, there was "an early diffuse decrease of gray matter volume and white matter volume together with a decrease of the over-activation in frontal regions" compared to controls.[41]

A longitudinal prospective functional MRI study of 28 breast cancer patients with and without chemotherapy compared with healthy age-matched controls at baseline, 1 and 12 months after chemotherapy found hyperactivation of the prefrontal cortex during working memory task when compared to controls, with reduced activation after 1 month and only partial return to baseline hyperactivation after 1 year. These findings suggest that early brain hyperactivation reflects neural compensation; however, long-term reduced activation may correspond to established deficits.[38]

RISK FACTORS AND PATHOGENESIS OF CANCER-RELATED COGNITIVE IMPAIRMENT IN PATIENTS WITH BREAST OR GYNECOLOGICAL CANCER

Multiple risk factors and mechanisms of pathogenesis associated with CRCI include the following variables

1. advanced age,
2. chemotherapy-induced cellular mechanisms that lead to accelerated aging,
3. direct neurotoxicity of chemotherapy,
4. hormonal therapies,

TABLE 20.1
Clinical Cognitive Domains, Functions, and Cancer-Related Cognitive Impairment (CRCI)–Related Symptoms

Cognitive Domains	Cognitive Functions	CRCI-Related Symptoms
Memory (verbal and visual)	Ability to register, encode, and retrieve verbal, visual, and spatial information; both in the short term (immediate) and long term (delayed)	Trouble remembering names, important dates, or appointments, what you have just read, details of conversations with others. Misplacing everyday items such as keys, wallet, and cell phone; difficulty navigating while driving; trouble remembering where parked
Visuospatial	Ability to analyze and synthesize abstract, nonverbal, visual material; fluid reasoning	Judging distance, rate of movement when driving, estimating how much water in a pot, reading a map or blueprint, putting a puzzle together
Working memory	Ability to temporarily hold (remember) information and manipulate it; ability to immediately process conscious perceptual and linguistic information	Difficulty taking notes in class, remembering a phone number long enough to dial it, mental arithmetic
Attention and concentration	Ability to tune into auditory and visual information; ability to sustain focus over time while effectively disregarding any competing distractions	Difficulty concentrating, short attention span, easily distracted, feel like they "space out," trouble completing tasks
Processing speed	Ability to process information (simple and complex) with speed, efficiency, and accuracy (without making mistakes)	Take longer amount of time to finish simple or routine tasks, complain of disorganized or slow thinking, less time and mental energy for understanding new information or "thinking on your feet"
Executive function	Ability to manage multiple tasks simultaneously, cognitive flexibility, novel problem-solving; decision-making, judgment and impulse control, short- and long-term planning	Difficulty multitasking, can only do one thing at a time; hesitancy in making decisions when that normally would not be the case; trouble "thinking outside the box"; trouble learning something new

TABLE 20.2
Neuroanatomical Correlates of Cancer-Related Cognitive Impairment in Breast Cancer Patients Treated With Chemotherapy

Neuroanatomy	Associated Cognitive Function
Frontal and parietal lobes	Attention, concentration
Prefrontal cortex (ventrolateral and dorsolateral areas)	Working memory, executive function
Prefrontal, anterior cingulate and orbitofrontal cortex	Emotional regulation, impulse control
Prefrontal cortex and subcortical white matter networks	Processing speed

5. low baseline cognitive reserve,
6. cytokine-mediated neuroinflammation driven by the systemic effects of the tumor microenvironment and cancer-related treatments, and
7. genetic vulnerability to cognitive impairment.

It is well established that there is a natural cognitive decline with age that has led to speculation by researchers that older adults may be more vulnerable to the cognitive effects of cancer treatment. A review by Ahles et al. states that "research suggests that biologic processes underlying cancer, the impact of cancer treatments, aging, neurodegeneration and cognitive decline are linked, leading to the hypothesis that cancer treatments may accelerate the aging process."[29,42] Specific biological processes by which chemotherapy accelerates aging include chemotherapy-induced neuronal injury with inadequate repair through oxidative DNA damage associated with neurodegenerative disease[43] and chemotherapy-induced shortening of telomeres in glial cells.[44,45]

Chemotherapy-induced direct neurotoxic effects on the brain have been shown in preclinical studies and clinical neuroimaging studies. Animal studies have found very minute leakage of chemotherapy can cause cell death and reduce cell division in the dentate gyrus of the hippocampus that is critical for memory.[46] Direct neurotoxic effects of methyltrexate include coagulative necrosis of the white matter, axonal swelling, and demyelinization.[47] In addition, 5 fluorouracil causes acute and delayed myelin damage.[48] Areas that are most affected by chemotherapy include brain hub regions such as the prefrontal cortex (executive function, processing speed, working memory), hippocampus (verbal and visual memory), and frontal/parietal lobes (attention, concentration, spatial/perceptual ability). In addition, brain network connectivity is also impacted.[27] In particular, platinum-based agents such as cisplatin, often used in the treatment of gynecological cancers, are highly neurotoxic.[49] According to Pendergrass et al., it has been estimated that "13–70% of patients receiving cancer chemotherapy have measurable cognitive impairment" and that adjunct endocrine therapy, as is often used in breast cancer treatment for several years, can result in cognitive impairment.[1]

A review of several studies found endocrine therapy significantly impacted cognitive function. Specifically, hormonal therapy was accompanied by deficits in verbal memory/fluency, motor speed, attention, and working memory.[34] In a prospective controlled study neuropsychological testing was administered to 300 postmenopausal women at two time points: before hormonal therapy and after 1 year on hormonal therapy. The sample included 180 breast cancer patients on maintenance hormonal therapy with no systemic therapy exposure compared to 120 healthy age-matched controls.[4] The study found that tamoxifen users ($N = 80$) had significant deterioration in verbal memory and executive function at 1 year compared to the healthy controls. In contrast, exemestane users ($N = 98$) did not have significant cognitive deficits at 1 year compared to the healthy controls.[4] This is clinically relevant as therapy compliance can be affected by the experience of CRCI for many women.

The role of baseline cognitive reserve is important when discussing the potential risk for developing CRCI. Cognitive reserve as defined by Ahles et al. "represents innate and developed cognitive capacity (influenced by education, occupational attainment and lifestyle)."[29] Baseline cognitive reserve was measured by the Wide Range Achievement Test (WRAT) reading subscale that measures baseline reading ability. This ability to read words is generally resistant to the effects of most types of cerebral dysfunction. A high cognitive reserve is associated with reduced cognitive decline. The promising aspect of this is that cognitive reserve potentially can be developed. More research is needed in this area.

Perhaps the most intriguing biological underpinning of CRCI includes cytokine-mediated neuroinflammation.[50–54] Cancer patients have increased circulating levels of proinflammatory cytokines associated with the tumor microenvironment, cell death, and tissue injury due to surgery, chemotherapy and radiotherapy, and physical and psychological distress.[50–52] A linear correlation has been found between an increase in peripheral cytokine levels (IL-6, MCP-1, IL-8) and cognitive dysfunction in breast cancer patients.[53,54] In contrast, increased levels of circulating TNF receptor 2 associated with CRCI and decreased levels at 1 year after chemotherapy were associated with improved cognitive performance.[51] In addition, reduced hippocampal volumes are associated with higher levels of proinflammatory cytokines, TNF-alpha, and IL-6, in breast cancer survivors exposed to chemotherapy as compared to age-matched controls.[52] Increased systemic inflammation driven by the tumor microenvironment and cancer treatments triggers neuroinflammation which in turn creates changes in neurotransmission and gray matter volume which impacts cognition.[54]

Polymorphisms of specific genes that regulate neural repair/plasticity and neurotransmission may predispose cancer patients to CRCI. Specifically, breast cancer survivors exposed to chemotherapy with the ApoE4 allele scored lower on visual memory.[55] COMT (catechol-*O*-methyltransferase) is an enzyme that metabolizes dopamine, a critical biogenic amine needed for cognition. COMT val + genotype carriers have increased COMT enzymatic activity that leads to decreased dopamine in the frontal networks interfering with cognitive performance. A COMT genotype study among breast cancer survivors with radiotherapy ($N = 59$) and/or chemotherapy ($N = 72$) found that COMT val + carriers scored significantly lower on verbal memory, attention, and motor speed as compared to COMT Met + homozygotes.[56] In contrast to CRCI high-risk breast cancer survivor genotyping studies, genotyping for polymorphisms that influence neuronal plasticity such as brain-derived neurotrophic factor (BDNF) may identify those patients protected against CRCI. In a study of 145 breast cancer survivors, those survivors with BDNF Met + /Met + homozygote genotyping were protected from chemotherapy-induced cognitive changes with preserved verbal memory and multitasking ability when compared to those with

BDNF val + carriers.[57] These studies highlight the role of genotyping to identify high-risk and low-risk patients with respect to CRCI and instituting this genotyping as a protocol to mitigate CRCI among breast cancer patients.

ASSESSMENT OF THE CANCER PATIENT WITH COGNITIVE IMPAIRMENT

1. Assessment of CRCI requires a comprehensive biopsychosocial evaluation with an emphasis on the medical workup for altered mental status and the required objective neuropsychological testing to identify the extent and nature of subtle deficits of CRCI. A complete history and clinical examination, with baseline laboratory and neuroimaging workup for cognitive deficits in a breast cancer or gynecological cancer patients, should include the following:
   - **a.** Laboratory studies (complete blood count, comprehensive metabolic panel, C-reactive protein, vitamin B12, folate, thyroid-stimulating hormone level): Additional relevant labs if CNS paraneoplastic syndrome suspected.
   - **b.** Brain MRI with/without contrast and diffusion tensor imaging study to assess for metastatic disease, CVA, white matter integrity.
   - **c.** Neuropsychiatric consultation to assess for premorbid/comorbid mood and anxiety disorders, alcohol/substance abuse, premorbid history of attention deficit disorder, sleep disorders, dementia, mild cognitive impairment, or traumatic brain injury. Although administering the Montreal Cognitive Assessment (MoCA) should be a routine portion of the neuropsychiatric evaluation for cognition, this screening tool is insufficient to diagnose or rule out CRCI and a normal MoCA score ≥26 should not preclude administering the neuropsychological testing battery. Standardized self-report measures of depression and anxiety such as the Beck Depression Inventory-II and the Beck Anxiety Inventory should be repeatedly administered to help quantify a patient's level of emotional distress as well as to monitor these distress levels over time.
   - **d.** Assess for antihistamine, antiemetic, benzodiazepine, and opiate-induced cognitive adverse effects.
2. The International Cognition and Cancer Task Force (ICCTF) was created in 2006 by experts in the neuroscience field to reach a consensus on how to assess, research, and treat CRCI. The task force determined that self-report alone was an inadequate measure of CRCI, and that objective neuropsychological testing was necessary. The proposed neuropsychological testing battery recommended by the ICCTF includes, at minimum, the following: Hopkins Verbal Learning Test-Revised (HVLT-R), Trail Making Tests A and B, and Controlled Oral Word Association (COWA) (see Table 20.3). These tests evaluate the cognitive functions typically affected by CRCI such as noncontextualized verbal memory, visual processing speed, executive function (mental flexibility), and word-finding fluency.[27] While this brief battery of tests provide valuable information, a more robust clinical picture of a patient's cognitive strengths and weaknesses occurs by adding the following neuropsychological tests: Working Memory (e.g., Digit Span and Arithmetic subtests from the WAIS-IV), Processing Speed (Coding and Symbol Search subtests from the WAIS-IV), Visual Spatial Ability (Block Design and Matrix Reasoning subtests from the WAIS-IV), Contextualized Verbal Memory and Visual Memory (e.g., Logical Memory I & II; Visual Reproduction I & II from the WMS-IV), and one or more abbreviated test versions of Executive Functioning (e.g., WCST-64, Stroop test, Halstead Category test). This additional testing does not require extensive time to administer (approximately 2.5 hours to complete the entire battery), and this testing is well tolerated by the vast majority of patients we have examined. The results can provide important additional information about a patient's cognitive capacity as well as provide a

TABLE 20.3 International Cognition and Cancer Task Force Neuropsychological Assessment Recommended Tests

Recommended Core Battery	Cognitive Domains Measured
HVLT-R	Learning and memory
TMT	Processing speed and executive function
COWA	Verbal fluency and executive function

COWA, Controlled Oral Word Association; *HVLT-R*, Hopkins Verbal Learning Test-Revised; *TMT*, Trail Making Test.

valuable blueprint identifying targets for cognitive rehabilitation. In addition, serial follow-up with these tests can provide objective evidence of cognitive recovery.

While subjective reports may not always be reliable, it is still an important component of a thorough assessment, as neuropsychological tests are simply a snapshot in time and done in an artificial environment. Cancer patients experiencing cognitive difficulties may describe difficulty multitasking, trouble concentrating/focusing, forgetfulness, and difficulty finding words, taking longer to process information and/or complete a task, among others.

TREATMENT OF COGNITIVE IMPAIRMENT IN BREAST AND GYNECOLOGICAL CANCER PATIENTS

According to the National Cancer Institute (NCI), "evidence-based interventions to manage cognitive impairment in cancer patients and survivors have not been firmly established. Several non-pharmacologic approaches have shown promise, including cognitive rehabilitation, exercise, and psychosocial interventions such as attention-restoring activities and meditation."[34] Cognitive rehabilitation can include education on brain function, cognitive deficits, and its impact on matters of daily life; education on compensatory strategies focused on learning new ways to adapt to current cognitive deficits (i.e., use of external aids such as cellular phones, calendars, or notebooks, minimizing distractions when performing a cognitive task); and cognitive training that involves "the use of repetitive, increasingly challenging tasks (often via computer) to improve, maintain, or restore cognitive function in the areas of attention, memory, processing speed and executive function."[34] Traditional cognitive rehabilitation is provided by a speech or occupational therapist and typically involves attending an in-person session twice per week, 30–45 minutes per session for 6–12 weeks. Alternatively, cognitive training done remotely via an online computer-based platform, such as BrainHQ by Posit Science, can also be an option. The typical recommended dose is 4 days/week, 20 minutes per session, for up to 12 weeks. For more information about the use of BrainHQ by Posit Science with cancer patients, visit the Research-Tested Intervention Programs (RTIPs) page on NCI's website at www.rtips.cancer.gov.

When assessing and planning intervention for CRCI, consideration should be given to where the patient is in terms of their treatment trajectory. Deficits identified during active chemotherapy treatment, for example, may benefit most from timing cognitive remediation after treatment ends whenever possible. The reason for this, in part, is the potential for worsening cognitive deficits and decreased mental and physical stamina during the remainder of the treatment, which could be addressed most adequately once treatment is complete.

The neuro-rehabilitation team is interdisciplinary and can include psychiatry (medical and psychological workup), neuropsychology (administration and interpretation of objective cognitive testing that help pinpoint areas for possible intervention as well as assist in making determinations about a patient's instrumental activities of daily living), in addition to speech pathology and occupational therapists (evaluation of cognitive deficits and provision of cognitive remediation therapy, typically in an outpatient setting).

At our institution, Miami Cancer Institute (MCI), we offer a Brain Fitness Lab that is dedicated to assessing, diagnosing, and treating CRCI (see Fig. 20.1). Currently, our team consists of psychiatrists, psychometricians, and a clinical neuropsychologist. We serve cancer patients of all ages, pediatric and adult, across all cancer types and all cancer treatment modalities. We also work closely with a team of speech pathologists and occupational therapists in our outpatient neuro-rehabilitation center.

In addition, we offer BrainHQ by Posit Science for patients who prefer to do cognitive training on their own. It is accessed via Internet, and therefore patients can log in remotely on any computer or smartphone application (currently apps are available for both iPhone and Androids), allowing for greater flexibility as users can train on days/times that are most convenient. This option can also be advantageous for patients who have financial, childcare, or transportation difficulties that may make going to traditional in-person therapy challenging, especially within the context of an often busy calendar comprised of other medical appointments and school/work/family life demands. However, it is important to also consider their reported level of motivation and self-discipline ability when choosing this rehabilitation option, as the key to obtaining the most benefit from a cognitive training program is regular, consistent practice over several weeks. In our clinical experience, many patients choose traditional therapy precisely because it is a scheduled appointment that they are accountable for attending (often reporting that it is

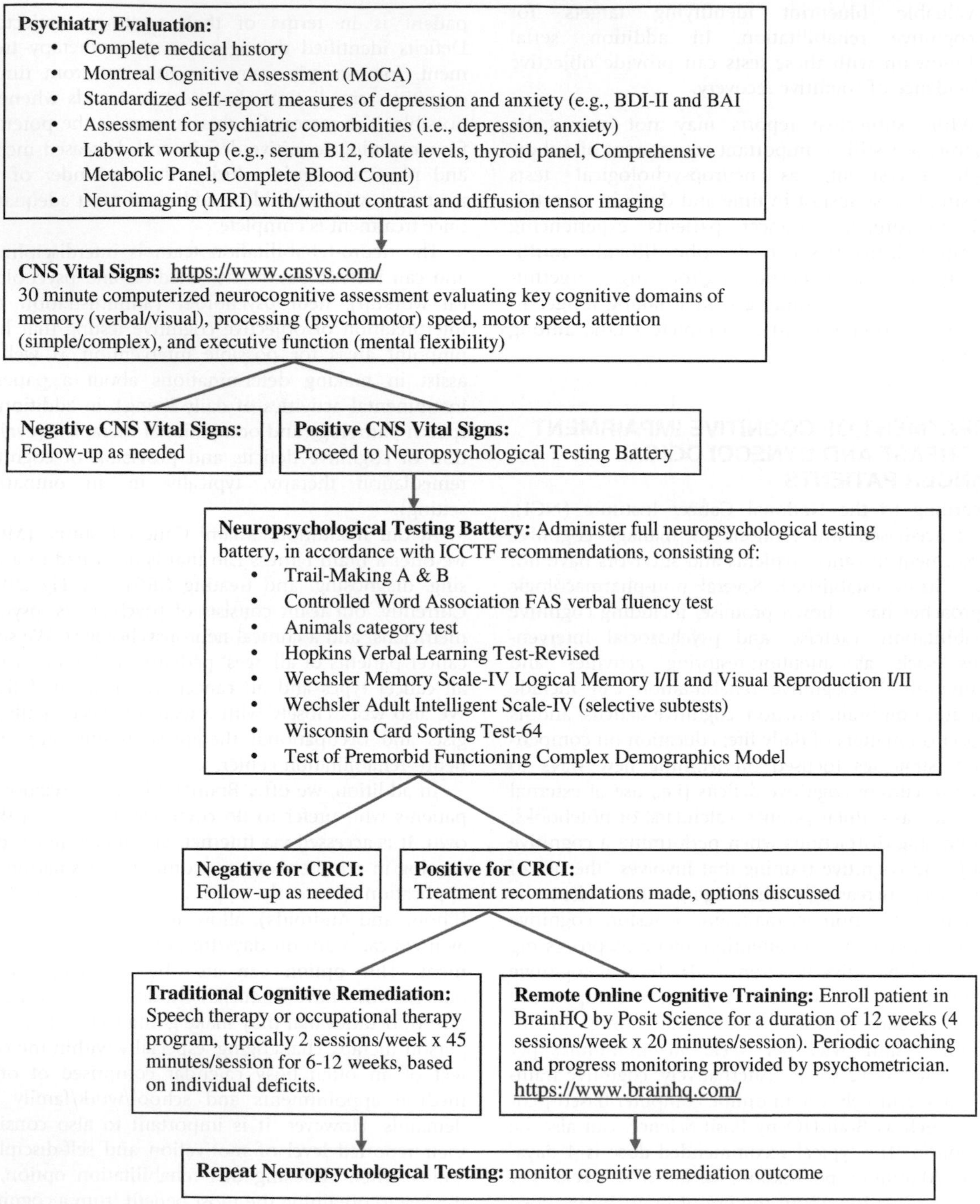
Psychiatry Evaluation:
Complete medical history
Montreal Cognitive Assessment (MoCA)
Standardized self-report measures of depression and anxiety (e.g., BDI-II and BAI
Assessment for psychiatric comorbidities (i.e., depression, anxiety)
Labwork workup (e.g., serum B12, folate levels, thyroid panel, Comprehensive Metabolic Panel, Complete Blood Count)
Neuroimaging (MRI) with/without contrast and diffusion tensor imaging
CNS Vital Signs: https://www.cnsvs.com/
30 minute computerized neurocognitive assessment evaluating key cognitive domains of memory (verbal/visual), processing (psychomotor) speed, motor speed, attention (simple/complex), and executive function (mental flexibility)
Negative CNS Vital Signs: Follow-up as needed
Positive CNS Vital Signs: Proceed to Neuropsychological Testing Battery
Neuropsychological Testing Battery: Administer full neuropsychological testing battery, in accordance with ICCTF recommendations, consisting of:
Trail-Making A & B
Controlled Word Association FAS verbal fluency test
Animals category test
Hopkins Verbal Learning Test-Revised
Wechsler Memory Scale-IV Logical Memory I/II and Visual Reproduction I/II
Wechsler Adult Intelligent Scale-IV (selective subtests)
Wisconsin Card Sorting Test-64
Test of Premorbid Functioning Complex Demographics Model
Negative for CRCI: Follow-up as needed
Positive for CRCI: Treatment recommendations made, options discussed
Traditional Cognitive Remediation: Speech therapy or occupational therapy program, typically 2 sessions/week x 45 minutes/session for 6-12 weeks, based on individual deficits.
Remote Online Cognitive Training: Enroll patient in BrainHQ by Posit Science for a duration of 12 weeks (4 sessions/week x 20 minutes/session). Periodic coaching and progress monitoring provided by psychometrician. https://www.brainhq.com/
Repeat Neuropsychological Testing: monitor cognitive remediation outcome

FIGURE 20.1 Neurocognitive assessment, diagnosis, and treatment protocol at Miami Cancer Institute.

less likely they would stick to a time to do it on their own), as well as a preference for having an in-person human connection with a therapist. While decreasing motivation levels and issues with compliance can be experienced with either cognitive remediation option, in our practice we observe more compliance problems with the remote cognitive training. We believe this may largely be due to the real challenge cancer patient's face in balancing ongoing multiple medical appointments with their personal lives (school/work/family/social) and while the flexibility of training on a convenient day/time of your choosing is appealing, the downside is that it is potentially easier to let other things take priority because you can always "get to it later." Another contributing factor is that confronting a cognitive deficiency can be emotionally invasive for some patients.

The majority of the adult patients seen in the Brain Fitness Lab are either in active treatment or survivors who have completed treatment, sometimes even years later. However, there is a percentage of patients who we see after diagnosis but prior to starting treatment, in order to establish a baseline of cognitive functioning. While this is the ideal scenario, it is often not feasible. One of the challenges of a prehabilitation cognitive assessment is the timing. Typically, at this early point of a patient's journey, they are faced with a multitude of medical appointments that may include specialist consultations, imaging, and/or procedures; in addition to dealing with the psychological, emotional, and social impact of a cancer diagnosis. As a result, many patients are overwhelmed and may not wish to address this aspect upfront. For some patients, there may also be a financial component that weighs into a decision to delay a cognitive assessment, unless needed down the line.

The elements needed to develop a state of the art clinical program dedicated to the diagnosis and management of CRCI include (1) a thorough medical workup, including history of medical comorbidities (of particular importance are hypertension, cardiac disease, dementia, stroke, diabetes, thyroid disease, hyperlipidemia), blood tests (CBC, CMP, folate, vitamin B levels, thyroid hormones), brain imaging studies (MRI with DTI studies) if indicated, and psychological comorbidities (mood disturbances such as anxiety or depression, chronic insomnia, premorbid attention difficulties and dementia); (2) clinicians with expertise in working with a diverse oncology patient population; (3) computerized neurocognitive screening that is cost- and time-efficient (a critique on the use of computerized neuropsychological testing is beyond the scope of this chapter; for an excellent review of this topic see Bauer et al.)[58]; (4) administration of individually tailored neuropsychological testing batteries based on presenting symptomatology, cancer history, and treatment received; (5) availability of cognitive rehabilitative options (including traditional cognitive therapy with a speech or occupational therapist, or computer-based cognitive training such as BrainHQ by Posit Science) based on neuropsychological test results and patient goals; (6) patient/family education on brain function, cognitive deficits, and relevant compensatory strategies; and (7) availability of cognitive behavioral psychological interventions to treat the emotional sequelae of CRCI.

Patients often seek guidance from their healthcare team on when to return to work or school, as many are eager to get back to their life before cancer. This is a personal decision that involves taking a look at several influencing aspects such as the type of work or demands of the job as well as the nature and severity of the identified cognitive deficits. For example, if someone has a processing speed deficit, a job where they are required to function under deadlines with tight turnaround times would be difficult. For those with a word-finding deficit, thinking on their feet when teaching a class or running a meeting, for example, may be challenging. For someone with an executive function deficit, a job requiring planning, novel problem-solving and multitasking, like that of a project manager, for example, might not be ideal. As a result, individuals may find themselves needing to request from their employer temporary accommodations to their work schedules or adjustment of specific job functions, either of which may not always be possible. This can sometimes lead patients to leave their jobs altogether which further impacts their lives.

In summary, a holistic, comprehensive, interdisciplinary approach to caring for the patient is key because cognitive dysfunction does not occur in a vacuum. In fact, frequently the cause of cognitive deficits is multifactorial in nature. CRCI is a devastating sequelae of cancer that negatively impacts quality of life. Assessment and treatment, as well as future research to elucidate risk factors and biological underpinnings of this syndrome, is critical. Patients may not always know how to bring up when they experience these types of cognitive symptoms, so it is equally important for clinicians to routinely assess for CRCI symptoms and quality-of-life concerns.

In some cases pharmacologic intervention may be appropriate. According to a review done by Pearre and Bota, modafinil, a psychostimulant, has been shown to improve cognitive performance and attention in breast cancer patients; and similar results have been shown with methylphenidate and donepezil in brain cancer patients.[49] Memantine has also been studied in reducing cognitive dysfunction induced by whole-brain radiation therapy.[34]

AREAS OF FUTURE RESEARCH

Future areas of research are needed to develop treatment options and prevention strategies of CRCI. Potential targets of CRCI research may include (1) the use of anti-inflammatory agents (TNF-alpha blockers) to identify inflammation in the pathogenesis of CRCI; (2) genotyping patients for specific genes that regulate neural repair/plasticity such as ApoE4 allele, BDNF Met/Met, and COMT Val+ in order to identify patients at high risk for cognitive impairment and tailor chemotherapy options to mitigate risk of CRCI; (3) the role of cognitive remediation prior to cancer treatment in order to mitigate negative cognitive impact; (4) the efficacy of cognitive rehabilitation in improving functional outcomes following CRCI; and (5) developing prevention models to increase cognitive reserve to mitigate the rise of CRCI.

CONCLUSION

The prevalence of CRCI and its negative impact on quality of life is inextricably woven into the fabric of cancer survivorship. Thus assessment and treatment for CRCI merits clinical attention for all cancer patients. As future research elucidates the biological underpinnings of CRCI, effective treatment and prevention strategies must be developed to mitigate these debilitating sequelae and inform cancer treatment selection in breast and gynecological cancer patients, whenever possible.

PATIENT RESOURCES

1. ASCO answers: Chemobrain (©2017 American Society of Clinical Oncology) https://www.cancer.net/sites/cancer.net/files/asco_answers_chemobrain.pdf
2. Chemobrain: What You Need To Know (©2016 CancerCare) https://media.cancercare.org/publications/original/72-fs_chemo_cognitive.pdf
3. Coping With Chemobrain: Keeping Your Memory Sharp (©2016 CancerCare) https://media.cancercare.org/publications/original/70-fs_chemo_memory.pdf
4. Improving Your Concentration: Three Key Steps (©2016 CancerCare) https://media.cancercare.org/publications/original/71-fs_chemo_concentration.pdf
5. National Cancer Institute's Cancer Information Service 1-800-4-CANCER (1-800-422-6237) https://www.cancer.gov
6. American Cancer Society's Cancer Helpline 1-800-227-2345 https://www.cancer.org
7. CancerCare's Hopeline 1-800-813-HOPE (1-800-813-4673) https://www.cancercare.org

REFERENCES

1. Pendergrass JC, Targum SD, Harrison JE. Cognitive impairment associated with cancer: a brief review. *Innov Clin Neurosci*. 2017;15(1–2):36–44.
2. Bradshaw ME, Wefel JS. The neuropsychology of oncology. In: Parsons MW, Hammeke TA, eds. *Clinical Neuropsychology: A Pocket Handbook for Assessment*. 3rd ed. Washington, DC: American Psychological Association; 2014:331–337.
3. Janelsins MC, Heckler CE, Peppone CK, et al. Cognitive complaints in survivors of breast cancer after chemotherapy compared with age-matched controls: an analysis from a nationwide, multicenter, prospective longitudinal study. *J Clin Oncol*. 2017;35(5):506–514.
4. Schilder CM, Seynaeve C, Beex LV, et al. Effects of tamoxifen and exemestane on cognitive functioning of postmenopausal patients with breast cancer: results from the neuropsychological side study of the tamoxifen and exemestane adjuvant multinational trial. *J Clin Oncol*. 2010;28(8):1294–1300.
5. Ahles TA, Saykin AJ, McDonald BC, et al. Longitudinal assessment of cognitive changes associated with adjuvant treatment for breast cancer: impact of age and cognitive reserve. *J Clin Oncol*. 2010;28(29):4434–4440.
6. Biglia N, Bounous VE, Malabaila A, et al. Objective and self-reported cognitive dysfunction in breast cancer women treated with chemotherapy: a prospective study. *Eur J Cancer Care (Engl)*. 2012;21(4):485–492.
7. Collins B, Mackenzie J, Stewart A, Bielajew C, Verma S. Cognitive effects of hormonal therapy in early stage breast cancer patients: a prospective study. *Psychooncology*. 2009;18(8):811–821.
8. Debess J, Riis JØ, Engebjerg MC, Ewertz M. Cognitive function after adjuvant treatment for early breast cancer: a population-based longitudinal study. *Breast Cancer Res Treat*. 2010;121(1):91–100.
9. Fan HG, Houédé-Tchen N, Yi QL, et al. Fatigue, menopausal symptoms, and cognitive function in women after adjuvant chemotherapy for breast cancer: 1- and 2-year follow-up of a prospective controlled study. *J Clin Oncol*. 2005;23(31):8025–8032.
10. Hedayati E, Alinaghizadeh H, Schedin A, Nyman H, Albertsson M. Effects of adjuvant treatment on cognitive

function in women with early breast cancer. *Eur J Oncol Nurs*. 2012;16(3):315–322.

11. Hermelink K, Untch M, Lux MP, et al. Cognitive function during neoadjuvant chemotherapy for breast cancer: results of a prospective, multicenter, longitudinal study. *Cancer*. 2007;109(9):1905–1913.
12. Hermelink K, Henschel V, Untch M, Bauerfeind I, Lux MP, Munzel K. Short-term effects of treatment-induced hormonal changes on cognitive function in breast cancer patients: results of a multicenter, prospective, longitudinal study. *Cancer*. 2008;113(9):2431–2439.
13. Hurria A, Goldfarb S, Rosen C, et al. Effect of adjuvant breast cancer chemotherapy on cognitive function from the older patient's perspective. *Breast Cancer Res Treat*. 2006;98(3):343–348.
14. Jansen CE, Cooper BA, Dodd MJ, et al. A prospective longitudinal study of chemotherapy-induced cognitive changes in breast cancer patients. *Support Care Cancer*. 2011;19(10):1647–1656.
15. Jenkins V, Shilling V, Deutsch G, et al. A 3-year prospective study of the effects of adjuvant treatments on cognition in women with early stage breast cancer. *Br J Cancer*. 2006;94(6):828–834.
16. Mehlsen M, Pedersen AD, Jensen AB, Zachariae R. No indications of cognitive side-effects in a prospective study of breast cancer patients receiving adjuvant chemotherapy. *Psychooncology*. 2009;18(3):248–257.
17. Quesnel C, Savard J, Ivers H. Cognitive impairments associated with breast cancer treatments: results from a longitudinal study. *Breast Cancer Res Treat*. 2009;116(1): 113–123.
18. Shilling V, Jenkins V, Morris R, Deutsch G, Bloomfield D. The effects of adjuvant chemotherapy on cognition in women with breast cancer—preliminary results of an observational longitudinal study. *Breast*. 2005;14(2):142–150.
19. Stewart A, Collins B, Mackenzie J, Tomiak E, Verma S, Bielajew C. The cognitive effects of adjuvant chemotherapy in early stage breast cancer: a prospective study. *Psychooncology*. 2008;17(2):122–130.
20. Vearncombe KJ, Rolfe M, Wright M, Pachana NA, Andrew B, Beadle G. Predictors of cognitive decline after chemotherapy in breast cancer patients. *J Int Neuropsychol Soc*. 2009;15(6):951–962.
21. Wefel JS, Lenzi R, Theriault RL, Davis RN, Meyers CA. The cognitive sequelae of standard-dose adjuvant chemotherapy in women with breast carcinoma: results of a prospective, randomized, longitudinal trial. *Cancer*. 2004;100(11):2292–2299.
22. Wefel JS, Saleeba AK, Buzdar AU, Meyers CA. Acute and late onset cognitive dysfunction associated with chemotherapy in women with breast cancer. *Cancer*. 2010;116(14):3348–3356.
23. Mandelblatt JS, Small BJ, Luta G, et al. Cancer-related cognitive outcomes among older breast cancer survivors in the thinking and living with cancer study. *J Clin Oncol*. 2018;36(32):3211–3222.
24. Tager FA, McKinley PS, Schnabel FR, et al. The cognitive effects of chemotherapy in post-menopausal breast cancer patients: a controlled longitudinal study. *Breast Cancer Res Treat*. 2010;123(1):25–34 [Erratum in *Breast Cancer Res Treat* 2011 Feb;126(1):271-2].
25. Bender CM, Sereika SM, Berga SL, et al. Cognitive impairment associated with adjuvant therapy in breast cancer. *Psychooncology*. 2006;15:422–430.
26. Schagen SB, Muller MJ, Boogerd W, et al. Change in cognitive function after chemotherapy: a prospective longitudinal study in breast cancer patients. *J Natl Cancer Inst*. 2006;98:1742–1745.
27. Janelsins MC, Kesler SR, Ahles TA, Morrow GR. Prevalence, mechanisms, and management of cancer-related cognitive impairment. *Int Rev Psychiatry*. 2014;26 (1):102–113.
28. Ahles TA, Saykin AJ, McDonald BC, et al. Cognitive function in breast cancer patients prior to adjuvant treatment. *Breast Cancer Res Treat*. 2008;110:143–152.
29. Ahles TA, Root JC, Ryan EL. Cancer- and cancer treatment-associated cognitive change: an update on the state of the science. *J Clin Oncol*. 2012;30: 3675–3686.
30. Wefel JS, Lenzi R, Teirault R, et al. Chemobrain in breast carcinoma? A prologue. *Cancer*. 2004;101:466–475.
31. Tannock IF, Ahles TA, Ganz PA, et al. Cognitive impairment associated with chemotherapy for cancer: report of a workshop. *J Clin Oncol*. 2004;22:2233–2239.
32. Wefel JS, Vardy J, Ahles TA, et al. International Cognition and Cancer Task Force recommendations to harmonise studies of cognitive function in cancer patients. *Lancet Oncol*. 2011;12:703–708.
33. Van Arsdale A, Rosenbaum D, Kaur G, et al. Prevalence and factors associated with cognitive deficit in women with gynecologic malignancies. *Gynecologic Oncol*. 2016; 141:323–328.
34. PDQ® Supportive and Palliative Care Editorial Board. *PDQ Cognitive Impairment in Adults With Non–Central Nervous System Cancers*. Bethesda, MD: National Cancer Institute. Available from: <https://www.cancer.gov/about-cancer/treatment/side-effects/memory/cognitive-impairment-hp-pdq> Accessed 09.01.19; updated 11.05.18. [PMID: 29112351].
35. Deprez S, Amant F, Smeets A, et al. Longitudinal assessment of chemotherapy-induced structural changes in cerebral white matter and its correlation with impaired cognitive functioning. *J Clin Oncol*. 2012;30(3): 274–281.
36. McDonald BC, Conroy SK, Ahles TA, West JD, Saykin AJ. Alterations in brain activation during working memory processing associated with breast cancer and treatment: a prospective functional magnetic resonance imaging study. *J Clin Oncol*. 2012;30(20):2500–2508.
37. McDonald BC, Conroy SK, Ahles TA, West JD, Saykin AJ. Gray matter reduction associated with systemic chemotherapy for breast cancer: a prospective MRI study. *Breast Cancer Res Treat*. 2010;123(3):819–828.
38. McDonald BC, Conroy SK, Smith DJ, West JD, Saykin AJ. Frontal gray matter reduction after breast cancer chemotherapy and association with executive symptoms: a

replication and extension study. *Brain Behav Immun.* 2013;30(suppl):S117–S125.
39. Inagaki M, Yoshikawa E, Matsuoka Y, et al. Smaller regional volumes of brain gray and white matter demonstrated in breast cancer survivors exposed to adjuvant chemotherapy. *Cancer.* 2007;109(1):146–156.
40. Saykin AJ, Ahles TA, McDonald BC. Mechanisms of chemotherapy-induced cognitive disorders: neuropsychological, pathophysiological, and neuroimaging perspectives. *Semin Clin Neuropsychiatry.* 2003;8(4):201–216. Review.
41. Simó M, Rifà-Ros X, Rodriguez-Fornells A, Bruna J. Chemobrain: a systematic review of structural and functional neuroimaging. *Neurosci Biobehav Rev.* 2013;37: 1311–1321.
42. Maccormick RE. Possible acceleration of aging by adjuvant chemotherapy: a cause of early onset frailty? *Med Hypotheses.* 2006;67:212–215.
43. Mariani E, Polidori MC, Cherubini A, Mecocci P. Oxidative stress in brain aging, neurodegenerative and vascular diseases: an overview. *J Chromatogr B Anal Technol Biomed Life Sci.* 2005;827(1):65–75.
44. Schröder CP, Wisman GB, de Jong S, et al. Telomere length in breast cancer patients before and after chemotherapy with or without stem cell transplantation. *Br J Cancer.* 2001;84(10):1348–1353.
45. Lahav M, Uziel O, Kestenbaum M, et al. Nonmyeloablative conditioning does not prevent telomere shortening after allogeneic stem cell transplantation. *Transplantation.* 2005; 80(7):969–976.
46. Dietrich J, Han R, Yang Y, Mayer-Pröschel M, Noble M. CNS progenitor cells and oligodendrocytes are targets of chemotherapeutic agents in vitro and in vivo. *J Biol.* 2006;5(7):22.
47. Vezmar S, Becker A, Bode U, Jaehde U. Biochemical and clinical aspects of methotrexate neurotoxicity. *Chemotherapy.* 2003;49(1–2):92–104.
48. Han R, Yang YM, Dietrich J, Luebke A, Mayer-Pröschel M, Noble M. Systemic 5-fluorouracil treatment causes a syndrome of delayed myelin destruction in the central nervous system. *J Biol.* 2008;7(4):12.
49. Pearre DC, Bota DA. Chemotherapy-related cognitive dysfunction and effects on quality of life in gynecologic cancer patients. *Expert Rev Qual Life Cancer Care.* 2018;3 (1):19–26.
50. Currier MB, Nemeroff CB. Depression as a risk factor for cancer: from pathophysiological advances to treatment implications. *Annu Rev Med.* 2014;65:203–221.
51. Ganz PA, Bower JE, Kwan L, et al. Does tumor necrosis factor-alpha (TNF-α) play a role in post-chemotherapy cerebral dysfunction? *Brain Behav Immun.* 2013;30 (suppl):S99–S108.
52. Kesler S, Janelsins M, Koovakkattu D, et al. Reduced hippocampal volume and verbal memory performance associated with interleukin-6 and tumor necrosis factor-alpha levels in chemotherapy-treated breast cancer survivors. *Brain Behav Immun.* 2013;30(suppl):S109–S116.
53. Janelsins MC, Mustian KM, Palesh OG, et al. Differential expression of cytokines in breast cancer patients receiving different chemotherapies: implications for cognitive impairment research. *Supp Cancer Care.* 2012;20(4): 831–839.
54. Wang XM, Walitt B, Saligan L, Tiwari AF, Cheung CW, Zhang ZJ. Chemobrain: a critical review and causal hypothesis of link between cytokines and epigenetic reprogramming associated with chemotherapy. *Cytokine.* 2015;72(1):86–96.
55. Ahles TA, Saykin AJ, Noll WW, et al. The relationship of APOE genotype to neuropsychological performance in long-term cancer survivors treated with standard dose chemotherapy. *Psychooncology.* 2003;12(6):612–619.
56. Small BJ, Rawson KS, Walsh E, et al. Catechol-*O*-methyltransferase genotype modulates cancer treatment-related cognitive deficits in breast cancer survivors. *Cancer.* 2011;117(7):1369–1376.
57. Ng T, Teo SM, Yeo HL, et al. Brain-derived neurotrophic factor genetic polymorphism (rs6265) is protective against chemotherapy-associated cognitive impairment in patients with early-stage breast cancer. *Neuro Oncol.* 2016;18(2):244–251.
58. Bauer RM, Iverson GL, Cernick AN, Binder LM, Ruff RM, Naugle RI. Computerized neuropsychological assessment devices: joint position paper of the American Academy of Clinical Neuropsychology and the National Academy of Neuropsychology. *Arch Clin Neuropsychol.* 2012;27: 362–373.

FURTHER READING

Boykoff N, Moieni M, Subramanian SK. Confronting chemobrain: an in-depth look at survivors' reports of impact on work, social networks, and health care response. *J Cancer Surviv.* 2009;3:223–232.
Hess LM, Huang HQ, Hanlon AL, et al. Cognitive function during and six months following chemotherapy for front-line treatment of ovarian, primary peritoneal or fallopian tube cancer: an NRG oncology/gynecologic oncology group study. *Gynecol Oncol.* 2015;139(3): 541–545.
Hutchinson AD, Hosking JR, Kichenadasse G, Mattiske JK, Wilson C. Objective and subjective cognitive impairment following chemotherapy for cancer: a systematic review. *Cancer Treat Rev.* 2012;38:926–934.
Janelsins MC, Kohli S, Mohile SG, Usuki K, Ahles TA, Morrow GR. An update on cancer- and chemotherapy-related cognitive dysfunction: current status. *Semin Oncol.* 2011;38(3):431–438.
Joly F, Giffard B, Rigal O, et al. Impact of cancer and its treatments on cognitive function: advances in research from the Paris International Cognition and Cancer Task Force Symposium and Update Since 2012. *J Pain Symptom Manage.* 2015;50(6):830–841.
Lange M, Joly F. How to identify and manage cognitive dysfunction after breast cancer treatment. *J Oncol Pract.* 2017;13(12):784–791.

Morean DF, O'Dwyer L, Cherney LR. Therapies for cognitive deficits associated with chemotherapy for breast cancer: a systematic review of objectives outcomes. *Arch Phys Med Rehabil.* 2015;96:1880–1897.

Von Ah D, Tallman EF. Perceived cognitive function in breast cancer survivors: evaluating relationships with objective cognitive performance and other symptoms using the functional assessment of cancer therapy-cognitive function instrument. *J Pain Symptom Manage.* 2015;49(4): 697–706.

Wieneke MH, Dienst ER. Neuropsychological assessment of cognitive functioning following chemotherapy for breast cancer. *Psychooncology.* 1995;4:61–66.

CHAPTER 21

Lymphedema in Breast and Gynecologic Oncology

MARY CROSSWELL PT DPT CLT • ADRIAN CRISTIAN, MD, MHCM

INTRODUCTION

Lymphedema is a common impairment and side effect of cancer treatment and is a significant survivorship issue reported by women after both breast and gynecologic cancers.[1,2] Advances in early diagnosis and medical treatments have led to the progressive increase in overall cancer survival rates. In 2019 it was estimated that there were 16.9 million cancer survivors in the United States, of which there are 3.8 million women living with breast cancer and over 1.6 million survivors of gynecologic cancer.[2] It is expected that there will be 22.1 million cancer survivors by 2030.[2] The Institute of Medicine in 2005 published the landmark report, From Cancer Patient to Cancer Survivor: Lost in Transition,[3] that identifies lymphedema as a relatively common late side effect of cancer treatment with medical and psychosocial consequences.[3] The public health burden of lymphedema can be expected to increase in concordance with increasing cancer survival rates.[1] The current incidence and prevalence of lymphedema are likely underestimated. In part, this may be attributable to a lack of a standardized definition of diagnostic thresholds and lack of consensus and certainty on the most efficient measurement tools for lymphedema detection.[4,5]

The majority of research has focused on the area of upper extremity lymphedema following breast cancer surgery. There is limited robust data addressing lymphedema in women with gynecologic cancer. Following breast cancer, uterine cancer is the second most prevalent cancer among female cancer survivors.[2] The Center for Disease Control (CDC) reports cancer of the uterus as one of the cancers with increasing incidence and mortality.[6]

DiSipio et al. in a systematic review and metaanalysis reported that more than one in five breast cancer survivors will develop lymphedema with an overall estimated incidence of 21.4%, with an increased incidence at least up to 24 months after surgery, and may continue at a slower rate beyond this period.[7] Lymphedema has been reported to develop years to decades later.[5]

Lymphedema occurs at appreciable rates in women undergoing gynecologic cancer treatment. Estimates of the risk of lymphedema in gynecologic cancer vary widely from 0% to 73%.[8] Incidence estimates are influenced by the type of cancer with the highest incidence associated with vulvar cancer. Cormier et al. in a metaanalysis reported the estimated lymphedema incidence for gynecologic cancer as 25% with specific incidences of 27%, 30%, and 1% for cervical, vulvar and endometrial cancers, respectively.[8] A large population-based study on endometrial cancer provides evidence that one in eight women (13%) treated for endometrial cancer will develop lymphedema within the first 2 years after surgery.[9] In a recent prospective longitudinal study, bioimpedance spectroscopy (BIS) was used to define lymphedema in patients with gynecologic cancer. Overall, 50% of women showed evidence of lymphedema within 2 years postgynecologic cancer with 60% of the cases persistent and 40% transient.[10]

Clinically, lymphedema most often affects the involved extremity but may also include the respective trunk areas, breast, and in the case of gynecologic cancer the abdomen and genitalia.[11] Lymphedema is a chronic progressive condition for which there is no cure, and although it is usually not life threatening, it often has a significant impact on the quality of life (QOL).[11–13] Compared to upper extremity lymphedema, lower extremity lymphedema is associated with a higher intensity and level of distress and fatigue $\geq 75\%$.[13] Studies have shown that cancer survivors diagnosed with lymphedema have a significantly lower health-related QOL score compared with survivors without lymphedema.[14,15] Fear and frustration are common emotions experienced by patients with lymphedema.[12,16] Women may experience pain, impaired mobility and function, loss of body image, decreased physical activity, fatigue and distress.[13,16]

Breast Cancer and Gynecologic Cancer Rehabilitation DOI: https://doi.org/10.1016/B978-0-323-72166-0.00021-9

ANATOMY OF THE LYMPHATIC SYSTEM

The lymphatic system plays a very significant role in immune system function and transport of immune cells, inflammation, fat absorption, and flow of interstitial fluid.[17] It is also important in the clearing of cellular debris and metabolic waste from the interstitium.[18]

In the dermis, there are lymphatic vessels made up of single layer lymphatic cells. Changes in tissue fluid content lead to a separation between these cells allowing interstitial fluid and cells to enter these lymphatic vessels. The fluid is subsequently transported into larger lymphatic vessels located in the subcutaneous tissue and deeper tissues. These larger lymphatic vessels have smooth muscles and unidirectional valves that help to propel lymphatic fluid forward.

Lymphatic vessels transport fluid from the interstitial tissues to venous circulation through a series of lymphatic capillaries, precollecting and collecting vessels located in the dermis and deeper tissues. There appear to be two parallel lymphatic collecting networks in extremities—one that collects lymph from the skin and subcutaneous system and another deeper collecting system that collects ground from muscle and bones. These two systems are believed to communicate with each other in the limbs and merge in the axilla and pelvis for the upper and lower extremity, respectively.[18] Daily lymph formation is between 2 and 3 L/day.[18]

Lymphatic fluid moves in the lymphatic vessels through a combination of muscle cell contractions in the walls of larger lymphatic vessels, presence of unidirectional valves, exercise, positional changes in hydrostatic pressure, response to tissue edema, temperature changes, respiration, gravity and vasoactive substances such as histamine and substance P.[18]

There are 600–700 lymph nodes in the human body, and they serve as filters of lymphatic fluid. They are commonly located in the axilla, inguinal region, thoracic mediastinum, and gastrointestinal mesentery.[18] Lymph enters the lymph node through afferent vessels and while there, lymphatic fluid is exposed to macrophages and B cells. Lymphatic fluid subsequently exits through efferent vessels and flows to the cisterna chyli, where it then continues as the thoracic duct. Ultimately, lymphatic fluid unites with venous circulation at the junction of the thoracic duct with the subclavian vein.[17,18] The lymph nodes of the upper extremities consist of a superficial and a deep set.

The lymph nodes of the upper extremity are divided into two groups—superficial and deep. The superficial nodes drain the third, fourth, and fifth fingers, ulnar portion of the hand, and the superficial forearm. The deep nodes are primarily located in the axilla. There are about 20 of them, and they tend to be large and are divided into lateral, anterior, posterior, central, and medial nodes. The lateral nodes drain the upper extremity, the anterior nodes drain the skin and muscle of the chest, and the posterior nodes drain the skin and muscles of the upper back. The anterior and posterior nodes drain into the central lymph nodes that subsequently drain into the medial nodes whose efferent vessels subsequently become the subclavian trunk. From here the lymphatic fluid enters the venous circulation at the junction of the internal jugular and subclavian veins[18] (Fig. 21.1).

In the lower extremity the inguinal lymph nodes are divided into superficial and subinguinal lymph nodes that are further divided into superficial and deep nodes. The superficial lymph nodes drain the perineum, buttock, and abdominal wall below the umbilicus. The superficial subinguinal lymph nodes drain lymph from the superficial lymphatic vessels and the perineum and buttock. The deep subinguinal lymph nodes receive lymphatic fluid from the clitoris and deeper lymphatic trunks[18] (Fig. 21.2).

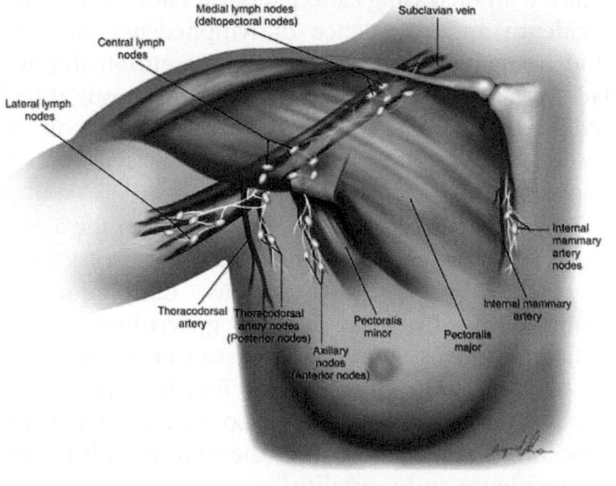

FIGURE 21.1 The anatomy of the axillary lymphatics illustrating the axillary lymph node groups that drain the upper extremity, chest and upper back. (Reprinted with permission from Rockson SG. Anatomy and structural physiology of the lymphatic system. In: Cheng MH, Chang DW, Patel KM, eds. *Principles and Practice of Lymphedema Surgery:* Elsevier: 2016.)[18]

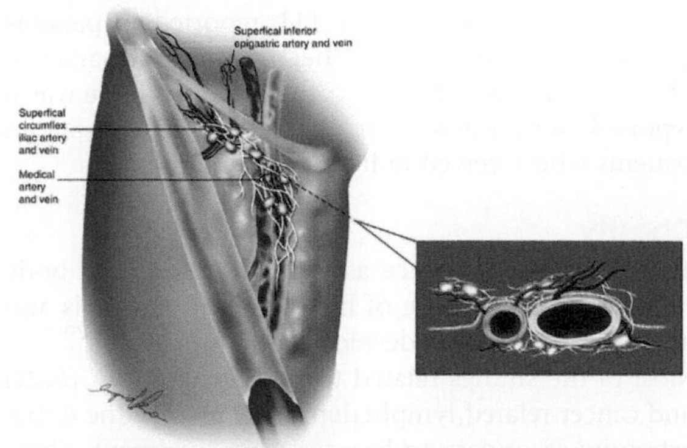

FIGURE 21.2 Lymphatic anatomy of the inguinal region illustrating lymph nodes in the deep and superficial planes. The superficial group of nodes drain mainly the perineum, buttock and abdominal wall below the umbilicus. (Reprinted with permission from Rockson SG. Anatomy and structural physiology of the lymphatic system. In: Cheng MH, Chang DW, Patel KM eds. *Principles and practice of lymphedema surgery*. Elsevier; 2016.)[18]

PATHOPHYSIOLOGY OF LYMPHEDEMA

The exact cause of lymphedema following breast or gynecologic cancer is not fully known. Lymphedema of the arm or leg can occur after an injury, such as lymphadenectomy or an obstruction of the lymphatic system. Injury to both superficial and deep lymphatic vessels leads to impairment in their ability to move interstitial fluid that leads to edema and an activation of inflammatory pathways.

Edema, deposition of fibroadipose tissue and sclerosis of lymphatic vessels can occur when radiation therapy is administered to the lymph nodes.[17] The fibrosis has been reported to be mediated by proliferation of CD4 + cells that differentiate into a type of T helper cell that produces cytokines (interleukin 4, 13) and promotes fibrosis.[17] Infections may also promote the development of lymphedema. Genetics may also play a factor in the development of lymphedema. Women with mutations in gene encoding for connexin 47 or hepatocyte growth factor were found to have an increased risk of developing lymphedema after mastectomy and axillary node dissection (ALND).[17] The presence of increased interstitial fluid has also been linked with increased deposition of adipocytes which in turn can worsen the lymphedema.[17]

RISK FACTORS

Risk factors with a strong level of evidence in breast cancer–related lymphedema (BCRL) are axillary lymph node dissection (ALND), adjuvant radiation, and being overweight or obese.[7,19–21] Similar lymphedema risk factor considerations apply to lower extremity gynecologic lymphedema, but the evidence is not equally strong due to fewer studies.[19] The association between lymphadenectomy and lymphedema is consistent in the literature for both breast and gynecologic cancers.[22] From a physiotherapeutic perspective, knowledge of incidence and risk factors for lymphedema helps the clinician to identify patients at high risk and, in conjunction with a screening model, provides the opportunity for early intervention that leads to better outcomes and prognosis.[23]

Breast Cancer

In breast cancer the extent of axillary surgery is an important prognostic factor for lymphedema. Both ALND and sentinel lymph node biopsy (SLNB) put patients at a lifelong risk for lymphedema. Disipio et al. estimated that the rate of arm lymphedema is about four times more likely with ALND as compared to SLNB (19.9% and 5.6%, respectively).[7]

Clinical studies have found that radiotherapy is a risk factor for the development of lymphedema with a synergistic effect when combined with ALND.[24] Shaitelman et al. in a recent metaanalysis concluded that the risk for lymphedema in breast cancer patients is significantly higher among patients treated with regional lymph node radiation (RLNR) as compared to those treated with whole breast radiation alone, with the highest risk associated with patients who receive RLNR following ALND.[24] The study calculates the pooled incidence of lymphedema as stratified by radiation targets with a pooled incidence of 7.4% for patients treated with breast/chest wall radiation and a range of 10.8%–15.5% for different combinations of RLNR. Further stratification was performed to include the extent of axillary surgery and radiation targets with a 4.1% pooled incidence for patients treated with SLNB and breast/chest wall radiation with an increase to 5.7% with the addition of RLNR to breast/chest wall radiation. For patients treated with ALND, there was an increased risk for lymphedema with a pooled incidence of 9.4% with ALND and breast/chest wall radiation with a significant increase in risk to 18.2% with the addition of RLNR to breast/chest wall radiation.[24]

It is suggested that breast cancer patients who undergo RLNR even without ALND ought to be considered as high risk for lymphedema.[23]

McDuff et al. in a recent large prospective cohort study of 2171 women estimated a 5-year cumulative incidence of 13.7% for lymphedema. The overall risk peaked between 12 and 30 months postoperatively depending on the treatment received. ALND was associated with early onset lymphedema, while late-onset lymphedema (>12 months) was associated with RLNR.[25] These findings can inform clinical practice and provide information that may be used for patient education and surveillance practices.[25]

Other Risk Factors

Evidence shows other BCRL risk factors, including chemotherapy with taxanes, cellulitis, subclinical edema, and lack of breast reconstruction.[23] There is growing evidence of genetics as a predisposing factor in the development of secondary lymphedema, with evidence of genetic mutations as a risk factor in lymphedema following breast cancer treatment.[26,27]

Gynecologic Cancer

For gynecologic cancers the risk of lower limb lymphedema (LLL) varies based on the extent of surgery and lymphadenectomy, the removal of specific nodes, radiotherapy treatment, and the disease site (endometrial, vulvar, ovarian, cervical).[28]

Inguinofemoral lymph node dissection as is often the case with vulvar cancer is correlated with the highest risk of LLL in gynecologic cancers, ranging from 30% to 70%, and includes most of the cases of genital lymphedema.[29] Cormier et al. estimate a lymphedema risk of 22% in patients undergoing pelvic dissection.[8] The removal of the circumflex iliac lymph nodes to the level of the distal external iliac node (CINDEIN) is associated with a significantly higher level of postoperative lower extremity lymphedema.[30] Lymphadenectomy of the pelvic and para-aortic lymph nodes are often involved in endometrial cancer with a variation in node dissection from a sampling of a few nodes to median of 10–30 nodes.[31] A 12-year retrospective study showed that removal of ≥10 nodes[32] and in another study ≥15 nodes[9] were indicative of an increased risk for LLL in women with endometrial cancer, however, Yost et al. in a large retrospective study did not find a lymphedema risk associated with the number of nodes removed.[33] SLNB is a safe and effective alternative to complete dissection in vulvar cancer. Promising evidence of SLNB in endometrial and cervical cancers continue to emerge.[34] While it is estimated that the overall incidence for gynecologic cancer is 25%,[8] Shaitelman et al. estimate an overall pooled incidence of 9% in patients who receive SLNB as part of their gynecologic cancer treatment.[35]

There is a higher risk of LLL reported in patients treated with adjuvant radiotherapy. In a metaanalysis of 1193 patients with gynecologic cancer, there was a reported 34% pooled incidence of lymphedema in patients who received radiation treatment [8]

Obesity

There is strong evidence associated with a high body mass index at the time of breast cancer diagnosis and an increased risk of developing lymphedema.[20,21,36] Most of the studies related to body mass index (BMI) and cancer-related lymphedema risk involve the upper extremity secondary to breast cancer treatment. These findings may also be applicable to patients at risk for LLL following inguinal lymphadenectomy.[37]

As early as 1957, from a study of 1007 postradical mastectomy cases, obesity was identified as a predisposing factor for lymphedema.[36] In a prospective study, Ridner et al. reported that breast cancer survivors with a BMI ≥30 at the time of diagnosis were 3.6 times more likely to develop lymphedema as compared to those patients with a BMI <30.[20] Jammallo et al. prospectively found a preoperative BMI ≥30 as an independent risk factor for lymphedema and an associated increased risk of BCRL with postoperative weight fluctuations with loss or gain of greater than 10 lb.[21]

Mehrara and Greene suggest evidence that obesity impairs lymphatic transport and a clear relationship between obesity and lymphedema, although the cellular mechanisms are currently not known.[37] In a randomized clinical trial, it was found that a weight reduction diet over a span of 12 weeks in patients with BCRL resulted in significant reduction in arm volumes relative to the control group that received no specific dietary interventions.[38] It is recommended that weight management and weight reduction efforts should be integrated into lymphedema management of patients at risk or with a diagnosis of lymphedema.[37,38]

THE ASSESSMENT OF THE PATIENT WITH LYMPHEDEMA

Medical Chart Review

A thorough chart review is an essential starting point in the assessment of the patient for lymphedema. It is important to review the patient's cancer history, including the location of the cancer, presence and location of metastatic disease, diagnostic testing results such as PET/CT scans, bone scans, CT of chest, abdomen, and pelvis if available. Since swelling of the affected limb can also be due to other causes such as deep vein thrombosis, results of venous ultrasound tests can also be beneficial.

Surgical treatment is often a part of the treatment of breast and gynecologic cancers. A review of the surgical report that includes information on whether or not lymph nodes were removed and if so, which ones (i.e., lymph node dissection) can be very helpful information.

If radiation therapy was part of the treatment, a review of the radiation therapy treatment plan or radiation oncology consultation report is important to determine which structures were irradiated, including lymph nodes as well as dose and number of fractions.

Lymphedema History

Pertinent information to gather from the patient includes (1) when and how long ago did they notice swelling of the extremity? (2) were there any associated circumstances around the time that the swelling was first noticed—cuts, bruises, redness of skin, trauma to limb, etc.? (3) did the swelling start gradually or suddenly? (4) is this the first time that the patient has noticed swelling of the limb or have there been other times as well? (5) was there a recent change in their cancer history such as progression of disease? (6) is the swelling present in one extremity or more? (7) has the patient experienced a perception of heaviness of the limb accompanied by difficulty wearing jewelry, a watch or a long sleeve shirt? (8) is there any associated weakness, numbness, or tingling sensation of the affected limb? It is also important to determine the impact of the limb swelling on the patient's function. In BCRL, does the patient have a difficult time performing self-care, household chores, work, childcare, or hobby activities due to the swelling of the limb? In LLL, does the patient have difficulty wearing pants, walking or has noticed an impaired balance, falls, or "near-falls" due to the swelling of the leg?

In patients with a history of lymphedema, other important information are to obtain: (1) is the current limb swelling different or worse than previous lymphedema flare-ups? (2) are there any other or new symptoms or signs such as weakness, pain in ipsilateral joints or muscles or sensory complaints? (3) recent history of weight gain? (4) history of treatment for the lymphedema, including manual lymphatic drainage (MLD), compression sleeves or bandage use, or intermittent pneumatic compression (IPC)?

Physical Examination

Inspection: (1) is the patient obese? (2) any cuts, bruises, erythema, skin changes such as cobblestoning, skin overgrowth, and wart-like changes indicative of more advanced disease deformities of the limb as well as distribution of the swelling. *Palpation*: tissue fibrosis, tender points, pitting versus nonpitting edema, presence of axillary cords, or regional lymphadenopathy (i.e., axillary or supraclavicular lymphadenopathy). *Range of motion*: any restrictions in the range of motion of proximal and/or distal joints in the affected extremity. In addition, circumferential measurements of the affected and nonaffected limb as well as assessment of muscle strength and sensory deficits are important components of the physical examination. Lastly, a functional assessment of the person's ability to use the affected limb can provide relevant information, for example, the ability of the person with BCRL to put on a shirt or the assessment of gait abnormality in person with LLL.

STAGING AND DIAGNOSIS

Staging

The International Society of Lymphology (ISL) describes a three stage scale (Stage 0/Ia–Stage III) for the classification of lymphedema.[39] (Table 21.1). It considers the extent of swelling and evidence or absence of pitting. It describes the progression from a latent state where there may be changes in tissue fluid with no apparent swelling to more advanced disease characterized by trophic skin changes, tissue hypertrophy, fibrosis, and fat deposition.[39] Based on the classification, Stage 0 signifies a latent or subclinical state where there is no overt swelling despite impaired lymph transport. Subjective symptoms may be present. This stage may persist for months or years. Stage I describes an early accumulation of high protein fluid that abates with limb elevation. Pitting may occur. Stage II is further classified into an early and late stage. In the early stage, elevation seldom reduces the swelling and pitting is manifest. In the later stage, there may be no pitting due to increasing fat and fibrotic tissue deposition. Stage III also described as lymphostatic elephantiasis is the most advanced stage of the disease where pitting is absent and the presence of pronounced skin changes, including acanthosis, thickening and loss of skin flexibility, and other dystrophic changes are evident. There is further deposition of fat and fibrotic tissue. A limb may

TABLE 21.1
Clinical staging according to the International Society of Lymphology Consensus Document. Adapted with permission from International Society of Lymphology[39]

Stage	Clinical Characteristics
0	A latent or subclinical stage. Lymphatic transport capacity reduced, but sufficient to manage lymph flow. Swelling is not yet apparent. May experience subjective complaints/symptoms
I	Early accumulation of high protein fluid. Pitting may occur. Swelling subsides with elevation
II	Limb elevation alone rarely reduces swelling, and pitting is manifest
Late Stage II	Pitting may or may not be present as excess subcutaneous fat, and tissue fibrosis is more evident
III	Lymphostatic elephantiasis. Pitting may be absent. Further deposition of fat and fibrotic tissue with thickening and loss of skin flexibility. Pronounced skin changes such as thickening, acanthosis, warty overgrowths

exhibit more than one stage affecting different lymphatic territories within the limb.[39]

A functional severity assessment utilizing volume differences is often used along with the ISL staging to provide another aspect of severity within each stage. Whereby a volume difference of >5–<20% increase is assessed as minimal, 20%–40% increase moderate, and >40% increase severe. The volume measurements are a gross measurement and do not define the composition of the swelling. Clinicians in describing severity may also include other factors such as extensiveness, erysipelas, and inflammation.[39]

The ISL recognizes the need for a more detailed and inclusive staging system that goes beyond describing only the physical condition of the extremities and to include other areas such as radiographic and pathogenic components of lymphedema, genetic considerations, disability, and QOL.[39,40]

Diagnosis

In most cases the diagnosis of lymphedema can be made based on a thorough clinical history and physical examination, including assessment of tissue quality and a measurement of increased limb volume along with a patient-reported symptom assessment.[39,41] The patient's risk status is also considered. The clinical signs and symptoms of lymphedema are influenced by the duration and severity of the disease.[42]

In the early stages the symptoms may be subtle and there may be mild swelling with pitting edema due to the increasing volume of fluid in the interstitial spaces. In a subclinical condition, swelling may not be evident despite impaired lymph transport.[39]

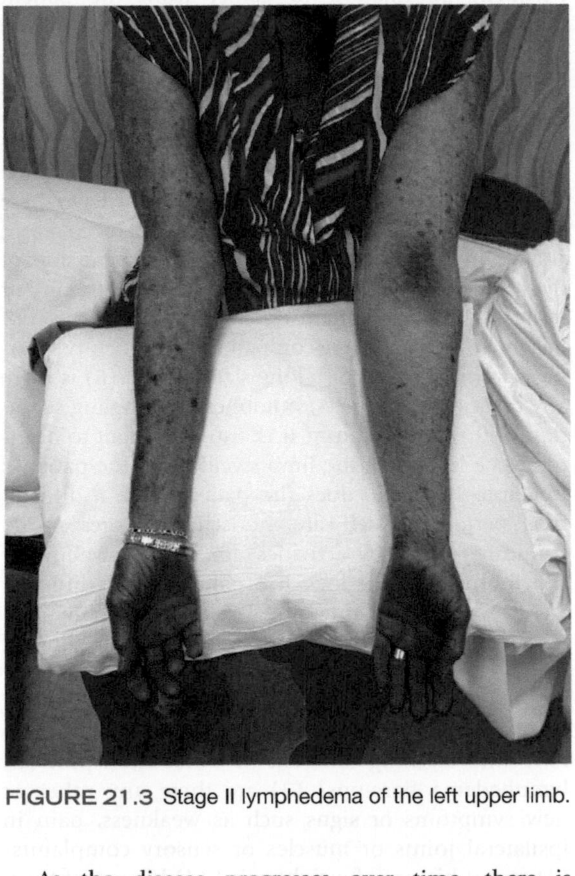

FIGURE 21.3 Stage II lymphedema of the left upper limb.

As the disease progresses over time, there is increased cellular proliferation, fibrosis, and adipose deposition that are associated with a nonpitting edema along with thickening and loss of flexibility of the skin.[39,42] (Fig. 21.3)

In the chronic/late stages, there are characteristic cutaneous changes that distinguish lymphedema from nonlymphatic forms of edema. There may be a positive Stemmer sign that is the inability to tent the skin at the base of digits. A positive sign is diagnostic of lymphedema of the extremities; however, the absence of a Stemmer sign does not rule out lymphedema.[43] Other characteristics distinguishing physical findings for late stage lymphedema may include peau d'orange, papillomatosis, cobblestone deformities, lymph cysts, and chronic inflammatory changes.[39,42]

Conditions such as morbid obesity, venous insufficiency, unrecognized trauma, and repeated infections may complicate the clinical presentation of lymphedema.[39]

Malignant lymphedema should always be considered where there is a possibility of cancer recurrence. Progression of cancer or metastases may obstruct or infiltrate the proximal lymphatics resulting in impaired lymph flow and development of lymphedema.[39,42] Clinically, malignant lymphedema is more likely to begin centrally with pronounced vascular changes, the development of symptoms is more rapid and progressive, the edema and tissues tend to be firm from the outset, and there may be more pain as compared to benign forms of lymphedema.[42]

Accurate and objective measurement techniques together with patient-reported symptoms are required not only for evaluation and diagnosis but also to track the progress or regression of both the disease and treatment interventions.[44]

BIS, water displacement, tape measurement, perometry, and imaging are current options of objective measures used in the diagnosis and monitoring of lymphedema.[41]

Water Displacement

Water displacement is a volume measurement and is considered the reference standard due to its excellent reliability and validity. It is accurate and inexpensive but is limited by clinical utility. It is time-consuming, and there are concerns for cross contamination in individuals with open wounds and skin breakdown.[41]

Circumferential Measurements

Circumferential measurements utilizing a measuring tape is the most common practice method for girth and volume measurements.[44] The American Physical Therapy Association (APTA) Clinical Practice Guidelines for the Diagnosis of Upper Quadrant Lymphedema[41] recommend that when circumferential measurements are used, the measurement of each limb should be calculated to a volume measurement. using a mathematical formula, with a summed truncated frustum cone formula as the preferred method. Calculated limb volumes derived from circumferential measurements show excellent interrater and intrarater reliability for the upper limb. A volume differential between sides of $\geq$200 mL will help rule in lymphedema, however values below 200 mL do not rule out lymphedema. The guidelines further specify that a 2 cm circumferential difference lacks accuracy and should not be used as a diagnostic standard for upper extremity lymphedema. A volume ratio of 1.04 of affected:unaffected limb may be indicative of upper limb lymphedema. If preoperative measurements were performed, a 5% volume change from the baseline measurement is a diagnostic criterion for lymphedema. Also to be considered, is that volume calculated circumferential measurements may not capture subclinical and early stage lymphatic transport deficits.[41]

Perometry

Perometry is a volume measurement that uses infrared light and optoelectronic sensors to create a three-dimensional silhouette of the limb from which limb volume is calculated. Perometry may be used for volume assessment in the early, moderate, and late stages of lymphedema. It has excellent inter/intrarater reliability and psychometric properties. The time to measure and setup is approximately 5 minutes, and the accompanying software enables easy documentation and comparison of results. It is highly reproducible, accurate and provides segmental volumes. Disadvantages include bulkiness, lack of portability, and expense of the equipment.[41,44,45]

Bioimpedance Spectroscopy

BIS is a noninvasive method for detection of early/subclinical stages of edema. The 2017 APTA Clinical Practice Guidelines for the Diagnosis of Upper Quadrant Lymphedema, recommends the use of BIS to detect subclinical/early stage lymphedema. It further suggests the use of BIS to assist in the diagnosis of early/subclinical lymphedema (stages 0 and 1) in patients at risk for BCRL. In 2008 the FDA approved the L- Dex U400 (ImpediMed, Limited) BIS device for clinical use.[41] By means of skin electrodes, it passes an alternating low-frequency current through the limb, and the impedance to the current is then used to detect and measure the extracellular fluid in a limb. It derives a lymphedema L-Dex value (L-Dex score) that measures the ratio of fluid differences between the affected and unaffected limb. For a patient without lymphedema, the L-Dex defines the normal range of −10 to 10. L-Dex values that lie outside the normal range or reflect a shift of +10 units from preoperative baseline measurements are regarded as clinically significant and may indicate subclinical lymphedema.[45] L-Dex scores of more than 7.1 is a diagnostic criterion when no preoperative assessment is available. A preoperative BIS measurement may improve the ability for earlier detection of post operative tissue fluid changes which may be indicative of lymphedema.[41]

The clinical utility advantages of BIS includes portability, is easily performed, takes less than 8 minutes and requires minimal technical training. The machine is relatively inexpensive; however, a new set of electrodes that are costly are required for each assessment.[45] Recently, a new BIS unit with L-Dex technology was introduced, which does not require electrodes. It is a standing unit with scanning technology that measures fluid status in seconds (Fig. 21.4).

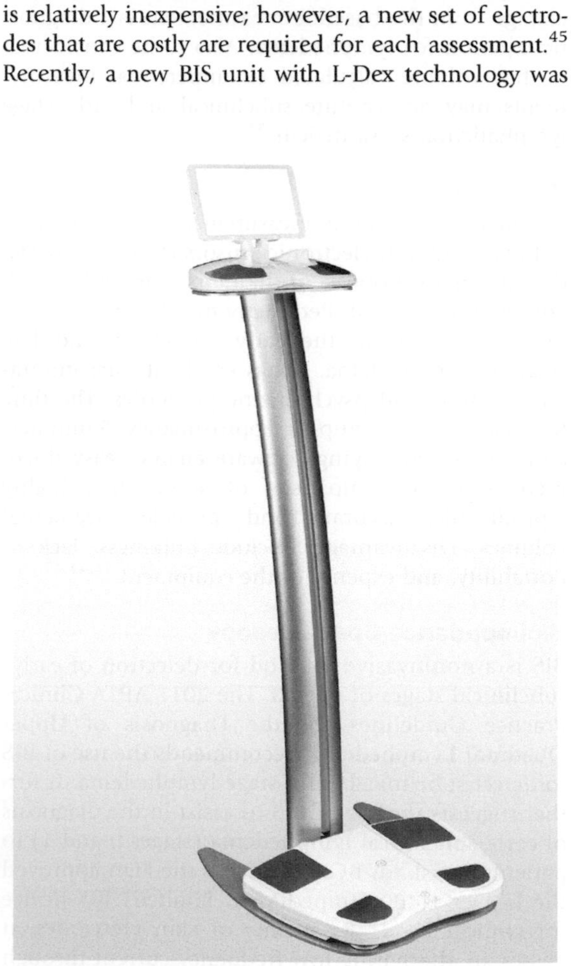

FIGURE 21.4 Bioimpedence spectroscopy device (Reprinted with permission from SOZO® Bioimpedance Spectroscopy Device, Copyright © ImpediMed Limited and ImpediMed Inc.)

BIS is sensitive, specific and noninvasive and is being increasingly utilized for detection of early stage edema and is also used in prospective screening for early/subclinical edema in patients at risk for lymphedema.[12] The BIS device however, measures fluid content only and does not capture the secondary tissue changes of fibrosis and adipose deposition that are characteristic in the moderate and later stages of lymphedema. It is therefore recommended that a volume measurement, for example, circumferential measurements should also be taken even though it may show no volume increase in the early/subclinical stage of the disease.[41] A baseline volume measurement is useful for ongoing monitoring to identify increased volume due to secondary tissue changes.[41]

Near-Infrared Fluorescent Lymphography

Near-infrared fluorescent (NIRF) lymphography or indocyanine green (ICG) lymphography, is gaining popularity as it enables visualization of superficial lymph flow in real time without radiation exposure.[46] The ICG dye is injected intradermally in the second web space of the extremity, illuminating the superficial lymphatic flow. The light emitted by ICG in the lymph vessels, is imaged using a specialized camera.[41]

It measures lymph pump function and dermal backflow. Dermal backflow is a sign unique to lymphedema and indicates lymphatic fluid congestion in the subcutaneous and dermal space secondary to the rerouting of the lymphatic fluid.[19]

There are various classification systems utilizing ICG lymphography. The MD Anderson ICG classification system has four stages based on ICG findings and the severity of dermal backflow. In Stage 1 the patient has several patent lymphatics and minimal dermal backflow; in Stage 2, there are a moderate number of patent lymphatics with segmental dermal backflow; in Stage 3, there are few patent lymphatics with extensive dermal backflow throughout the arm; and lastly, in Stage 4, there are no patent lymphatics and severe dermal backflow of the entire arm and hand[47] (Fig. 21.5). The Pathophysiological Severity Staging System is another ICG classification system that includes the extremities, the genitals, and the lower abdominal area. ICG lymphography patterns change from a normal linear pattern with no dermal backflow (Stage 0) to abnormal dermal backflow patterns (Stages I–V) ranging from splash (Stage I mild

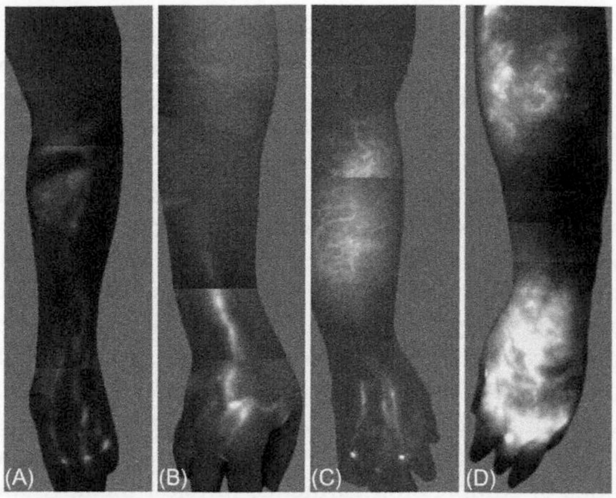

FIGURE 21.5 MD Anderson lymphedema ICG classification system. *ICG*, Indocyanine green. (A) Stage 1: many patent lymphatic vessels, with minimal, patchy dermal backflow. (B) Stage 2: moderate number of patent lymphatic vessels, with segmental dermal backflow. (C) Stage 3: few patent lymphatic vessels, with extensive dermal backflow involving the entire arm. (D) Stage 4: no patent lymphatic vessels, with severe dermal backflow involving the entire arm and extending to the dorsum of the hand. (Reprinted with permission from Chang DW, Suami H, Skoracki R. A prospective analysis of 100 consecutive lymphovenous bypass cases for treatment of extremity lymphedema. *Plast Reconstr Surg*. 2013; 132(5): 1305–1314.)[47]

dermal backflow), stardust (Stages II–IV moderate dermal backflow), and diffuse (Stage V severe dermal backflow) patterns.[46]

NIRF lymphography provides information that can be useful in the decision-making for lymphedema evaluation and a guide to determine conservative, surgical, or combined treatments.[5,46,47]

Self-Report/Subjective Symptoms

Patients at risk or who have lymphedema may present with symptoms such as heaviness, fatigue, perceived sensations of swelling, tingling, pain, sensory changes, and changes in fit of clothing.[48,49] Patient-reported symptoms are important as these may indicate volume and pressure changes in the interstitial space before there are measurable volume changes.[50] Patients are often the first to describe symptoms in their limb before physical or detectable volume changes occur. Self-reported measures may therefore assist with the identification of subclinical or early lymphedema and also a trigger for further examination and objective measures.[41]

There are several self-report assessment tools available. The APTA Clinical Practice Guidelines suggest the Norman Questionnaire and the Morbidity Screening Tool (MST) should be considered. Other assessment tools reported in the guidelines include the Lymphedema and Breast Cancer Questionnaire (LBCQ), the Visual Analogue Scale (VAS), and The Lymphedema Symptom Intensity and Distress Survey (LSIDS).[41]

For evaluation of LLL in gynecologic patients the Gynecologic Cancer Lymphedema Questionnaire (GCLQ) is a self-reporting assessment tool analyzing physical function and symptoms of numbness, swelling, heaviness, and aching.[29,51]

A recent study of 100 patients with a history of breast cancer showed that symptoms of perceived arm swelling, along with differences in tissue texture determined by a patient-administered basic self-assessment forearm pinch test, were associated with and sensitive to BIS-detected BCRL. The findings support the use of self-assessment to help identify the early development of BCRL, and an indication for the patient to seek further professional evaluation.[52]

Additional Diagnostic Measures

As discussed, the diagnosis of lymphedema in most cases can be determined clinically through observation, the patient's history, physical examination, an objective measurement, and self-reported symptoms. If there is unclear etiology or need for further clarification, there are other imaging diagnostic measures that may be utilized which are able to detect tissue quality, visualize edema, or evaluate structural lymphatic transport capacity.[41] These measures include lymphoscintigraphy, magnetic resonance imaging, ultrasonography, CT, and NIRF spectroscopy. Lymphoscintigraphy is regarded as a standard investigation technique in lymphedema diagnosis.[5] In a study of 227 patients (454 limbs), lymphoscintigraphy was found to be very sensitive (96%) and specific (100%) for lymphedema. It is useful in confirming the diagnosis of lymphedema in patients with an equivocal clinical diagnosis, can verify normal lymphatic function, and can document the severity of lymphatic dysfunction.[53] Magnetic resonance imaging is being considered more for diagnosis of lymphedema. A recent small population study reported greater sensitivity with MRI (100%) for depiction of lymph vessels as compared to lymphoscintigraphy (83.3%). The study also demonstrated concordance in the MRI and lymphoscintigraphy results for axillary lymph node enhancement and lymphatic drainage in the upper extremities.[54] Venous duplex ultrasound is a simple, noninvasive imaging technique. It should be performed on patients with lymphedema to assess the venous system for possible deep vein thrombosis which could also present with limb swelling. Ultrasound may be used in the later stages of lymphedema to detect underlying tissue changes. It is able to detect fluid collection, subcutaneous tissue thickness, and fibrosis.[41] There is a potential advantage for ultrasound to be used to measure areas such as the chest wall, breast, or genitalia.[44] Tonometry evaluates tissue tension, the tissue resistance to pressure. It is not a volume measurement. It assesses compliance of the dermis and is an index of fibrotic induration.[41,45] Tissue dielectric constant (TDC) assesses localized skin to fat tissue water changes. It uses a high-frequency electromagnetic wave via a probe to the skin to measure the water content in the tissue. TDC is a clinically efficient procedure, measurement takes approximately 10 seconds at multiple sites, and it can be used to measure at almost any body site.[41,55] Mayrovitz et al. in a study of 80 women treated for breast cancer demonstrated that with TDC a greater number of patients were found to have interarm ratio increases exceeding 10% that were not identified using BIS ratios. This may suggest a greater sensitivity to localized tissue water changes[55] and may play a role in detection of subclinical edema.

Screening and Prevention

There has been a shift in the diagnosis and surveillance of lymphedema away from the traditional impairment-based model with a now growing consensus for a preventative, prospective screening model.[23] This approach facilitates the detection of subclinical lymphedema that is thought to be associated with more effective treatment and prevention of disease progression. However, there needs to be further research to lend support to this theory. Nevertheless, recognized practice guidelines recommend prospective surveillance. The ISL supports a prospective surveillance model and early lymphedema detection and intervention as strategies for greater success with treatment and potential cost savings.[39] The National Lymphedema Network (NLN) position paper on screening and early detection of BCRL contends that a screening model for early detection and treatment of lymphedema, even in the subclinical stage, may reverse the progression to chronic lymphedema.[56]

Although large randomized control trials (RCTs) are lacking, there is mounting evidence in the research literature that surveillance leads to subclinical detection, earlier diagnosis, and subsequent earlier treatment interventions that may prevent progression to a more advanced stage of lymphedema.

Stout et al. prospectively screened via perometry 196 patients for BCRL. Patients diagnosed with subclinical lymphedema were prescribed a compression garment intervention for 4 weeks (in this study the diagnosis of lymphedema was defined as an increase >3% in arm volume compared to preoperative measurements). After the 4 weeks of compression, there was a significant volume reduction, and this was maintained at an average follow-up of 4.8 months after the completion of the intervention.[57] In another prospective study by Soran et al., 186 patients with breast cancer and ALND were screened with either BIS or circumferential measurements. Patients with a diagnosis of subclinical lymphedema received interventions of compression garments, physical therapy, and education. In the BIS surveillance group, 33% of patients were diagnosed with subclinical lymphedema, of which only 4.4% developed clinical lymphedema over an average of 20 months follow-up, whereas in the control group, there was a 36.4% incidence of clinical lymphedema.[58]

Prospective screening and early intervention may also have implications for health-care costs. Stout et al. by estimating costs from the Medicare 2009 physician fee schedule found the cost per year per patient to manage early stage BCRL through prospective surveillance was $636.19 as compared to $3124.92 per year to manage late stage BCRL using a traditional model of care.[59]

Important components that should be considered in a surveillance program for lymphedema include (1) *a reliable and valid objective measurement instrument* such as circumferential measurements, perometry, and BIS. Whichever tool is chosen, it should be used consistently, they are not interchangeable, and accuracy will be improved if a standardized measurement protocol is established;[23,60] (2) *baseline preoperative measurements*,[23,60] Sun et al. analyzed 1028 patients and reported that without a preoperative baseline measurement diagnosis of subclinical and clinical lymphedema are missed 40%–50% of the time. The study further reported that approximately half of lymphedema cases that are diagnosed without a baseline measurement are most likely overdiagnoses as arms are rarely symmetrical at baseline;[61] (3) an *ongoing serial follow up measurement protocol at regular intervals*[23,60] Ostby et al. proposed a prospective surveillance program for BCRL (PROSURV-BCRL), whereby assessment and measurements are coordinated with doctors' visits at intervals of 1, 3, 6, 9, 12 months followed by semiannual visits for 1–3 years;[62] (4) *the use of measurement methods/formulas that factors in natural arm asymmetry and weight changes*. Recommended quantification formulas include the relative volume change equation for patients with unilateral breast surgery and the weight change–adjusted equation for patients with bilateral breast surgery;[60] and finally, (5) *patient symptom report* should always be used together with objective measures and can be invaluable in identifying subclinical lymphedema.[48,62]

TREATMENT

Complete Decongestive Therapy

Complete decongestive therapy (CDT) is a combination therapy for the management of lymphedema that includes MLD, compression, exercise, skin care, patient education, and self-management.[63] CDT is a two-phase therapy: Phase I may be considered as the reduction phase that is aimed at volume reduction, mobilizing high protein interstitial fluid and reduction of increased connective tissue[64] utilizing MLD, short-stretch compression wrappings, exercise to promote lymph flow and skin care. Phase II is described as the maintenance or self-management phase aimed at optimizing and preserving the gains made in Phase I. Interventions are based on the stage of lymphedema and may include the use of compression garments, MLD, and ongoing exercise and skin care.[64] CDT has long been considered the standard of care and is recognized as the therapy of choice by several organizations, including the ISL.[39] CDT can effectively reduce limb volume and provide long-term benefits of an enhanced transport capacity of the lymph vascular system and removal of accumulated protein from the interstitium.[65] The goal of CDT as described by Földi et al. is to improve lymphatic function and lymph drainage, soften fibrotic tissue, decrease collagen deposition, and skin care to reduce the risk of opportunistic infections.[64] Lasinski et al. in a systematic review evaluated 27 studies on the effectiveness of CDT and concluded that CDT was effective in limb volume reduction and was beneficial in mild, moderate, or severe lymphedema.[66] The majority of research is focused on CDT in its totality, but the relative contribution and efficacy of each of the components of CDT is not well understood.[67] There are some less robust studies that suggest the benefit of techniques such as MLD as possible monotherapies especially in the subclinical and early stages of lymphedema.[39] The efficacy of the individual components of CDT in lymphedema management is relevant especially with the current shift toward prevention, subclinical diagnosis, early intervention, and consideration of treatment costs. The ISL 2016 consensus document acknowledges compression garments alone as treatment for subclinical and early stage lymphedema particularly in BCRL. It recognizes published reports supporting MLD as a monotherapy but underlines the need for further research and convincing evidence.[39]

Manual Lymphatic Drainage

MLD is a specialized manual therapy technique centered on the anatomy of the lymphatic system. The light tissue compression used in the course of MLD is aimed at reducing swelling through improved lymphatic contractility, uptake of interstitial fluid, rerouting of lymph into nonobstructed lymphatics, and development of accessory lymph collectors.[65]

MLD is regarded as an important component of CDT. However, in the literature, there is discussion and debate on the function and efficacy of MLD with a lack of supporting objective data. A recent Cochrane review of trials concluded that MLD is safe and well tolerated and beneficial to patients with mild-to-moderate BCRL. It further demonstrated that MLD may offer benefit when added to compression bandaging. Compression bandaging alone resulted in a significant reduction in volume of 30%–38.6% with a further gain of 7.11% reduction with the addition of MLD. In addition, it was found that those with mild-to-moderate BCRL may be the ones who benefit from adding MLD to compression bandaging versus individuals with moderate-to-severe BCRL.[68] The authors suggest that there should be more trials that include volumetric outcomes in truncal and breast lymphedema. MLD may play an important role in truncal/chest wall or breast swelling, areas that may not be as amenable to compression therapy.[68]

Tan et al. used NIRF imaging to compare lymphatic contractile function pre- and post-MLD treatment in both the symptomatic and asymptomatic limbs of 10 patients with Stages I or II lymphedema.[69] The research showed an increase in the average lymph velocity in both the affected and unaffected limbs of 23% and 25%, respectively. The study also included a control group of 12 healthy participants with a reported 28% increase in lymph velocity post-MLD.[69]

In an RCT of 120 patients, Torres Lacomba et al. showed that early physical therapy, including MLD, could be effective in preventing secondary lymphedema for at least 1 year in women following breast cancer surgery and ALND.[70] In the study the control group received education only and the intervention group MLD, scar massage, and shoulder exercises. Risk factors for lymphedema were similar between groups. At 1 year follow-up the difference was significant ($P = .01$). In the control group, 25% developed lymphedema compared to 7% in the intervention group. It may be argued in the study MLD was combined with other therapy modalities so there was no clear contribution from MLD.[70]

There is an emerging new approach using fluroroscopy guided MLD to enable more specific application of MLD treatment. In a recent study Suami et al. developed a prospective protocol using ICG fluorescent lymphography to identify lymphatic drainage pathways in patients with BCRL. The protocol is intended to assist with the diagnosis and treatment interventions of BCRL including ICG- directed MLD. In the imaging procedures for the protocol MLD is performed by a therapist to facilitate movement of ICG through the lymphatics. The study cohort included 103 upper limbs examined in 100 patients of which ALND was performed in 99 limbs. The ICG lymphographic findings of the study demonstrate that MLD can advance the transit of ICG by way of dermal backflow and lymph vessels; it identified various lymphatic drainage pathway patterns including the ipsilateral axilla, clavicular, parasternal and contralateral axilla regions; although the majority of patients had undergone ALND, the ipsilateral axilla drainage pathway was found to be the the most commonly used pathway in 67% of the upper limbs, suggesting that there are patent lymph vessels that traverse the axilla and provided drainage in over 2/3 of the patients in the study.[71] The MD Anderson ICG classification/staging system[47] (Fig. 21.5) was incorporated into the study to investigate the correlation between the identified lymphatic drainage pathways and the severity. As the severity of the disease increased there was a decrease in ipsilateral axilla drainage and increased drainage to the parasternal and contralateral axilla as found in Stage 4 of the MD Anderson ICG staging. MLD is a central component of lymphedema management. The ICG lymphograpy protocol identifies the individuals lymphatic drainage pathways enabling a personalized approach to MLD which may potentially improve MLD application and techniques.[71]

The relative contribution of MLD to complete decongestive therapy (CDT) should be further examined. This would address the question as to whether MLD alone would be of benefit especially in participants with mild BCRL.[68]

Compression

Compression is an important and indispensable component of CDT and is necessary for both initial and long-term lymphedema management. It is considered a cornerstone of lymphedema treatment.[72,73]

Compression modalities most commonly used in lymphedema treatment are compression bandages (CBs), Adjustable Velcro compression devices (AVCDs), and compression garments.

Compression therapy is always included in CDT. Studies have been conducted to unbundle compression from the other components of CDT to determine the efficacy and contribution of compression as a first-line therapy in the management of lymphedema. This is relevant as CDT is both labor intensive and costly to both the patient and health-care sector.[66,67] In a small randomized controlled study McNeely et al. assessed 50 women with BCRL and demonstrated that 4 weeks of CB reduced arm volume effectively with or without the addition of MLD.[74] Andersen et al. conducted an RCT of 42 patients with mild or early onset BCRL and found that MLD was not a significant factor contributing to further reduction in volume compared to compression alone.[75] Another trial by Dayes et al. randomly assigned 103 women with lymphedema to either CDT (daily MLD, bandaging, followed by compression garments) or compression garments alone. The study demonstrated no significant difference in volume reduction, arm function, and QOL measures between the two groups.[76] Study results suggest that a subgroup of patients with a diagnosis of lymphedema exceeding 1 year benefited more from CDT compared to compression garments alone. Conversely, women with a history of lymphedema of less than 1 year the treatment benefit was almost identical in both groups.[76] Finally, Zasadzka et al. in a recent randomized trial in elderly patients with unilateral LLL, compared CDT to CB alone. The study measured 103 patients, 50 treated with CDT, and 53 with CB, reduction in swelling in both groups, were achieved but with no significant difference in volume reduction between the two groups.[77]

These studies provide data that suggest CB as a possible first line therapy in the management of lymphedema. However, although most of the studies are RCTs the findings are limited due to small sample sizes.

In a consensus document a classification system for compression was introduced to describe the deciding characteristics of compression bandaging. Pressure, LAyers, Components, and Elastic properties (PLACE) as the primary variables to consider when applying a CB.[78] The elastic properties of a bandage may be inelastic (rigid bandages or short-stretch bandages) or elastic (long-stretch bandages). The static stiffness index (SSI) may be a helpful parameter to specify stiffness for CBs, including multicomponent multilayer short-stretch compression bandaging.[78] The SSI is the subbandage pressure when changing from a supine to standing position. This is measured at approximately 12 cm above the medial malleolus. A pressure >10 mm Hg is considered a stiff product (inelastic) and <10 mm Hg marks elasticity.[78]

Short-stretch bandages are the preferred choice in the management of lymphedema especially during the reduction phase of therapy due to its low resting pressure that is comfortable at rest and a high working pressure that will maximize the pressure generated with muscle contraction during movement. This allows for a reduction in limb volume and a massaging effect on the tissues and softening of fibrosclerotic skin areas. The use of special padding materials may be added to the bandages to provide a local massaging effect to indurated tissue. The most significant volume reduction usually occurs during the first week of treatment.[79]

In many studies over the years a strong pressure was defined from 40 to 60 mm Hg and very strong as greater than 60 mm Hg with high stiffness, but the compression was not often measured.[72] There is now a debate in the literature of optimal pressure for edema reduction, stiffness, and other variables related to efficacy and comfort. Mosti and Cavezzi in a recent review of the literature describe a trend toward the use of lower pressure for both upper and lower extremities with a range of 20–30 mm Hg in arm lymphedema and 40–60 mm Hg for LLL as effective parameters and suggest that high stiffness may not be an essential prerequisite.[72] A randomized controlled trial compared the effect of low (20–30 mm Hg) versus high pressure (44–58 mm Hg) short stretch, multilayer CBs in patients with moderate-to-severe BCRL. In the first 24 hours the lower pressure bandages were shown to be better tolerated and were equally effective as bandages applied at a higher pressure.[80]

Short-stretch, multilayered CBs are an essential component of CDT and are a mainstay in lymphedema management particularly in the acute treatment phase. However, there is a pressure drop that will occur with short-stretch bandages requiring reapplication of bandages on a regular basis often on a daily basis in order to maintain optimal pressure. AVCDs can be used in both the initial and maintenance phase of treatment (Fig. 21.6). These adjustable devices were once recommended for the maintenance treatment phase only; however, research studies have shown them to be also effective in the initial treatment phase.[81,82] Damstra and Partsch conducted a randomized controlled trial comparing AVCDs to CBs during the initial treatment of leg lymphedema and demonstrated significant leg volume reduction with the use of the AVCDs as compared to conventional bandaging.[81] In a recent RCT, Mosti et al. demonstrated AVCDs to be effective in reducing venous edema in the initial treatment phase. The study demonstrated that both compression systems (AVCDs and CBs) achieved a significant reduction of total lower leg volume as compared to baseline measurements; however, in comparing effects of both devices the AVCD group showed a significant

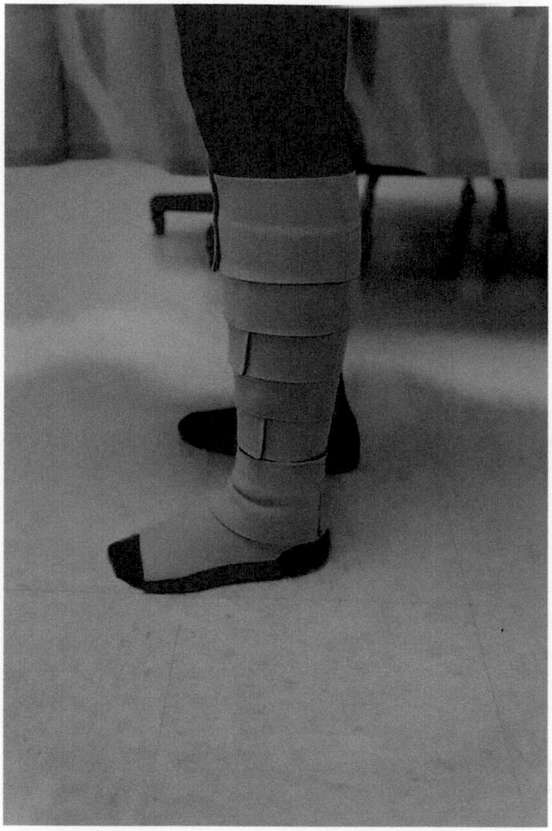

FIGURE 21.6 AVCD for the (left) lower extremity. *AVCD* Adjustable Velcro compression device.

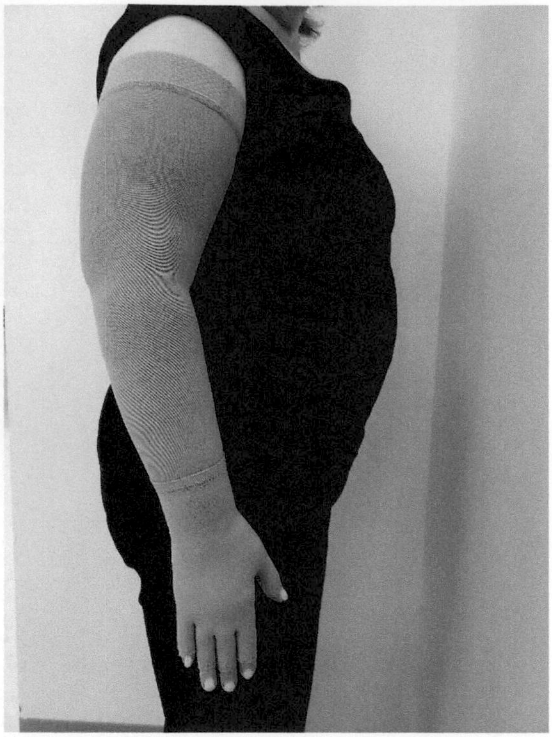

FIGURE 21.7 Compression sleeve and glove for the (right) upper limb.

volume reduction after both 1 and 7 days as compared to the CB group ($P < .001$).[82] The authors concluded AVCDs to be an effective and well-tolerated option in both the initial and maintenance phase of treatment.[82] Advantages of AVCDs include the ease and handling of the device by the patient or caregiver, and if there is a pressure loss, it can be readjusted by the patient according to subjective sensations.[82] Patients were also found to avoid the use of unacceptable high and low pressures during self-application or readjustment of the devices.[83]

Compression Garments

Compression garments are an integral part of lymphedema management and are the mainstay for control and maintenance of volume decongestion (Fig. 21.7). Preliminary research findings suggest that early diagnosis and initiating compression in the subclinical phase may reduce development of clinical lymphedema.[57,84] An expert consensus document examining prophylaxis and early intervention after breast cancer treatment shows supportive evidence for early intervention and compression to prevent progression to chronic lymphedema. The panel recommends that these findings need to be verified by further research, including large-scale controlled trials.[85]

There are studies, including small RCTs, providing supportive evidence for compression garments as first-line intervention for BCRL. Stout et al. in a prospective study with women newly diagnosed with stage 1-111 breast cancer found that wearing a compression sleeve and gauntlet (20–30 mm Hg) for a 4 week period successfully treated subclinical lymphedema.[57]

In an RCT, Ochalek et al. suggest that compression sleeves in conjunction with an exercise program may be a safe and efficient option to prevent postsurgical arm swelling and development of lymphedema. In the study, 45 postoperative breast cancer patients with axillary lymph node interventions were preoperatively randomized to either a group wearing compression sleeves (15–21 mm Hg) in combination with a standardized physical exercise program or a control group with a standardized exercise program without compression. The compression group showed significantly lower mean affected arm volumes between 3 and 12 months after ALND as compared with the group without compression.[84] In a recent posttrial follow-up of this RCT, it was found that at 2 years the findings were consistent with the previous study with a significantly lower mean affected arm volume in the exercise and compression group compared to the control group of exercise without compression ($P = .023$). There was also a significant improvement in QOL parameters, including function, pain, arm, and breast symptoms.[86]

Intermittent Pneumatic Compression

IPC is another method of compression therapy for patients with lymphedema and is often used as an adjunct to the other components of CDT[87] (Fig. 21.8).

Since the early 1950s, pneumatic compression systems have been used in the management of swelling. Over the past decades, the technology has improved substantially. The initial pneumatic compression pumps were single chamber nonsegmented, nonprogrammable, pumps providing a single uniform compression to the limb. Over time, there has been an evolution in design with progression to segmented multichamber pumps that allow for pressure gradients. The technology continues to evolve and in recent years, more sophisticated advanced pneumatic systems have been introduced that aim to mechanically mimic the effects of MLD. The expanded IPC devices have equipment and digital programming capabilities that can deliver low pressure, phasic

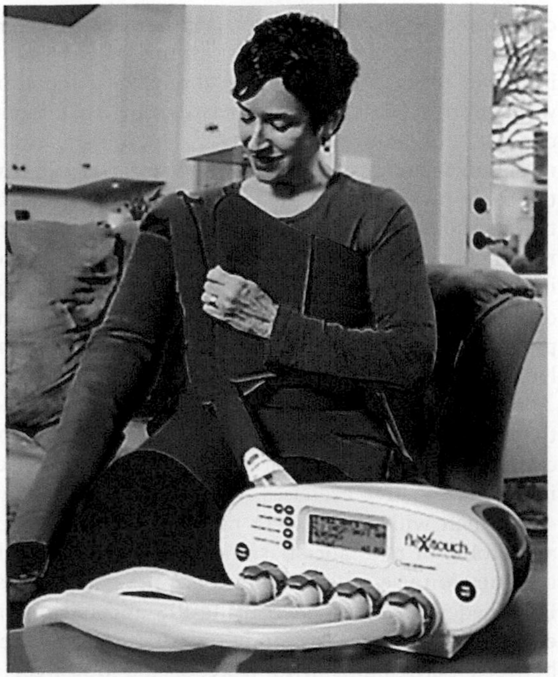

FIGURE 21.8 Intermittent pneumatic compression system for the (right) upper limb. (Reprinted with permission from Tactile Medical).

compression and promote fluid clearance from the trunk as well as the limbs.[88] IPC therapy is able to effectively decrease excess fluid from the extremity, and this is ideally achieved with the use of advanced multichamber pumps. However, there are reports in the literature of theoretical concerns associated with IPC, including damage to the skin lymphatics due to application of high pressures from the devices, and another concern is with the displacement of fluid more proximally that may result in genital edema and also possible development of a fibrosclerotic ring above the proximal border of the IPC garment.[39,87] The ISL consensus document recommends careful judicious observation to avoid these adverse effects.[39]

In a metaanalysis of 7 published randomized controlled studies, Shao et al. assessed IPC efficacy in patients with BCRL and found no significant differences between routine management of lymphedema with or without the use of IPC.[89] However, some studies have shown the benefits of IPC as an addition to a multimodality lymphedema treatment regimen. In a study to examine the adjunctive role of IPC in BCRL, 23 patients with untreated BCRL were randomized to receive either CDT alone or CDT with added IPC (applied 30 minutes daily for 10 days with a standard pressure setting of 40–50 mm Hg). The addition of IPC to CDT resulted in an additional mean volume reduction during the initial decongestive phase of treatment (45.3% vs 26%; $P \leq .05$).[90] In a second arm of the study, 27 additional BCRL patients were assessed during the maintenance phase of therapy; IPC (self-administered 60 minutes daily with a pressure setting of 40–50 mm Hg) was added to CDT versus CDT alone. At 6–12 months, there was a statistically significant mean volume reduction in the group that received CDT and adjunctive IPC as compared to a mean volume increase in the group that received CDT alone.[90] The study concluded that adjunctive IPC improved the therapeutic response in both the initial and maintenance phases of treatment, and overall was well tolerated without apparent complications.[90] In a recent study, lymph movement was assessed in patients with both primary and cancer-related LLL using NIRF lymphatic imaging. During a single 1 hour treatment session, it was demonstrated that sequential pneumatic compression enabled lymph to move proximally away from edematous regions through functional lymphatic vessels when available, or through interstitial spaces with modest tissue volume reductions.[91] In addition, Zaleska et al. in a study of LLL presented some preliminary evidence that IPC compression may contribute to the development of tissue channels that may provide pathways for drainage of edema fluid.[92]

Overall, there is a lack of consensus in regard to the optimal treatment parameters or dosage pertaining to the use of IPC. Recent published evidence in a systematic review suggests a dosage time of 45–60 minutes, applying pressures between 30 and 60 mm Hg using multicell, sequential IPC programs for individuals with lymphedema. There was little available evidence for application of specific IPC dosage for a particular limb.[93]

IPC technology has improved significantly over the past few decades but remains controversial as a component in the therapeutic management of lymphedema. It has been suggested that IPC may be considered as an adjunct to treatment in both the initial and maintenance phase and can be incorporated into a multimodal, therapeutic program.[87] The guidelines for patient and device selection along with parameters for frequency, duration, and pressures continue to evolve.[87,93]

Exercise

Exercise is integral in the management of patients at risk or with a diagnosis of lymphedema. The basic exercise modes are applicable in the management of lymphedema: range of motion; stretching flexibility exercises to increase or maintain range of motion and minimize scar tissue and joint stiffness that may decrease lymph flow; resistance or weight lifting; aerobic conditioning; and lymphedema remedial/decongestive exercises combined with compression.[94] In lymphedema, the intrinsic lymph pump that relies on the phasic contractions of the smooth muscle layers of the collecting lymphatic vessels may be compromised and lymph flow may become more dependent on the extrinsic lymph pump mechanism. The extrinsic pump relies on the cyclical compression and expansion of lymphatics related to the action of external forces that may include physical movement, arterial pulsations, respiration, muscle contractions, manual massage, and tissue compression that may all impact lymph flow.[95,96]

Previously strength training and weight lifting of the at-risk limb were not recommended. Patients were advised through various cancer web sites and guidelines to avoid lifting children, heavy bags, and objects. These recommendations at the time were intended to prevent harm but could consequently lead to limitations with physical recovery, employment, and activities of daily living.[97]

In addition, clinical guidelines suggested that women with or at risk for lymphedema should protect and avoid overuse of the affected arm, these restrictions potentially could limit activity and lead to deconditioning of the limb with an increased risk for injury from regular activities of daily living.[98]

In 2009 there was a seminal, Level 1 RCT by Schmitz et al., 141 patients with stable BCRL were randomized to a weight lifting or a control group. After 1 year, there was no significant difference in limb swelling between groups, with a reduced incidence of lymphedema exacerbations and increased strength in the weight lifting cohort. The exercise program for the weight lifting group included upper body exercises of seated rows, chest press, lateral or front raises, bicep curls, and tricep pushdowns first introduced with minimal resistance with a gradual progressive strengthening approach with no upper limit for the amount of weight used.[97] It is recommended that exercise training should initially be supervised starting with a low dose with gradual progression according to symptom response.[99] These findings are important for both patients and clinicians as it provides high-level evidence to support safe functional use and strengthening of the affected limb. Several other studies have been performed which corroborate the evidence.[100,101] Furthermore, there is clinical evidence that weight lifting significantly improves tissue composition in the affected limbs of women with BCRL, with increased lean mass, bone density, and reduced arm fat.[102] Singh et al. in a recent metaanalysis and systematic review evaluated the current literature on the effects of exercise irrespective of mode (aerobic, resistance, mixed, and other) in patients with upper and lower limb cancer-related lymphedema.[103] The research confirms that individuals with secondary lymphedema can safely perform progressive, regular exercise without worsening of lymphedema and related symptoms.[103]

In regards to the use of compression garments, there have been recent studies that query the use of compression during various modes of exercise, including resistive exercises.[104,105] In a recent study, 41 women with BCRL were randomized into either an aerobic or resistance-based exercise program with compression use at the discretion of the participants. Lymphedema was assessed using BIS and circumference measurements. The study reported no difference between participants who wore or did not wear a compression garment.[104] However, Singh et al. in their review and metaanalysis conclude that there is insufficient evidence to support or refute the use of compression garments during exercise and suggest the use of garments be considered on an individual basis with consideration of factors such as the stage and stability of lymphedema, climate, and patient adherence.[103] It is noted that earlier RCTs that demonstrated safety and efficacy of exercise in patients with cancer-related lymphedema required the use of compression garments for those individuals with a diagnosis of lymphedema.[97,100]

Once survivors have completed their cancer treatments, it is recommended that they continue to maintain a healthy lifestyle of physical activity and optimal weight. Many survivors can safely begin a low-to-moderate-intensity exercise program such as walking without supervision or an exercise specialist evaluation.[106] For patients proceeding to more vigorous exercise or with increased risk for complications, exercise testing and prescription is warranted before progressing to a community-based program.[106] For patients with or at risk for lymphedema, ongoing physical activity and maintaining a healthy life style are important as obesity and weight fluctuations are risk factors for lymphedema,[21] as well as a poor prognostic factor with regard to lymphedema treatment.[107] The American College of Sports Medicine (ACSM) provides exercise guidelines for cancer survivors, including breast and gynecologic cancers. The recommendations are weekly aerobic activity of 150 minutes of moderate-intensity exercise or 75 minutes of vigorous-intensity exercise or an equivalent combination and two-to-three weekly sessions of progressive strengthening exercises. The guidelines recommend that survivors avoid inactivity.[106]

In recent years, there is growing interest and research on the effects of more nontraditional methods of exercise, including Pilates, yoga, tai chi, and qigong. A recently published metaanalysis investigated the effects of exercise as an intervention for BCRL, including nontraditional forms of exercise, such as Pilates, yoga, and qigong, and concluded that they may be safe in the management of individuals with or at risk for BCRL. Additional research is needed to further examine efficacy and safety.[108] Fisher et al. showed that when six women with a diagnosis of BCRL participated in a yoga program three times per week for 8 weeks, there was significant reduction in arm volume while QOL and self-reported arm function remained stable.[109] In another study, 60 patients with BCRL were randomized to a clinical Pilates group and a control group of standard lymphedema exercises three times a week for 8 weeks. In the Pilates group, there was significant improvement in pain, severity of lymphedema, grip strength shoulder range of motion, and QOL.[110]

Aqua lymphatic therapy (ALT) is another mode of exercise used in the maintenance phase of cancer-related lymphedema. It utilizes the physical properties of water, self-massage, exercise, and the hydrostatic pressure of water that provides a compression element as a method to control lymphedema. In ALT the recommended water temperature range is between 31°C and 33.5°C.[111] In a randomized study, 25 women with BCRL were assigned to either an ALT program plus homeland-based exercise versus a homeland-based exercise program alone. Those that received ALT after 12 weeks showed a significant improvement in QOL, reduction in pain, and improved arm function. But there was no change in limb volume in either group.[112] Conversely, a prospective study showed that an aquatic exercise protocol reduced limb volume significantly in chronic LLL.[113] However, a recently published systematic review and metaanalysis concluded that there was no significant benefit of ALT over standard land-based care in upper extremity lymphedema.[114]

The abovementioned discussion is focused on lymphedema treatment; however, there needs to be a comprehensive approach to the rehabilitation of patients with breast and gynecologic cancer-related lymphedema. Patients may present with multiple cancer-related treatment deficits. For example, a patient with a breast cancer diagnosis may be referred for lymphedema but also present with other deficits, including pain, shoulder dysfunction, upper body weakness, osteoporosis, and balance deficits due to neuropathy. Besides lymphedema-specific treatment, the patient needs a comprehensive integrated program to address specific impairments while avoiding exacerbation of lymphedema symptoms. For instance, decreased shoulder mobility and pain if not addressed will inhibit the extrinsic muscle pump needed for lymph flow. A progressive exercise program is an essential component for optimal outcomes. The patient's goals and preferences should be considered in deciding on the exercise mode as this will have an impact on compliance.

Low-Level Laser Therapy

Low-level laser therapy (LLLT) also known as cold laser is a noninvasive form of phototherapy that utilizes wavelengths of light in the visible to near-infrared range of 670–950 nm.[115] Low power or cold lasers usually between 5 and 500 mW[115] have a nonthermal stimulatory effect on the tissues impacting cellular change.[116] The specifics of the wavelength are important as it determines the depth penetration within the tissues and should be appropriate and specific to the condition being treated.[117] In 2006 the FDA approved LLLT as a therapeutic intervention to treat lymphedema using the LTU 904 laser unit.[117] The 904-nm wavelength recommended for lymphedema is able to penetrate cutaneous and subcutaneous tissues without an increase in temperature and may impact tissues up to a depth of 5 cm.[118] LLLT is now used in rehabilitation to treat a variety of conditions. One device cannot effectively treat all diagnoses. It is important that the correct device with the appropriate wavelength is utilized. Usually, the wavelength cannot be adjusted on the device, the wavelength may be inherent to the specific laser device.[117] For example, the device used to treat a musculoskeletal injury may not be the optimal wavelength required for lymphedema management.[117] There are different types of units for LLLT application. Handheld units with a probe are used for specific spot treatment applications as compared to scanning units which deliver LLLT over a larger area.[115]

Basic experimental studies on LLLT have shown a range of modifying biochemical and cellular effects on macrophages, lymphocytes, mitochondria, increased or decreased fibroblast activity, increased vascular endothelial growth factor, and endothelial cell proliferation.[119] Several studies on the use of LLLT in lymphedema management suggest both subjective and objective benefits, including softening of fibrotic and scar tissue, wound healing, and reduction in pain and swelling.[115,120–122] LLLT is postulated to benefit the lymphatic system by increasing the lymphatic flow through lymphangiogenesis, stimulation of lymphatic motoricity, and reduction or softening of lymphostatic tissue fibrosis.[115,121] Purportedly, LLLT may also be helpful in preventing tissue fibrosis.[123] More recently, an experimental study showed both antiinflammatory and lymphangiogenic effects with the use of low-level laser in lymphedema.[124] Several studies have been conducted to assess the efficacy of LLLT in BCRL.[118,120–122] Carati et al. in a double-blind single crossover RCT measured changes in volume and extracellular fluid via perometry and BIS, respectively. The study found that following two cycles of LLLT 33% of patients demonstrated a clinically significant decrease in limb volume 3 months after treatment. There was also reported reduction in dermal tissue hardness as measured by tonometry.[120] Omar et al. in a small RCT compared LLLT combined with exercise, education, and compression garments to a placebo laser group also, including exercise, education, and use of compression garments. The findings suggest that LLLT combined with other treatment interventions may be effective in reducing arm circumference, increased handgrip, and shoulder mobility in women with BCRL.[125] Ridner et al. in an RCT of 46 women with BCRL demonstrated that a 20-minute treatment of LLLT followed by compression bandaging may be as effective in arm volume reduction relative to more prolonged treatment times associated with MLD or combined MLD/LLLT followed by compression.[121] Dirican et al. in a small single-group study of 17 women with BCRL concluded that LLLT when used in conjunction with conventional treatments resulted in improved scar mobility and increased shoulder range of motion along with reduced limb circumference and pain.[122]

Further research is needed to define the optimal treatment parameters for LLLT treatments.[126] In a meta-analysis of nine studies, it was found that the treatment parameters for LLLT most commonly used in patients with BCRL included a dosage of 1.5 J/cm^2, $3 \times$/week for 3–4 weeks for approximately 17 minutes per treatment session. The most common wavelength used was 904 nm, and the most common site of application was the axillary region.[115] The antecubital fossa and forearm are also often used as an application site.[126]

Evidence suggests that LLLT may be a feasible adjunct to lymphedema treatment.[117] Baxter et al. in a recent systematic review of low-level laser for BCRL submit that LLLT may be an effective treatment modality for women with BCRL.[126] However, the authors underline the need for further high-quality trials in this area.[126]

Kinesiology Taping

Kinesiology taping (KT) was first developed in Japan in the 1970s by Dr. Kenzo Kase and is a commonly used intervention in physical therapy and the rehabilitation community for managing musculoskeletal and sport injuries. More recently, KT has emerged as a treatment option in the management of lymphedema. It is a thin elastic tape designed to be similar to the skin's weight and thickness and is capable of stretching 30%–40% of its resting length.[127] The tape is permeable to air allowing the skin to breathe, and the patient may shower and the tape will remain effective and comfortable for 3–5 days.[127]

It is proposed that KT facilitates lymphatic drainage by enabling the upper layers of the skin to be lifted away from muscle fascia creating convolutions in the skin therein opening up lymphatic channels and facilitating vascular and lymphatic flow. It is further suggested that it aids myofascial release and increases reabsorption of lymph in surrounding tissues.[127,128]

In lymphedema management, KT is of interest and may be considered as a desirable alternative to compression as it is lightweight and does not limit movement or function and the muscle activity further encourages lymphatic flow. Moreover, compression is difficult to apply to the trunk and breast, and KT is a useful option for the treatment of lymphedema in these areas.[128]

There have been several studies examining the efficacy of KT in the treatment of lymphedema, particularly BCRL. Some of the outcome measures/indicators considered in the research include volumetric measurements, range of motion, pain, QOL, and function.[128]

Tsai et al. randomized 41 women with BCRL, including patients with Stages I, II, and III lymphedema. The intervention group received CDT with compression bandaging and the control group CDT with the use of KT instead of compression bandaging. There was significant reduction in circumferential and volume measurements in both groups with no significant difference between groups.[129] However, there was better compliance reported in the KT group.

Interestingly, the study found that compression bandaging resulted in a significant reduction in the circumference of the lower part of the upper arm while KT significantly decreased the circumference in the forearm. The findings suggest KT as an alternative to compression bandaging.[129] Conversely, Taradaj et al. in a randomized study also assessed the efficacy of KT in BCRL and concluded that it was not effective in the reduction of Stages II and III lymphedema and at this time should not replace CDT.[130] A recent randomized trial in women with Stages II and III BCRL demonstrated that 3 weeks of KT in the maintenance phase of CDT were more effective than compression garments in volume reduction. In addition, there were improvements in grip strength and overall QOL with taping as compared to the compression garment group.[131] KT was also found to be beneficial in reducing the severity and duration of seroma following axillary clearance for breast cancer treatment.[132] A metaanalysis of six RCTs comparing compression bandaging to KT concluded there was no statistically significant difference in volume reduction between the two interventions. Although no significant difference was found with metaanalysis, in four of the five studies, there was a greater volume reduction in the compression group. Lymphedema-related symptoms showed greater improvement with KT as compared to bandaging.[133] There was an increased risk of skin complications with KT affecting between 10% and 21% of patients.[133]

More research is needed with larger sample sizes and follow-up to provide stronger evidence to support conclusions regarding the efficacy of KT in BCRL.

SURGICAL TREATMENT FOR LYMPHEDEMA

Whereas the current gold standard for lymphedema care is CDT, surgical treatment for lymphedema can be an alternative when this treatment is not effective. The indications for surgical treatment of lymphedema are to (1) reduce weight in the affected extremity, (2) prevent progression of the lymphedema, (3) reduce the frequency of infections, and (4) improve cosmetics and function.[134] Types of surgical treatments include excision of tissues through liposuction and debulking procedures with skin grafting.

Liposuction involves the removal of adipose tissue that is increased in tissues with excessive lymphatic fluid. A disadvantage of this procedure is in the need for continuous use of compression garments to minimize the reaccumulation of fluid.[134] It has been recommended for severe late stage BCRL that is unresponsive to conservative management.[135] Debulking procedures remove skin and subcutaneous tissues and require skin grafting; however, these types of procedures have been associated with increased morbidity and risks such as infections and hematoma.

In lymphatic to lymphatic bypass, veins or healthy lymphatics from other parts of the body such as the medial thigh are used as conduits across an area with injured lymphatics and anastomosed to existing lymphatic vessels.[134] Bypass grafting can also be performed directly linking lymph vessels with venous vessels in lymphovenous bypass and lymphovenous anastomosis (LVA). According to Teng, LVA may be best used in patients with mild arm lymphedema and minimal irreversible tissue fibrosis.[134]

In vascularized lymph node transfers (VLNT), vascularized lymph nodes are harvested from different regions of the body and then transplanted to an affected region such as the axilla for arm lymphedema and ankle and groin for lower extremity lymphedema. These procedures have been reported as being generally safe; however, complications such as donor site lymphedema, seroma, infections, and impaired wound healing can occur.[134] VLNT is best considered in early stages of lymphedema before onset of fibrosis of lymphatic vessels or adipose deposition occurs.[134,135]

EDUCATION

Patient education is an important strategy in the management of lymphedema. The National Comprehensive Cancer Network (NCCN) Breast Cancer Panel in its standard for surveillance and follow-up recommends to "educate, monitor, and refer for lymphedema management."[136]

The American Society of Breast Surgeons recommended goals for patient education include instruction on the lifetime risk for lymphedema particularly in 3–5 years after surgery; education on the early signs and symptoms of lymphedema that may include ipsilateral heaviness, achiness, fullness, stiffness, tight clothing or jewelry, or patient perceived swelling; education on risk reduction strategies; and contact information for a specialist in the event that the patient experiences onset of symptoms.[137]

Educating patients on self-reported symptoms that may include perceived swelling, heaviness, tingling, pain, sensory changes and changes in fit of clothing is important, as these symptoms may occur before the onset of visible swelling and indicate subclinical lymphedema enabling an opportunity for early intervention and treatment.[48,50,52,138]

Patient education may reduce lymphedema risk and related symptoms. In a study of 136 breast cancer survivors, Fu et al. demonstrated that patients who received lymphedema education were more knowledgeable of BCRL and reported significantly less symptoms.[139] Findings from several studies suggest that education, and early treatment intervention, may prevent progression of lymphedema.[57,58,70]

A recent study examining barriers to BCRL self-management identified lack of education about lymphedema treatment and risk reduction as one of the main barriers to self-management.[140] Patient education should begin preoperatively and be incorporated at time points throughout the continuum of care into survivorship. There is a need for patient educational standards and further research to improve BCRL educational programs that provide practical, accessible, and evidence-based information.[137]

RISK REDUCTION BEHAVIORS

As discussed previously, risk factors of lymphedema include lymphadenectomy, radiation and high BMI along with other associated treatment-related risk factors. It is not fully understood why some patients develop lymphedema and others do not despite similar cancer treatment interventions and demographics.[141,142] To establish an individualized risk profile for BCRL is challenging as there are several variables to be considered. These include cancer treatment-related risk factors and non-treatment related risk factors such as genetic predisposition, individual anatomy and physiology, and behavior/lifestyle associated factors.[7,137] Due to the inconsistency of risk factors, clinicians continue to recommend precautionary measures/risk reduction behaviors in an effort to decrease lymphedema risk.[143]

There are several resources that provide information on lymphedema and guidelines on behavioral practices (Table 21.2). The NLN is internationally recognized and regularly cited in the literature. It has a series of position papers with recommendations for patients at risk or with a confirmed diagnosis of lymphedema.[144] A summary of these recommendations include meticulous skin care, making sure that the skin is kept in good condition by keeping it clean and dry, applying moisturizer daily to prevent chapped skin and use of sunscreen and insect repellant, maintaining a healthy lifestyle of optimal weight, healthy diet, and exercise with a gradual buildup of the intensity and duration of exercise. There are further recommendations to try to avoid possible triggers such as extreme temperatures; prolonged sitting or standing for leg lymphedema; avoidance of limb constriction such as tourniquets, blood pressure cuffs, tight clothing; avoidance of injections, blood draws, and intravenous sticks; a compression sleeve is advised for individuals with a confirmed diagnosis of lymphedema while those at risk for lymphedema should make a decision to wear compression based on their individual risk factors. Compression garments for the arm should include a handpiece of either a glove or gauntlet. Garments should be well fitted and worn well in advance of air travel to ensure proper fit.[144]

These precautionary measures and recommendations are intended to decrease stress on the lymphatics of the at risk extremity and prevent lymphatic overload. Clinical experience suggests that factors that increase capillary filtration such as infection, inflammation, and skin injury are precipitating for edema.[5] It is acknowledged that

TABLE 21.2
Online Lymphedema Information Resources

NLN: https://www.lymphnet.org
LE&RN: https://lymphaticnetwork.org
NCCN: https://www.nccn.org/patients/resources/life_with_cancer/managing_symptoms/lymphedema.aspx
NCI: https://www.cancer.gov/about-cancer/treatment/side-effects/lymphedema/lymphedema-pdq
American Cancer Society: https://www.cancer.org/treatment/treatments-and-side-effects/physical-side-effects/lymphedema.html

LE&RN, Lymphatic Education & Research Network; *NCCN*, National Comprehensive Cancer Network; *NCI*, National Cancer Institute; *NLN*, National Lymphedema Network.

many of these recommendations lack supporting or refuting high-level scientific evidence and are primarily based on knowledge of the pathophysiology and decades of clinical experience by experts in the field.[143–145]

In recent years a new generation of studies have emerged that question many of these routine recommendations.[141,145,146] There is concern that the conventional guidelines have not kept pace with ongoing surgical and treatment advances.[145] Also suggested is that some of the measures may be burdensome to patients and a source of anxiety along with avoidance of activities. Ferguson et al. screened, via perometry, 632 patients (760 at risk arms) in patients undergoing breast cancer treatment and showed no significant association between lymphedema and change in arm volume in patients with a history of air travel, blood draws, and blood pressure readings. Of note, 80% of the patient population for the study was comprised of women who had no axillary surgery or had sentinel lymph node biopsy only. The study also showed that BMI $\geq 25\ \text{lb/in}^2$ at the time of diagnosis, ALND, RLNR, and cellulitis was all significantly associated with arm swelling.[141] Kilbreath et al. in a large cohort prospective study on risk factors for lymphedema in women with breast cancer found that air travel, arm trauma, medical procedures, and arm usage did not increase risk of lymphedema in women with ≥ 5 nodes removed.[146] A recent systematic review of 12 studies concluded that air travel is not associated with worsening of lymphedema.[147] Asdourian et al. demonstrated similar findings in a prospective cohort of 327 patients (654 at risk arms) who underwent bilateral breast cancer surgery with a median follow-up time of 27 months (range, 6–68 months). The study showed no significant association between lymphedema and change in arm volume with regard to blood pressure readings, blood draws, injections, and air travel. Nonetheless, the research authors emphasize, that these findings provide insufficient data to change clinical practice in respect to risk reduction patient education. Pending high-level research, the authors propose a risk-adjusted approach in the application of guidelines.[145]

The 2016 ISL consensus document suggests that there is substantially less risk of secondary lymphedema associated with conservative breast cancer treatments such as lumpectomy and sentinel lymph node biopsy and further submits that some of the restrictions included in risk reduction practices may not be appropriate and may subject patients to therapies that are unsupported.[39]

An expert panel of the American Society of Breast Surgeons in their recommendations for risk-reducing behaviors propose an early detection and surveillance program, including baseline and ongoing assessments; the use of the ipsilateral arm for IVs or blood pressure that they conclude as not contraindicated; and individualized risk reduction guidelines as opposed to widespread application of practices.[135,137]

In the literature, there is ongoing dialogue and debate regarding routine use of conventional precautionary measures/guidelines. In response to recent studies on risk reduction behaviors, there has been editorial commentary in professional journals, by practitioners and experts in the field suggesting that with the lack of definitive evidence, there should be caution in abandoning or discounting conventional risk reduction behaviors.[148]

Conversely, there is consensus and strong evidence supporting exercise, physical activity, and optimal body weight as areas for potential risk reduction strategies and the management of lymphedema.[7,20,21,23,99] Obesity is a major risk factor for lymphedema and weight management should be considered as a risk reduction strategy.[7,20,21,23,37] Shaw et al. in a RCT demonstrated that weight loss can reduce BCRL significantly.[38] In the past, guidelines discouraged use of the affected arm, including restrictions with lifting to less than 5–15 lb as a risk reduction practice for lymphedema.[99] There is now strong evidence that exercise, including weight lifting is safe, with an ameliorating effect for patients at risk and for those with a diagnosis of lymphedema.[97,98,100–102]

In summary, there is uncertainty regarding the effectiveness of some of the conventional recommended lymphedema risk reduction practices, including avoidance of blood pressure measurements, venipuncture in the affected arm, and minimizing air travel.[5,141,145] The professional guidelines from the ISL[39] and the American Society of Breast Surgeons[135,137] place emphasis on surveillance, exercise to reduce risk, weight management, and recommend an individualized approach in the application of guidelines and strategies.

CONCLUSION

Lymphedema is common in persons treated for breast and gynecologic cancers. A prospective surveillance approach with focus on education, preoperative assessment, identification of early/subclinical lymphedema, ongoing monitoring, and early intervention, may reduce risk or slow progression of the disease.[57,58,60-62] BIS technology is increasingly being used for prospective detection of early/subclinical lymphedema.[12,58] CDT, MLD, compression, weight management strategies, and exercise are the cornerstones of an effective lymphedema management program. There is evidence to support the use of compression garments worn for a period of time as an effective treatment for subclinical BCRL and may also assist in reducing disease progression.[57] There is also an increasing use of surgical treatments for lymphedema. There are a variety of imaging techniques that may be used to confirm a diagnosis of lymphedema. Research in recent decades has led to increased understanding of lymphatic biology and function, with recognition of the need for more research on the pathophysiology and treatment of this disabling condition.

REFERENCES

1. Lee MJ, Rockson SG. Lower extremity cancers. In: Lee BB, Rockson SG, Bergan J, eds. *Lymphedema: A Concise Compendium of Theory and Practice*. 2nd ed. Cham, Switzerland: Springer; 2018:887–897.
2. American Cancer Society. Cancer treatment and survivorship statistics. 2019:2021 https://www.cancer.org/content/dam/cancer-org/research/cancer-facts-and-statistics/cancer-treatment-and-survivorship-facts-and-figures/cancer-treatment-and-survivorship-facts-and-figures-2019-2021.pdf. 2019 Accessed December 2, 2019.
3. Institute of Medicine and National Research Council. *From Cancer Patient to Cancer Survivor: Lost in Transition*. Washington, DC: The National Academies Press; 2006. Available from: https://doi.org/10.17226/11468.
4. Dylke ES, Schembri GP, Bailey DL, et al. Diagnosis of upper limb lymphedema: development of an evidence-based approach. *Acta Oncol*. 2016;55(12):1477–1483.
5. Rockson SG. Lymphedema after breast cancer treatment. *N Engl J Med*. 2018;379(20):1937–1944.
6. Henley SJ, Miller JW, Dowling NF, Benard VB, Richardson LC. Uterine cancer incidence and mortality - United States, 1999-2016. *MMWR Morb Mortal Wkly Rep*. 2018;67(48):1333–1338. Available from: https://doi.org/10.15585/mmwr.mm6748a1. Published 2018 Dec 7.
7. DiSipio T, Rye S, Newman B, Hayes S. Incidence of unilateral arm lymphoedema after breast cancer: a systematic review and meta-analysis. *Lancet Oncol*. 2013;14(6):500–515.
8. Cormier JN, Askew RL, Mungovan KS, Xing Y, Ross MI, Armer JM. Lymphedema beyond breast cancer: a systematic review and meta-analysis of cancer-related secondary lymphedema. *Cancer*. 2010;116(22):5138–5149.
9. Beesley VL, Rowlands IJ, Hayes SC, et al. Incidence, risk factors and estimates of a woman's risk of developing secondary lower limb lymphedema and lymphedema-specific supportive care needs in women treated for endometrial cancer. *Gynecol Oncol*. 2015;136(1):87–93.
10. Hayes SC, Janda M, Ward LC, et al. Lymphedema following gynecological cancer: Results from a prospective, longitudinal cohort study on prevalence, incidence and risk factors. *Gynecol Oncol*. 2017;146(3):623–629.
11. Tiwari P, Coriddi M, Salani R, Povoski SP. Breast and gynecologic cancer-related extremity lymphedema: a review of diagnostic modalities and management options. *World J Surg Oncol*. 2013;11:237.
12. Rockson SG. General considerations. In: Lee BB, Rockson SG, Bergan J, eds. *Lymphedema: A Concise Compendium of Theory and Practice*. 2nd ed. Cham, Switzerland: Springer; 2018:3–7.
13. Stolldorf DP, Dietrich MS, Ridner SH. Symptom frequency, intensity, and distress in patients with lower limb lymphedema. *Lymphat Res Biol*. 2016;14(2):78–87.
14. Ridner S, Deng J, Rhoten BA. Adherence and quality of life. In: Lee BB, Rockson SG, Bergan J, eds. *Lymphedema: A Concise Compendium of Theory and Practice*. 2nd ed. Cham, Switzerland: Springer; 2018:493–501.
15. Ahmed RL, Prizment A, Lazovich D, Schmitz KH, Folsom AR. Lymphedema and quality of life in breast cancer survivors: the Iowa Women's Health Study. *J Clin Oncol*. 2008;26(35):5689–5696.
16. Taghian NR, Miller CL, Jammallo LS, O'Toole J, Skolny MN. Lymphedema following breast cancer treatment and impact on quality of life: a review. *Crit Rev Oncol Hematol*. 2014;92(3):227–234.
17. Kataru RP, Wiser I, Baik JE, et al. Fibrosis and secondary lymphedema: chicken or egg? *Transl Res*. 2019;209:68–76. Available from: https://doi.org/10.1016/j.trsl.2019.04.001.
18. Rockson SG. Anatomy and structural physiology of the lymphatic system. In: Cheng MH, Chang DW, Patel KM, eds. *Principles and Practice of Lymphedema Surgery*. Elsevier; 2016.
19. Rockson SG, Keeley V, Kilbreath S, Szuba A, Towers A. Cancer-associated secondary lymphoedema. *Nat Rev Dis Primers*. 2019;5(1):22. Available from: https://doi.org/10.1038/s41572-019-0072-5.
20. Ridner SH, Dietrich MS, Stewart BR, Armer JM. Body mass index and breast cancer treatment-related lymphedema. *Support Care Cancer*. 2011;19(6):853–857.
21. Jammallo LS, Miller CL, Singer M, et al. Impact of body mass index and weight fluctuation on lymphedema risk in patients treated for breast cancer. *Breast Cancer Res Treat*. 2013;142(1):59–67.
22. Beesley V, Janda M, Eakin E, Obermair A, Battistutta D. Lymphedema after gynecological cancer treatment: prevalence, correlates, and supportive care needs. *Cancer*. 2007;109(12):2607–2614.
23. Gillespie TC, Sayegh HE, Brunelle CL, Daniell KM, Taghian AG. Breast cancer-related lymphedema: risk

factors, precautionary measures, and treatments. *Gland Surg*. 2018;7(4):379–403.
24. Shaitelman SF, Chiang YJ, Griffin KD, et al. Radiation therapy targets and the risk of breast cancer-related lymphedema: a systematic review and network meta-analysis. *Breast Cancer Res Treat*. 2017;162(2):201–215.
25. McDuff SGR, Mina AI, Brunelle CL, et al. Timing of lymphedema after treatment for breast cancer: When are patients most at risk? *Int J Radiat Oncol Biol Phys*. 2019;103(1):62–70.
26. Finegold DN, Baty CJ, Knickelbein KZ, et al. Connexin 47 mutations increase risk for secondary lymphedema following breast cancer treatment. *Clin Cancer Res*. 2012;18(8):2382–2390.
27. Finegold DN, Schacht V, Kimak MA, et al. HGF and MET mutations in primary and secondary lymphedema. *Lymphat Res Biol*. 2008;6(2):65–68.
28. Horst L, Chen JJ. Radiation considerations. In: Lee BB, Rockson SG, Bergan J, eds. *Lymphedema: A Concise Compendium of Theory and Practice*. 2nd ed. Cham, Switzerland: Springer; 2018:899–909.
29. Biglia N, Zanfagnin V, Daniele A, Robba E, Bounous VE. Lower body lymphedema in patients with gynecologic cancer. *Anticancer Res*. 2017;37(8):4005–4015.
30. Yamazaki H, Todo Y, Takeshita S, et al. Relationship between removal of circumflex iliac nodes distal to the external iliac nodes and postoperative lower-extremity lymphedema in uterine cervical cancer. *Gynecol Oncol*. 2015;139(2):295–299.
31. Lindqvist E, Wedin M, Fredrikson M, Kjølhede P. Lymphedema after treatment for endometrial cancer – a review of prevalence and risk factors. *Eur J Obstet Gynecol Reprod Biol*. 2017;211:112–121.
32. Abu-Rustum NR, Alektiar K, Iasonos A, et al. The incidence of symptomatic lower-extremity lymphedema following treatment of uterine corpus malignancies: a 12-year experience at Memorial Sloan-Kettering Cancer Center. *Gynecol Oncol*. 2006;103(2):714–718.
33. Yost KJ, Cheville AL, Al-Hilli MM, et al. Lymphedema after surgery for endometrial cancer: prevalence, risk factors, and quality of life. *Obstet Gynecol*. 2014;124(2 Pt 1): 307–315.
34. Robison K, Holman LL, Moore RG. Update on sentinel lymph node evaluation in gynecologic malignancies. *Curr Opin Obstet Gynecol*. 2011;23(1):8–12.
35. Shaitelman SF, Cromwell KD, Rasmussen JC, et al. Recent progress in the treatment and prevention of cancer-related lymphedema. *CA Cancer J Clin*. 2015;65 (1):55–81.
36. Treves N. An evaluation of the etiological factors of lymphedema following radical mastectomy; an analysis of 1,007 cases. *Cancer*. 1957;10(3):444–459.
37. Mehrara BJ, Greene AK. Lymphedema and obesity: is there a link? *Plast Reconstr Surg*. 2014;134 (1):154e–160e. Available from: https://doi.org/10.1097/PRS.0000000000000268.
38. Shaw C, Mortimer P, Judd PA. A randomized controlled trial of weight reduction as a treatment for breast cancer-related lymphedema. *Cancer*. 2007;110 (8):1868–1874.
39. Executive Committee. The diagnosis and treatment of peripheral lymphedema: 2016 Consensus Document of the International Society of Lymphology. *Lymphology*. 2016;49(4):170–184.
40. Endicott K, Laredo J, Lee BB. Combined clinical and laboratory lymphoscintigraphic staging. In: Lee BB, Rockson SG, Bergan J, eds. *Lymphedema: A Concise Compendium of Theory and Practice*. 2nd ed. Cham, Switzerland: Springer; 2018:187–196.
41. Levenhagen K, Davies C, Perdomo M, Ryans K, Gilchrist L. Diagnosis of upper-quadrant lymphedema secondary to cancer: clinical practice guideline from the oncology section of APTA. *Phys Ther*. 2017;97(7):729–745.
42. Rockson SG. Clinical diagnosis, General overview. In: Lee BB, Rockson SG, Bergan J, eds. *Lymphedema: A Concise Compendium of Theory and Practice*. 2nd ed. Cham, Switzerland: Springer; 2018:155–163.
43. Zuther JE, Cormier JN, Cromwell KD, et al. Pathology lymphedema. In: Zuther JE, Norton S, eds. *Lymphedema Management: The Comprehensive Guide for Practitioners*. 3rd ed. Stuttgart, Germany: Thieme; 2013:46–74.
44. Johnson KC, Kennedy AG, Henry SM. Clinical measurements of lymphedema. *Lymphat Res Biol*. 2014;12 (4):216–221.
45. Perdomo M, Davies C, Levenhagen K, Ryans K. Breast cancer edge task force outcomes. Assessment measures of secondary lymphedema in breast cancer survivors. *Rehabil Oncol*. 2014;32(1):22–35.
46. Yamamoto T. Near-infrared fluorescent lymphography. In: Lee BB, Rockson SG, Bergan JJ, eds. *Lymphedema: A Concise Compendium of Theory and Practice*. 2nd ed. Cham, Switzerland: Springer; 2018:345–355.
47. Chang DW, Suami H, Skoracki R. A prospective analysis of 100 consecutive lymphovenous bypass cases for treatment of extremity lymphedema. *Plastic Reconstr Surg*. 2013;132(5):1305–1314.
48. Armer JM, Radina ME, Porock D, Culbertson SD. Predicting breast cancer-related lymphedema using self-reported symptoms. *Nurs Res*. 2003;52(6):370–379.
49. Hayes S, Janda M, Cornish B, Battistutta D, Newman B. Lymphedema secondary to breast cancer: how choice of measure influences diagnosis, prevalence, and identifiable risk factors. *Lymphology*. 2008;41(1):18–28.
50. Kosir MA, Rymal C, Koppolu P, et al. Surgical outcomes after breast cancer surgery: measuring acute lymphedema. *J Surg Res*. 2001;95(2):147–151.
51. Carter J, Raviv L, Appollo K, Baser RE, Iasonos A, Barakat RR. A pilot study using the Gynecologic Cancer Lymphedema Questionnaire (GCLQ) as a clinical care tool to identify lower extremity lymphedema in gynecologic cancer survivors. *Gynecol Oncol*. 2010;117 (2):317–323.

52. Svensson BJ, Dylke ES, Ward LC, Black DA, Kilbreath SL. Screening for breast cancer-related lymphoedema: self-assessment of symptoms and signs (published online ahead of print October 22, 2019). *Support Care Cancer*. 2019. Available from: https://doi.org/10.1007/s00520-019-05083-7.
53. Hassanein AH, Maclellan RA, Grant FD, Greene AK. Diagnostic accuracy of lymphoscintigraphy for lymphedema and analysis of false-negative tests. *Plast Reconstr Surg Glob Open*. 2017;5(7):e1396. Available from: https://doi.org/10.1097/GOX.0000000000001396.
54. Bae JS, Yoo RE, Choi SH, et al. Evaluation of lymphedema in upper extremities by MR lymphangiography: comparison with lymphoscintigraphy. *J Magn Reson Imaging*. 2018;49:63–70.
55. Mayrovitz HN, Weingrad DN, Lopez L. Patterns of temporal changes in tissue dielectric constant as indices of localized skin water changes in women treated for breast cancer: a pilot study. *Lymphat Res Biol*. 2015;13(1):20–32.
56. National Lymphedema Network. National lymphedema network position statement: Screening and early detection of breast cancer-related lymphedema: The Imperative. Available from: https://lymphnet.org/position-papers. Accessed December 21, 2019.
57. Stout Gergich NL, Pfalzer LA, McGarvey C, Springer B, Gerber LH, Soballe P. Preoperative assessment enables the early diagnosis and successful treatment of lymphedema. *Cancer*. 2008;112(12):2809–2819.
58. Soran A, Ozmen T, McGuire KP, et al. The importance of detection of subclinical lymphedema for the prevention of breast cancer-related clinical lymphedema after axillary lymph node dissection; a prospective observational study. *Lymphat Res Biol*. 2014;12(4):289–294.
59. Stout NL, Pfalzer LA, Springer B, et al. Breast cancer-related lymphedema: comparing direct costs of a prospective surveillance model and a traditional model of care. *Phys Ther*. 2012;92(1):152–163.
60. Brunelle C, Skolny M, Ferguson C, Swaroop M, O'Toole J, Taghian AG. Establishing and sustaining a prospective screening program for breast cancer-related lymphedema at the Massachusetts general hospital: lessons learned. *J Pers Med*. 2015;5(2):153–164.
61. Sun F, Skolny MN, Swaroop MN, et al. The need for preoperative baseline arm measurement to accurately quantify breast cancer-related lymphedema. *Breast Cancer Res Treat*. 2016;157(2):229–240.
62. Ostby PL, Armer JM, Dale PS, Van Loo MJ, Wilbanks CL, Stewart BR. Surveillance recommendations in reducing risk of and optimally managing breast cancer-related lymphedema. *J Pers Med*. 2014;4(3):424–447.
63. Gebruers N, Verbelen H, De Vrieze T, et al. Current and future perspectives on the evaluation, prevention and conservative management of breast cancer related lymphoedema: a best practice guideline. *Eur J Obstet Gynecol Reprod Biol*. 2017;216:245–253.
64. Földi E, Földi M, Rockson SG. Complete decongestive physiotherapy. In: Lee BB, Rockson SG, Bergan J, eds. *Lymphedema: A Concise Compendium of Theory and Practice*. 2nd ed. Cham, Switzerland: Springer; 2018:403–411.
65 Rockson SG. Lymphedema. *Am J Med*. 2001;110(4):288–295.
66. Lasinski BB, McKillip Thrift K, Squire D, et al. A systematic review of the evidence for complete decongestive therapy in the treatment of lymphedema from 2004 to 2011. *PM R*. 2012;4(8):580–601.
67. Sayegh HE, Asdourian MS, Swaroop MN, et al. Diagnostic methods, risk factors, prevention, and management of breast cancer-related lymphedema: past, present, and future directions. *Curr Breast Cancer Rep*. 2017;9(2):111–121.
68. Ezzo J, Manheimer E, McNeely ML, et al. Manual lymphatic drainage for lymphedema following breast cancer treatment. *Cochrane Database Syst Rev*. 2015;(5) CD003475. Available from: https://doi.org/10.1002/14651858.CD003475.pub2.
69. Tan IC, Maus EA, Rasmussen JC, et al. Assessment of lymphatic contractile function after manual lymphatic drainage using near-infrared fluorescence imaging. *Arch Phys Med Rehabil*. 2011;92(5):756–764.e1.
70 Torres Lacomba M, Yuste Sanchez MJ, Zapico Goni A, et al. Effectiveness of early physiotherapy to prevent lymphoedema after surgery for breast cancer: randomised, single blinded, clinical trial. *BMJ (Clinical research ed.)*. 2010;340:b5396.
71. Suami H, Heydon-White A, Mackie H, Czerniec S, Koelmeyer L, Boyages J. A new indocyanine green fluorescence lymphography protocol for identification of the lymphatic drainage pathway for patients with breast cancer-related lymphoedema. *BMC Cancer*. 2019;19(1):985.
72. Mosti G, Cavezzi A. Compression therapy in lymphedema: between past and recent scientific data. *Phlebology*. 2019;34(8):515–522.
73. Lee B, Andrade M, Bergan J, et al. Diagnosis and treatment of primary lymphedema. Consensus document of the International Union of Phlebology IUP-2009. *Int Angiol*. 2010;29(5):454–470.
74. McNeely ML, Magee DJ, Lees AW, Bagnall KM, Haykowsky M, Hanson J. The addition of manual lymph drainage to compression therapy for breast cancer related lymphedema: a randomized controlled trial. *Breast Cancer Res Treat*. 2004;86(2):95–106.
75. Andersen L, Højris I, Erlandsen M, Andersen J. Treatment of breast-cancer-related lymphedema with or without manual lymphatic drainage—a randomized study. *Acta Oncol*. 2000;39(3):399–405.
76. Dayes IS, Whelan TJ, Julian JA, et al. Randomized trial of decongestive lymphatic therapy for the treatment of lymphedema in women with breast cancer. *J Clin Oncol*. 2013;31(30):3758–3763.
77. Zasadzka E, Trzmiel T, Kleczewska M, Pawlaczyk M. Comparison of the effectiveness of complex decongestive therapy and compression bandaging as a method of treatment of lymphedema in the elderly. *Clin Interv Aging*. 2018;13:929–934.

78. Partsch H, Clark M, Mosti G, et al. Classification of compression bandages: practical aspects. *Dermatol Surg*. 2008;34(5):600–609.
79. Partsch H, Rockson S. Compression therapy. In: Lee BB, Rockson SG, Bergan JJ, eds. *Lymphedema: A Concise Compendium of Theory and Practice*. 2nd ed. Cham, Switzerland: Springer; 2018:431–441.
80. Damstra RJ, Partsch H. Compression therapy in breast cancer-related lymphedema: a randomized, controlled comparative study of relation between volume and interface pressure changes. *J Vasc Surg*. 2009;49 (5):1256–1263.
81. Damstra RJ, Partsch H. Prospective, randomized, controlled trial comparing the effectiveness of adjustable compression Velcro wraps versus inelastic multicomponent compression bandages in the initial treatment of leg lymphedema. *J Vasc Surg Venous Lymphat Disord*. 2013;1(1):13–19.
82. Mosti G, Cavezzi A, Partsch H, Urso S, Campana F. Adjustable Velcro Compression Devices are more effective than inelastic bandages in reducing venous edema in the initial treatment phase: a randomized controlled trial. *Eur J Vasc Endovasc Surg*. 2015;50 (3):368–374.
83. Lee BB, Andrade M, Antignani PL, et al. Diagnosis and treatment of primary lymphedema. Consensus document of the International Union of Phlebology (IUP)-2013. *Int Angiol*. 2013;32(6):541–574.
84. Ochalek K, Gradalski T, Partsch H. Preventing early postoperative arm swelling and lymphedema manifestation by compression sleeves after axillary lymph node interventions in breast cancer patients: a randomized controlled trial. *J Pain Symptom Manage*. 2017;54 (3):346–354.
85. Partsch H, Stout N, Forner-Cordero I, et al. Clinical trials needed to evaluate compression therapy in breast cancer related lymphedema (BCRL). Proposals from an expert group. *Int Angiol*. 2010;29(5):442–453.
86. Ochalek K, Partsch H, Gradalski T, Szygula Z. Do compression sleeves reduce the incidence of arm lymphedema and improve quality of life? two-year results from a prospective randomized trial in breast cancer survivors. *Lymphat Res Biol*. 2019;17(1):70–77.
87. Rockson SG. Intermittent pneumatic compression therapy. In: Lee BB, Rockson SG, Bergan J, eds. *Lymphedema: A Concise Compendium of Theory and Practice*. 2nd ed. Cham, Switzerland: Springer; 2018:443–448.
88. Feldman JL, Stout NL, Wanchai A, Stewart BR, Cormier JN, Armer JM. Intermittent pneumatic compression therapy: a systematic review. *Lymphology*. 2012;45 (1):13–25.
89. Shao Y, Qi K, Zhou QH, Zhong DS. Intermittent pneumatic compression pump for breast cancer-related lymphedema: a systematic review and meta-analysis of randomized controlled trials. *Oncl Res Treat*. 2014;37 (4):170–174.
90. Szuba A, Achalu R, Rockson SG. Decongestive lymphatic therapy for patients with breast carcinoma-associated lymphedema. A randomized, prospective study of a role for adjunctive intermittent pneumatic compression. *Cancer*. 2002;95(11):2260–2267.
91. Aldrich MB, Gross D, Morrow JR, Fife CE, Rasmussen JC. Effect of pneumatic compression therapy on lymph movement in lymphedema-affected extremities, as assessed by near-infrared fluorescence lymphatic imaging. *J Innov Opt Health Sci*. 2017;10 (2):1650049. Available from: https://doi.org/10.1142/S1793545816500498.
92. Zaleska M, Olszewski WL, Cakala M, Cwikla J, Budlewski T. Intermittent pneumatic compression enhances formation of edema tissue fluid channels in lymphedema of lower limbs. *Lymphat Res Biol*. 2015;13 (2):146–153.
93. Phillips JJ, Gordon SJ. Intermittent pneumatic compression dosage for adults and children with lymphedema: a systematic review. *Lymphat Res Biol*. 2019;17(1):2–18.
94. National Lymphedema Network. Position statement on exercise. Available from: https://lymphnet.org/position-papers. 2012. Accessed December 21, 2019.
95. Zawieja DC. Contractile physiology of lymphatics. *Lymphat Res Biol*. 2009;7(2):87–96.
96. Mukherjee AHJ, Dixon JB. Physiology: lymph flow. In: Lee BB, Rockson SG, Bergan J, eds. *Lymphedema: A Concise Compendium of Theory and Practice*. 2nd ed. Cham, Switzerland: Springer; 2018:91–111.
97. Schmitz KH, Ahmed RL, Troxel A, et al. Weight lifting in women with breast-cancer-related lymphedema. *N Engl J Med*. 2009;361(7):664–673.
98. Schmitz KH, Troxel AB, Cheville A, et al. Physical activity and lymphedema (the PAL trial): assessing the safety of progressive strength training in breast cancer survivors. *Contemp Clin Trials*. 2009;30(3):233–245.
99. Schmitz KH. Balancing lymphedema risk: exercise versus deconditioning for breast cancer survivors. *Exerc Sport Sci Rev*. 2010;38(1):17–24.
100. Ahmed RL, Thomas W, Yee D, Schmitz KH. Randomized controlled trial of weight training and lymphedema in breast cancer survivors. *J Clin Oncol*. 2006;24(18):2765–2772.
101. Cormie P, Pumpa K, Galvao DA, et al. Is it safe and efficacious for women with lymphedema secondary to breast cancer to lift heavy weights during exercise: a randomised controlled trial. *J Cancer Surviv*. 2013;7 (3):413–424.
102. Zhang X, Brown JC, Paskett ED, Zemel BS, Cheville AL, Schmitz KH. Changes in arm tissue composition with slowly progressive weight-lifting among women with breast cancer-related lymphedema. *Breast Cancer Res Treat*. 2017;164(1):79–88.
103. Singh B, Disipio T, Peake J, Hayes SC. Systematic review and meta-analysis of the effects of exercise for those with cancer-related lymphedema. *Arch Phys Med Rehabil*. 2016;97(2):302–315.

104. Singh B, Buchan J, Box R, et al. Compression use during an exercise intervention and associated changes in breast cancer-related lymphedema. *Asia Pac J Clin Oncol*. 2016;12(3):216–224.
105. Singh B, Newton RU, Cormie P, et al. Effects of compression on lymphedema during resistance exercise in women with breast cancer-related lymphedema: a randomized cross-over trial. *Lymphology*. 2015;48(2):80–92.
106. Schmitz KH, Courneya KS, Matthews C, et al. American College of Sports Medicine roundtable on exercise guidelines for cancer survivors. *Med Sci Sports Exerc*. 2010;42(7):1409–1426.
107. Shaw C, Mortimer P, Judd PA. Randomized controlled trial comparing a low-fat diet with a weight-reduction diet in breast cancer-related lymphedema. *Cancer*. 2007;109(10):1949–1956.
108. Panchik D, Masco S, Zinnikas P, et al. Effect of exercise on breast cancer-related lymphedema: what the lymphatic surgeon needs to know. *J Reconstr Microsurg*. 2019;35(1):37–45.
109. Fisher MI, Donahoe-Fillmore B, Leach L, et al. Effects of yoga on arm volume among women with breast cancer related lymphedema: a pilot study. *J Bodyw Mov Ther*. 2014;18(4):559–565.
110. Şener HÖ, Malkoç M, Ergin G, Karadibak D, Yavuzşen T. Effects of clinical pilates exercises on patients developing lymphedema after breast cancer treatment: a randomized clinical trial. *J Breast Health*. 2017;13 (1):16–22.
111. Tidhar D, Drouin J, Shimony A. Aqua lymphatic therapy in managing lower extremity lymphedema. *J Support Oncol*. 2007;5(4):179–183.
112. Letellier ME, Towers A, Shimony A, Tidhar D. Breast cancer-related lymphedema: a randomized controlled pilot and feasibility study. *Am J Phys Med Rehabil*. 2014;93(9):751–759.
113. Gianesini S, Tessari M, Bacciglieri P, et al. A specifically designed aquatic exercise protocol to reduce chronic lower limb edema. *Phlebology*. 2017;32 (9):594–600.
114. Yeung W, Semciw AI. Aquatic therapy for people with lymphedema: a systematic review and meta-analysis. *Lymphat Res Biol*. 2018;16(1):9–19.
115. Smoot B, Chiavola-Larson L, Lee J, Manibusan H, Allen DD. Effect of low-level laser therapy on pain and swelling in women with breast cancer-related lymphedema: a systematic review and meta-analysis. *J Cancer Surviv*. 2015;9(2):287–304.
116. Chung H, Dai T, Sharma SK, Huang YY, Carroll JD, Hamblin MR. The nuts and bolts of low-level laser (light) therapy. *Ann Biomed Eng*. 2012;40(2):516–533.
117. Bell L, Stout NL. Using low-level light laser in your lymphedema practice: benefits and cautions. *Rehabil Oncol*. 2018;36(1):70–72.
118. Piller NB, Thelander A. Treatment of chronic postmastectomy lymphedema with low level laser therapy: a 2.5 year follow-up. *Lymphology*. 1998;31(2):74–86.
119. Lawenda BD, Mondry TE, Johnstone PA. Lymphedema: a primer on the identification and management of a chronic condition in oncologic treatment. *CA Cancer J Clin.*. 2009;59(1):8–24.
120. Carati CJ, Anderson SN, Gannon BJ, Piller NB. Treatment of postmastectomy lymphedema with low-level laser therapy: a double blind, placebo-controlled trial. *Cancer*. 2003;98(6):1114–1122.
121. Ridner SH, Poage-Hooper E, Kanar C, Doersam JK, Bond SM, Dietrich MS. A pilot randomized trial evaluating low-level laser therapy as an alternative treatment to manual lymphatic drainage for breast cancer-related lymphedema. *Oncol Nurs Forum*. 2013;40(4):383–393.
122. Dirican A, Andacoglu O, Johnson R, McGuire K, Mager L, Soran A. The short-term effects of low-level laser therapy in the management of breast-cancer-related lymphedema. *Support Care Cancer*. 2011;19(5):685–690.
123. Assis L, Moretti AI, Abrahao TB, de Souza HP, Hamblin MR, Parizotto NA. Low-level laser therapy (808 nm) contributes to muscle regeneration and prevents fibrosis in rat tibialis anterior muscle after cryolesion. *Lasers Med Sci*. 2013;28(3):947–955.
124. Jang DH, Song DH, Chang EJ, Jeon JY. Anti-inflammatory and lymphangiogenetic effects of low-level laser therapy on lymphedema in an experimental mouse tail model. *Lasers Med Sci*. 2016;31(2):289–296.
125. Ahmed Omar MT, Abd-El-Gayed Ebid A, El Morsy AM. Treatment of post-mastectomy lymphedema with laser therapy: double blind placebo control randomized study. *J Surg Res*. 2011;165(1):82–90.
126. Baxter GD, Liu L, Petrich S, et al. Low level laser therapy (Photobiomodulation therapy) for breast cancer-related lymphedema: a systematic review. *BMC Cancer*. 2017;17(1):833.
127. Finnerty S, Thomason S, Woods M. Audit of the use of kinesiology tape for breast oedema. *J Lymphoedema*. 2010;5(1):38–44.
128. Tremback-Ball A, Harding R, Heffner K, Zimmerman A. The efficacy of kinesiology taping in the treatment of women with post–mastectomy lymphedema: a systematic review. *J Womens Health Phys Ther*. 2018;42(2):94–103.
129. Tsai HJ, Hung HC, Yang JL, Huang CS, Tsauo JY. Could Kinesio tape replace the bandage in decongestive lymphatic therapy for breast-cancer-related lymphedema? A pilot study. *Support Care Cancer*. 2009;17(11):1353–1360.
130. Taradaj J, Halski T, Rosinczuk J, Dymarek R, Laurowski A, Smykla A. The influence of kinesiology taping on the volume of lymphoedema and manual dexterity of the upper limb in women after breast cancer treatment. *Eur J Cancer Care (Engl)*. 2016;25(4):647–660.
131. Tantawy SA, Abdelbasset WK, Nambi G, Kamel DM. Comparative study between the effects of Kinesio taping and pressure garment on secondary upper extremity lymphedema and quality of life following mastectomy: a randomized controlled trial. *Integr Cancer Ther*. 2019;18. Available from: https://doi.org/10.1177/1534735419847276.

132. Bosman J, Piller N. Lymph taping and seroma formation post breast cancer. *J Lymphoedema*. 2010;5(2):12–21.
133. Gatt M, Willis S, Leuschner S. A meta-analysis of the effectiveness and safety of kinesiology taping in the management of cancer-related lymphoedema. *Eur J Cancer Care (Engl)*. 2017;26(5). Available from: https://doi.org/10.1111/ecc.12510.
134. Teng E, Chang DW. Overview of surgical techniques. In: Cheng MH, Chang DW, Patel KM, eds. *Principles and Practice of Lymphedema Surgery*. Elsevier; 2016.
135. McLaughlin SA, DeSnyder SM, Klimberg S, et al. Considerations for clinicians in the diagnosis, prevention, and treatment of breast cancer-related lymphedema, recommendations from an expert panel: Part 2: preventive and therapeutic Options. *Ann Surg Oncol*. 2017;24(10):2827–2835. Available from: https://doi.org/10.1245/s10434-017-5964-6. Epub 2017 Aug 1.
136. National Comprehensive Cancer Network. Breast Cancer, Version 1.2015 update. Available from: https://www.nccn.org/about/news/ebulletin/ebulletindetail.aspx?ebulletinid=498. Accessed December 4, 2019.
137. McLaughlin SA, Staley AC, Vicini F, et al. Considerations for clinicians in the diagnosis, prevention, and treatment of breast cancer-related lymphedema: recommendations from a multidisciplinary expert ASBrS Panel: Part 1: Definitions, assessments, education, and future directions. *Ann Surg Oncol*. 2017;24(10):2818–2826.
138. Fu MR, Axelrod D, Cleland CM, et al. Symptom report in detecting breast cancer-related lymphedema. *Breast Cancer (Dove Med Press)*. 2015;7:345–352.
139. Fu MR, Chen CM, Haber J, Guth AA, Axelrod D. The effect of providing information about lymphedema on the cognitive and symptom outcomes of breast cancer survivors. *Ann Surg Oncol*. 2010;17(7):1847–1853.
140. Ostby PL, Armer JM, Smith K, Stewart BR. Patient perceptions of barriers to self-management of breast cancer-related lymphedema. *West J Nur Res*. 2018;40(12):1800–1817.
141. Ferguson CM, Swaroop MN, Horick N, et al. Impact of ipsilateral blood draws, injections, blood pressure measurements, and air travel on the risk of lymphedema for patients treated for breast cancer. *J Clin Oncol*. 2016;34(7):691–698.
142. Shaitelman SF, Cromwell KD, Rasmussen JC, et al. Recent progress in the treatment and prevention of cancer-related lymphedema. *CA Cancer J Clin*. 2015;65(1):55–81.
143. McLaughlin SA, Bagaria S, Gibson T, et al. Trends in risk reduction practices for the prevention of lymphedema in the first 12 months after breast cancer surgery. *J Am Coll Surg*. 2013;216(3):380–389.
144. National Lymphedema Network. Lymphedema risk reduction practices (Internet). Available from https://lymphnet.org/position-papers. Accessed December 19, 2019.
145. Asdourian MS, Swaroop MN, Sayegh HE, et al. Association between precautionary behaviors and breast cancer-related lymphedema in patients undergoing bilateral surgery. *J Clin Oncol*. 2017;35(35):3934–3941.
146. Kilbreath SL, Refshauge KM, Beith JM, et al. Risk factors for lymphoedema in women with breast cancer: a large prospective cohort. *Breast*. 2016;28:29–36.
147. Co M, Ng J, Kwong A. Air travel and postoperative lymphedema—a systematic review. *Clin Breast Cancer*. 2018;18(1):e151–e155.
148. Nudelman J. Debunking lymphedema risk-reduction behaviors: risky conclusions. *Lymphat Res Biol*. 2016;14(3):124–126.

CHAPTER 22

Peripheral Nervous System Involvement in Breast and Gynecologic Cancers

FRANCHESCA KÖNIG, MD • CHRISTIAN M. CUSTODIO, MD

INTRODUCTION

In its simplest form a peripheral nervous system injury is described as a lesion or damage to one or more of the nerves located outside of the brain and spinal cord. Causes are extensive and presentations may be highly variable. There are known congenital, nutritional, metabolic, and traumatic etiologies, among others. In the realm of oncology, peripheral nerve injuries are a widely recognized, but still likely underreported, complication of both the cancer itself and its treatment. Prompt diagnosis and subsequent management is of utmost importance, as these types of nerve injuries may have a detrimental effect on both function and quality of life. While no cancer type is necessarily exempt, this chapter will focus on nerve injuries as they relate to breast cancer and its treatment.

Patients with breast and gynecological cancers may experience damage to the nerves as a result of a number of different mechanisms. Direct neuromuscular effects may occur due to direct tumor compression or leptomeningeal disease (LMD). Paraneoplastic syndromes, such as stiff-person syndrome, occur as an immune response triggered by the cancer. Treatment may ultimately affect the nervous system as well. Chemotherapeutic treatments may cause length-dependent neuropathies. Radiation has the potential to cause an inflammatory state within the radiation field, which, in turn, may cause brachial or lumbosacral plexopathies depending on the location. Surgical procedures, including mastectomies and debulking surgeries, may also potentially cause some form of nerve damage.

Physicians specialized in cancer rehabilitation assist with the diagnosis and treatment of these types of injuries, among others. A detailed history along with a neurologic examination and further workup, including blood values, specialized neuroimaging, and electrodiagnostic studies, are warranted in the evaluation of nerve injuries. The importance of a clear diagnosis is twofold, both in providing a functional prognosis and subsequent management, including treatment and determining if oncologic management requires modification. In this vein, cancer rehabilitation specialists collaborate closely with oncologists, therapists, and other health-care professionals. Early intervention, including prevention, identification, and treatment, can reduce the occurrence of functional limitations.

DIRECT NEUROMUSCULAR EFFECTS

Mononeuropathy

Focal mononeuropathies related to cancer may occur as a result of direct compression or infiltration from a primary tumor or metastases. Tumors arising from nerve components are typically benign, such as schwannomas and neurofibromas. Metastases to individual nerves are rare. Clinical presentation is dependent upon the individual nerves being affected. In patients with breast and gynecological cancers, mononeuropathies more commonly result as an indirect complication from the cancer or treatment, such as rapid weight loss resulting in a peroneal nerve compression neuropathy or median neuropathy arising from lymphedema.

Plexopathy

It has been estimated that neoplastic (tumor) brachial plexopathies occur with a frequency of approximately 0.43% in patients with cancer, most commonly occurring in those with lung (37%) and breast (32%) cancers.[1] These types of plexopathies are divided into primary and secondary. Primary neoplastic plexopathies are rare and most commonly benign in nature.

Breast Cancer and Gynecologic Cancer Rehabilitation DOI: https://doi.org/10.1016/B978-0-323-72166-0.00022-0

Of these, schwannomas are the most common (83%), followed by neurofibromas (9%). Less commonly, these tumors are malignant, such as malignant peripheral nerve sheath tumors (9%).[2] Secondary neoplastic plexopathies are considered malignant and tend to occur as a late-stage complication of cancer.[3] They occur as an extension and infiltration of either the primary tumor or metastases causing compression. Similarly, malignant lumbosacral plexopathies may also occur. While still rare, literature suggests that neoplastic lumbosacral plexopathies occur more frequently in patients with prostate cancer (through proliferation through the plexus) and less frequently in ovarian cancer (which tends to involve pressure on the lumbosacral plexus).[4]

Clinically, pain is the most common presenting symptom (75%–98%), followed by the development of weakness and sensory deficits. Distribution of symptoms is dependent on the anatomic location of the lesion. MRI, CT, and positron emission tomography (PET) scans all serve diagnostic purposes, with MRI scans providing the best anatomic detail. While tumor plexopathies may involve the whole plexus, electrodiagnostic studies have shown involvement of the lower trunk and medial cord occurring more commonly.[5] Treatment commonly involves local radiation therapy with improvement of pain in approximately 46%–86% of patients.[1] Patients may benefit from early intervention utilizing a multimodal approach, including physical and occupational therapy, bracing evaluation, analgesics, and specialized procedures, such as regional nerve blocks.

Radiculopathy

Osseous metastatic disease in breast cancer may present as osteoblastic, osteolytic, or mixed lesions to the bone and can increase the risk for skeletal-related events, defined as pathological fractures, spinal cord or nerve root compression, and bone pain or impending fracture requiring radiation therapy or surgery. In patients with breast cancer, approximately 5% present with metastases at the time of their initial diagnosis, with bone being the most common site.[6] Postmortem evaluation has demonstrated evidence of metastatic osseous disease in up to 70% of patients.[7] There appears to be a predilection for the spine, accounting for two-thirds of osseous metastases in patients with breast cancer. Furthermore, one-third of these lesions to the spine become symptomatic, resulting in pain and neurologic deficits.[8] While they may occur, osseous metastases are much less common in gynecologic cancers. Literature suggests the incidence of primary bone metastases in endometrial cancer is less than 1%.[9] Complications may involve spinal cord compression and pathologic fractures. Prognosis is typically poor, and patients are usually treated with palliative radiation for pain control and improved quality of life.[10]

Any patient with cancer presenting with new onset back or neck pain warrants a thorough, detailed evaluation. Pain in the thoracic spine is more suspicious for metastatic disease as symptomatic degenerative disease more commonly involves the cervical and lumbar regions. After spinal stenosis and disk disease, tumors involving the spine are the most common causes of radiculopathy[11] and result in compression or irritation of individual nerve roots via tumor infiltration. Radicular pain is commonly described as shooting pain along the dermatomal distribution of a nerve root. As in nonmalignancy-related radiculopathies, weakness and sensory deficits may also occur. MRI of the spine is the gold-standard diagnostic modality, while PET and CT scans may also play a role depending on the type of osseous lesion. Treatment may consist of physical therapy with an emphasis on core and spine extensor strengthening, neuromodulators, radiation therapy, and surgical nerve root decompression.[8]

Leptomeningeal Disease

LMD refers to the infiltration of the meninges surrounding the brain and spinal cord by malignant tumor cells. Along with lung and melanoma, breast cancer is among the most common types of cancers associated with LMD. It has been shown to occur in approximately 10%–25% of patients with breast cancer who have developed metastases to the central nervous system (CNS). Furthermore, an increased incidence has been found in patients with triple-negative breast cancer (approximately 30%–40% of breast LMD), suggesting the presence of tumor-specific biological risk factors. Dissemination is believed to be secondary to hematogenous spread through arterial or venous circulation or lymphatic system spread. Tumor cell extension into the cerebrospinal fluid (CSF) from adjacent CNS disease is also thought to play a role.[12] As with osseous metastases, LMD in gynecologic malignancies is considered rare.

Diagnosis may be difficult as patients can present with a highly variable constellation of symptoms, including both radicular and focal pain, paresthesias, weakness, areflexia, upper motor neuron signs, and cranial nerve involvement (most commonly oculomotor, facial, and auditory nerves).[13] Clinical symptoms are thought to be related to disease infiltration of neurologic tissue. Patients may also exhibit nausea, vomiting, positional headaches, and altered mental status secondary to obstructive hydrocephalus increasing intracranial pressure. Up to 80% of patients are symptomatic at the moment of diagnosis.[14] Furthermore, patients may exhibit a rapidly progressive neurologic decline depending on disease burden.

There is currently no gold-standard diagnostic evaluation. If there is a clinical suspicion for LMD, MRI with gadolinium contrast of both brain and spine, CSF cytology, and a detailed neurologic evaluation are all warranted. MRI findings may include enhancing nodules of the leptomeninges and sulcal, linear ependymal, and cranial nerve root enhancement. Imaging abnormalities have been found in approximately 70%–80% of patients. CSF studies may reveal the presence of tumor cells. While the sensitivity of these studies is limited, repeating CSF cytology increases sensitivity to above 90%.[14] In addition to a neurologic evaluation, electrodiagnostic studies serve as an extension to the physical examination and can reveal findings consistent with a polyradiculopathy.[13]

Similar to diagnostic evaluation, there is no generally accepted standard of care in the treatment of LMD. Treatment is personalized and dependent on disease burden, functional status, and associated medical comorbidities. Both radiation therapy and chemotherapy (intrathecal and systemic) can be utilized; however, overall prognosis is poor, for which treatment often times is considered more palliative than curative.

PARANEOPLASTIC SYNDROMES

Paraneoplastic neurological syndromes (PNS) are a group of nonmetastatic syndromes affecting any part of the central and peripheral nervous system occurring in patients with cancer. They are not caused by direct invasion, rather thought to be induced by antigens expressed by tumor cells, or as an immune response triggered by the cancer. PNS are extremely rare and are estimated to occur in 0.01% of all patients with cancer.[15] Among the most common malignancies associated with PNS are small-cell lung cancer (associated with Lambert–Eaton myasthenic syndrome), thymoma (associated with myasthenia gravis), and breast cancer (which may be associated with stiff-person syndrome). Gynecologic malignancies may also be associated with paraneoplastic syndromes. For instance, the incidence paraneoplastic subacute sensory neuropathy may occur in up to 33.3% of patients with ovarian cancer. Lambert–Eaton myasthenic syndrome, although as above, is more commonly associated with small-cell lung cancer and has also been associated with uterine leiomyosarcoma and small-cell carcinoma of the cervix.[16]

Given that any component of the neuraxial continuum may be affected, clinical presentation is highly variable, and diagnosis may be challenging. Patients usually present with symptoms occurring over weeks to months, producing significant and progressive functional disability. PNS usually present in patients with no known cancer history, for which early identification is crucial. It has been estimated that in up to 80% of patients, cancer is diagnosed within months to years.[15] One study demonstrated that the median time from neurologic symptom onset to diagnosis of breast cancer was 4 weeks.[17] Diagnostic workup, including MRI of the brain and spine, CSF cytology, serum paraneoplastic antibodies, and electrodiagnostic studies, is recommended in patients with clinical suspicion for PNS. Treatment is focused on effective control of the underlying malignancy.

Peripheral Neuropathy

While chemotherapy-induced peripheral neuropathy (CIPN) is a more common manifestation of peripheral neuropathy in breast cancer, paraneoplastic neuropathies have also been described. Paraneoplastic sensory neuronopathies usually present as an acute or subacute onset of asymmetric pain and sensory loss more common in the upper extremities. Sensory ataxia and pseudoathetoid movements have been described; however, motor deficits are typically absent.[13] As opposed to platin-induced peripheral neuropathy that predominantly affects proprioception and spares small-fiber modalities, paraneoplastic sensory neuronopathy examination reveals sensory loss to all modalities.[18] Subacute sensory neuronopathy is thought to occur secondary to destruction of the dorsal root ganglion by cytotoxic T lymphocytes. It is described as the classic paraneoplastic peripheral neuropathy and while it may occur in breast cancer, it is more commonly seen in small-cell lung cancer with evidence of anti-Hu antibodies.[15]

Some of the earliest reports of paraneoplastic sensorimotor neuropathy as a presenting symptom in breast cancer date back to the 1990s. Sensorimotor polyneuropathies may be more difficult to diagnose as the pattern of involvement may mimic polyneuropathy seen as a result of chemotherapy and other underlying medical conditions, such as diabetes mellitus. Clinical presentation is consistent with paresthesias, numbness, pain, and weakness in a stocking–glove distribution. The only differentiating factor may be a more rapid progression of clinical signs and symptoms compared to nonparaneoplastic polyneuropathy.[13] Paraneoplastic sensorimotor polyneuropathy occurs more commonly with plasma cell dyscrasia, such as multiple myeloma; however, it may also be seen in association with both breast and lung cancers. Antineuronal antibodies, most commonly anti-Hu, anti-Yo, and anti-Ri, have been detected in approximately 85% of cases.[19]

Stiff-Person Syndrome

Previously known as stiff-man syndrome, this syndrome of hyperactivity has both nonparaneoplastic and paraneoplastic variants. The nonparaneoplastic variant is associated with glutamic acid decarboxylase antibodies and is seen in patients with autoimmune diseases, such as diabetes mellitus type 1. While also considered an autoimmune phenomenon, the paraneoplastic variant is most commonly associated with antibodies against amphiphysin and more commonly detected in patients with breast cancer, although cases in patients with lung carcinoma and Hodgkin's lymphoma have also been described. Stiff-person syndrome is classically characterized by the gradual onset of painful axial and proximal lower extremity muscle stiffness and rigidity. Muscle contraction may be sustained, resulting in abnormal posturing. Symptoms may be precipitated by certain triggers, such as emotional upset or a loud noise. While not entirely understood, pathogenesis is thought to include a B cell–mediated process.[18] Electrodiagnostic evaluation is normal, with the exception of continuous motor unit activity on needle electromyography.[13] Treating the underlying malignancy is essential. Additional symptomatic treatment may also include antispasmodics.

TREATMENT RELATED

Chemotherapy

Chemotherapy-Induced Peripheral Neuropathy

CIPN is a common and often times disabling toxicity associated with the administration of chemotherapy. While CIPN is a well-recognized phenomenon, it is likely underreported. Understanding the epidemiology of CIPN is vital as the onset and progression of symptoms may ultimately require modification or discontinuation of chemotherapeutic protocols.

A wide variation of CIPN prevalence exists, owing largely to the utilization of numerous different measurement tools and scales. These may include the National Cancer Institute Common Terminology Criteria for Adverse Events, CIPN Assessment Tool, Total Neuropathy Scale, and the Patient Neurotoxicity Questionnaire. Despite this wide variability, literature has shown that both prevalence and incidence continue to be high. One study, utilizing the European Organization for Research and Treatment of Cancer Quality of Life Questionnaires C30 in patients with breast cancer, demonstrated CIPN prevalence of 73%.[20] Other studies have shown prevalence ranging from 53% to 97%.[21,22] Despite such high statistics, prevalence has been shown to decrease after completion of chemotherapy—approximately 68% 1 month after completion of treatment, decreasing to 60% at 3 months, and down to 30% at 6 months.[23] In regard to incidence, literature has shown that both the percentage of patients exhibiting symptoms related to CIPN and the severity of the symptoms increases with cumulative dosing.[23,24]

While nearly all chemotherapeutic agents have been associated with peripheral neuropathies, there are specific groups that are notorious for expressing neurotoxic effects. Among these are the platinum-based antineoplastics (such as cisplatin and oxaliplatin), the vinca alkaloids (vincristine, vinblastine, vinorelbine), the taxanes (paclitaxel, docetaxel), proteasome inhibitors (such as bortezomib), and immunomodulatory drugs (such as thalidomide). Patients with breast cancer commonly undergo neoadjuvant or adjuvant treatment with taxanes. Patients with gynecologic cancers, including ovarian, endometrial, cervical, and uterine cancers, typically receive both platinum-based and taxane treatments. The mechanism of neurotoxic action is diverse and includes DNA and microtubular targets, causing cell division arrest and, ultimately, apoptosis. Altered microtubule function may disrupt vesicular axonal transport, leading to axonal loss via Wallerian degeneration. In addition to this, neurotoxic chemotherapeutic agents may cause oxidative stress, altered calcium homeostasis, membrane remodeling, immune processes, and neuroinflammation.[25]

CIPN commonly presents as a symmetric, length-dependent, sensory more than motor polyneuropathy. As such, a typical stocking–glove pattern is seen with the majority of agents. Alternatively, a glove–stocking pattern may be seen with platinum compounds in the setting of direct cytotoxic effects causing neurotmesis. Patients describe a wide range of predominantly sensory symptoms including paresthesias, numbness, allodynia, and hypersensitivity to temperature. Loss of proprioception and vibration may also occur, causing difficulty with fine motor tasks and gait. Symptom onset may be acute to subacute during chemotherapy. A phenomenon described as "coasting" has also been observed with vinca alkaloids and platinum-based compounds, in which symptoms either continue to progress despite completion of treatment or patients who were previously asymptomatic start to develop new symptoms.[26] Risk factors include underlying or preexisting peripheral neuropathies, duration of treatment, dosing and frequency of treatment, and coadministration with other neurotoxic agents.[27] Obesity, insomnia, and mood disorders (such as depression and anxiety) have also been described as risk factors.[28]

There is currently no standardized approach for the diagnosis of CIPN. Evaluation should be tailored to each individual patient and should begin with a detailed neurologic examination with close attention to sensation, strength, proprioception, vibration, gait, and balance. A neuropathy panel is valuable to evaluate for reversible causes of peripheral neuropathy, including diabetes mellitus, thyroid abnormalities, and nutritional deficiencies. Although not strictly necessary, electrodiagnostic studies may provide further diagnostic insight if presentation is atypical. Neuroimaging of the peripheral nerves is typically not indicated; however, if a compounding central cause is suspected, an MRI of brain and spine may be warranted.

Similarly, there are no standard preventative measures for CIPN. Cryotherapy has shown promising results with patient reported outcomes demonstrating a statistically significant reduction in patient reported outcomes.[29] Studies, however, have been limited. Trials studying the neuroprotective effect of anticonvulsants, such as pregabalin have been inconclusive.[30,31] Vitamins, such as alpha-lipoic acid and vitamin E, have also been studied. The majority of trials to date have predominantly offered a small sample size and low statistical power and have not provided significant conclusive evidence for clinically preventative measures. As of 2014, the American Society of Clinical Oncology clinical practice guidelines have not recommended any agents for the prevention of CIPN.

The treatment approach for CIPN is multimodal. Physical and occupational therapy should focus on individual deficits and impairments but typically includes focus on fine motor skills, nerve gliding techniques, strengthening, proprioception, and gait and balance training. Medications may also be used. Duloxetine has been shown to result in greater reduction in pain compared to placebo for painful CIPN.[32,33] It should be noted, however, that SSRIs, such as duloxetine, may reduce the concentration of Tamoxifen via the CYP2D6 pathway, for which concurrent use is generally avoided.[34] Neuromodulators, such as gabapentin and pregabalin, have been used anecdotally; however, supporting studies are limited. These medications may provide relief for positive symptoms (i.e., painful paresthesias, burning, sharp pain); however, they may provide little to no relief for negative symptoms (i.e., numbness).

Radiation

Radiation-Induced Brachial Plexopathy

Radiation-induced brachial plexopathy (RIBP) is a delayed, nontraumatic brachial plexus injury following radiotherapy to adjacent areas, including the chest wall, axilla, and neck. Frequency has been estimated to be between 1.8% and 4.9% in treated patients.[1] A percentage of 40 to 75 of reported cases have been found to be associated with radiation therapy for cancers of the breast, followed by lung cancer, and then lymphoma.[35] There does appear to be a correlation between the total dose of radiation and the risk of developing RIBP, with higher doses increasing the risk. Literature has shown that RIBP incidence has ranged from 66% in the 1960s when 60 Gy in 5 Gy fractions was the preferred dosing regimen to less than 1% with 50 Gy in 2 Gy fractions today.[36]

While RIBP is a well-recognized phenomenon, the pathophysiology remains less understood. Radiation may cause direct neurotoxic damage to the mature nerve, including the axon and vasa nervorum, from ionizing radiation with additional secondary and progressive microvascular injury.[1,37] Nerve trunk fibrosis with components of demyelination and axon loss has been found during surgery and at postmortem evaluation.[35] Risk factors may be either treatment-related or patient-related. Treatment-related factors include total dose of radiation, dose per fraction, and treatment schedule. Chemotherapy, especially when dosed concomitantly, has been suggested to increase the risk as well.[38] Patient-related factors may include advanced age, obesity, and underlying medical conditions such as hypertension, dyslipidemia, diabetes mellitus, and peripheral neuropathy.[36]

There appears to be a delayed onset of neurological symptoms with median time to onset typically described at 1.5 years, however, ranging from 6 months to 20 years after completion of radiation therapy.[39] Patients classically present with symptoms of paresthesias, which may decrease as numbness develops. Distribution of symptoms depends on the level of injury. Pain is typically less common. Weakness may develop later on, tends to be progressive, and may eventually result in paralysis of the affected upper extremity. Lymphedema may also be present, however, may concurrently develop as a result of ipsilateral lymph node dissection. Neurologic deficits tend to progressively worsen over the span of several years to the point of significant functional impairment in approximately two-thirds of patients. Spontaneous neurologic recovery at this point is much less likely.[35]

It may be challenging to clinically distinguish neoplastic versus RIBP. In fact, both conditions may occur simultaneously. Classically, neoplastic brachial plexopathy has been described as more painful and having a predilection for the lower trunk while RIBP has been described as less painful and typically affecting the upper portion of the plexus. Plexus involvement, however, may be more diffuse than previously thought. Electrodiagnostic studies demonstrate myokymia on electromyography in approximately 60% of patients.[1] It should be noted that while myokymia by itself is not pathognomonic for radiation-induced injury, it is assumed that this is in fact the etiology when it is present in patients who have received radiotherapy. It should be noted, however, that the absence of myokymia on electrodiagnostic studies does not rule out the possibility of radiation-induced injury. MRI of the brachial plexus remains useful in further evaluation of compressive or infiltrative lesions. In cases of RIBP, brachial plexus MRI may demonstrate linear areas of high signal intensity suggesting fibrosis.[37] More proximal imaging of the cervical spine should also be considered to rule out confounding involvement of the cervical nerve roots.

When developing a treatment plan, expectations should be set given the known clinical trajectory and depending on the patient's individual severity of symptoms. Physical therapy should focus on cervical, shoulder, and scapular range of motion and stretching exercises, chest expansion exercises, shoulder girdle and spine extensor strengthening, and myofascial release. Occupational therapy may also be beneficial for neuromuscular reeducation and fine motor skills. Intermittent bracing may be necessary to prevent development or progression of glenohumeral joint subluxation. If the patient is experiencing pain, neuropathic agents or a short course of prednisone may be considered. In addition, if the patient is experiencing lymphedema, it is reasonable to start a course of complex decongestive therapy and evaluation for compression garments.

Radiation-Induced Lumbosacral Plexopathy

Lumbosacral plexopathy secondary to radiation may also occur in patients with gynecologic malignancies. While this phenomenon tends to be rare, it has been shown to occur from 0.8% to 3.0% of patients with cervical cancer.[40] Similar to RIBP, risk increases with radiation fraction dose, concomitant chemotherapy, and individual risk factors. Symptom onset may occur acutely during the course of irradiation, subacutely within 6 months of completion of treatment, or even years later, with sources citing up to 30 years from completion of course.[40] The exact pathophysiology remains unclear, again, thought to be related to a state of direct neurotoxic damage. Of the few cases described, Georgiou et al. noted the predominant neurologic symptom is deficits of strength in the lower extremities.[41] Diagnosis and subsequent management parallels that of RIBP.

Surgery

Postmastectomy Pain Syndrome

Breast cancer surgery typically includes breast-conserving surgery (lumpectomy) or mastectomy. The overall rate of mastectomies is on the uptrend, with data suggesting a 21% increase between 2005 and 2013.[42] Mastectomies, however, are only one type of breast surgery. Others surgical procedures include lumpectomies (or breast-conserving surgery), axillary/sentinel lymph node dissection, reconstruction, and augmentation. Postmastectomy pain syndrome (PMPS) is a misnomer, as this chronic pain syndrome may occur with these other types of breast surgeries as well. PMPS is essentially a diagnosis of exclusion and is defined as pain developing postoperatively at or near the surgical site and persisting more than 3 months after all other causes of pain, including recurrence, have been ruled out.[43] Incidence has been shown to range from approximately 20% to 68% of patients.[44] This wide variation of incidence rates may be in part due to the absence of a consensus for the definition or diagnostic criteria of PMPS.

The pathophysiology is still not entirely understood. PMPS has traditionally been thought to be a neuropathic condition, specifically due to surgical damage to the intercostobrachial, medial pectoral, lateral pectoral, thoracodorsal, or long thoracic nerves.[45] Neuromas and phantom breast pain may also contribute. Risk factors may include pain in other parts of the body, young age, history of axillary lymph node dissection, and adjuvant radiation therapy.[46] Psychosocial factors, including depression, anxiety, and insomnia, may also increase the risk of PMPS.[47]

Patients present with pain most commonly in the axilla, shoulder, arm, and area of the scar.[44] Symptoms may begin acutely in the postoperative period or several months after the surgery, lasting beyond the expected timeframe for surgical recovery.[48] Patients may describe lancinating or burning pain and hypersensitivity around the operative site. The severity of PMPS has been described as moderate and studies have shown that approximately 22% of patients reported pain impacting daily life.[44] Given PMPS is a diagnosis of exclusion, diagnostic studies include those that assist in ruling out other etiologies. PET/CT scans may be useful if tumor recurrence is suspected. MRI of the neck, shoulder, or brachial plexus may rule out cervical radiculopathy, musculoskeletal causes, or injury to the plexus, respectively. Furthermore, electrodiagnostic studies may assist with potential diagnosis of cervical radiculopathy, brachial plexopathy, or peripheral neuropathy. Diagnostic interventional procedures may also be considered, such as intercostobrachial nerve block under ultrasound guidance. Other etiologies, such as infection and rib/sternal fractures, should also be ruled out.

There is currently no standard preventative measure; however, one randomized control study suggested perioperative oral pregabalin starting at the morning of surgery and continued for 1 week significantly reduced neuropathic pain in patients undergoing elective breast cancer surgery.[49] Treatment is multimodal and includes physical therapy with focus on myofascial mobilization, early desensitization techniques, range of motion (neck, shoulder, and scapula), stretching (notably the latissimus dorsi and pectoralis musculature), and strengthening of the shoulder girdle and spine extensors. Pharmacologic interventions may also be indicated, including nonsteroidal antiinflammatories (when medically indicated) and coanalgesics such as neuromodulators, including gabapentin or pregabalin, and selective serotonin reuptake inhibitors, such as duloxetine. Interventional procedures, including intercostobrachial nerve block, stellate ganglion block, paravertebral block, and serratus plane block, may be beneficial. Surgical resection for painful neuromas may also be considered.

Debulking Surgery

Surgical debulking is a surgical procedure in which a surgically incurable malignant tumor is partially removed without curative intent, but instead to make adjuvant treatment with chemotherapy or radiation therapy more effective.[50] In patients who may not be surgical candidates to begin with, whether it be due to stage of gynecologic disease or other medical contraindications, neoadjuvant chemotherapy followed by interval debulking surgery (IDS) may be an option.

Women undergoing primary debulking or IDS may also be at risk for peripheral nerve injury. One large multiinstitutional cooperative group study comparing operative morbidity of primary and IDS for advanced stage ovarian cancer demonstrated that patients who received IDS with chemotherapy had a significantly higher risk of peripheral neuropathy than women who received chemotherapy alone.[51] Mononeuropathy may also occur. One case report described a rare case of obturator nerve diagnosed ultimately by electrodiagnosis in a patient with left thigh weakness after primary debulking surgery for left-sided ovarian cancer.[52]

INDIRECT NERVE INJURIES

Patient with both breast and gynecologic malignancies may also experience indirect involvement of the peripheral nervous system. Preexisting medical conditions, such as diabetes mellitus and thyroid disease, may cause an underlying peripheral neuropathy. Patients with cancer are often times immunocompromised and, as such, are at higher risk for secondary infections. Herpes zoster may become reactivated and cause postherpetic neuralgia. Toxic neuropathy may also develop as a result of extended use of antibiotic treatment for infections. Fluoroquinolones, linezolid, metronidazole, and nitrofurantoin, among others, have been shown to cause peripheral neuropathy. Critical illness itself may also cause peripheral neuropathy. Usually presenting as flaccid and symmetric weakness, it has been estimated to occur in 25%–45% of patients admitted to the intensive care unit.[53] Weight loss as a complication of malignancy may also cause neuropathy as seen in compression neuropathy of the peroneal nerve at the fibular head. Malnutrition, in turn, may cause vitamin B12 deficiency, ultimately causing demyelination of sensory nerve fibers.

CONCLUSION

With an estimated 3.1 million survivors in the United States alone, breast cancer is the most common noncutaneous cancer diagnosed in females. The American Cancer Society's current estimates suggest that there will be approximately 270,000 new cases of breast cancer diagnosed in the United States in 2019.[53] While gynecologic cancers are far less common than breast cancer, the CDC estimated that between 2012 and 2016, approximately 94,000 women were diagnosed with gynecologic cancers per year.[54]

Given these and statistics for other types of cancer, it can easily be suggested that, regardless of subspecialty training, the majority of clinicians will treat patients who have or have had some form of cancer. It is crucial for clinicians to have at least a basic understanding of neurologic complications of both cancer and its treatment. As demonstrated with paraneoplastic neurologic syndromes, the majority of cases occur in patients without a prior diagnosis of cancer, thus making early recognition and intervention a pivotal component of the evaluation.

It is equally important for clinicians to educate their patients on potential neurologic complications related to their cancer and treatment. Patients should be aware that certain chemotherapeutic agents, such as taxanes and platins in breast and gynecologic cancers, may cause peripheral neuropathy. Clinicians should be able to manage expectations in regard to radiation therapy and educate their patients on potential lifelong complications related to radiation-induced injuries. Patients should also be educated on expectations in regard to pain management and early intervention after surgical treatments to minimize postoperative pain and dysfunction. Patient education, management of expectations, and reassurance are undoubtedly vital components of the treatment plan in patients with breast cancer.

REFERENCES

1. Jaeckle KA. Neurologic manifestations of neoplastic and radiation-induced plexopathies. *Semin Neurol.* 2010; 30(3):254–262.
2. Shanina E, et al. Brachial plexopathies: update on treatment. *Curr Treat Options Neurol.* 2019;21(5):24.
3. Kamenova B, et al. Effective treatment of the brachial plexus syndrome in breast cancer patients by early detection and control of loco-regional metastases with radiation or systemic therapy. *Int J Clin Oncol.* 2009; 14(3):219–224.
4. Ehler E, et al. Painful lumbosacral plexopathy: a case report. *Medicine (Baltimore).* 2015;94(17):e766.
5. Ko K, et al. Clinical, electrophysiological findings in adult patients with non-traumatic plexopathies. *Ann Rehabil Med.* 2011;35(6):807–815.
6. Jensen AO, et al. Incidence of bone metastases and skeletal-related events in breast cancer patients: a population-based cohort study in Denmark. *BMC Cancer.* 2011;11:29.
7. Coleman RE. Clinical features of metastatic bone disease and risk of skeletal morbidity. *Clin Cancer Res.* 2006;12 (20 Pt 2):6243s–6249s.
8. Ju DG, et al. Diagnosis and surgical management of breast cancer metastatic to the spine. *World J Clin Oncol.* 2014;5(3):263–271.
9. Uccella S, et al. Bone metastases in endometrial cancer: report on 19 patients and review of medical literature. *Gynecol Oncol.* 2013;130(3):474–482.
10. Foerster R, et al. Spinal bone metastases in gynecologic malignancies: a retrospective analysis of stability, prognostic factors and survival. *Radiat Oncol.* 2014;9:194.
11. Shelerud RA, Paynter KS. Rarer causes of radiculopathy: spinal tumors, infections, and other unusual causes. *Phys Med Rehabil Clin N Am.* 2002;13(3):645–696.
12. Figura NB, et al. Breast leptomeningeal disease: a review of current practices and updates on management. *Breast Cancer Res Treat.* 2019;177(2):277–294.
13. Custodio CM. Neuromuscular complications of cancer and cancer treatments. *Phys Med Rehabil Clin N Am.* 2008;19(1):27–45. v–vi.
14. Franzoi MA, Hortobagyi GN. Leptomeningeal carcinomatosis in patients with breast cancer. *Crit Rev Oncol Hematol.* 2019;135:85–94.
15. Toothaker TB, Rubin M. Paraneoplastic neurological syndromes: a review. *Neurologist.* 2009;15(1):21–33.
16. Viau M, et al. Paraneoplastic syndromes associated with gynecological cancers: a systematic review. *Gynecol Oncol.* 2017;146(3):661–671.
17. Murphy BL, et al. Breast cancer-related paraneoplastic neurologic disease. *Breast Cancer Res Treat.* 2018;167(3): 771–778.
18. Darnell RB, Posner JB. Paraneoplastic syndromes affecting the nervous system. *Semin Oncol.* 2006;33(3): 270–298.
19. Fanous I, Dillon P. Paraneoplastic neurological complications of breast cancer. *Exp Hematol Oncol.* 2015;5:29.
20. Simon NB, et al. The prevalence and pattern of chemotherapy-induced peripheral neuropathy among women with breast cancer receiving care in a large community oncology practice. *Qual Life Res.* 2017;26(10): 2763–2772.
21. Shah A, et al. Incidence and disease burden of chemotherapy-induced peripheral neuropathy in a population-based cohort. *J Neurol Neurosurg Psychiatry.* 2018;89(6):636–641.

22. Tanabe Y, et al. Paclitaxel-induced peripheral neuropathy in patients receiving adjuvant chemotherapy for breast cancer. *Int J Clin Oncol*. 2013;18(1):132–138.
23. Seretny M, et al. Incidence, prevalence, and predictors of chemotherapy-induced peripheral neuropathy: a systematic review and meta-analysis. *Pain*. 2014;155(12): 2461–2470.
24. Dougherty PM, et al. Taxol-induced sensory disturbance is characterized by preferential impairment of myelinated fiber function in cancer patients. *Pain*. 2004; 109(1–2):132–142.
25. Starobova H, Vetter I. Pathophysiology of chemotherapy-induced peripheral neuropathy. *Front Mol Neurosci*. 2017;10:174.
26. Cavaletti G, et al. Chemotherapy-induced neuropathy. *Curr Treat Options Neurol*. 2011;13(2):180–190.
27. Tzatha E, DeAngelis LM. Chemotherapy-induced peripheral neuropathy. *Oncology (Williston Park)*. 2016;30(3): 240–244.
28. Bao T, et al. Long-term chemotherapy-induced peripheral neuropathy among breast cancer survivors: prevalence, risk factors, and fall risk. *Breast Cancer Res Treat*. 2016;159(2):327–333.
29. Hanai A, et al. Effects of cryotherapy on objective and subjective symptoms of paclitaxel-induced neuropathy: prospective self-controlled trial. *J Natl Cancer Inst*. 2018;110(2):141–148.
30. Shinde SS, et al. Can pregabalin prevent paclitaxel-associated neuropathy?—an ACCRU pilot trial. *Support Care Cancer*. 2016;24(2):547–553.
31. de Andrade DC, et al. Pregabalin for the prevention of oxaliplatin-induced painful neuropathy: a randomized, double-blind trial. *Oncologist*. 2017;22(10):1154–e1105.
32. Smith EM, et al. Effect of duloxetine on pain, function, and quality of life among patients with chemotherapy-induced painful peripheral neuropathy: a randomized clinical trial. *JAMA*. 2013;309(13):1359–1367.
33. Sideras K, et al. Coprescription of tamoxifen and medications that inhibit CYP2D6. *J Clin Oncol*. 2010;28(16): 2768–2776.
34. Dropcho EJ. Neurotoxicity of radiation therapy. *Neurol Clin*. 2010;28(1):217–234.
35. Delanian S, et al. Radiation-induced neuropathy in cancer survivors. *Radiother Oncol*. 2012;105(3):273–282.
36. Qayyum A, et al. Symptomatic brachial plexopathy following treatment for breast cancer: utility of MR imaging with surface-coil techniques. *Radiology*. 2000;214(3): 837–842.
37. Markiewicz DA, et al. The effects of sequence and type of chemotherapy and radiation therapy on cosmesis and complications after breast conservation therapy. *Int J Radiat Oncol Biol Phys*. 1996;35(4):661–668.
38. Fathers E, et al. Radiation-induced brachial plexopathy in women treated for carcinoma of the breast. *Clin Rehabil*. 2002;16(2):160–165.
39. Steiner CA, Weiss AJ, Barrett ML, Fingar KR, Davis PH. Trends in bilateral and unilateral mastectomies in hospital inpatient and ambulatory settings, 2005–2013. In: *HCUP Statistical Brief #201*. 2016. Rockville, MD: Agency for Healthcare Research and Quality.
40. Malgorzata K, et al. Radiotherapy-induced lumbosacral plexopathy in a patient with cervical cancer: a case report and literature review. *Contemp Oncool*. 2012;16(2): 194–196.
41. Georgiou A, et al. Radiation induced lumbosacral plexopathy in gynaecologic tumors: clinical findings and dosimetric analysis. *Int J RAdiat Oncol Biol Phys*. 1993;26:479–482.
42. Meijuan Y, et al. A retrospective study of postmastectomy pain syndrome: incidence, characteristics, risk factors, and influence on quality of life. *ScientificWorldJournal*. 2013;2013:159732.
43. Vilholm OJ, et al. The postmastectomy pain syndrome: an epidemiological study on the prevalence of chronic pain after surgery for breast cancer. *Br J Cancer*. 2008; 99(4):604–610.
44. Brackstone M. A review of the literature and discussion: establishing a consensus for the definition of post-mastectomy pain syndrome to provide a standardized clinical and research approach. *Can J Surg*. 2016;59(5): 294–295.
45. Mejdahl MK, et al. Persistent pain and sensory disturbances after treatment for breast cancer: six year nationwide follow-up study. *BMJ*. 2013;346:f1865.
46. Belfer I, et al. Persistent postmastectomy pain in breast cancer survivors: analysis of clinical, demographic, and psychosocial factors. *J Pain*. 2013;14(10):1185–1195.
47. Wisotzky E, et al. Deconstructing postmastectomy syndrome: implications for physiatric management. *Phys Med Rehabil Clin N Am*. 2017;28(1):153–169.
48. Reyad RM, et al. The possible preventive role of pregabalin in postmastectomy pain syndrome: a double-blinded randomized controlled trial. *J Pain Symptom Manage*. 2019;57(1):1–9.
49. Silberman AW. Surgical debulking of tumors. *Surg Gynecol Obstet*. 1982;155(4):577–585.
50. Interval debulking surgery for advanced epithelial ovarian cancer. *Cochrane Database Syst Rev*. 2016;(1):CD006014.
51. Lee C. Temporary obturator neuropathy suspected as a result of obturator fossa edema after debulking surgery. *Taiwan J Obstet Gynecol*. 2005;44(4):378–380.
52. Zhou C, et al. Critical illness polyneuropathy and myopathy: a systematic review. *Neural Regen Res*. 2014;9(1): 101–110.
53. Siegel RL, et al. Cancer statistics, 2019. *CA Cancer J Clin*. 2019;69(1):7–34.
54. Centers for Disease Control and Prevention. Gynecologic Cancer Incidence, United States – 2012-2016. In: *USCS Data Brief, No. 11*. Atlanta, GA: Centers for Disease Control and Prevention, US Department of Health and Human Services; 2019.

CHAPTER 23

Inpatient Rehabilitation for Breast and Gynecologic Cancer Patients

TERRENCE MACARTHUR PUGH, MD • VISHWA S. RAJ, MD •
CHARLES MITCHELL, DO

INTRODUCTION

As the number of oncology patients grows in the United States, rehabilitation professionals are asked to be involved in the care at various points before, during, and after treatment. Rehabilitation services can be delivered in numerous postacute care settings; however, as value becomes increasingly important, cost and outcome measures within the various settings will help determine where the care is delivered.[1] Only 2.4% of all oncology patients utilize inpatient rehabilitation services.[2] High-quality rehabilitation services have been shown to be a key component in the oncologic care spectrum,[3] and some of these patients are best managed in inpatient rehabilitation facilities (IRFs).

EPIDEMIOLOGY

Cancer survival from breast and gynecologic malignancies is becoming more prevalent as early screening, better diagnostic techniques, and improved treatment regimens are utilized more frequently. Female breast cancer is the most commonly diagnosed malignancy in the United States accounting for an estimated 268,600 new cases in 2019, which comprises 15.2% of all new cancer diagnoses.[4] Less commonly, uterine cancer accounts for 61,880 cases (3.5% of new cancer diagnoses),[5] ovarian cancer with 22,530 cases (1.3%),[6] and 13,170 people with (0.7%) new cervical cancer diagnoses in 2019.[7] Vulvar cancer accounts for only 6070 (0.3%) of new cancer diagnoses over the same time span.[8] Given focused screening leading to early identification followed by more comprehensive chemotherapy/hormonal therapeutic options, surgical techniques, and radiation protocols, 5-year survival for these malignancies ranges from 47.6% (ovarian) to 89.9% (breast).[4,6]

REASON FOR ADMISSION TO ACUTE INPATIENT REHABILITATION

To be considered for admission to an acute IRF, a patient must meet several criteria (Table 23.1). The Centers for Medicare and Medicaid Services (CMS) also mandates that supporting documentation, including preadmission screens, postadmission physician evaluations, and individualized overall plans of care, be included for compliant IRF admission.[9] The 60% rule requires that IRF admits no less than 60% of patients that can be identified as having 1 out of 13 specific conditions.[10] Although cancer is not explicitly stated within the 60% rule, several cancer diagnoses may be consistent with the listed conditions, that is, metastatic brain tumor patients representing nontraumatic brain injuries or spinal cord lesions as nontraumatic spinal cord injuries (Table 23.2).[11] However, in skilled nursing facilities, CMS is initiating the Patient-Driven Payment Model starting on October 1, 2019, which will include cancer as a compliant diagnosis which, if successful, could provide a model for compliant IRF admission of oncology patients in the future.[12]

Breast and gynecological cancer patients comprise between 3% and 5% of an inpatient rehabilitation population[13] with admissions generally related to impairments due to the spread of the cancer beyond the primary site or sequelae of treatment. The most common sites of metastasis in patients with breast cancer are bone, lung, brain, and liver.[14] Endometrial carcinoma typically demonstrates localized metastasis, but can also spread to the lungs. Less commonly endometrial cancer manifests in the bone, brain, liver, and adrenals.[15] Patients with ovarian cancer often demonstrate localized spread within the peritoneum, retroperitoneum, and even distant sites of metastasis.[16] Multidisciplinary teams within IRF, including physiatrists, advanced-care practitioners,

Breast Cancer and Gynecologic Cancer Rehabilitation DOI: https://doi.org/10.1016/B978-0-323-72166-0.00023-2

TABLE 23.1
Admission Criteria for Inpatient Rehabilitation Facility Programs

- Requirement for active and ongoing intervention from multiple therapy disciplines (including PT, OT, SLP, or prosthetics and orthotics)
- Intensive rehabilitation program consisting of either
  3 h of therapy per day for at least 5 days/week
  15 h of intensive rehabilitation therapy within a 7-consecutive day period beginning with the day of admission (in certain well-documented cases)
- Intensive rehabilitation therapy program for which the patient's condition and functional status allow for the patient to make reasonably expected and measurable improvement within a prescribed period of time that will be of practical value to improve the patient's functional capacity or adaptation to impairments
- Face-to-face visits for at least 3 days/week by a rehabilitation physician to address medical and functional needs and modify the course of treatment as needed
- Intensive and coordinated interdisciplinary team approach

OT, Occupational therapists; *PT*, physical therapists; *SLP*, Speech-language pathologist.
From *Centers for Medicare and Medicaid Services*. <https://www.cms.gov/Outreach-and-Education/Medicare-Learning-Network-MLN/MLNProducts/downloads/Inpatient_Rehab_Fact_Sheet_ICN905643.pdf> Accessed 22.11.19.

TABLE 23.2
Conditions Compliant With the 60% Rule for Inpatient Rehabilitation Facility (IRF)

Stroke Congenital deformity Major multiple trauma Brain injury	Spinal cord injury Amputation Fracture of femur (hip) Burns With evidence that less intensive treatments were attempted and failed to improve the patient's condition before admission to IRF
• Arthropathies that have led to the functional impairments of ambulation and ADLs, including active polyarticular rheumatoid arthritis psoriatic arthritis seronegative arthropathies	Systemic vasculitides with joint inflammation leading to the functional impairments of ambulation and ADLs
• Severe or advanced osteoarthritis with the following conditions: involvement of two or more weight-bearing joints with joint deformity atrophy of muscles surrounding the joint significant functional impairment of ambulation and ADLs *Joint cannot be counted if it has a prosthesis	• Neurological disorders including multiple sclerosis motor neuron disease polyneuropathy muscular dystrophy Parkinson's disease
• Knee or hip joint replacement (or both) during an acute care hospitalization immediately preceding IRF stay and meeting one of the following criteria: Patient underwent bilateral hip or bilateral knee joint replacement surgery during the acute care hospitalization and immediately preceding IRF admission Patient is extremely obese with body mass index of at least 50 at the time of admission to IRF Patient is 85 years or older at the time of admission to IRF	

ADLs, Activities of daily living.
From *Centers for Medicare and Medicaid Services*. <https://www.cms.gov/Medicare/Medicare-Fee-for-Service-Payment/InpatientRehabFacPPS/Criteria> Accessed 22.11.19.

physical and occupation therapists, speech language pathologists, rehabilitation nurses, social workers, clinical nutritionists, case management, pastoral care, and psychologists, are often well equipped to manage people with various disease-related conditions. The following sections will discuss inpatient rehabilitation management of these patients and impairments associated with the treatment.

INPATIENT REHABILITATION MANAGEMENT

Localized Surgical Resection

The goal of surgical intervention for breast and gynecological cancers is to minimize risk of local recurrence while simultaneously minimizing patient morbidity. Surgical planning involves identifying and removing tissues that have visible tumor or are at risk for microscopic tumor infiltration, determining which tissues can be spared and which locally advanced tumors are amenable to resection. Wide local excision has long been the strategy, but tumor recurrence rates remain high with this technique. An analysis of cervical cancers after surgical resection has been recently used to help model tumor growth and to improve outcomes for patients undergoing wide local excisions. By achieving more complete resection of a tumor initially, patients have better response to adjuvant treatments.[17]

Early in the 20th century, radical mastectomy was the surgical intervention of choice for patients with breast cancer; however, currently breast conservation techniques are utilized more frequently. Periareolar incisions and localized lumpectomies are used for tumors that are not as large and are less than 2 cm from the areola. For patients undergoing mastectomy, whether electively or out of medical necessity, the need for reconstruction is discussed in the preoperative and the surgical approached is tailored to the needs of the patient.[18] Furthermore, sentinel lymph node dissection (SLND) has replaced axillary lymph node dissection (ALND) as the primary method of staging in part not only because of its diagnostic utility but also because of decreased risk of postmastectomy lymphedema.[19]

Breast surgical complications, including wound infections, axillary seromas, axillary paresthesia, lymphedema, and brachial plexus injury, can be seen at higher rates in SLND plus ALND when compared to SLND alone.[19] These surgical complications can oftentimes be managed in an IRF. Wound care nursing along with antibiotic therapy (if indicated) can enhance wound healing. The patients with brachial plexus injuries can have significant impairment of the affected limb. A comprehensive rehabilitation therapy program with physical and occupational therapy can help to restore function.

Patients in an IRF population can admit secondary to complications from a surgical procedure adding to the medical necessity required for inpatient rehabilitation admission. Enhanced recovery programs in acute care hospitals have been shown to decrease inpatient length of stay and minimize surgical complications, including hemorrhage, wound dehiscence, anastomotic leakage, abscess, or small bowel obstruction.[20] These complications may lead to patient transfer to a postacute care setting sooner after surgical intervention to further facilitate recovery before returning home.

In patients with endometrial cancer, deoxyribonucleic acid damaging agents such as platinum-based chemotherapies have been used as an adjunctive treatment to surgical debulking.[21] Ovarian cancer has a much higher mortality rate than most other gynecologic cancers due to its advanced stage (75% of cases) at the time of diagnosis. Localized spread occurs to the uterus and fallopian tubes, but there can also be contiguous spread to the colon, bladder, and peritoneum.[22] First-line chemotherapy for metastatic ovarian cancer also involves utilization of platinum-based compounds and taxanes.[23] Neoadjuvant chemotherapy reduces the rate of patients needing to undergo multiple bowel resections, which also minimizes the risk of surgical complications.[24] To maximize disease-free survival in patients with advanced ovarian cancer, these patients often undergo modified pelvic exenteration with adjuvant chemotherapy (paclitaxel/carboplatin plus/minus bevacizumab) and as a result these patients sometimes have a new colostomy or an ileostomy.[25] Wound care and ostomy nursing care within an IRF are often needed to help patients and families manage a new colostomy or an ileal conduit for locally invasive metastatic disease amenable to resection. Patients with ovarian cancer who are more frail tend to have more surgical complications, shorter disease-free survival and increased mortality than those who do not meet the frailty index independent of patient age.[26] The inpatient rehabilitation team can often intervene during the pre- or postoperative period to minimize this risk.

Intracranial Metastatic Disease

A percentage of 25 to 30 of brain tumors admitted to IRFs are due to metastatic disease.[27] These are diagnosed with computed tomography or magnetic resonance imaging when neurologic symptoms manifest. Breast cancer is one of the most common primary sites for metastatic spread to the brain.[28] Seventy percent of these patients with metastatic breast cancer present with hormone receptor–positive disease[29] with endocrine therapy as the first-line treatment.[30] There is a higher incidence of cerebellar metastases in patients with breast carcinoma.[31] The location of the lesion corresponds to the symptoms that manifest within the patient. Patients with cerebellar lesions may demonstrate ataxia that can increase risk for falls. Physical therapy interventions, including balance and postural training, gait training, and the use of orthotics, can minimize this risk.[32] Nearly all patients with a metastatic intracranial lesion receive steroids during their disease. However, there is not a standardized method of dosing or weaning.[33] The physician overseeing the care initiates a taper in effort to obtain the minimum effective dosage of the steroid. Glucocorticoid-induced myopathy (GIM) is a serious complication noted with long-term steroid use. Sixty percent of those with GIM have proximal muscle weakness that can negatively impact activities of daily living (ADLs).[34] Maximizing functional independence with ADLs is often a goal for patients within an IRF. Considerations must also be made by the provider regarding the management of seizure prophylaxis and venous thromboembolism prophylaxis/treatment.[35]

Surgical resection of brain tumors may also be considered for patients who have significant disease burden and to minimize symptoms. Several randomized trials have recommended the use of surgery for single brain metastatic disease to increase survival. Although targeted radiation therapy is favorable, in patients with metastatic disease may receive whole-brain radiation therapy (WBRT).[36]

Ninety percent of patients receive WBRT complaining of cognitive impairment.[37] Physiatrists may use neurocognitive stimulant medications to improve functional outcomes in patients with metastatic breast or gynecologic cancer. For example, memantine, in addition to hippocampal avoidance, has been shown to reduce neurocognitive side effects in patients receiving WBRT and targeted stereotactic radiation surgery.[38] Methylphenidate and modafinil are also reasonable options, given their favorable side effect profiles.[35]

Spinal Metastatic Disease

The spine is the most common site of bony metastatic disease, which is thought to be due, in part, to its high vascularity with antegrade arterial spread and retrograde spread via Batson's plexus. The majority, 70%, of spinal metastases are found in the thoracic spine with 22% in the lumbosacral spine and 8% in the cervical spine.[39] With most of these lesions in the thoracic and lumbar spine, the patients often manifest with paraplegia as opposed to tetraplegia. Metastatic disease to the spine accounts for up to 30% of patients at the time of initial diagnosis[40] leading to epidural spinal cord compression.[41] For these patients with spinal cord compression, initial management is with steroids[42] followed by surgical resection, spine stabilization, and radiation therapy.[43] Early on these patients may demonstrate a flaccid paralysis, but eventually upper motor neuron dysfunction predominates. This can manifest as hyperreflexia or hypertonicity (spasticity or dystonia). Treatment of spasticity and dystonia can include therapeutic intervention, exercises, bracing, oral antispasmodic medications, botulinum toxin injections, neurolytic agents (i.e., phenol), and/or intrathecal baclofen.[44] The rehabilitation team must also manage and prevent other associated conditions such as neurogenic bowel/bladder, pressure ulcers, venous thromboembolism, restrictive lung disease, and pain.[45] Patients undergoing spinal stabilization surgery have been shown to have improvements in ADLs, quality of life (QoL), and disease-related life expectancy with implementation of a multidisciplinary team approach.[46]

Bony Metastatic Disease/Pathologic Fractures

The multidisciplinary rehabilitation team must also manage patients with bony metastatic disease outside of the spinal column. Lower extremity bony metastatic disease, excluding the spine, occurs more often than upper extremity metastatic disease (76% vs 24%, respectively). Within the appendicular skeleton the femur is the most common site of metastatic disease followed by the humerus and the tibia, respectively.[47] Patients with bony metastatic disease, who are surgical candidates, often undergo tumor resection followed by intramedullary nailing in long bones or plate and screw fixation when appropriate. Radiation therapy can also be used as an adjunctive treatment or as primary palliative therapy. Survivability in these cases is related to premorbid performance status and site of primary cancer.[48] Patients with metastatic bone disease can also present with hypercalcemia due to bone destruction of the associated malignancy. Healthy bone has endocrinologic-mediated osteoblast and osteocyte signaling, which ensures the integrity of the bony matrix. In patients with metastatic breast cancer the breast cancer cells secrete factors that enhance osteoclastic activity causing bone resorption. This, in turn, increases the release of signaling factors, that is, TGF-β, from the matrix, which enhances tumor invasion and growth. Further tumor invasion leads to more bone destruction, which can manifest as a fracture or pain and can also cause nerve compression.[49] Bisphosphonates such as zoledronic acid and pamidronate have been used to prevent progression or delay skeletal complications in breast cancer patients. In patients that have hypercalcemia or osteolytic lesions, zoledronic acid has been proven to be superior to pamidronate.[50]

When treating patients with bony metastatic disease, the rehabilitation team must consider sites of known metastasis and weight-bearing restrictions when developing the rehabilitation plan. General precautions for patients with bone metastases include limiting manual muscle testing and avoiding progressive resistance training in the affected limb. Therapists also encourage the use of assistive devices to offload the affected limb. For spinal metastases, patients should avoid excessive spinal flexion, extension, or rotation while monitoring for worsening pain.[51] Mirels' criteria can be used to predict the risk of pathologic fracture.[52] The interdisciplinary team within an IRF implements a plan of care to maximize function while minimizing risk of adverse skeletal events.

OTHER COMMON IMPAIRMENTS

Chemotherapy-Induced Peripheral Neuropathy

As stated earlier, taxanes and platinum-based chemotherapies are used as first-line agents to treat many gynecologic cancers. Unfortunately, platinum-based compounds (70%–100%) and taxanes (11%–87%) have the highest rates inducing chemotherapy-induced peripheral neuropathy (CIPN).[53] CIPN usually manifests as a small fiber, sensory neuropathy that can also be associated with motor or autonomic dysfunction. With electrodiagnostic testing a primarily axonal, sensorimotor polyneuropathy is seen.[54] The development of the symptoms often occurs late in the chemotherapy course, which makes it difficult to determine if dose adjustments can mitigate risk; however, once symptoms begin, oncologists often adjust treatment. Patients usually complain of a stocking/glove distribution of the neuropathy, and patients can also complain of numbness, tingling, paresthesias, dysesthesias, or allodynia.[55] A combination of anticonvulsant medications such as gabapentin, carbamazepine, oxcarbazepine, lamotrigine, and topiramate along with antidepressants such as amitriptyline, nortriptyline, venlafaxine, and duloxetine has been shown to be effective in treating neuropathic pain.[56]

In addition to pain, balance deficits can be seen in patients with CIPN, which can increase his or her risk for falls. Fall risk has been noted to be two to three times more likely in patients with CIPN.[57] Balance exercises have been shown to improve symptoms, including pain, and maximize function.[58] When balance training is combined with endurance training, functional status improves while also improving the QoL.[59] Breast cancer patients with CIPN of the hands noted significant difficulty in their ability to return to work up to 1 year after the completion of treatment, which also negatively impacts health-related QoL.[60] A comprehensive rehabilitation program with physical and occupational therapy to address these issues is important in both inpatient and outpatient settings. Physiatrists may order electrodiagnostic testing to rule out any other peripheral nerve injuries that could be impacting a person's ability to function. Therapists may also utilize modalities such as fluidotherapy or scrambler therapy to treat pain in patients with CIPN.[61]

Lymphedema

The pathophysiology of lymphedema is not well understood; however, any disruption to a normal functioning lymphatic system can predispose a person to the development of lymphedema. With any disruption (surgery, radiation, injury, etc.), there is an increase in intralymphatic fluid pressure distal to the obstruction, which causes lymphatic vessels to dilate, making the valves incompetent. This in turn makes the cellular junctions incompetent and causes the development of lymphedema.[27] Patients who undergo ALND, regional radiation therapy, and/or sentinel lymph node biopsy for breast cancer diagnosis and treatment are at an increased lifetime risk for developing lymphedema. The exact incidence is hard to determine due to the many types of surgical and radiation treatment protocols; however, it is thought to be between 5% and 50%.[62] The average time to the onset of symptoms is 14.4 months after the completion of treatment.[63] In addition to treatment-related effects, patients with a body mass index ≥ 25 kg/m^2 are at increased risk of developing lymphedema.[62,63]

Patients with gynecologic malignancies are also at risk for developing lymphedema. Surgical treatment for patients with ovarian cancer often involves sampling or resection of lymph vessels and lymph nodes in the pelvic sidewall and the para-aortic area, increasing the risk for the development of lower extremity lymphedema.[64] Since surgical intervention for gynecologic cancer involves bilateral lymph node dissection, patients often have bilateral lower limb lymphedema.[65] The prevalence of lower extremity lymphedema in this population is thought to be between 7% and 38%.[64]

In an IRF, physicians, therapists, and nurses may encounter patients with lymphedema. It is important for rehabilitation professionals to be able to identify lymphedema and determine how it can potentially impact the patient's ability to maximize functional progress. Other causes of peripheral edema should also be ruled out, including, but not limited to, venous thrombosis, edema related to renal or hepatic dysfunction, or hypoalbuminemia. The gold standard for measuring lymphedema is to be either performed by a trained lymphedema specialist or by a perometer.[66] Lymphedema massage and kinesiology taping can be performed in IRFs, which have shown to decrease limb volume.[67] Patients may also utilize compression garments, including thromboembolic disease hose or Tubigrip to minimize edema in inpatient rehabilitation settings. By reducing limb volume, patients can experience improvement in gait quality, minimize fall risk, and make safe stair navigation more feasible.

Patients and the rehabilitation team may have questions about specialized precautions for the affected limb. Weight training has not been shown to exacerbate or improve lymphedema in breast cancer survivors.[68] Similarly, exercise does not exacerbate lower limb lymphedema in patients with ovarian cancer.[64] The nursing staff often restricts blood pressure measurements or blood draws on a lymphedematous limb over concerns about exacerbating the swelling. Two recent analyses showed that neither ipsilateral blood pressure checks, venipuncture, air travel nor extreme temperatures increased the risk of lymphedema in patients with breast cancer. Patient education regarding limb hygiene and infection prevention should be provided as cellulitis can exacerbate or increase the risk of developing lymphedema.[62,63]

Additional Symptoms/Conditions

Rehabilitation professionals may also provide other supportive services for the cancer survivor. Opioid-induced constipation can be present in 70%–100% or patients with cancer-related pain.[69] Bowel management with medications such as stool softeners, colonic irritants, osmotic agents, promotility agents, suppositories, or enemas in combination or individually can improve these symptoms. In addition, 25% of patients who received radiation therapy for cervical cancer complain of urinary frequency for up to 2 years after treatment.[70] Timed toileting programs with the addition of anticholinergic mediations or α-blockers may help improve continence. Indwelling Foley catheters may be utilized for medically complex patients or for those transitioning to the end-of-life comfort care. Patients receiving anthracyclines for treatment of breast cancer or those undergoing chest radiation therapy may have cardio/pulmonary toxicity; however, active breath coordination during radiation may minimize this risk.[71] Active breath coordination involves using the deep inspiration breath hold technique when a person is getting chest radiation for breast cancer. When a patient takes a deep breath, the diaphragm flattens, expands the chest cavity, and moves the heart out of the radiation field thus limiting damage to cardiac tissue.[72] Early identification and management of these treatment sequelae can help the patient maximize function during rehabilitation stay. Herceptin (trastuzumab), which can be used in the treatment of certain types of breast cancer, and certain taxanes have been known to cause pancytopenia.[51] Transfusion parameters to minimize bleeding risk should be discussed with the primary oncology team prior to transfer to IRF. Granulocyte colony–stimulating factors can be administered to combat leukopenia and neutropenia. Therapists should be mindful of blood counts and adjust plan of care accordingly (Table 23.3). Fatigue is also seen in 60%–90% of cancer survivors and is multifactorial in nature. Dopamine agonists have been shown to be effective in managing fatigue. Methylphenidate is the drug of choice to improve opioid-induced sedation, cognitive decline, and fatigue.[73]

THERAPEUTIC INTERVENTIONS

Systemic therapy with chemotherapy, immunotherapy, or hormonal therapy is oftentimes initiated by the medical oncologist depending on the type of cancer and if the patient's performance status is high enough to tolerate it. Oncologists gauge performance status with the Eastern Cooperative Oncology Group (Table 23.4) or the Karnofsky (Table 23.5) scale, while rehabilitation professionals often use the Functional Independence Measure (Table 23.6). Although there are limitations with all of the scales, functional status is used to determine whether or not a person is able to continue with cancer treatment. Multidisciplinary inpatient

TABLE 23.3
General Rehabilitation Considerations in the Context of Hematological Compromise[13,16,19]

Blood Count	Rehabilitation Considerations
White blood cells	$>11.0 \times 10^9$/L: symptom-based approach, monitor for fever $<4.0 \times 10^9$/L: symptom-based approach, monitor for fever $<1.5 \times 10^9$/L (neutropenia): symptom-based approach, neutropenic precautions based on facility guidelines Mild $<1.5 \times 10^9$/L Moderate $0.5-1.0 \times 10^9$/L Severe $<0.5 \times 10^9$/L
Platelets	<150,000 cells/μL (thrombocytopenia): symptom-based approach, monitor tolerance to activity >50,000 cells/μL: progressive exercise as tolerated, aerobic, and resistive with monitoring for symptoms associated with bleeding >30,000 cells/μL: active range-of-motion exercises, moderate exercise, aquatic therapy based on immune status >20,000 cells/μL: light exercise, walking, activities of daily living without strenuous effort; assess fall risk and implement safety plan for falls prevention <20,000 cells/μL: understand transfusion status or plan of care, walking, light activities of daily living, symptom monitoring, precaution for falls
Hemoglobin	Reference values Male: 14–17.4 g/dL Female: 12–16 g/dL <11 g/dL (anemia): establish baseline vital signs; may be tachycardic or present with orthostatic hypertension; symptom-based approach to intervention, monitoring self-perceived exertion <8 g/dL (severe anemia): close monitoring of symptoms and vital signs with intervention; transfusion may or may not be indicated based on individual presentation; short periods of intervention, symptom-limited; education for energy conservation

From Maltser S, Cristian A, Silver JK, et al. A focused review of safety considerations in cancer rehabilitation. *PM R*. 2017;9:s415–s428.

TABLE 23.4
Eastern Cooperative Oncology Group (ECOG) Performance Status

Grade	ECOG Performance Status
0	Fully active, able to carry on all predisease performance without restriction
1	Restricted in physically strenuous activity but ambulatory and able to carry out work of a light or sedentary nature, e.g., light house work or office work
2	Ambulatory and capable of all self-care, but unable to carry out any work activities; up and about more than 50% of waking hours
3	Capable of only limited self-care, confined to bed or hair more than 50% of waking hours
4	Completely disable, cannot carry on any self-care, totally confined to bed or chair
5	Dead

From Oken MM, Creech RH, Tormey DC, et al. Toxicity and response criteria of the Eastern Cooperative Oncology Group. *Am J Clin Oncol*. 1982;5(6):654.[74]

rehabilitation teams are tasked with implementing individualized care plans to help patients recover after treatment or help them reach a performance status to tolerate the next phase of treatment.[77] In IRFs, physiatrists coordinate care between the oncology providers and the rehabilitation team in an effort to help maximize function before, during, or after treatment.

Improvements in breast cancer treatment has increased survivability, but patients often experience impairments such as pain, fatigue, anxiety, functional limitations, and lack of participation in daily activities. Occupational therapists (OT) are instrumental in helping patients develop problem-solving strategies to maximize functional independence with basic ADLs and

TABLE 23.5
Karnofsky Performance Status Scale

Score	Karnofsky Performance Status
100	Normal, no complaints; no evidence of disease
90	Able to carry on normal activity; minor signs or symptoms of disease
80	Normal activity with effort, some signs or symptoms of disease
70	Cares for self but unable to carry on normal activity or to do active work
60	Requires occasional assistance but is able to care for most personal needs
50	Requires considerable assistance and frequent medical care
40	Disabled; requires special care and assistance
30	Severely disabled; hospitalization is indicated, although death not imminent
20	Very ill; hospitalization and active supportive care necessary
10	Moribund
0	Dead

From Karnofsky D, Burchenal J. The clinical evaluation of chemotherapeutic agents in cancer. In: MacLeod C, ed. *Evaluation of Chemotherapeutic Agents*. New York: Columbia University Press; 1949:p. 196.[75]

TABLE 23.6
Functional Independence Measure

Score	Description
No Helper Required	
7	Complete independence
6	Modified independence (patient requires use of a device, but no physical assistance)
Helper (Modified Independence)	
5	Minimal contact assistance (patient can perform ≥75% of task)
4	Modified independence (patient requires use of a device, but no physical assistance)
3	Moderate assistance (patient can perform 50%–74% of task)
Helper (Complete Dependence)	
2	Maximal assistance (patient can perform 25%–49% of tasks)
1	Total assistance (patient can perform <25% of the task or requires >1 person to assist

From *Rehabilitation Measures Database*. FIM® instrument (FIM); FIM® is a trademark of the Uniform Data System for Medical Rehabilitation. Available from: <http://rehabmeasures.org/lists/rehabmeasures/dispform.aspx?id = 889> Accessed 30.09.19. Keith RA, Granger CV, Hamilton BB, Sherwin FS. The functional independence measure: A new tool for rehabilitation. Adv Clin Rehabil. 1987;1:6-18.[77]

instrumental ADLs. Patients, for instance, may have difficulty with dressing, bathing, and functional mobility. As the person achieves improvements in these areas and/or develops strategies to accommodate for deficits, patients also note improvements in fatigue and depression.[78] Patients with breast or gynecologic cancer may also discuss returning to work once the inpatient rehabilitation stay is completed. If appropriate, patients may be referred for vocational rehabilitation or for work hardening programs after IRF admission. Rehabilitation interventions have been shown to positively impact a patient's ability to return to work.[79]

Physical therapists (PT) also play an instrumental role in impacting a patient's functional status. Transfer and gait training are incorporated into the rehabilitation plan of care. Therapists help determine the type of transfer and other equipment needed to ensure a safe transition home. Considerations of the patient's strength, balance, and prognosis are accounted for in the management of cancer patients. Family education is provided by the multidisciplinary team to the cancer survivor and caregivers to ensure safety upon discharge. Transfer training includes bed mobility, transfers into and out of bed or wheelchair, toilet transfers, shower transfers, car transfers, and floor transfers. Various assistive devices, including mechanical lifts and transfer boards, may be utilized to further ensure safety.[80] A home exercise program should be given to patients prior to discharge home as recreational physical activity has been shown to reduce rates of fatigue, neuropathy, depression, anxiety, sleep quality, and QoL and may also reduce the risk of some types of ovarian cancer.[81] Patients with chronic medical conditions, including cancer, are encouraged to participate in 150–300 minutes of moderate-intensity aerobic exercise or 75–150 minutes of high-intensity aerobic exercise or an equivalent combination of the two spread over the week. Patients are also encouraged to engage in muscle-strengthening exercises, involving all muscle groups, 2 or more days per week if he or she is physically able.[82] Exercise has also been shown to improve anxiety, depression, fatigue, health-related QoL, lymphedema, and physical functioning in cancer survivors. Physiatrists can help determine a frequency, intensity, type, and time prescription to guide exercise after discharge from IRF.[83] However, individual exercise prescriptions may have to be adapted if the person has other medical and physical limitations.

Patients undergoing chemotherapy for the treatment of breast cancer may experience cognitive dysfunction and fatigue that may significantly impact QoL.[84] As patients self-describe this phenomenon, it has become known as "chemo brain" or "chemo fog."[85] Cancer-related cognitive impairment can affect up to half of breast cancer survivors with symptoms noted up to 10 years after treatment. Patients can have deficits in attention, memory, psychomotor speed, and executive functioning.[86] Speech and language pathologists develop plans of care to help patients accommodate for deficits while also providing patients and caregivers strategies and cognitive aids to maximize cognitive function. Cancer can cause reactive oxidization in healthy brain tissue, which can alter norepinephrine production in the brain causing mood disturbances and depression.[87] Psychology and pastoral care may also be consulted during the rehabilitation stay in an effort to address these issues and maintain spiritual health.

Minority women and women with lower incomes are more likely to have advanced breast cancer at the time of diagnosis and have poorer outcomes overall. This, in part, is due to the lack of access to facilities that perform screening. Patient navigation efforts have been shown to positively impact patients in these communities. Organizations such as the Susan G. Komen Foundation, through grant funding, may also have programs available to help address health-care disparities.[88] Survivorship care plans, when provided, offer ovarian cancer patients information and resources as patients progress out of active treatment.[89] Social workers and case managers within IRFs are important in helping patients address issues, financial, or otherwise, to help patients successfully transition out of an inpatient rehabilitation setting.

CONCLUSION

People with breast and gynecologic malignancies are increasingly becoming a part of an inpatient rehabilitation population. Admission often occurs when the malignancy has spread beyond the primary site. The interdisciplinary rehabilitation team can treat disease-related complications and impairments to maximize the functional status of those impacted by this group of diagnoses. Regular communication with the medical, surgical, and radiation oncology providers is necessary for clarification of prognostic information and ensuring that the postrehabilitation course is successful and patient needs are addressed before discharge. This will minimize readmission risk and ensure the best patient outcome.

REFERENCES

1. Raj VS, Pugh TM. Inpatient care for the cancer survivor: opportunities to develop and deliver standards for care. *Am J Phys Med Rehabil.* 2018;97:595–601.
2. Mix JM, Granger CV, LaMonte MJ, et al. Characteristics of cancer patients in inpatient rehabilitation facilities: a retrospective cohort study. *Arch Phys Med Rehabil.* 2017;98(5):971–980.
3. Silver JK, Raj VS, Fu JB, et al. Cancer rehabilitation and palliative care: critical components in the delivery of high-quality oncology services. *Support Care Cancer.* 2015;23(12):3633–3643.
4. National Cancer Institute. Surveillance, Epidemiology and End Results Program, 2019. <https://seer.cancer.gov/statfacts/html/breast.html> Accessed 12.08.19.
5. National Cancer Institute. Surveillance, Epidemiology and End Results Program, 2019. <https://seer.cancer.gov/statfacts/html/corp.html> Accessed 12.08.19.
6. National Cancer Institute. Surveillance, Epidemiology and End Results Program, 2019. <https://seer.cancer.gov/statfacts/html/ovary.html> Accessed 19.08.19.
7. National Cancer Institute. Surveillance, Epidemiology and End Results Program, 2019. <https://seer.cancer.gov/statfacts/html/cervix.html> Accessed 12.08.19.
8. National Cancer Institute. Surveillance, Epidemiology and End Results Program, 2019. <https://seer.cancer.gov/statfacts/html/vulva.html> Accessed 19.08.19.
9. Department of Health and Human Services; Centers for Medicare & Medicaid Services. Inpatient rehabilitation therapy services: complying with documentation requirements. <https://www.cms.gov/Outreach-and-Education/Medicare-Learning-Network-MLN/MLNProducts/

downloads/inpatient_rehab_fact_sheet_icn905643.pdf>; 2012 Accessed 10.09.19.
10. Shay PD, Ozcan YA. Freestanding inpatient rehabilitation facility performance following the 60 percent rule: a matter of fit. *Med Care Res Rev: MCRR*. 2013;70(1):46–67.
11. Department of Health and Human ServicesCenters for Medicare & Medicaid Services. Inpatient rehabilitation facility prospective payment system. <https://www.cms.gov/Outreach-and-Education/Medicare-Learning-Network-MLN/MLNProducts/downloads/InpatRehabPaymtfctsht09-508.pdf>; 2017 Accessed 10.09.19.
12. Department of Health and Human ServicesCenters for Medicare & Medicaid Services. Patient Driven Payment Model, 2019. <https://www.cms.gov/Medicare/Medicare-Fee-for-Service-Payment/SNFPPS/PDPM.html#fact> Revision 30.08.19; Accessed 10.09.19.
13. Shin KY, Guo Y, Konzen B, et al. Inpatient cancer rehabilitation: the experience of a national comprehensive cancer center. *Am J Phys Med Rehabil*. 2011;90(5 suppl 1):S63–S68. Available from: https://doi.org/10.1097/PHM.0b013e31820be1a4.
14. Patanaphan V, Salazar OM, Risco R. Breast cancer: metastatic patterns and their prognosis. *South Med J*. 1988;81(9):1109–1112.
15. Kurra V, Krajewski K, Jagannathan J, et al. Typical and atypical metastatic sites of recurrent endometrial carcinoma. *Cancer Imaging*. 2013;13(1):113–122. Available from: https://doi.org/10.1102/1470-7330.2013.0011.
16. Kenda Suster N, Virant-Klun I. Presence and role of stem cells in ovarian cancer. *World J Stem Cell*. 2019;11(7):383–397. Available from: https://doi.org/10.4252/wjsc.v11.i7.383.
17. Kubitschke H, Wolf B, Morawetz E, et al. Roadmap to local tumor growth: insights from cervical cancer. *Sci Rep*. 2019;9(1):12768. Available from: https://doi.org/10.1038/s41598-019-49182-1.
18. McDonald ES, Clark AS, Tchou J, et al. Clinical diagnosis and management of breast cancer. *J Nucl Med*. 2016;57(1):9S–16S.
19. Lucci A, McCall LM, Beitsch PD, et al. Surgical complications associated with sentinel lymph node dissection (SLND) plus axillary lymph node dissection compared with SLND alone in the American College of Surgeons Trial Z0011. *J Clin Oncol*. 2007;25:3657–3663.
20. Wilk L, Udumyan R, Pache B, et al. International validation of enhanced recovery after surgery society guidelines on enhanced recovery for gynecologic surgery. *Am J Obstet Gynecol*. 2019;221(3):237e1–237e11.
21. Bi J, Areecheewakul S, Li Y, et al. MTDH/AEG-1 downregulation using pristimerin-loaded nanoparticles inhibits Fanconi anemia proteins and increases sensitivity to platinum-based chemotherapy. *Gynecol Oncol*. 2019;. Available from: https://doi.org/10.1016/j.ygyno.2019.08.014. pii: S0090-8258(19)31466-0.
22. Lyngyel E. Ovarian cancer development and metastases. *Am J Pathol*. 2010;177(3):1053–1064. Available from: https://doi.org/10.2353/ajpath.2010.100105.
23. Otsuka I. Cutaneous metastases in ovarian cancer. *Cancers (Basel)*. 2019;11(9). Available from: https://doi.org/10.3390/cancers11091292. pii: E1292.
24. Tozzi R, Casarin J, Baysal A, et al. Morbidity of multiple bowel resection compared to single bowel resection after debulking surgery for ovarian cancer. *Eur J Obstet Gynecol Reprod Biol*. 2019;240:215–219. Available from: https://doi.org/10.1016/j.ejogrb.2019.07.011.
25. Szymankiewicz M, Dziobek K, Sznajdorwska M, et al. An analysis of the influence of infection on overall survival rates, following modified pelvic exenteration for advanced ovarian cancer. *Ginekol Pol*. 2018;89(11):618–626. Available from: https://doi.org/10.5603/GP.a2018.0106.
26. Kumar A, Langstraat CL, DeJong SR, et al. Functional not chronologic age: frailty index predicts outcomes in advanced ovarian cancer. *Gynecol Oncol*. 2017;147(1):104–109. Available from: https://doi.org/10.1016/j.ygyno.2017.07.126.
27. Stubblefield MD, O'Dell MW. *Cancer Rehabilitation: Principles and Practice*. New York: Demos Medical; 2009 [Chapter 43].
28. American Brain Tumor Association. Metastatic brain tumors, 2019. <http://www.abta.org/secure/metastatic-brain-tumor.pdf> Accessed 12.09.19.
29. Lobbezoo D, van Kampen R, Voogd AC, et al. Prognosis of metastatic breast cancer subtypes: the hormone receptor/HER2-positive subtype is associated with the most favorable outcome. *Breast Cancer Res Treat*. 2013;141(3):507–514.
30. Cardoso F, Costa A, Senkus E, et al. 3rd ESO-ESMO international consensus guidelines for advanced breast cancer (ABC 3). *Ann Oncol*. 2017;28(12):3111.
31. Kyeong S, Cha YJ, Ahn SG, et al. Subtypes of breast cancer show different spatial distributions of brain metastases. *PLoS One*. 2017;12(11):e0188542. Available from: https://doi.org/10.1371/journal.pone.0188542.
32. Kelly G, Shanley J. Rehabilitation of ataxic gait following cerebellar lesions: applying theory to practice. *Physiother Theory Pract*. 2016;32(6):430–437.
33. Schwarzrock C. Collaboration in the presence of cerebral edema: the complications of steroids. *Surg Neurol Int*. 2016;7(suppl 7):S185–S189. Available from: https://doi.org/10.4103/2152-7806.179228.
34. Batchelor TT, Taylor LP, Thaler HT, et al. Steroid myopathy in cancer patients. *Neurology*. 1997;48:1234–1238.
35. Schiff D, Lee EQ, Nayak L, et al. Medical management of brain tumors and the sequelae of treatment. *Neuro Oncol*. 2015;17(4):488–504. Available from: https://doi.org/10.1093/neuonc/nou304.
36. Tsao MN. Brain metastases: advances over the decades. *Ann Palliat Med*. 2015;4(4):225–232. Available from: https://doi.org/10.3978/j.issn.2224-5820.2015.09.01.
37. Crossen JR, Garwood D, Glatstein E, et al. Neurobehavioral sequelae of cranial irradiation in adults: a review of radiation-induced encephalopathy. *J Clin Oncol*. 1994;12(3):627–642.

38. Tanguturi S, Warren LEG. The current and evolving role of radiation therapy for central nervous system metastases from breast cancer. *Curr Oncol Rep*. 2019;21(6):50. Available from: https://doi.org/10.1007/s11912-019-0803-5.
39. Sayed D, Jacobs D, Sowder T, et al. Spinal radiofrequency ablation combined with cement augmentation for painful spinal vertebral metastasis: a single-center prospective study. *Pain Physician*. 2019;22(5):E441–E449.
40. Tatsui H, Onomura T, Morishita S, Oketa M, Inoue T. Survival rates of patients with metastatic spinal cancer after scintigraphic detection of abnormal radioactive accumulation. *Spine (Phila Pa 1976)*. 1996;21:2143–2148.
41. Mak KS, Lee LK, Mak RH, et al. Incidence and treatment patterns in hospitalizations for malignant spinal cord compression in the United States, 1998-2006. *Int J Radiat Oncol Biol Phys*. 2011;80(3):824–831.
42. Loblaw DA, Mitera G, Ford M, et al. A 2011 updated systematic review and clinical practice guideline for the management of the malignant extradural spinal cord compression. *Int J Radiat Oncol Biol Phys*. 2012;84 (2):312–317.
43. van den Bent MJ. Surgical resection improves outcome in metastatic epidural spinal cord compression. *Lancet*. 2005;366(9486):609–610.
44. Fu J, Gutiérrez C, Bruera E, et al. Use of injectable spasticity management in a cancer center. *Support Care Cancer*. 2013;21(5):1227–1232.
45. Paralyzed Veterens of America. Consortium for spinal cord injury medicine. Clinical practice guidelines, 2008. <http://www.pva.org/publications/clinical-practice-guidelines> Accessed 01.10.19.
46. Uei H, Tokuhashi Y, Maseda M, et al. Clinical results of multidisciplinary therapy including posterior spinal stabilization surgery and postoperative adjuvant therapy for metastatic spinal tumor. *J Orthop Surg Res*. 2018;13 (1):30. Available from: https://doi.org/10.1186/s13018-018-0735-z.
47. Ratasvouri M, Wedin R, Keller J, et al. Insight opinion to surgically treated metastatic bone disease: scandinavian sarcoma group skeletal metastasis registry report of 1195 operated skeletal metastasis. *Surg Oncol*. 2013;22 (2):132–138.
48. Wisanuyotin T, Sirichativapee W, Sumnanoont C, et al. Prognostic and risk factors in patients with metastatic bone disease of an upper extremity. *J Bone Oncol*. 2018;13:71–75. Available from: https://doi.org/10.1016/j.jbo.2018.09.007.
49. Reagan JN, Mikesell C, Reiken S, et al. Osteolytic breast cancer causes skeletal muscle weakness in an immunocompetent syngeneic mouse model. *Front Endocrinol (Lausanne)*. 2017;8:358. Available from: https://doi.org/10.3389/fendo.2017.00358.
50. Goldvaser H, Amir R. Role of bisphosphonates in breast cancer therapy. *Curr Treat Options Oncol*. 2019;20 (4):26. Available from: https://doi.org/10.1007/s11864-019-0623-8.
51. Maltser S, Cristian A, Silver JK, et al. A focused review of safety considerations in cancer rehabilitation. *PM R*. 2017;9:s415–s428.
52. Mirels H. Metastatic disease in long bones. A proposed scoring system for diagnosing impending pathologic fractures. *Clin Orthop Relat Res*. 1989;249:256–264.
53. Banach M, Juranek JK, Zygulska AL. Chemotherapy-induced neuropathies—a growing problem for patients and health care providers. *Brain Behav*. 2016;7:e00558.
54. Azhary H, Farooq MU, Bhanushali M, Majid A, Kassab MY. Peripheral neuropathy: differential diagnosis and management. *Am Fam Phys*. 2010;81:887–892.
55. Zajaczkowska R, Kocot-Kepska M, Leppert W, et al. Mechanisms of chemotherapy induced peripheral neuropathy. *Int J Mol Sci*. 2019;20(6). Available from: https://doi.org/10.3390/ijms20061451. pii: E1451.
56. Starobova H, Vetter I. Pathophysiology of chemotherapy-induced peripheral neuropathy. *Front Mol Neurosci*. 1744;201:10.
57. Wildes TM, Dua P, Fowler SA, et al. Systematic review of falls in older adults with cancer. *J Geriatr Oncol*. 2015;6:70–83.
58. Streckmann F, Hess V, Blotch W, et al. Individually tailored whole-body vibration training to reduce symptoms of chemotherapy-induced peripheral neuropathy: a study protocol of a randomized controlled trial – VANISH. *BMJ Open*. 2019;9(4):e024467. Available from: https://doi.org/10.1136/bmjopen-2018-024467.
59. Kneis S, Wehrle A, Muller J, et al. It's never too late – balance and endurance training improves function performance, quality of life and alleviates neuropathic symptoms in cancer survivors suffering from chemotherapy-induced peripheral neuropathy: results of a randomized control trial. *BMC Cancer*. 2019;19(1):414. Available from: https://doi.org/10.1186/s12885-019-5522-7.
60. Zanville VR, Nudelman KN, Smith DJ, et al. Evaluating the impact of chemotherapy-induced peripheral neuropathy symptoms (CIPN-sx) on perceived ability to work in breast cancer survivors during the first-year post treatment. *Support Care Cancer*. 2016;24(11):4779–4789. Available from: https://doi.org/10.1007/s00520-016-3329-5.
61. Majithia N, Smith TJ, Coyne PJ, et al. Scrambler therapy for the management of chronic pain. *Support Care Cancer*. 2016;24(6):2807–2814.
62. Asdourian MS, Skolny MN, Brunelle C, et al. Precautions for breast cancer-related lymphoedema: risk from air travel, ipsilateral arm blood pressure measurements, skin puncture, extreme temperatures and cellulitis. *Lancet Oncol*. 2016;17:e392–e405.
63. Ferguson CM, Swaroop MN, Horick N, et al. Impact of ipsilateral blood draws, injections, blood pressure measurements, and air travel on the risk of lymphedema for patients treated for breast cancer. *J Clin Oncol*. 2016;34:691–698.
64. Iyer NS, Cartmel B, Friedman L, et al. Lymphedema in ovarian cancer survivors: assessing diagnostic methods and the

effect of physical activity. *Cancer*. 2018;124(9):1929–1937. Available from: https://doi.org/10.1002/cncr.31239.

65. Lockwood-Rayerman S. Lymphedema in gynecologic cancer survivors: an area for exploration? *Cancer Nurs*. 2007;30:E11–E18.
66. Stanton AWB, Northfield JW, Holroyd B, et al. Validation of an optoelectronic limb volumeter (perometer). *Lymphology*. 1997;39:77–97.
67. Gatt M, Willis S, Leuschner S, et al. A meta-analysis of the effectiveness and safety of kinesiology taping in the management of cancer-related lymphoedema. *Eur J Cancer Care (Engl)*. 2017;26(5). Available from: https://doi.org/10.1111/ecc.12510.
68. Schmitz KH, Ahmed RL, Troxel A, et al. Weight lifting in women with breast-cancer-related lymphedema. *N Engl J Med*. 2009;361:664–673.
69. Coyne KS, Sexton C, LoCasale RJ, et al. Opioid-induced constipation among a convenience sample of patients with cancer pain. *Front Oncol*. 2016;6:131.
70. Klee M, Thranov I, Machin Prof D. The patients' perspective on physical symptoms after radiotherapy for cervical cancer. *Gynecol Oncol*. 2000;76(1):14–23.
71. Kunheri B, Kotne S, Nair SS, et al. A dosimetric analysis of cardiac dose with or without active breath coordinator moderate deep inspiratory breath hold in left sided breast cancer radiotherapy. *J Cancer Res Ther*. 2017;13(1):56–61.
72. Cleveland Clinic. Deep inspiration breath hold in breast cancer treatment. <https://my.clevelandclinic.org/health/treatments/16711-deep-inspiration-breath-hold-in-breast-cancer-treatment> Accessed 21.11.19. Last reviewed 1/7/19.
73. Qu D, Zhang Z, Yu X, et al. Psychotropic drugs for the management of cancer-related fatigue: a systematic review and meta-analysis. *Eur J Cancer Care*. 2016;25(6):970–979.
74. Oken MM, Creech RH, Tormey DC, et al. Toxicity and response criteria of the Eastern Cooperative Oncology Group. *Am J Clin Oncol*. 1982;5(6):654.
75. Karnofsky D, Burchenal J. The clinical evaluation of chemotherapeutic agents in cancer. In: MacLeod C, ed. *Evaluation of Chemotherapeutic Agents*. New York: Columbia University Press; 1949:196.
76. Raj VS, Silver JK, Pugh TM, Fu JB. Palliative care and physiatry in the oncology care spectrum: an opportunity for distinct and collaborative approaches. *Phys Med Rehabil Clin N Am*. 2017;28:35–47. Available from: https://doi.org/10.1016/j.pmr.2016.08.006.
77. Keith RA, Granger CV, Hamilton BB, Sherwin FS. The functional independence measure: A new tool for rehabilitation. *Adv Clin Rehabil*. 1987;1:6–18.
78. Sahin S, Uyanik M. The impact of occupation-based problem-solving strategies training in women with breast cancer. *Health Qual Life Outcomes*. 2019;17(1):104. Available from: https://doi.org/10.1186/s12955-019-1170-5.
79. Noeres D, Park-Simon T-W, Grabow J, et al. Return to work after treatment for primary breast cancer over a 6-year period: results from a prospective study comparing patients with the general population. *Support Care Cancer*. 2013;21:1901–1909. Available from: https://doi.org/10.1007/s00520-013-1739-1.
80. Cheville A. Rehabilitation of patients with advanced cancer. *Cancer*. 2001;92:1039–1048. 10.1002/1097-0142(20010815)92:4 + < 1039::AID-CNCR1417 > 3.0.CO;2-L.
81. Cannioto RA, Moysich KB. Epithelial ovarian cancer and recreational physical activity: a review of the epidemiological literature and implications for exercise prescription. *Gynecol Oncol*. 2015;137(3):559–573. Available from: https://doi.org/10.1016/j.ygyno.2015.03.016.
82. Office of Disease Prevention and Health Promotion. Physical activity guidelines, 2018. <https://health.gov/paguidelines/second-edition/pdf/Physical_Activity_Guidelines_2nd_edition.pdf> Accessed 07.10.19.
83. Campbell K, Winters-Stone KM, Wiskemann J, et al. Exercise guidelines for cancer survivors: consensus statement from international multi-disciplinary roundtable. *Med Sci Sports Exerc*. 2019;51(11):2375–2390. Available from: https://doi.org/10.1249/MSS.0000000000002116.
84. Ahles TA. Brain vulnerability to chemotherapy toxicities. *Psychooncology*. 2012;21:1141–1148. Available from: https://doi.org/10.1002/pon.3196.
85. Kaiser J, Bledowski C, Dietrich J. Neural correlates of chemotherapy-related cognitive impairment. *Cortex*. 2014;54:33–50. Available from: https://doi.org/10.1016/j.cortex.2014.01.010.
86. Kovalchuk A, Ilnytskyy Y, Rodriguez-Juarez R, et al. Chemo brain or tumor brain – that is the question: the presence of extra-cranial tumors profoundly affects molecular processes in the prefrontal cortex of TumorGraft mice. *Aging (Albany NY)*. 2017;9(7):1660–1676. Available from: https://doi.org/10.18632/aging.101243.
87. Bayer JL, Spitz DR, Christensen D, et al. Biobehavioral and neuroendocrine correlates of antioxidant enzyme activity in ovarian carcinoma. *Brain Behav Immun*. 2015;50:58–62. Available from: https://doi.org/10.1016/j.bbi.2015.04.019.
88. Thompson B, Hohl HD, Molina Y, et al. Breast cancer disparities among women in underserved communities in the USA. *Curr Breast Cancer Rep*. 2018;10(3):131–141. Available from: https://doi.org/10.1007/s12609-018-0277-8.
89. Thomas TH, Nauth-Shelley K, Thompson MA, et al. The needs of women treated for ovarian cancer: results from a #gyncsm Twitter chat. *J Patient Cent Res Rev*. 2018;5(2):149–157. Available from: https://doi.org/10.17294/2330-0698.1592.

CHAPTER 24

Palliative Care and Symptom Management in Breast and Gynecological Cancers

SULEYKI MEDINA, MD • MARIANA KHAWAND-AZOULAI, MD

The World Health Organization (WHO) defines palliative care as "an approach that improves the quality of life of patients and their families facing the problems associated with life-threatening illness, through the prevention and relief of suffering by means of early identification and impeccable assessment and treatment of pain and other problems, physical, psychosocial and spiritual."[1]

Patients with breast and gynecological cancers face numerous obstacles and sequelae from their illness as well as from treatment side effects that can be effectively addressed by palliative care specialists. Currently, the American Society of Clinical Oncology (ASCO) recommends that patients with advanced cancer should be referred to interdisciplinary palliative care teams in a consultative model, early in the course of disease and alongside active treatment of their cancer.[2] Patients with early-stage disease, but high symptom burden, can also benefit from comanagement with a palliative care team.

Palliative care provides an added layer of support for relief of pain, symptoms, and stress for individuals with serious illness. Specialty palliative care teams are composed of palliative care-certified physicians, nurses, social workers, chaplains, and individuals from other disciplines that provide expert consultation and/or comanagement.

Palliative medicine specialists can treat a wide array of symptoms related to cancer and cancer treatments, including, but not limited to, cancer-related pain, chemotherapy-induced peripheral neuropathy, nausea, vomiting, diarrhea, appetite disturbances, constipation, fatigue, insomnia, and mood disorders such as depression and anxiety.

In addition to symptom management, palliative medicine clinicians provide assistance in assessing the patient's illness understanding and documenting patient preferences, including advance directives (ADs). Palliative medicine clinicians use open-ended questions to assess patient and family expectations of the illness and treatment plan. This is especially crucial in patients with advanced illness or poor prognosis. The physician works hand-in-hand with the other specialties—medical oncology, radiation oncology, surgical oncology, physical medicine, and rehabilitation—to understand the patient's illness and overall prognosis.

The team then uses this information to guide patients in their advance care planning (ACP).

The palliative medicine team also provides psychosocial and spiritual support to patients, families, and caregivers via the collaboration of social workers and chaplains certified in palliative care.

When patients are referred in a timely manner, palliative medicine specialists can address these issues early in the course of illness.

Benefits of early palliative care include[3]

- better patient and family understanding of what to expect;
- relief of pain and other symptoms;
- increased life expectancy (in some populations);
- increased family and caregiver support; and
- decreased crises, 911 calls, ED visits, and hospitalizations.

While palliative care is a medical subspecialty, the principles and the practices of palliative care can and should be employed by all clinicians that work with seriously ill patients. This is known as primary palliative care. Specialty palliative care is delivered by an interdisciplinary team, usually headed by a board-certified palliative medicine specialist.

Palliative care is often confused for hospice care; however, the two approaches have important distinguishing factors (Table 24.1). While hospice is a "palliative care

Breast Cancer and Gynecologic Cancer Rehabilitation DOI: https://doi.org/10.1016/B978-0-323-72166-0.00024-4

TABLE 24.1
Palliative Care vs Hospice Care

Palliative Care	Hospice
Based on patient and family need, not prognosis	
Concurrent with disease treatment	Certified prognosis of <6 months
Appropriate at any stage of serious illness from disease onset to bereavement for families	Patient agrees to give up insurance coverage of disease treatment
Concurrent with all appropriate treatments and services	Life expectancy ≤6 months, and bereavement for families
Widely available in hospitals; limited but growing access in community settings	Must forego "curative" care for terminal illness as condition of enrollment
	Widely available in community and institutional settings (>5500 programs in the United States)

only" approach, palliative care begins at diagnosis and can be delivered alongside curative or life-prolonging therapies. In order to receive hospice benefit, a patient must have a certified prognosis of less than 6 months if the illness runs its natural course. In addition, once enrolled in hospice services, a patient agrees to forfeit insurance coverage for their "hospice-qualifying diagnosis." Finally, while receiving hospice care, a patient must forego "curative" or life-prolonging therapies, whereas palliative care services are appropriately delivered concurrently with all appropriate treatments and services.

It is important to note that *all hospice care is palliative care, but not all palliative care is hospice*.

Both palliative care and hospice care are underutilized. According to the Center to Advance Palliative Care, as of 2017, only 48% of Medicare deaths are preceded by hospice care. Among enrollees, 54% receive hospice care for less than 30 days, and 28% receive hospice care for a week or less.

Near the end of life, palliative care teams often assist in the patient and family decisions to enroll in hospice care and can ease the transition from receiving aggressive treatment to focusing solely on comfort.

Palliative care delivered early on, through the course of a serious illness such as cancer, can improve patients' symptoms, satisfaction with care, and quality of life. Excellent palliative care delivery begins with a detailed patient assessment.

COMPREHENSIVE PATIENT ASSESSMENT

A comprehensive palliative care assessment is essential to the management of cancer patients. Uncontrolled symptoms such as pain and fatigue often result in worsening well-being, psychological symptoms, and ultimately quality of life for patients and their families. Symptom assessment tools are widely available in the field of palliative care to ensure timely screening and diagnosis of symptoms and syndromes, resulting in their timely management. The palliative care domains important to assess are physical symptoms, performance status; psychological/psychiatric symptoms; social and economic needs of the patient, family, caregiver; and religious, spiritual, and existential issues.[4]

One effective tool to screen for palliative care needs is the National Comprehensive Cancer Network (NCCN) distress thermometer which is effective and well validated to evaluate untreated distress in the physical, social, or psychological domains. Patients can rate distress from 0 to 10 and designate particular areas of concern that may merit a palliative care consultation.[5]

The Edmonton Symptom Assessment System (ESAS) and the Memorial Symptom Assessment Scale (MSAS) are reliable, validated tools used to assess physical symptoms in the clinical setting. The ESAS assesses 10 common symptoms (pain, fatigue, nausea, depression, anxiety, drowsiness, shortness of breath, appetite, feeling of well-being, and other symptoms) over the past 24 hours.[4] Other less commonly reported symptoms such as pruritus, xerostomia, hiccups, and muscle spasms are also inquired about. Performance status tools used in palliative care include the Karnofsky Performance Status (KPS), Eastern Cooperative Oncology Group (EGOG), and Palliative Performance Scale (PPS). Both the KPS and the ECOG performance status have been validated in patients with cancer and correlate with survival. For example, a KPS of 40 or/and ECOG score of greater than 3 are associated with survival of 3 months or less.[5]

Palliative care clinicians also use a multitude of assessment tools to assess psychological, psychiatric, and cognitive domains; these include ESAS, MDAS

(Memorial Delirium Assessment Scale), and PHQ-9. There are also assessment tools used to assess the spiritual domain; these include FICA (faith, importance, community, action), HOPE (sources of hope, organized religion, personal spirituality and practices, effects on medical care, and end-of-life issues), and SPIRIT (spiritual belief system, personal spirituality, integration with a spiritual community, ritualized practices and restrictions, implications for medical care, and terminal event planning). Only FICA has been validated.[4]

PAIN MANAGEMENT

Pain is defined as "an unpleasant sensory and emotional experience associated with actual or potential tissue injury or damage. The intensity of pain varies with the degree of injury, disease, or emotional impact."[6] Pain is one of the main symptoms experienced by cancer patients during both curative and palliative therapy. Numerous national and international surveys have found that 30%–50% of cancer patients in active therapy and as many as 60%–90% with advanced disease have pain.[4] Although pain management and the alleviation of suffering are core clinical competencies for all clinicians treating seriously ill patients, in reality pain is frequently undertreated. There are many barriers to pain management which include physicians' lack of knowledge, lack of availability of opioid medications, governmental regulations, physicians' fear of regulations, diversion of medications, and fear of addiction.[4]

In 2016 the American Society of Clinical Oncology (ASCO) issued a statement reflecting that cancer patients should be largely exempt from measures taken to halt the epidemic of opioid abuse and addiction, on the grounds that cancer patients are a "special population." Their statement also reflected that cancer patients should be exempt from regulations that limit their access to appropriate medical opioid therapy given the unique nature of cancer, its treatment, and potentially the lifelong adverse health effects from having had cancer. ASCO also recognized the need to balance public health concerns regarding abuse and misuse of prescription opioids with the need to ensure access to appropriate pain management to cancer patients and survivors. Emphasis should be placed on safe opioid prescribing principles, including appropriate utilization, storage, and disposal of prescription pain medications. Regularly consulting your state's prescription monitoring program, which enables clinicians to access patients' controlled substance prescription history, is also highly recommended.[7]

There are multiple etiologies of cancer pain. For example, there is pain associated with direct tumor involvement (infiltration of bone, nerves, and viscera) that occurs in 65%–85% of patients with advanced cancer. Pain can also occur indirectly via tumor release of inflammatory mediators. Treatments aimed at cure or palliation can also cause significant pain in approximately 15%–25% of patients receiving chemotherapy, surgery, or radiation therapy.[4]

Therapeutic choices for pain management are often guided by pathophysiology. Pain syndromes are generally divided into two categories: acute versus chronic. Pain that occurs in the acute setting is mainly related to cancer therapeutic interventions. Chronic pain is subdivided into nociceptive (somatic vs visceral) and neuropathic. *Nociceptive* pain is associated with ongoing tissue damage. *Somatic* pain occurs as a result of activation of cutaneous and deep tissue receptors, and it is roughly described as sharp, well localized, throbbing, and gnawing. *Visceral* pain results when distention, stretching, and inflammation activate nociceptors. It is described as dull, poorly localized, cramping, or pressure. Neuropathic pain is described as tingling, shooting, stabbing, burning, electric like, and numb, and results from damage to nerves.[4]

Breakthrough pain is common in cancer patients and is defined by Yennuranjalingam and Bruera as a "transitory exacerbation of pain that occurs on a background of otherwise stable persistent pain." Breakthrough pain may be caused by activity or end-of-dose failure (a situation in which a patient experiences pain before their medication therapeutic time is expected to end); it can also occur spontaneously.[4]

A thorough pain history requires eliciting information about anatomic regions and organ systems, temporal characteristics (pattern of occurrence), intensity, time of onset of pain, and etiology.[8] A helpful pneumonic to elicit a pain history is the PQRST mnemonic that stands for provocative factors, quality, region and radiation, severity, and temporal factors.[9] A thorough history should also be followed by a physical exam, review of the medical record, including labs and imaging.[8]

The intensity of pain should be measured on a 0 (no pain) to 10 (extreme severe pain) scale, and this intensity should be quantified over time to identify any underlying patterns and to assess treatment efficacy. Mild levels of pain (less than 4/10) are not disabling and allow a more normal function and engagement. Moderate pain levels of 4–6 on a 10-point scale and tend to interfere with normal function and sleep, while severe pain levels of 7/10–10/10 significantly affect the patient's ability to perform instrumental activities of daily living (IADLs). It is important to remember that psychological, social, spiritual, and financial problems can affect a patient's perception and tolerance of pain.[8]

Opioids are the basis for the management of cancer-related pain as they are the most effective and fastest acting analgesics to target this condition. The treatment of cancer-related pain should also involve a multidimensional approach that includes the optimization of nonpharmacologic treatments and the expertise of specialists when necessary.[4]

There are no strict rules to follow when choosing between strong opioids (i.e., morphine, hydromorphone, methadone, and fentanyl) to treat cancer-related pain. Generic morphine is a reasonable initial choice because of its efficacy, relatively low cost, familiarity by physicians, wide availability, and variety of formulations. Initial choice of opioid therapy should also be guided by patient factors such as the presence of renal and hepatic insufficiency, and older age.[8]

Renal impairment generally increases a drug's half-life through a decrease in renal elimination. Since opioids are renally cleared, dose reductions, dose interval increases, or a different drug may be necessary for patients with renal insufficiency. Generally, morphine, codeine, meperidine, and tramadol should be avoided in this setting. Preferred short-acting medications include hydromorphone and oxycodone. Methadone and fentanyl are not dialyzable and therefore should be used with caution in patients on dialysis.[8]

Hepatic impairment may result in decreased metabolism, decreased drug clearance, and increased bioavailability, which may lead to drug accumulation. Fentanyl, hydromorphone, oxycodone, morphine, and methadone can be used with caution. Dosage reductions or increased dosing intervals are warranted in this setting. Codeine and meperidine should be avoided because of the potential for accumulation of metabolites.[8]

Older adults who have reduced renal function need careful choice and dosing of analgesics. However, opioids should not be withheld from older adults in pain. The general approach is to "start low and go slow," titrating gradually using small increments and monitoring adverse effects, including changes in mental status, excessive sedation, or constipation.[8]

GENERAL GUIDELINES FOR PHARMACOLOGICAL PAIN MANAGEMENT

The goal of pain management from a clinical standpoint is to improve quality of life and improve function. Assessment of activities of daily living (ADLs) and instrumental activities of daily living (IADLs) as well as calculating performance status with ECOG or PPS, should be performed routinely to assess efficacy of therapy.

The first step to pharmacological pain management is to define goals of therapy and setting patients' expectations. Analgesics should be chosen based on etiology of pain, pathophysiologic mechanism of pain, analgesic responsiveness, potency of analgesic, and side effect profile.

The World Health Organization endorses a three-step ladder approach to analgesic prescribing. For mild pain, acetaminophen and/or nonsteroidal antiinflammatory drugs (NSAIDs) can be initiated with care not to exceed recommended max dose in 24 hours. For moderate-to-severe pain a combination product such as Acetaminophen/Oxycodone (Percocet) may be used, although these products have a ceiling dose for analgesia governed by the nonopioid component. Conversely, one may start a single agent (opioid) and titrate to achieve analgesia prior to adding or switching to another opioid.

The least invasive route should be chosen whenever possible. The oral route is the most convenient and cost-effective. Other available routes include intravenous, subcutaneous, transdermal, per rectum (inconvenient), intramuscular (painful), sublingual, and intrathecal (most invasive).

Clinician should choose a dosing schedule that is simple and individualized, based on temporal patterns. For example, for episodic or breakthrough pain, short-acting opioids every 4 hours as needed may be used. For continuous pain, short-acting opioids dosed every 4 hours around clock (ATC) may be chosen until steady state is reached at approximately 24 hours.

Patients with chronic and severe pain can benefit from long-acting opioids given around the clock because they allow the achievement of more consistent blood levels, reduce pain recurrence, improve adherence to treatment, and reduce dependence.[7] Conversion to a long-acting opioid may start after 24 hours of continuous ATC dosing of immediate release opioid. A short acting opioid (10% of 24 hour total dose) should be added for rescue (for breakthrough pain).

Opioid doses can then be titrated to achieve patient's preferred goal, only after steady state is reached at 48–72 hours. When a basal dose is increased, the rescue dose should also be increased.

An opioid may be rotated (switched) to a different opioid if there is no response to current regimen, if patient requires a different route of administration (i.e., a patient with dysphagia), or if patient develops intolerable side effects. Rotation should also be considered after nonopioid analgesics have also been tried.

When converting from one opioid to another, it is recommended the equianalgesic dose be reduced by one-third to one-half due to increased sensitivity to a new opioid when switching opioids.

Always treat opioid-related side effects that include nausea with or without vomiting, sedation, myoclonus, delirium, urinary retention, or other intolerable side effects. Usually, the first step in treating adverse effects is to decrease opioid dose or increase dosing frequency. Rapid cessation of opioids may result in opioid withdrawal, which is a syndrome characterized by yawning, sweating, lacrimation, rhinorrhea, anxiety, restlessness, dilated pupils, piloerection, nausea/vomiting, abdominal pain, diarrhea, and muscle aches. The Clinical Opiate Withdrawal Scale (COWS) is an 11-item scale administered by a clinician in the inpatient or outpatient setting, to determine the severity of withdrawal and a patient's dependence on opioids.[10]

Naloxone (Narcan), an opioid antagonist, should only be used in emergencies. It reverses respiratory depression, sedation, as well as analgesia.

Clinicians should remain vigilant in identifying and responding to warning signs of opioid misuse, which include asking for early refills, lost prescriptions, repeated requests for dose escalation, and obtaining prescriptions from multiple sources.[8] If addiction is suspected, it may be helpful to consult an addiction specialist for guidance.

Nonopioid adjuvants have analgesic properties and are frequently used for specific pain syndromes, alongside opioids. Sometimes, they are recommended as first-line agents in cancer pain management. They are recommended at every step of the WHO ladder. The main categories include tricyclic antidepressants, antiepileptic drugs, steroids, bisphosphonates, and selective serotonin and norepinephrine inhibitors. Other adjuvants such as NSAIDs may be added to treat bone pain/metastases, while others such as gabapentin can alleviate neuropathic pain. Dexamethasone is helpful to reduce pain arising from liver capsule distention. Cannabinoids may also be used in pain syndromes (see the section on medical marijuana later in this chapter).

Many patients have also reported improved pain relief from nonpharmacological methods such as massage therapy, distraction, pet therapy, acupuncture, and local heat or cold, although there is little systemic research to guide their use.[8] Nonetheless, these methods are often used alongside pharmacologic methods.

Psychological techniques such as biofeedback, relaxation, hypnosis, and cognitive and operant approaches can enable a patient to accept the responsibility of managing their pain so they can begin to cope and function more effectively.[8]

There may be instances in which an existing pain regimen may fail to provide relief, such as in the setting of cancer progression. A pain crisis is defined as an event in which a patient reports intense, uncontrolled pain that is causing severe personal or family distress. This event represents an acute change in the patient's condition or it may result from gradually increasing pain that crosses a threshold. Severe pain, usually rated in the range of 7/10–10/10 tends to dominate all other experiences. An acute pain crisis is considered a palliative care emergency. The first step in managing this emergency is to assess the patient. The extent of the workup required to treat it will be guided by the patient's underlying disease, prognosis, prior functional status, preferences, and past pain experiences and behaviors.

A comprehensive history and physical exam needs to be performed. If the pain results in an abrupt change in clinical status, evaluation may include diagnostic procedures, especially if the results will lead to potentially effective treatments that would improve the patient's quality of life. While the patient is being evaluated for a specific intervention, an opioid bolus of 10% of the patient's total daily dose can be given. Efficacy should be assessed every 10–15 minutes. If pain is still present, a higher dose can be administered; for example, rescue dose can be increased by 25% to 50%. Subsequent doses can be administered every 15 minutes until adequate analgesia is obtained. Once the effective dose is found, it can be scheduled to be given every 4 hours.[8] If patient-controlled analgesia (PCA) is required, the hourly basal rate should be calculated after the latest 24 hour total opioid requirement. Rescue doses are typically 50% of the hourly basal rate. These rescue doses may be given in intervals of 15 minutes or up to four rescue doses per hour.[7] A clinician activated dose can also be provided. It is generally 100%–200% of the hourly b; for example, rescue dose can be increased by 25% to 50%.asal rate every 2–4 hours as needed. Expert consultation with an inpatient palliative care service is recommended in an acute pain crisis.

Cancer-related pain management also incorporates procedural methods that can provide pain relief, which may include nerve blocks, spinal infusions, external beam radiation, and radiopharmaceuticals.

Expert pain management is essential to the success of breast and gynecological cancer patients participating in a rehabilitation program, as untreated or poorly controlled pain, could limit rehabilitation potential and could further diminish performance status.

NAUSEA

Nausea and vomiting (N/V) whether acutely related to chemotherapy, other chronic condition, or cancer complications, often results in significant distress, decreased social interaction, and poor quality of life.[7] The prevalence of N/V is as high as 70% among patients with cancer.

It is also a consequence of metabolic derangements, medication side effects, changes in gastric and bowel motility, and central nervous system disorders.[11] Chemotherapy-induced nausea and vomiting (CINV) is subdivided into three types depending on the onset of symptoms: anticipatory, acute, or delayed. Other causes may be directly related to chemicals (medications, toxins), impaired gastric emptying (opioids, ascites), visceral causes (bowel obstruction, peritoneal carcinomatosis), cortical (intracranial tumor), and vestibular (motion sickness). Nausea and vomiting interferes with patients' ability to take medications. It also limits oral intake often leading to dehydration, anorexia, weight loss, electrolyte disturbance, and diminished quality of life.[11] These complications also interfere with patients' ability to receive life-prolonging or palliative chemotherapy, as well as rehabilitative therapy.

The vomiting center is considered the final common pathway in emesis.[7] The vomiting center receives input directly from the cerebral cortex, thalamus, higher brain stem, hypothalamus, sensory organs, and the vestibular apparatus in the inner ear. Indirect stimulation of the vomiting center arrives from the chemoreceptor trigger zone (CTZ) that is located on the floor of the fourth ventricle. Stimulation of the CTZ occurs via noxious stimuli such as chemotherapy, medications, and metabolic disturbances. The CTZ then stimulates the vomiting center via dopamine, serotonin, histamine, vasopressin, and substance P, ultimately resulting in emesis.[7] The most common mechanism implicated in CINV is via direct stimulation of the CTZ within the area postrema.

The assessment of nausea and vomiting requires a careful history and a focused physical examination to identify specific physical and psychological contributors. In the palliative care setting, the causes are almost always multifactorial.

Diagnostic workup will depend in part on the stage of the patient's illness and the patient's goals of care. Workup may include blood draws to check electrolytes and drug levels. Radiologic imaging may be necessary to rule out potential medical complications including increased intracranial pressure, gastroparesis, ileus, gastric outlet obstruction, and bowel obstruction. Intraabdominal sources are common in gynecological and gastrointestinal cancer patients and often present with an obstructive component. The goal is to rapidly identify and treat underlying reversible causes. Empiric pharmacologic treatment is usually needed to control symptoms. A strategic approach in the management of nausea and vomiting is to target several implicated receptors simultaneously for a synergistic effect in order to achieve optimal control of symptoms.[11]

Presently, the management of acute chemotherapy-induced nausea and vomiting (CINV) due to chemotherapy with high emetogenic potential includes a combination of a 5-HT3 (5-hydroxytryptamine) receptor antagonist, corticosteroids, a neurokinin-1-receptor antagonist, and olanzapine. Olanzapine is excluded if CINV is due to chemotherapy with moderate emetogenic potential.[12]

The treatment of delayed CINV due to chemotherapy with high emetogenic potential is dexamethasone on days 2–4, plus Aprepitant. For moderate emetogenic chemotherapy, the treatment for delayed CINV is Aprepitant on days 2 and 3.[12]

Treatment for anticipatory CINV includes an effective antiemetic regimen prior to chemotherapy. Short-acting benzodiazepines (alprazolam, lorazepam) are also useful. Nonpharmacologic strategies include relaxation, music therapy, and acupuncture.[11]

For breakthrough CINV, antipsychotics such as metoclopramide can substitute 5-HT3 antagonists. For refractory symptoms or failure to respond to conventional antiemetics, cannabinoids such as dronabinol and nabilone may be added. The atypical antipsychotic Olanzapine has potential antiemetic properties because of its effects on multiple receptor sites implicated in the nausea and vomiting pathway.[11]

When treating nausea and vomiting from other causes, a nonpharmacological approach can be helpful. For example, environmental factors should be identified and eliminated (i.e., fragrances, strong cooking smells) prior to initiating a pharmacological regimen.

The treatments for other conditions contributing to nausea and vomiting should also be implemented.

Antiemetics can be started using a case-based or empirical approach. Antiemetics should be taken when best tolerated, either spread throughout the day or after meals. They can also be taken prophylactically or on a regular basis. Treating nausea and vomiting effectively and aggressively is vital to optimizing a patient's rehabilitation potential.

CONSTIPATION

Constipation is prevalent in the palliative care population and in end-of-life care. It involves a complex interaction of anatomic, neurologic, and iatrogenic factors. Constipation may be caused by low intake of food, fluid and fiber, immobility, and drugs used to treat other conditions that impair gut motility such as opioids, antiemetics, anticholinergics, and NSAIDs. Cancer-related complications such as bowel obstruction, hypercalcemia, intraabdominal, and pelvic disease; cord compression; and cauda equina syndrome are other contributing factors. Constipation is defined as infrequent or absent bowel movements; decrease of BM volume; difficulty or pain with defecation; incomplete defecation, abdominal distention, oozing liquid stool; or hard stool.[7] It should be treated quickly and aggressively.

Assessment includes taking a careful history about bowel habits, stool frequency and consistency, laxative use, and associated environmental factors such as lack of privacy or a long distance to the toilet and performing a physical exam (including a digital rectal exam). Bowel obstruction must be ruled out prior to any further investigation.

The treatment of constipation in the palliative care setting is based on limited research evidence. Most patients will need both a scheduled medication regimen and the use of rescue medications for episodes of constipation. Patients on regular doses of opioid therapy should receive a regularly scheduled laxative, and most will benefit from a stimulant or osmotic laxative administered as needed (PRN).[8]

Bulk-forming fiver agents (e.g., psyllium and methylcellulose) should be avoided because of their tendency to form impactions when patients stop taking adequate amounts of fluids. Approach to management of constipation is mainly pharmacological, but nonpharmacological options should also be considered. Drug choice should be individualized.

Drug classes frequently used to treat constipation include stool softeners, stimulants, osmotic agents, enemas, antipsychotics, and opioid antagonists. One senna tablet daily is a common starting point, although it may require titration to a maximum of four tabs twice a day. Additional medications can be added in a stepwise fashion.[11]

Polyethylene glycol a commonly used osmotic laxative that is tasteless, odorless, and generally well tolerated by patients. It has been found to be effective for opioid-induced constipation, and there is evidence that it may be more effective than lactulose for chronic constipation.[8]

Rectal suppositories and enemas may be used when constipation is severe. Oral medications should limit the need for their use if the bowel regimen if used efficiently. Common side effects include bloating, flatulence, disliked taste, and diarrhea. Tolerance to stimulant laxatives is uncommon. Bowel obstruction may be a contraindication to stimulant laxatives, as laxatives may increase colic. Increased activity, ambulation, and exercise can also improve constipation.

MALIGNANT BOWEL OBSTRUCTION

Malignant bowel obstruction is a common complication of gastrointestinal and ovarian cancers. It usually occurs in the advanced stages of illness. The average life expectancy is about 80 days at the time of presentation, as evidenced by a recent prospective study.[11] The pathogenesis of bowel obstruction may be directly related to cancer lesions. There are several types observed clinically. One type is the intraluminal obstruction that leads to impaired peristalsis and occlusion of the lumen. Extramural obstructions are generally caused by mesenteric lesions, omental masses, and adhesions.[11] Complications of cancer treatments such as surgical adhesions and intraperitoneal chemotherapy are also causes of obstruction. Obstructions can be partial or complete. The absence of feces or flatus suggests a complete obstruction while incomplete obstruction may present with overflow incontinence. Common symptomatology includes nausea with or without vomiting and periumbilical, colicky abdominal pain that travels in waves.[8] The pathophysiology is described next.

At the onset of obstruction, there is significant damage that occurs to the gut epithelium. This damage triggers an inflammatory response marked by release of inflammatory mediators such as prostaglandins, vasoactive peptide, and other secretagogues. This inflammatory cascade ultimately stimulates a large influx of fluid into the gut lumen with concomitant decreased reabsorption of water and electrolytes. Eventually, bowel dilation and edema ensue, leading to colicky pain, nausea, and vomiting. This cycle is viciously repeated as the gut continues to contract.[11] Complications of malignant bowel obstruction include dehydration, electrolyte disturbances, and ultimately perforation. Diagnosis is confirmed via imaging (i.e., abdominal XR revealing air-fluid levels and distended loops of bowel).

Although most bowel obstructions are partial obstructions and can be managed effectively with medications, surgical intervention, venting gastrostomy, or metallic stenting should also be considered as part of palliative care management plans. Venting gastrostomy may be helpful for high-grade proximal obstructions, eliminating the necessity of nasogastric (NG) tube suctioning and IV fluids for symptom control.[11] In addition, self-expanding metallic stents (SEMS) are possible alternatives for individuals with esophageal gastric outlet, proximal bowel, and large bowel obstructions.[11] Late complications of SEMS placement can be as high as 50% and include migration, obstruction, perforation, and tenesmus.[11]

Surgical interventions may or may not be practical, especially if there are multiple sites of obstruction present. Patient selection is critical, as patients with advanced disease carry significant perioperative morbidity and mortality.[11] Generally, patients with a life expectancy of 2 months or less and patients with poor performance status should forgo surgery.

Successful symptom control can also be achieved with a combination of analgesic, anticholinergic, and antiemetic drugs, thought to reduce intestinal secretions and intraluminal hypertension, working synergistically.

For intractable symptoms and in the setting of partial obstruction, combinations of opioids, dexamethasone, haloperidol, and metoclopramide may be needed. Octreotide has been used to reduce gastrointestinal secretions in malignant obstructions, although a recent systematic review suggested that its efficacy on key clinical outcomes may be limited.[8] Timely treatment increases the possibility of return to normal bowel function, which is instrumental in allowing eating, improved quality of life, and possibly survival.[11]

ANOREXIA CACHEXIA SYNDROME

Anorexia, or loss of appetite, is frequently encountered in the cancer-palliative care setting. Cachexia, which frequently accompanies anorexia, is among the most debilitating and life-threatening aspects of cancer progression, occurring in about 80%–90% of patients with advanced cancer.[6] Cachexia is usually associated with significant patient and family distress. It is associated with poor prognosis and occurs in a spectrum (precachexia, cachexia, refractory cachexia).

This is a multifactorial syndrome characterized by ongoing loss of skeletal muscle mass (with or without the loss of fat mass) that cannot be fully reversed by conventional nutritional support and leads to progressive functional impairment.[13]

Nutritional impact symptoms and a proinflammatory response are two of several interrelated mechanisms responsible for the anorexia cachexia syndrome. The role of nutritional impact symptoms, such as dental problems, severe pain, mouth sores, altered taste, dry mouth, fatigue, early satiety, constipation, and nausea and vomiting, are well established.[6] These ultimately lead to decreased oral intake and malnutrition. A proinflammatory response mainly involving IL-6 (interleukin 6), IFN (interferon), and TNF (tumor necrosis factor) ultimately result in muscle wasting. Proinflammatory cytokines are thought to induce catabolism; this may explain the inability of artificial feeding techniques to improve the cachexia associated with terminal illness.[7]

In the evaluation of anorexia–cachexia, it is important to take a careful history, including a nutritional history and a medication history. It is also important to assess for other contributing symptoms via the ESAS tool and to screen for nutritional impact symptoms leading to poor oral intake.

The objective assessment includes documenting weight loss of $\geq$5% in 6 months or weight loss of >2% in patients showing decreasing BMI or decrease in muscle mass within 6 months, physical exam and body composition, serial measurement of body weight and oral intake, and imaging and labs.[6]

Generally, the management of anorexia–cachexia is challenging (even with involvement of palliative care specialists) due to current lack of effective treatments. If cachexia does not respond to treatments aimed at reversing treatable causes, the treatment approach becomes a multidisciplinary one. The goals of therapy may include decreasing family distress, improving appetite, increasing social interaction, and improving physical function as recovery of muscle is less likely. The treatment approach may include best supportive care/palliative care, psychosocial support, incorporating an exercise program, incorporating nutritional support/dietary counseling, managing nutritional impact symptoms, and incorporating pharmacological management to increase appetite.

The established therapies in the cancer population include megestrol acetate (160 mg/day titrated to

800 mg/day), glucocorticoids (prednisone 20–40 mg/day) or equivalent doses of dexamethasone (3–4 mg/day in divided doses). Cannabinoids have not demonstrated any activity against anorexia and cachexia in patients with advanced cancer. Cyproheptadine (serotonin and histamine antagonist) 8 mg three times daily is a good option for patients with carcinoid syndrome who have anorexia/cachexia. Miscellaneous treatments include mirtazapine and olanzapine. Mirtazapine is a tetracyclic antidepressant–inducing weight gain and food intake. Definitive proof of benefit requires randomized, placebo-controlled trial.[14]

Data suggests that olanzapine adds to the already established benefits of megestrol acetate in reducing the severity of cancer-associated anorexia and increasing nonfluid weight gain, but results were not considered definitive due to single-institution study.[14]

Artificial nutrition is generally not recommended for cancer cachexia–anorexia syndrome, as systematic reviews suggest that parenteral nutrition is harmful when provided to patients undergoing radiation or chemotherapy for cancer. Artificial nutrition and hydration has not been shown to prolong life.

It is important to educate and counsel patients and families in distress. It is helpful to explain that anorexia is part of the advanced disease process and a natural part of life coming to an end. It is important to note that patients are not starving and can live comfortably for long periods on minimal food or water. On the contrary, force-feeding causes patient discomfort, nausea, aspiration, and potentially respiratory distress.

Control should be placed back on the patients, and they should be encouraged to choose their favorite foods, quantities, and eating schedules. Dietary restrictions should be liberalized.

DEPRESSION AND ANXIETY

Psychological distress is a significant cause of suffering among patients with advanced cancer and is highly associated with decreased quality of life. More than 60% of patients with cancer report experiencing distress. Differentiating these causes of normative distress associated with illness from other psychiatric disorders is essential to the implementation of appropriate treatment plans and to prevent any further threats to patients' physical, psychological, social, and spiritual well-being.[11]

Depression is a significant distressing emotional experience for patients and their families. In the context of a serious illness such as cancer, it can be amplified by physical symptoms, fear of dying, family distress, and as death approaches.[8] It also decreases patient's ability to feel pleasure and connectedness.[11] Depression is also associated with decreased adherence to treatments, prolonged hospital stays, and reduced quality of life. It is also an independent risk factor for suicide and requests for hastened death. Depression has been increasingly recognized to affect survival in several cancers. Symptoms of depression have been reported in up to 58% of the patients with cancer. Rates of major depression range as high as 38% among these patients.[11]

Anxiety is an expected, normal, transient response to stress. An excessive response to an unidentified internal stressor is considered pathological. Anxiety symptoms are often physical (diaphoresis, dizziness), emotional (feeling of impending doom), behavioral (psychomotor agitation), and cognitive (worry, fear). Anxiety symptoms are thought to occur in more than 70% of medically ill patients, especially those with cancer or those approaching the end of life.[11] Anxiety often cooccurs with adjustment disorders. An adjustment disorder is a psychological response to an identifiable stressor that results in the development of clinically significant emotional or behavioral symptoms but does not qualify for a diagnosis of anxiety disorder. Many people with serious medical illnesses may have trouble adjusting psychologically to their diagnosis, prognosis, or treatment regimens.

The following two questions have been found to have good sensitivity to screen for depression. A more formal exploration is indicated if the patient has a positive answer to either of these questions: Are you depressed? Do you have much interest or pleasure in doing things?[8]

Clinical depression is associated with hopelessness, helplessness, worthlessness, and guilt. Clinically depressed terminally ill patients are at higher risk of suicide and suicidal ideation, and they may have increased desires and requests for hastened death. Because many of the symptoms of severe illness overlap with symptoms of depression (fatigue, anorexia, sleep disturbance, poor concentration, social withdrawal, hopelessness), consultation with an experienced psychiatrist and/or psychologist may be helpful in complex situations.

Performing a history and physical exam in addition to identifying treatable and reversible medical complications are essential first steps. Special attention should be placed on concomitant symptoms such as physical, psychological, social, and spiritual pain.

Anxiety symptoms may be triggered by a range of medical transitions such as the initial diagnosis of a serious illness, a recurrence, treatment side effects or failure, or discussion of hospice. Other fears or anxiety triggers less often brought to the attention of the clinician include uncontrolled pain, isolation, abandonment, loss of control, worrying about a spouse or child, being a burden, death, and dying. Anxiety disorder is very treatable when recognized.

The need to medically treat depression and anxiety depends on their intensity, persistence, and disruption of basic life functioning. Treatment should be considered when these effects dominate other emotions and interfere with the ability to enjoy other aspects of life.

The treatment of anxiety and depression in cancer patients incorporates antidepressant medications, supportive psychotherapy, and patient and family education.[11] Drugs classes include psychostimulants such as methylphenidate, selective serotonin receptor inhibitors (SSRIs), selective serotonin–norepinephrine receptor inhibitors (SSNRIs), tricyclic antidepressants (TCAs), and bupropion. Pharmacological therapy for anxiety also includes benzodiazepines, buspirone, and atypical antipsychotics. Potential nonpharmacological interventions include psychotherapy, meaning-centered therapy, mindfulness meditation, and relaxation.[11] Palliative care specialists work hand-in-hand with mental health professionals such as psychiatrists, psychologists, and licensed clinical social workers to comanage mood disorders.

MEDICAL CANNABIS

Medical cannabis is a novel modality used in palliative care for a multitude of physical and psychological symptoms. Cannabis is an investigational new drug in the United States. Although it is classified as a schedule I controlled substance in the United States, in recent decades an increasing number of states have legalized cannabis for medical purposes via state medical cannabis programs.

For cancer pain a multicenter randomized controlled trial (RCT) involving 360 patients investigated oral cannabis to treat breakthrough cancer pain in subjects who were started on long-acting opioids. It showed analgesic efficacy in the low- and medium-dose ranges that were also well tolerated. Three additional RCTs, including 100 subjects in total of inhaled cannabis for chronic intractable neuropathic pain due to multiple etiologies, showed efficacy for smoked and vaporized cannabis.[15]

The cannabis plant, which comes in different strains, produces resins with varying ratios of pharmacologically active cannabinoids, principally tetrahydrocannabinol (THC) and cannabidiol (CBD), along with terpenoids, flavonoids, and other molecules. The majority of the effects of THC from cannabis are mediated through partial agonism of central and peripheral cannabinoid receptors CB1 and CB2. THC is excreted via hepatic and renal mechanisms. In setting of hepatic and renal impairment, it is expected to cause side effects that are more exaggerated or prolonged. Cannabinoids are highly protein bound in the blood and are not expected to be removed by hemodialysis.[15]

Dosing depends on individual patient needs and tolerance of side effects. A general principal of dosing is to start low and go slow. Routes of delivery include oral route, mucosal, topical, rectal, and inhalation. Vaporization has the advantage of rapid onset of effects and easy titration. Oral ingestion of cannabis has a delayed onset of action, compared to other routes, so titration is more difficult. In the palliative care setting, cannabinoids are generally used to treat pain, nausea/vomiting, anorexia, insomnia, fatigue, and neuropathy. Common side effects include xerostomia, drowsiness, dizziness, nausea, confusion, dysphoria, anxiety, and acute psychosis. Cannabis ingestion increases the risk of motor vehicle accidents (MVAs).[15]

It is important to screen patients for marijuana use in a nonjudgmental manner. Whether patients are using it recreationally or medically, it is a potent drug and has clinical side effects, in addition to drug–drug interactions.[8] More research studies are required in order to expand and standardize its therapeutic use.

SPIRITUAL ISSUES AND EXISTENTIAL DISTRESS

Periyajoil et al. define spirituality as "a dynamic and intrinsic aspect of humanity through which persons seek ultimate meaning, purpose, and transcendence in relationship to self, family, community, society, nature, and the significant, or sacred, expressed via beliefs, values, traditions, and practices."[8] In contrast, religions are belief systems that provide a framework for making sense of life, death, and suffering cannabinoids. They involve beliefs and rituals shared by a community in the context of a relationship with the transcendent. During the course of an illness, both spiritual and religious rituals may be a source of support for patients.

Spiritual or existential distress has been defined as the distress brought about by the actual or perceived threat to the integrity or continued existence of the whole person. Spiritual and existential distress are common in the cancer population. Spiritual distress is reported in more than one-half of patients with advanced cancer receiving palliative care.[8] Although patients place high value on these issues and often want to discuss it with health-care professionals, it is often unrecognized by clinicians and is generally a neglected area of cancer care.[11]

Sources of spiritual and existential distress may include hopelessness, lack of purpose or meaning, grief, loss, guilt, anger, and abandonment by God or others. It is the duty of all health-care providers to address every aspect of suffering—psychosocial, spiritual, and physical—as spiritual and existential well-being. The World Health Organization has emphasized the importance of palliative care and the integration of psychological and spiritual care in order to help patients live as meaningfully as possible until death.

The following two questions are useful to screen for spiritual issues: (1) Is spirituality or religion important for you? and (2) Are your spiritual or religious beliefs helping you right now?[8] A yes/no combination answer to these questions triggers a referral to a board-certified chaplain.[7]

There are several tools available to elicit a spiritual history: (1) FICA (faith, importance, community, action), (2) HOPE (sources of hope, organized religion, personal spirituality and practices, effects on medical care and end-of-life issues), and (3) SPIRIT (spiritual belief system, personal spirituality, integration with a spiritual community, ritualized practices and restrictions, implications for medical care and terminal event planning). Only FICA has been validated.[8]

Board-certified chaplains integrate spirituality into the treatment care plan. Spiritual care interventions can vary from communication techniques, to therapy, or self-care. Communication techniques such as life review are helpful to gain insight about a patient's life and his/her story.

Some specific approaches include meaning-centered therapy, which helps a patient address the unique meaning of his or her life, and dignity therapy, which addresses what a patient finds most meaningful and helps them to identify a personal history they want to be remembered by.[8]

ADVANCE CARE PLANNING AND END-OF-LIFE

Understanding patients' goals in the context of their cancer diagnosis enhances the clinician's ability to align the care that is delivered to patients with what is most important to them. Frequent discussions about patients' goals, values, and what matters to them, also promote good decision-making, patient-centered are, and earlier end-of-life planning.[16] These high quality discussions are often missing in the process of completing an advance directive (AD)—a document a patient completes while still in possession of decisional capacity, and reflects how treatment decisions should be made on her or his behalf in the event she or he loses the capacity to make such decisions.[17]

Prior to completing an advance directive, a clear understanding of an evolving medical problem is needed, frequent conversations about patients' goals of care in the context of their illness are also required, as well as patients and providers willingness to discuss patients' care preferences. For these reasons ADs are less frequently completed, even less frequently executed.

These shortcomings of the advance directive pushed for a more comprehensive approach that focuses on communication, rather than merely completing a form. The advance care planning (ACP) process extends beyond completing an advance directive because it stresses ongoing conversations among patients, their families, caregivers, and healthcare providers. It reflects on the exploration of goals, values, beliefs, illness understanding, medical care/treatment options, and plans for the future. It also promotes the documentation of these conversations in the electronic medical record. Ideally these conversations are integrated into routine care, are often revisited throughout the disease trajectory or natural course of the illness. ACP should also be held during important transition points such as prior to embarking on a potentially life threatening or risky treatment or procedure (i.e. a new chemotherapy regimen, high-risk surgery, or hematopoietic cell transplantation) and in the presence of evidence-based indicators for limited life expectancy (Stage IV status at cancer diagnosis, cancer progression). A patient's primary care physician or a specialist such as an oncologist who has been following a patient longitudinally for their cancer treatment, are the most appropriate persons to initiate goals of care discussions. Specialty Palliative Care consultations should be requested for complex goals of care and/or in depth advance care planning.

When ACP discussions are held, patients and families report a higher satisfaction with care, as well as lower risks of stress, anxiety, and depression. ACP is also associated with better patient outcomes. When these discussions occur routinely, providers also benefit by enhanced trust between patient and providers and lessening of conflict among family members and the health care team.

Given that one of the identified barriers to ongoing ACP among providers includes lack of training or experience in having these conversations, strategies and tools have been developed to assist clinicians with these tasks. At VitalTalk.org, a stepwise approach to goals of care discussions, such as REMAP—Reframe, Expect emotion and Empathize, Map the future, Align with the patient's values, Plan medical treatments that match patient's values—is available. The 2017 guideline from the American Society of Clinical Oncology also provides some recommendations about how to optimize communication about goals of care, treatment options, and prognosis.

THE ROLE OF REHABILITATION IN THE PALLIATIVE CARE SETTING

Palliative care specialists work hand-in-hand with rehabilitation specialists synergistically with overall goals to alleviate suffering and promote the best quality of life for patients and their families.[7] Rehabilitation has a definitive role in the management of cancer patients receiving palliative care. Rehabilitation services play an indisputable role in pain management, in maximizing function, independence, and well-being and improving quality of life. Physiatrists may be able to identify other drivers of pain that could intensify a patient's pain experience in the setting of newer acute or chronic cancer-related pain.

Synergistically, expert symptom assessment and management by palliative care specialists are critical to optimize a patient for a rehabilitation program.

CONCLUSION

Palliative care is specialized, whole-person care, delivered in an interdisciplinary fashion, and aimed at relieving suffering due to a serious illness. Palliative care is appropriate at any age or stage of a serious illness such as cancer, as evidence suggests that while provided concurrently with active cancer treatment, it can improve quality of life and potentially have a measurable mortality benefit.[18] Integration of palliative care is becoming the new standard of care in oncology care. The early provision of palliative care minimizes suffering, improves quality of life, and helps elucidate patient preferences and goals of care. Palliative care teams can also assist patients, families, and caregivers in the transition from receiving aggressive medical therapies to a more comfort based approach when appropriate.

PATIENT RESOURCES

1. Getpalliativecare.org
2. Caregiver.org—Understanding Palliative/Supportive Care: What Every Caregiver Should Know
3. Fivewishes.org

Analgesics used in cancer pain management

Medication/Drug Class	Advantages	Disadvantages/ Adverse Effects
Acetaminophen	Available OTC Rapid onset	Hepatotoxic at high doses. Max dose 3000 mg/day Monitor liver function/disease Ceiling effect for analgesia
NSAIDs (i.e. ibuprofen, celecoxib)	Rapid onset Effective for bone pain	Ceiling effect for analgesia GI/renal/cardiac toxicity Avoid in older adults
Corticosteroids	Rapid onset Effective for bone pain Benefit for other symptoms (n/v, anorexia, etc.)	Discouraged with immunotherapy Short-term AE: thrush, impaired glucose control, insomnia, delirium Long-term AE: myopathy, aseptic necrosis
Opioids (i.e. morphine, hydromorphone, methadone)	Rapid onset No ceiling effect Helpful for somatic, visceral, and neuropathic pain	Constipation Sedation, confusion, delirium Cognitive side effects Nausea/vomiting Tolerance Addiction
Antiepileptic drugs (i.e. gabapentin, pregabalin)	Minimal drug–drug Interactions Well tolerated Helpful for neuropathic pain and mucositis	Slow acting. May take weeks to reach analgesia Dose adjustment needed for renal dysfunction sedation, dizziness, ataxia
Tricyclic antidepressants	Helpful for neuropathic pain	Slow acting. May take weeks to reach analgesia Sedation, anticholinergic AE, cardiac arrhythmia

SSNRIs (i.e. duloxetine, venlafaxine)	Helpful for neuropathic pain	Slow acting. May take weeks to reach analgesia Drug–drug interactions SSNRIs may decrease effect of tamoxifen Fentanyl and SSNRI, increase risk of serotonin syndrome avoid if renal impairment
Topical analgesics (i.e lidocaine, capsaicin)	Helpful for neuropathic pain	Localized skin reaction, not practical for diffuse pains

AE, Adverse effects; *GI*, gastrointestinal; *N/V*, nausea/vomiting; *NSAIDs*, nonsteroidal antiinflammatory drugs; *OTC*, over the counter; *SSNRI*, selective serotonin and norepinephrine reuptake inhibitor.

REFERENCES

1. <www.who.int/cancer/palliative/definition/en>.
2. Ferrell B, Temel J, Temin S, Alesi E, Balboni T. Integration of palliative care into standard oncology care. American Society of Clinical Oncology Clinical Practice Guidelines Update. *J Clin Oncol*. 2017;35:96–112.
3. An in-depth look at palliative care and its services. <https://www.capc.org/training/an-in-depth-look-at-palliative-care-and-its-services> Accessed 14.09.19.
4. Yennuranjalingam S, Bruera E. *Oxford American Handbook of Hospice and Palliative Medicine*. New York: Oxford University Press; 2011.
5. Goldstein N, Morrison R. *Evidence-Based Practice of Palliative Medicine*. Philadelphia, PA: Elsevier; 2013.
6. Bruera E, Dalal S. *The MD Anderson Supportive and Palliative Care Handbook*. Houston, TX: UT Printing & Media Services. The University of Texas Health Science Center at Houston; 2015.
7. Stubblefield M. *Cancer Rehabilitation, Principles and Practice*. New York: Springer Publishing Company; 2019.
8. Periyakoil V, Denney-Koelsch E, White P, Zhuvosky D. *Primer of Palliative Care*. Chicago, IL: American Academy of Hospice and Palliative Medicine; 2019.
9. Davis M, Dalal S, Goforth H, McPherson M. *Essential Practices in Hospice and Palliative Medicine: UNIPAC 3*. Chicago, IL: American Academy of Hospice and Palliative Medicine; 2017.
10. <www.drugabuse.gov/nidamed-medial-health-professionals>.
11. Goldstein N, Morrison R. *Evidence-Based Practice of Palliative Medicine*. Philadelphia, PA: Elsevier; 2013.
12. Hesketh P, Mark G, Basch E. Antiemetics: American Society of Clinical Oncology clinical practice guideline update. *J Clin Oncol*. 2017;35(28):3240–3261.
13. Fearon K, Strasser F, Anker S. Definition and classification of cancer cachexia: an international consensus. *Lancet*. 2011;12(5):489–495.
14. Loprinzi C, Jatoi A. *Pharmacologic Management of Cancer Anorexia/Cachexia*. June 2018.
15. Aggarwal S, Blinderman C, Craig D. Cannabis for symptom control. In: *Fast Fact #279*. 2013.
16. <http://coalitioncc.org/what-we-do/advance-care-planning>; 2017. Accessed 28.04.17.
17. Detering K, Silveria M. *Advance Care Planning and Advance Directives*. 2018 June.
18. Temel J, Greer J, Muzikansky A. Early palliative care for patients with metastatic non-small cell lung cancer. *N Engl J Med*. 2010;363(8):733–742.

CHAPTER 25

Fertility Preservation in the Setting of Breast and Gynecologic Cancers and Cancer Treatment

ELINA MELIK-LEVINE, ARNP • JOHN P. DIAZ, MD, FACOG

INTRODUCTION

A significant proportion of reproductive-aged women are affected by a breast or gynecologic cancer diagnosis in the United States. In 2019 there will be an estimated 268,600 new cases of invasive breast cancers with 15% occur under the age of 45.[1] The percentages for newly diagnosed uterine, ovarian, and cervical cancers under the age of 45 are 6.5%, 12%, and 36.5%, respectively.[2] Over the last several decades the number of women having their first child after the age of 35 has increased. In addition to reproductive aging and cancer treatments, fertility concerns have become more prevalent and complicated for women diagnosed with cancer. This population is faced with difficult considerations: their new cancer diagnosis, treatment options, prognosis, and impact on future fertility. Standard treatment for these cancers, in particular, gynecologic malignancies results in the removal and ablation of the reproductive organs, and the importance of preserving fertility has become more apparent. Health-care providers need to be familiar with fertility options and provide timely and appropriate referrals.

Treatment for cancer often consists of a combination of surgery, chemotherapy, and radiotherapy. Alkylating agents, platinum derivatives, taxanes, anthracyclines, and antimetabolites are the most commonly used antineoplastic drugs for breast and gynecologic cancers. However, these treatments can harm healthy tissues and organs. Following chemotherapy and radiotherapy women are at increased risk of premature ovarian failure and early menopause.[3] The extent of the impact on the reproductive organs, particularly the ovaries, depends on several factors, including age of diagnosis, cumulative dose of chemotherapy, radiation, and type of chemotherapy. When abdominal and pelvic radiation doses are kept to less than 4 Gy, there does not appear to be an impact on ovarian or uterine function. Among chemotherapy treatments, alkylating agents such as cyclophosphamide pose the highest risk for ovarian toxicity and infertility. A chemotherapy combination containing cyclophosphamide is often used in the management of breast cancer. It is rarely used in the upfront management of gynecologic malignancies. The preferred regimen for the management of gynecologic cancers consists of a platinum and taxane doublet. Clinical trials have demonstrated that these agents pose relatively moderate-to-low risk for infertility.[4]

To preserve fertility while treating gynecological cancers requires the use of techniques that have been proven to have efficacious oncologic outcomes while preserving fertility. There are several fertility techniques such as ovarian transposition, in vitro fertilization, oocyte freezing, and cryopreservation of ovarian tissue that have been evaluated.[5] The patient and her partner should be informed of these options by a fertility specialist who specializes in oncofertility.

Organ-sparing surgical treatment aimed at preserving the uterus and at least one ovary has gained acceptance in the management of early stage gynecological cancers in selected patients of childbearing age. The aim is to preserve the functionality of the reproductive organs by reducing the radicality of the surgical procedure, thereby allowing the possibility of a future pregnancy. The option of fertility-sparing surgical treatment is reserved only for selected cases that are defined by the stage, histology, grade, and prognostic factors of the disease.

Breast Cancer and Gynecologic Cancer Rehabilitation DOI: https://doi.org/10.1016/B978-0-323-72166-0.00025-6

HOW DOES CANCER THERAPY AFFECT FERTILITY?

Female fertility refers to the ability of a woman to become pregnant and bear a child. At the time of birth a female's ovaries contain hundreds of thousands to one million eggs or oocytes.[6] Eggs grow and mature inside of ovaries within fluid-filled sacs known as follicles. Upon the onset of menarche, several immature oocytes are released from the ovaries. Usually, only one egg will dominate in growth and become a mature oocyte. The mature oocyte is released from the ovary into the fallopian tube through a process called ovulation. The mature oocyte is then either fertilized by sperm to create an embryo or if sperm does not fertilize the egg, the egg breaks down and menstruation will occur. Over a lifetime, approximately 1% of all oocytes are ovulated.[6] This process occurs with every month's menstrual cycle until menopause takes place and accounts for the natural decline in a female's ovarian reserve.[7]

Follicles or oocytes that are not fully developed are vulnerable in the setting of anticancer treatment. The damages imposed on the gametes by such treatment manifest as short-term or long-term infertility.[8] Gynecological surgery impacts a patient directly due to removal of part, or all, of the female reproductive system. In addition, gynecological surgeries performed to treat cancers could result in scar tissue formation, making it challenging for female patients to carry a pregnancy to term.[8] Chemotherapy and radiotherapy have a direct gonadotoxic effect by destructing ovarian follicles or damaging the DNA of existing oocytes that impact normal ovulatory function and the ability to become pregnant, respectively.[9–12] Finally, antihormone therapies used to treat breast cancer patients have both direct and indirect consequences to fertility and ovarian function.[13]

SYSTEMIC TREATMENTS: CHEMOTHERAPY, TARGETED THERAPY AND IMMUNOTHERAPY, ANTIHORMONAL THERAPY

Chemotherapy

Chemotherapy targets all cells in the body that divide quickly. Many cells in our bodies are quickly dividing, including the gametes. When these cells are damaged by the cytotoxic effects of chemotherapy, infertility could occur.[3] The exact impact that a chemotherapy agent has on future fertility is almost impossible to predict. This is especially true for patients receiving multiple chemotherapy agents to treat cancer. There are some risk factors that are used to help health-care providers predict the risk that agents pose to fertility; however, these are only meant to be used a guide. These risk factors include the patient's age at the time she receives her treatment, the drug used, and the dose.

- Age: Since younger female patients have more eggs in their reserve, they have a higher chance of retaining fertility throughout the cytotoxic damage from chemotherapy. Women who are treated for cancer before they are 35 have the best chance of becoming pregnant after treatment.
- Drug: Some drugs are more likely to impact fertility than others. Alkylating agents and conditioning chemotherapies in preparation for bone marrow transplants are considered to pose the highest risk to future fertility. However, the exact degree to which fertility may be impacted in the future is very difficult to predict. This is especially true when treating patient with multiple chemotherapy agents.[5,10,15–18]
- Dose: Higher doses and longer duration of the chemotherapy have greater potential negative impact on fertility.

Targeted Therapy and Immunotherapy

Some targeted therapy may cause ovarian failure, however, there is limited research available regarding other targeted treatments and immuno-therapies on fertility.[19]

Antihormonal Therapy

Endocrine therapy, or antihormone therapy, is a common treatment for patients with hormone-sensitive tumors. Although hormone therapy may not impact fertility directly, many patients are prescribed these medications for anywhere from 5 to 10 years consecutively. Due the natural decline of ovarian reserve over time, the patient's age at the completion of therapy could make it increasingly difficult to achieve pregnancy. In addition, patients are advised to avoid pregnancy during the time that they are taking antihormone therapy because the medication poses a high risk of birth defect to a developing fetus.[13] It is important to educate patients that menstruation may be irregular or cease while on treatment. However, it may still be possible to become pregnant. For this reason, birth control should be implemented to prevent pregnancy.[13]

Radiation Therapy

Damage to fertility due to radiation therapy depends on the dose of radiation, the area of the body treated, and the woman's age at time she is receiving treatment. Radiation directed at the ovaries threatens the health of oocytes as they are considered sensitive to radiation therapy. Radiation directed at the uterus could lead to decreased uterine volume and endometrial atrophy. Total body radiation also poses high risk to future fertility.[10]

Age: Younger women are likely to have a higher ovarian reserve and, as a result, are less likely to enter permanent menopause at the time of therapy.[11,12]

Dose: A dose of only 5 or 6 Gy can cause ovarian failure in a woman over 40, but doses 14–20 Gy can cause ovarian failure in women under 35.

Location: Radiation therapy to the abdomen or pelvis can cause harm to the female reproductive organs. Radiation directed at the uterus and/or cervix could result in the inability to carry a pregnancy to term, a higher risk for miscarriage, preterm labor, and low birth weight babies.[12,22]

Radiation therapy to the brain can also disrupt fertility. The pituitary gland is responsible for regulation of the hormones luteinizing hormone (LH) and Follicle-stimuating hormone (FSH), which control ovulation. When the pituitary gland is in the field of brain radiation therapy, there is a risk that normal hormonal function, hence, ovulatory function is disrupted that can lead to infertility.[11,12]

OPTIONS FOR FERTILITY PRESERVATION

A referral to a reproductive endocrinologist (RE) is appropriate for any female patient that is at risk for future infertility as a result of cancer treatment. If the patient is interested in fertility preservation, all measures must be taken prior to the start of her cancer treatment and as soon as possible after initial diagnosis in an effort to delay the start of treatment as some fertility-sparing measures take 2–4 weeks. A patient that may need gynecological surgery may be candidates for fertility-sparing surgery. Egg or embryo cryopreservation is the standard of care for fertility preservation in female patients. At this time, ovarian suppression and ovarian tissue cryopreservation are fertility-sparing options that are considered to be experimental.

Fertility-Sparing Surgery

In this section the role of fertility-sparing surgery and nonsurgical treatment is discussed for endometrial, cervical, and ovarian cancers.

ENDOMETRIAL CANCER

Endometrial cancer is the most common gynecologic malignancy in the United States.[24] The standard-of-care treatment is total hysterectomy and bilateral salpingo-oophorectomy (BSO), with selective use of sentinel lymph node (SLN) mapping or pelvic and/or para-aortic lymph node dissection when appropriate, depending on the risk factors and apparent cancer staging.[25] Approximately 14% of the affected women with the disease will be of the childbearing age. The fertility-preserving (FP) treatment for patients with endometrial cancer is currently limited to hormonal treatment. The ideal candidate for FP treatment is a person with (1) grade 1 (well differentiated) tumor on dilation and curettage, (2) absence of lymphovascular space invasion (LVSI) on adequate curettage specimen, (3) no myometrial invasion on magnetic resonance imaging or ultrasound, and (4) no evidence of suspicious or metastatic disease on imaging.[26]

Currently, for patients with endometrial cancer, treatments involve the use of progesterone either orally or delivered by levonorgestrel-releasing intrauterine device (IUD). Megestrol acetate (160 mg daily or 80 mg bis in die (BID)) or medroxyprogesterone acetate (600 mg daily) are the two most commonly used oral regimens. Levonorgestrel-releasing intrauterine system is the only progesterone containing IUD that has been studied in endometrial cancer patients. Prospective studies have shown that levonorgestrel-releasing IUD is associated with greater regression of histology, lower relapse rates, and lower rates of hysterectomy.[27] Metaanalysis on quality-of-life data showed superiority of levonorgestrel releasing compared to oral progesterone, with reduced weight gain, sleep disorders, headaches, and mood disorders. It is recommended to provide continuous treatment for 3 months, followed by reevaluation with hysteroscopy and/or endometrial sampling.

Relapse can occur in up to 50% of cases,[28] but a second cycle of progesterone treatment has been associated with good response rate in up to 89% of patients.[29] Women who experience a remission are encouraged to pursue immediate conception. Timely referral to a RE is crucial to minimize the time to conception, as these patients tend to have other factors that may contribute to infertility such as obesity, polycystic ovary syndrome, and advancing age. The use of metformin has also demonstrated in improve outcomes in women with endometrial cancer. A meta-analysis demonstrated that the oncologic outcomes were 81% (regression rate) with obstetrical outcomes of 47% (live births).[30] Following completion of childbearing, women are recommended to undergo definitive hysterectomy.

CERVICAL CANCER

Cervical cancer is the second most common gynecologic malignancy in the United States, with an estimated 13,240 new cases and 4170 deaths in the year 2018.[24] Forty-three percent of patients diagnosed with cervical cancer are under the age of 45 and potentially desire to preserve fertility. Traditionally, the treatment for early, cervical cancer that is defined as stage I–IIA disease is radical hysterectomy. Microinvasion disease defined as International Federation of Gynecology and Obstetrics (FIGO) stage IA1 with <3 mm stromal invasion can be managed with conization, either a loop electrosurgical excisional procedure (LEEP) or a cold knife cone (CKC) biopsy.

Candidates for a fertility-sparing option include women with clinically early stage cervical cancer. Those with stage IA1 disease (microinvasion) are appropriate candidates for CKC if there is no evidence of LVSI, negative endocervical curetting after excision, and negative endocervical margins. If the patient meets all of the criteria defined earlier, the risk of recurrence is <0.5%.[31]

In the absence of margin status, patients with stage IA1 and negative LVSI have recurrence rate of approximately 7%, with over 80% of the recurrences occurring within the first 36 months.[32] Hence, close follow-up is paramount, and patients should be counseled to undergo definitive surgical management as soon as childbearing is complete. The LVSI status is an important prognostic factor for lymph node involvement, recurrence risk, and overall survival.

In cases of stage IA1 with positive LVSI, the recurrence risk increases up to 9%, and therefore a conization (with negative margins) with laparoscopic pelvic SLN mapping is a reasonable strategy.[33] Patients who undergo a CKC or LEEP procedure are at a small but known increased risk of preterm delivery, premature rupture of membranes, and low birth weight.[31] Adenocarcinoma in situ presents a more challenging clinical situation. Unlike the squamous cell lesions, adenocarcinoma is a glandular lesion and is considered multifocal. Up to 13% of patients have foci of the disease separated by 2-mm of stromal mucosa known as "skip lesions." Bisseling et al.[34] reported about 16 patients with stage IA1 disease who were managed with conization; and after 72 months none of the patients recurred.

For women with a stage IA2–IB1 cervical cancer, a FP radical trachelectomy (FPRT) is a reasonable option in selected cases.[35] The FPRT procedure comprises three main steps, that is, dividing the uterus proximal to the cervical isthmus, excising the entire cervix and surrounding parametria, and then suturing the uterus to the vagina. Once tumor-free margins have been achieved, many surgeons insert a cerclage suture around the lower uterine segment, in anticipation of future pregnancy. Assessment for lymph node metastases is critical for any patient with > 3 mm depth of invasion (i.e., >stage IA1) or other high-risk features (e.g., LVSI and high-risk histology) on a biopsy specimen. Frozen section may be utilized to assess for nodal metastases and positive surgical margins, in which case fertility-sparing surgery may be aborted, or the surgical procedure altered (e.g., complete ipsilateral pelvic and para-aortic lymphadenectomy). Candidates for an FPRT are (1) women desiring preservation of fertility, (2) are compliant with the expected follow-up, (3) have squamous cell or adenocarcinoma histology, (4) FIGO stage IA1 with LVSI or IA2/IB1 with tumor <2 cm in diameter, and (5) no evidence of pelvic lymph node metastases.

Patients with cervical tumors >2 cm have an increased risk of positive lymph nodes, deep infiltration, and LVSI. Selected centers offer FPRT for patients with lesions > 2 cm via the abdominal approach that allows for a wider surgical margin. In the United States, most fertility-sparing procedures are performed via the abdominal approach due to surgeon preference and comfort. Cervical factors such as stenosis, short length, and the lack of mucus to facilitate sperm migration are considered the main causes of infertility after trachelectomy. Rob et al.[35] noted that during trachelectomy at least 1 cm of cancer-free cervical stroma should be saved, as this increases the chance of pregnancy.

Bentivegna et al.[36] performed a systematic review of the literature comparing these methods. A total of 2488 patients submitted to FP, and 944 ensuing pregnancies were analyzed. One hundred and six (4.2%) recurrences were reported. The overall fertility, live birth, and prematurity rates for these procedures were, respectively, 55%, 70%, and 38%. There was no difference between the live birth rates according to the five FP procedures, but abdominal RT had overall higher prematurity rate (57%) compared to conization (15%), vaginal RT (39%), and minimally invasive RT (50%).[36]

OVARIAN CANCER

Epithelial ovarian cancer accounts for approximately 80% of ovarian malignancies. Most patients present at advanced stages (III, IV) of the disease, and rarely prior to the age of 40 years. The borderline/low-malignant potential (LMP), stage I, and germ cell tumors are more common in women of reproductive ages.

Thirty-four percent of cases of borderline ovarian tumors occur in women less than 40 years of age. For the early stage disease, survival is estimated to be around 99%. Therefore the standard of care is fertility preservation if desired by the patient. Ovarian cystectomy is reasonable, but there could be approximately 30% risk of recurrence in the affected ovary. Unilateral salpingo-oophorectomy (USO) carries an approximately 8% risk of recurrence. If there is bilateral ovarian involvement and complete resection can be achieved, ovarian cystectomy is the treatment of choice.[38] Surgeons must keep in mind that approximately 25% of the borderline tumors on frozen pathologic evaluation are upgraded to invasive on final pathologic assessments. About 20% of the patients may have noninvasive as well as invasive metastatic implants. Complete surgical staging (including exploration of the entire abdominal cavity, peritoneal washings, infracolic omentectomy, and multiple peritoneal biopsies) is essential.[37]

Traditionally, the management of invasive epithelial ovarian cancer (IEOC) includes hysterectomy, BSO, abdominal/pelvic washings, biopsies, and full lymphadenectomy. This is followed by adjuvant chemotherapy in all cases aside from completely staged, IA grade 1 and IB grade 1 lesions. However, in patients with well differentiated, encapsulated, unilateral lesions without adhesions or ascites, FP surgery may be a reasonable option. Surgical treatment of FP approaches includes (1) exploration, (2) USO, (3) pelvic and para-aortic lymphadenectomy, (4) omentectomy, (5) washings, and (6) peritoneal biopsies. Approximately 20% of the patients may have noninvasive or invasive implants. If the contralateral ovary appears grossly normal, the risk of occult malignancy is <3%. Therefore biopsy of a normal-appearing contralateral ovary should be avoided as this can result in diminished fertility either due to adhesion formation or diminished ovarian reserve. Of the 328 cases of fertility conserving surgery in the peer-reviewed literature, there were 119 pregnancies and a 96% live birth rate.[38] Overall, the FP staging among the IEOC cases resulted in reasonable obstetrics outcomes (36% pregnancies, 87% live births) and oncologic outcomes (13% recurrences). Per Version 2.2018 of the NCCN guidelines (Ovarian Cancer), USO (preserving uterus and contralateral ovary) or BSO (preserving uterus) can be considered for patient whose disease appears early stage or low risk such as LMP, malignant germ cell, mucinous, or malignant sex cord-stromal tumors. Comprehensive surgical staging even in these cases remains necessary.

Oocyte or Embryo Cryopreservation

In order to achieve oocyte or embryo cryopreservation, patients must undergo the process of ovarian stimulation followed by egg retrieval with a RE. At the initial consultation the RE often orders laboratory studies to assess blood hormone levels and may perform a transvaginal ultrasound to visualize the ovaries and follicles. The laboratory studies in combination with the ultrasound can provide some guidance regarding the status of the patient's ovarian reserve. If deemed an appropriate candidate for fertility preservation by the RE, the process of ovarian stimulation and egg retrieval is initiated.

Ovarian Stimulation

Female patients with normal ovarian function typically develop and mature one egg per month with each menstrual cycle. The goal of ovarian stimulations is to develop and mature the maximum amount of eggs available for cryopreservation.[19] The patient is prescribed a series of hormone injections that stimulate the ovaries to develop and mature multiple eggs in a short time frame. The RE carefully regulates each hormone dose and monitors the patient's follicular development via ultrasound scans and blood tests throughout this process. Special consideration is taken for patient with hormone-sensitive cancer in the setting of exogenous hormone treatments. In those particular cases the course of injections that the RE uses may be modified and/or oral antihormone therapy may be added during this time period.[19,23] The total time for this process is approximately 2–4 weeks.

Oocyte Retrieval

Once the RE identifies that the eggs have reached full maturity, the next step includes a transvaginal egg retrieval. This is an outpatient procedure that is performed under conscious sedation or light anesthesia. The physician uses vaginal ultrasound to direct a needle through the vaginal wall to extract mature eggs from the ovarian follicles. The amount of eggs that each female can produce varies and is dependent on her ovarian reserve.

Once the eggs are extracted from the ovaries, the female can cryopreserve the oocytes. If she chooses to use these eggs in the future, they would have to be fertilized with sperm after thawing to create embryos that would then be transferred to her uterus. If she chooses to create an embryo at the time of egg retrieval, the mature egg would be fertilized with sperm and the resulting embryo will be frozen. Those embryos could then be thawed and transferred into the uterus when the patient is ready to become pregnant.[19]

Ovarian Tissue Freezing

Although this measure is considered experimental, it may be the best option for patients who are not candidates for oocyte harvesting and cryopreservation because either the patient has not reached puberty or cannot delay the start of cancer treatment for 2–4 weeks due to the severity of her disease.

Ovarian tissue cryopreservation involves removal of all or part of one ovary prior to the start of cancer therapy. The ovarian cortex, or outer layer of the ovary that contains the eggs, is isolated and cryopreserved for future use.[39,40] Once the ovarian tissue is removed and frozen, the intention is for the patient to initiate cancer treatment and achieve remission from her disease. Once the patient is ready to use her cryopreserved specimen, the thawed ovarian tissue is placed into her body. This is performed by transplanting the tissue either directly back in the pelvis or in a different part of the body. Once implanted, the ovarian tissue matures and produces oocytes. These oocytes can be harvested and collected by the same means as ovarian stimulation and oocyte harvesting as previously mentioned.[40]

A number of pregnancies have come from using frozen tissue; however, this technique is considered investigational as implantation of previously frozen and thawed ovarian tissue may present a risk of reintroducing cancer into a patient in remission. Research on methods to perfect this technique is needed in order to determine its safety.

Ovarian Suppression

Ovarian suppression or gonado-protection may be another method to preserve fertility in some cases per ASCO guidelines. This is based on the theory that administering medication to temporarily shut down the ovaries can protect them from the gonadotoxic damage of chemotherapy. This can be done with long-acting hormone medications called gonadotropin-releasing hormone (GnRH) agonists. This method may help maintain fertility for some women, but the mechanism of action and efficacy remains a topic of research at this time.[41] In addition, there is no evidence to suggest that using GnRH agonists help to improve rate of pregnancy. Since this treatment is considered experimental at this time, it should be done so in combination with other nonexperimental methods of fertility preservation if used. However, a recent metaanalysis suggests a statistically significant benefit for using GnRH agonists for the prevention of premature ovarian failure.[41] The use of GnRH agonists should only be offered to patients when other standard-of-care methods to fertility preservation are not available.

Assessment of Ovarian Function After Therapy

Menstrual cycles can cease during or after treatment but have the potential to return. However, even if a woman's menstrual cycle resumes after cancer treatment is completed, her fertility is still uncertain. Females that resume menses after treatment are still risk for early menopause.[3] In the case the patient is interested in learning the status of her fertility postcancer treatment, she has the option to perform blood tests to measure hormone levels in the bloodstream. These blood tests are the best way to interpret the status of the ovarian reserve at the present time and can provide some guidance regarding the impact of the patient's treatment on her fertility. Ovarian reserve test results should be analyzed by a RE at which point the patient would be counseled regarding treatment options based on the results.[3]

SEXUAL EDUCATION DURING AND POSTCANCER TREATMENT

Patients must be educated that it is not safe to become pregnant while on cancer treatment due to high risk of birth defects. It is recommended that patients use two forms of birth control to avoid pregnancy while on anticancer treatment. Once treatment is completed, it may be possible to attempt pregnancy naturally. However, pregnancy must be discussed with the patient's oncology team as the timing of safe conception following cancer treatment is not clearly defined based on current research. Safe timing of pregnancy following cancer treatment is thought to anywhere from 6 months to 2 years.[5,13]

It is common for cancer patients to question whether they are at an increased risk of conceiving a child with birth defects due to exposure of oocytes to anticancer therapy. Current evidence does not suggest that there is an increased rate of birth defects in children of cancer survivors. Particularly for breast cancer patients with hormone-positive tumors, there are concerns that pregnancy after cancer treatment could increase the risk of recurrence of the cancer; however at this time, studies suggest that pregnancy does not increase the chance of cancer recurrence.

CONCLUSION

It is the choice of the patient whether or not she should proceed with fertility preservation prior to the start of cancer treatment. Making a decision about whether or not to preserve fertility is influenced by many factors, including the importance of having a biological child, the likelihood of success in having a child from eggs collected, the patient's acceptance of the uncertainties involved, and her financial resources. The role of the health-care provider is to provide patients with all resources regarding fertility preservation in order for the patient to make an independent, informed decision.

Discussion regarding infertility due to anticancer treatment and subsequent measures to preserve fertility is a multidisciplinary approach. All health-care providers in the oncology setting must be prepared to notify their patients that infertility is a potential risk associated with cancer therapy. This discussion should take place as soon as possible after initial cancer diagnosis is made and prior to the start of the patient's oncological plan of care. Although many patients may not express interest in fertility preservation at the onset of diagnosis, evidence suggests that discussions about fertility are of great importance to cancer patients. In addition, studies suggest that patients can benefit from discussing fertility with providers at any phase of her cancer journey.[44] Patients that express interest in fertility preservation or are ambivalent about the subject should be referred to a fertility expert as early as possible upon initial cancer diagnosis to assure that the patient has access to all possible fertility-sparing measures.

REFERENCES

1. Hankey BF, et al. Trends in breast cancer in younger women in contrast to older women. *J Natl Cancer Inst Monogr*. 1994;(16)7–14.
2. Bhasin S, et al. The implications of reproductive aging for the health, vitality and economic welfare of human societies. *J Clin Endocrinol Metab*. 2019;104(9):3821–3825.
3. Bedoschi G, et al. Chemotherapy-induced damage to ovary: mechanisms and clinical impact. *Future Oncol (London, Engl)*. 2016;12(20):2333–2344. Available from: https://doi.org/10.2217/fon-2016-0176.
4. Taylan E, et al. Current state and controversies in fertility preservation in women with breast cancer. *World J Clin Oncol*. 2017;8:241–248.
5. Fertility concerns and preservation for women. *Cancer. Net*, 13 Dec. 2019. <https://www.cancer.net/navigating-cancer-care/dating-sex-and-reproduction/fertility-concerns-and-preservation-women>.
6. Forabosco A, et al. Morphometric study of the human neonatal ovary. *Anat Rec*. 1991;231(2):201–208. Available from: https://doi.org/10.1002/ar.1092310208.
7. Soules MR, et al. Ovarian aging: mechanisms and clinical consequences. *OUP Acad*. 2009;. Available from: https://doi.org/10.1210/er.2009-0006. 1 Aug.
8. Lee SJ, et al. American Society of Clinical Oncology recommendations on fertility preservation in cancer patients. *J Clin Oncol*. 2006;24(18):2917–2931. Available from: https://doi.org/10.1200/jco.2006.06.5888.
9. Morgan S, et al. How do chemotherapeutic agents damage the ovary? *Hum Reprod Update*. 2012;18 (5):525–535. Available from: https://doi.org/10.1093/humupd/dms022.
10. Sanders JE, et al. Pregnancies following high-dose cyclophosphamide with or without high-dose busulfan or total-body irradiation and bone marrow transplantation. *Blood*. 1996;87(7):3045–3052. Available from: https://doi.org/10.1182/blood.v87.7.3045.bloodjournal8773045.
11. Wallace W, Hamish B, et al. Predicting age of ovarian failure after radiation to a field that includes the ovaries. *Int J Radiat Oncol Biol Phys*. 2005;62(3):738–744. Available from: https://doi.org/10.1016/j.ijrobp.2004.11.038.
12. Wallace WHB, et al. The radiosensitivity of the human oocyte. *Hum Reprod*. 2003;18(1):117–121. Available from: https://doi.org/10.1093/humrep/deg016.
13. Peccatori FA, et al. Cancer, pregnancy and fertility: ESMO clinical practice guidelines for diagnosis, treatment and follow-up. *Ann Oncol*. 2013;24:vi160–vi170. Available from: https://doi.org/10.1093/annonc/mdt199.
14. Anderson RA, Hamish W, Wallace B. Antimüllerian hormone, the assessment of the ovarian reserve, and the reproductive outcome of the young patient with cancer. *Fertil Steril*. 2013;99(6):1469–1475. Available from: https://doi.org/10.1016/j.fertnstert.2013.03.014.
15. *Chemotherapy*. Chemotherapy | Fertility Risks from Treatment. <https://www.allianceforfertilitypreservation.org/fertility-risks-from-treatment/chemotherapy>.

16. *Chemotherapy*. American Cancer Society. <https://www.cancer.org/treatment/treatments-and-side-effects/treatment-types/chemotherapy.html>.
17. Kalich-Philosoph L, et al. Cyclophosphamide triggers follicle activation and 'burnout'; AS101 prevents follicle loss and preserves fertility. *Sci Transl Med*. 2013;5(185). Available from: https://doi.org/10.1126/scitranslmed.3005402.
18. Ajala T, Rafi J, Larsen-Disney P, Howell R. Fertility preservation for cancer patients: a review. *Obstet Gynecol Int*. 2010;2010. Article ID 160386.
19. Kort JD, Eisenberg ML, Millheiser LS, Westphal LM. Fertility issues in cancer survivorship. *CA Cancer J Clin*. 2014;64:118–134. Available from: https://doi.org/10.3322/caac.21205.
20. Kim SS, et al. Breast cancer and fertility preservation. *Fertil Steril*. 2011;95(5):1535–1543. Available from: https://doi.org/10.1016/j.fertnstert.2011.01.003.
21. Mahajan N. Fertility preservation in female cancer patients: an overview. *J Hum Reprod Sci*. 2015;8(1):3–13. Available from: https://doi.org/10.4103/0974-1208.153119.
22. Critchley HOD. Impact of cancer treatment on uterine function. *J Natl Cancer Inst Monogr*. 2005;2005(34):64–68. Available from: https://doi.org/10.1093/jncimonographs/lgi022.
23. Loren AW, et al. Fertility preservation for patients with cancer: American Society of Clinical Oncology clinical practice guideline update. *J Clin Oncol*. 2013;31(19):2500–2510. Available from: https://doi.org/10.1200/jco.2013.49.2678.
24. Siegel RL, et al. Cancer statistics, 2018. *CA Cancer J Clin*. 2018;68:7–30.
25. Seagle BA. Prognosis and treatment of positive peritoneal cytology in early endometrial cancer. *Am J Obstet Gynecol*. 2018;329.
26. Ramierz PT, et al. Hormonal therapy for the management of grade 1 endometrial adenocarcinoma: a literature review. *Gynecol Oncol*. 2001;95:133.
27. Abu-Hashim H, et al. Levonorgestrel-releasing intrauterine system vs oral progestins for non-atypical endometrial hyperplasia: a systemic review and metaanalysis of randomized trials. *Am J Obstet Gynecol*. 2015;469.
28. Gallos ID, et al. LNG-IUS versus oral progestogen treatment for endometrial hyperplasia: a long-term comparative cohort study. *Hum Reprod*. 2013;28:2966.
29. Park JY, et al. Hormonal therapy for women with stage IA endometrial cancer of all grades. *Obstet Gynecol*. 2013;122:7.
30. Wei J, et al. Comparison of fertility-sparing treatments in patients with early endometrial cancer and atypical complex hyperplasia: a meta-analysis and systematic review. *Medicine (Baltimore)*. 2017;96:e8034.
31. Kyrgiou M, et al. Fertility and early pregnancy outcomes following conservative treatment for cervical intraepithelial neoplasia and early cervical cancer. *JAMA*. 2011;1496.
32. Hartman CA, et al. Analysis of conservative surgical treatment and prognosis of microinvasive squamous cell carcinoma of the cervix stage IA1: results of follow up to 20 years. *Int J Gynecol Cancer*. 2017;27:357–363.
33. Rob L, et al. Less radical fertility-sparing surgery than radical trachelectomy in early cervical cancer. *Int J Gynecol Cancer*. 2007;304.
34. Bisseling K, et al. Treatment of microinvasive adenocarcinoma of the uterine cervix: a retrospective study and review of the literature. *Gynecol Oncol*. 2007;107:424–430.
35. Rob L, et al. Fertility-sparing surgery in patients with cervical cancer. *Lancet Oncol*. 2011;12:192–200.
36. Diaz JP, et al. Oncologic outcome of Fertility-sparing radical trachelectomy versus radical hysterectomy for stage IB1 cervical carcinoma. *Gynecol Oncol*. 2008;111:225–260.
37. Bentivegna E, et al. Fertility results and pregnancy outcomes after conservative treatment of cervical cancer: a systematic review of the literature. *Fertil Steril*. 2016;106:1195–1211.e5.
38. Gershenson DM, et al. Ovarian serous borderline tumors with invasive peritoneal implants. *Cancer*. 1998;82:1096–1103.
39. Winter WE, et al. Surgical staging in patients with ovarian tumors of low malignant potential. *Obstet Gynecol*. 2002;100:671–676.
40. Eskander R, et al. Fertility preserving options in patients with gynecologic malignancies. *Am J Obstet Gynecol*. 2011;205:103–110.
41. Ben-Aharon I, et al. Optimizing the process of fertility preservation in pediatric female cancer patients – a multidisciplinary program. *BMC Cancer*. 2016;16(620). Available from: https://doi.org/10.1186/s12885-016-2584-7.
42. Oktay K, Buyuk E. Ovarian transplantation in humans: indications, techniques and the risk of reseeding cancer. *Eur J Obstet Gynecol Reprod Biol*. 2004;113(suppl 1):S45–S47.
43. Del Mastro, et al. Gonadotropin-releasing hormone analogues for the prevention of chemotherapy-induced premature ovarian failure in cancer women: systematic review and meta-analysis of randomized trials. *Cancer Treat Rev*. 2014;40:675–683.
44. Langagergaard V. Birth outcome in women with breast cancer, cutaneous malignant melanoma, or Hodgkin's disease: a review. *Clin Epidemiol*. 2010;3:7. Available from: https://doi.org/10.2147/clep.s12190.
45. Azim HA, et al. Prognostic impact of pregnancy after breast cancer according to estrogen receptor status: a multicenter retrospective study. *J Clin Oncol*. 2013;31(1):73–79. Available from: https://doi.org/10.1200/jco.2012.44.2285.
46. Rosen A, et al. Psychosocial distress in young cancer survivors. *Semin Oncol Nurs*. 2009;25(4):268–277. Available from: https://doi.org/10.1016/j.soncn.2009.08.004.

CHAPTER 26

Oncology Massage Therapy in Breast and Gynecologic Cancers

KRISTEN M. GALAMAGA, LMT • ADRIAN CRISTIAN, MD, MHCM

INTRODUCTION

Massage therapy is the scientific, systematic, manual, or mechanical manipulation of the soft tissues of the body for the purpose of normalizing those tissues. It employs manual techniques that include applying fixed or movable pressure, holding, and/or causing movement of, or, to the body. Movements such as rubbing, kneading, pressing, rolling, stroking, and tapping, for therapeutic purposes, promote circulation of the blood and lymph, relaxation of muscles, relief from pain, restoration of metabolic balance, and other benefits both physically and mentally.[1]

Touch is the foundation and cornerstone of massage therapy and has a long history of use as a healing tool.[2] Both Eastern and Western civilizations found that touch can aid in the natural healing process, relieve pain, and prevent and cure symptoms of different illnesses. In addition, the touch of the massage therapist reduces stress and produces deep relaxation. While massage can be described in terms of the type of techniques performed, touch is not used only in a mechanistic way in massage therapy.[2] This is especially important when performing an oncology massage. An oncology massage is a form of touch that causes no pain. Oncology massage therapy (OMT) is individualized to the unique needs and circumstances of the person with cancer. It takes into account the location of the cancer as well as its treatment to ensure the safety of the person being treated.[3]

OMT should only be provided by a massage therapist who has received specialized training in the specifics of cancer and cancer treatment.[3] This specialized training is more about cancer, cancer treatment and their impact on the body, and less about massage. During an oncology massage, the patient receives traditional, established massage therapy techniques that have been adapted to account for one's unique health situation. The changes that might be made to massage that make it an "oncology massage" can fall under any number of categories, but typically, they will be related to primarily the pressure used, (i.e., a noninvasive, compassionate touch); the direction of the strokes (always toward the heart, never away from it); the length of the session; and positioning of the body, including areas of specific concern.[3]

HISTORY

Massage is one of the earliest remedial practices of humankind, dating back thousands of years in ancient cultures that believed in its medical benefits. As one of the oldest health-care practices reported in history, it is described as the most natural and instinctive means of relieving pain and discomfort. The first written records of massage therapy are found in treatises from China and Egypt. Hippocrates wrote in the 4th century BCE: "The physician must be acquainted with many things and assuredly with rubbing." The ancient Greek term for massage was "rubbing."[4]

While massage therapy began as a sacred system of natural healing, cultural shifts rendered it a disreputable form of indulgence for extensive periods of history. However, between the period of 1600 and 1800, numerous physicians and scientists observed and documented the benefits of massage. It was not until the 19th century that different techniques in massage were advanced by western practitioners.

Per Henrik Ling was a Swedish physician who developed the Swedish Gymnastic Movement System. This system incorporated medical gymnastics, physiology, and massage. The massage consisted of various manual techniques such as stroking, striking, pressure, and squeezing that will be described later in the chapter. The massage method he created is commonly known as Swedish massage.[3] Today, massage is one of the most popular healing modalities, being used by

Breast Cancer and Gynecologic Cancer Rehabilitation DOI: https://doi.org/10.1016/B978-0-323-72166-0.00026-8

both conventional and alternative medical practitioners. Some believe that some of the roots of physical therapy are outgrowths of massage and its various techniques.[5]

COMPLEMENTARY VERSUS ALTERNATIVE THERAPY

The terms "complementary" and "alternative" are often used as though they mean the same thing. And although they are sometimes combined into one phrase—complementary and alternative therapies—they are different. Complementary therapies are used alongside conventional treatments and medicines, usually to manage side effects. Alternative therapies are used instead of conventional treatments. Many complementary therapies are being scientifically researched for use in people with cancer, while alternative therapies are unlikely to have been tested in this way.[6] Massage therapy is a complementary therapy.

OMT is based on the premise that each person is unique and is to be treated as such. It is an art expressed through the hands of a skilled therapist, with an ever so gentle touch, to be able to work with the superficial lymphatic system and the muscular system of the oncology patient.

BENEFITS OF ONCOLOGY MASSAGE THERAPY

The benefits of massage therapy in breast cancer were reviewed in a systematic review from 1990 to 2015 by Greenlee et al. in 2017. Massage therapy was noted to have a beneficial role in reducing anxiety, stress and improving mood disturbance, as well as in reducing pain and promoting relaxation.[7] Aromatherapy massage was found to have a beneficial effect on reducing anxiety in another metaanalysis, although it was unclear if the addition of aromatherapy to the massage therapy added a significant additional benefit.[8] In a large metaanalysis performed on the role of massage therapy in cancer pain, massage therapy was found to significantly reduce cancer pain when compared to no massage therapy or conventional care. It was reported to be especially beneficial for surgery-related pain. Foot reflexology appeared to be more effective when compared to other types of massage.[9] In a large prospective, nonrandomized, observational study, short-term symptom scores for pain, fatigue, stress, anxiety, nausea, and depression are declined by approximately 50% following massage therapy. Swedish and light touch were reported to be better than foot massage.[10] Massage therapy may also be useful for the prevention and treatment of neuropathic pain,[11,12] chronic localized pain and decreased upper extremity mobility after breast cancer surgery,[13] improvement of quality of life and reduction of physical complaints in survivors of gynecologic cancer,[14] and following autologous tissue reconstruction after mastectomy for breast cancer.[15]

For someone who is receiving treatment for cancer or recovering from it, massage can also provide additional benefits, including improvements in mental clarity, alertness, sleep, and meaningful social interactions.

CONTRAINDICATIONS TO MASSAGE THERAPY

OMT is generally considered to be safe, and complications are rare when treatment is rendered by skilled massage therapists.[16] The contraindications to massage therapy are based on the therapist's knowledge of the patient, the cancer and its metastatic sites, as well as the treatments used to treat the cancer—chemotherapy, radiation therapy, and surgery. Massage therapy should not be performed (1) directly over a surgical site until the surgical scar is fully healed with no evidence of infection; (2) directly over a mediport access site; (3) directly over skin that is actively treated with radiation therapy and deep pressure therapy; (4) over areas with known lymphedema, lymphatic involvement of cancer, or bone metastasis; (5) in patients with coagulation disorders complicated by hemorrhage, low platelet counts, or on medications such as warfarin or heparin; (6) over skin with infection; and (7) on days when the patient is receiving chemotherapy.[6,17,18]

Even though massage therapy is generally safe, patients may experience local bruising, local increase of muscle pain, swelling of massaged muscles or allergic reaction to skin lotions.

It is important to know that massage therapy is not flatly contraindicated for an oncology patient.[19] Massage has not been demonstrated to directly spread cancer.[20,21] While some types of massage therapy are contraindicated for a patient with cancer, knowledgeable, skilled touch, in some form, is rarely contraindicated. It is true that cancer limits certain massage techniques; however, within those limitations, there are techniques used by trained oncology massage therapists, which will help a patient forget that they are a patient and, psychologically, feel that they are not broken. With their skilled hands, an oncology massage therapist can help a person feel whole again and reduce pain, nausea, and fatigue, all of which enables the patient to regain hope, provide a forum for expressing feelings in an informal setting, reestablish a positive body image, rebuild hope, and enable the patient to receive a moment of pure relaxation that is greatly needed.[22]

Oncology patients need to never be denied compassionate, loving touch. A light, relaxing massage can safely be given to people in all stages of cancer. It goes without saying that a tumor or treatment site should not be massaged. Deep traumatic massage to any part of the body is contraindicated for anyone with active cancer, as the patient can bruise much easier due to chemotherapy, radiation, or medication. Injury to tissues causes the immune response to be activated. Again, while each person is unique and is to be treated as such, the pressure to be used throughout the treatment is an extremely light one, no matter which technique is used.

MASSAGE TECHNIQUES

There are five main passive techniques of massage: effleurage, petrissage, friction, tapotement, and vibration. Effleurage refers to the use of long and slow gliding strokes applied with light pressure using the fingers or palm. Petrissage refers to a kneading motion using the thumb and fingers. Friction is a technique in which greater forces are applied using the tips of fingers or thumb to reach deeper muscular tissues to break up areas of local fibrosis. Tapotement utilizes repeated blows utilizing the fingers, fists, or sides of palms of hands. This latter technique should not be applied to the areas of recent inflammation, contusions, or over internal organs such as the kidneys. Vibration is a technique in which the massage therapist uses the hands in a technique that is similar to strumming a guitar string between the fingers.[5]

There are several other different styles of massage and other touch therapies that can be used by an oncology massage therapist, including acupressure, aromatherapy, myofascial release, reflexology, shiatsu, trigger point therapy, and craniosacral therapy.[23]

One fundamental theory of massage therapy is based on the concept that the body functions at its best when arterial, venous, and lymphatic flows are unimpeded. When there is interruption of the flow of these fluids in muscles, changes occur in the muscles and overlying fascia and skin, which can contribute to the development of localized fibrosis, restrictions, and pain. Massage techniques are utilized to reestablish good fluid dynamics in skin, fascia, and muscle.[5]

PATIENT ASSESSMENT

Most people who are coming for an oncology massage session are very open and willing to tell the massage therapist about themselves and their cancer journey. It is imperative for the massage therapist to be completely present and listen very closely to the person receiving the massage about the cancer, its treatment, and the impact of both on their body. That information can subsequently help the therapist guide the treatment session to maximize benefit and minimize harm.[18]

The oncology massage therapist also reviews the medical chart of the person with cancer prior to the treatment session to understand the type of cancer, stage of cancer, and the treatment rendered. In breast and gynecological cancers, this treatment commonly includes surgery, radiation therapy, and chemotherapy.

This is followed by a physical assessment of the patient's skin to identify any surgical scars and their integrity, wounds and areas of potential skin infection as marked by erythema and access mediports for delivery of chemotherapy, lymphedema, skin bruises, and areas treated by radiation therapy. Muscles are examined for atrophy and bones for deformities. Palpation is an essential component of the assessment and muscles are palpated for tender points and tightness. It is also important to briefly assess for any insensate areas or areas of altered sensation as a result of chemotherapy.[18]

PRECAUTIONS IN ONCOLOGY MASSAGE THERAPY

Adverse effects can often be prevented with awareness, modification of touch and pressure, and changes to positioning. The Society for Integrative Oncology recommends the use of massage for cancer pain and anxiety but cautions against the use of deep or intense pressure near cancer lesions or enlarged lymph nodes, radiation field sites, intravenous catheters and medical devices, and anatomic distortions, or in patients with a bleeding tendency.[6]

It is true that cancer and cancer treatments can put people at risk for complications from massage, so it is important to take some precautions. Because of the different contraindications for massage in this population, it is very important for the massage therapist who is treating a person with a history of cancer—either currently or in the past—to have specialized training in oncology massage, as well as being a licensed massage therapist.

Caution should always be used for patients with cancer-related pain. Massage will not resolve pain resulting from pressure of the tumor on surrounding sites, nerve impingement (radiating pain), or bone pain from metastases. Light touch massage can reduce anxiety or distress, whereas deep massage can worsen the pain by increasing inflammation or potentially causing fragile bones to break. No oils or lotions should be used on the field of treatment, during the course of radiation. Rocking motions should be avoided with patients who are experiencing nausea.[22] Practicing diligent handwashing and using clean equipment and linens will reduce the risk of infection.[23] It is also important to use extra caution during a massage session to avoid the carotid artery, suboccipital triangle, supraclavicular fossa, posterior knee, femoral triangle, and abdominal cavity.[5]

MASSAGE TREATMENT SESSION

To maximize the benefits of the oncology massage therapy session, it is important to make sure that the patient is comfortable, relaxed, and warm. The ambiance in the massage therapy room should be conducive to a positive experience for the patient. Proper positioning with the use of bolsters and pillows is essential to ensure a comfortable position during the treatment session. Patient may be supine or prone on a massage therapy table or seated on a chair depending on the goals of the treatment session. Areas of the body not being massaged should be covered with blankets or sheets for warmth and modesty.

CONCLUSION

Oncology massage therapy provides significant benefits to persons with cancer and cancer survivors in both pain and stress reduction. A thorough understanding of the cancer location, metastasis, as well as cancer treatments such as chemotherapy, surgery, and radiation therapy is essential to maximizing the benefits and minimizing the risks. A well-trained, experienced oncology massage therapist can be an integral member of a cancer treatment team.

REFERENCES

1. Beck MF. *Milady's Theory and Practice of Therapeutic Massage.* Milady; 1994:3.
2. <https://medical-dictionary.thefreedictionary.com/massage + therapy>.
3. <https://www.s4om.org/clients-and-patients/clients-patients-faq>.
4. Thompson G. *Massage Therapy Gale Encyclopedia of Alternative Medicine.* 2nd ed. Farmington Hills: Thompson/Gale; 2005:1297–1301.
5. Micozzi MS. *Massage and manual therapies: principles of bodywork and manual healing. Fundamentals of Complementary and Alternative Medicine.* Saunders; 2015:15–16.
6. Deng GE, Frenkel M, Cohen L, et al. Evidence based clinical practice guidelines for integrative oncology: complementary therapies and botanicals. *J Soc Integr Oncol.* 2009;7(3):85–120.
7. Greenlee H, DuPont-Reyes MJ, Balneaves LG, et al. Clinical practice guidelines on the evidence-based use of integrative therapies during and after breast cancer treatment. *CA Cancer J Clin.* 2017;67(3):194–232. Available from: https://doi.org/10.3322/caac.21397. Epub 2017 Apr 24.
8. Fellowes D, Barnes K, Wilkinson S. Aromatherapy and massage for symptom relief in patients with cancer. *Cochrane Database Syst Rev.* 2004;(2)CD002287.
9. Lee SH, Kim JY, Yeo S, et al. Meta-analysis of massage therapy on cancer pain. *Integr Cancer Ther.* 2015;14(4):297–304. Available from: https://doi.org/10.1177/1534735415572885. Epub 2015 Mar 17.
10. Cassileth BR, Vickers AJ. Massage therapy for symptom control: outcome study at a major cancer center. *J Pain Symptom Manage.* 2004;28(3):244–249.
11. Izgu N. Effect of Aromatherapy Massage on chemotherapy-induced peripheral neuropathy and fatigue in patients receiving oxaliplatin: an open label quasi randomized controlled pilot study. *Cancer Nurs.* 2019;42(2):139–147.
12. Izgu N. Prevention of chemotherapy-induced peripheral neuropathy with classical massage in breast cancer patients receiving paclitaxel: an assessor-blinded randomized controlled trial. *Eur J Oncol Nurs.* 2019;40:36–43.
13. Massingill J. Myofascial massage for chronic pain and decreased upper extremity mobility after breast cancer surgery. *Int J Ther Massage Bodyw.* 2018;11(3):4–9.
14. Dion LJ. Massage therapy alone and in combination with meditation for breast cancer patients undergoing autologous tissue reconstruction: a randomized pilot study. *Complement Ther Clin Pract.* 2016;23:82–87.
15. Donoyama N. Effects of anma therapy (Japanese massage) on health related quality of life in gynecologic cancer survivors: A randomized controlled trial. *PLoS One.* 2018;13(5):e0196638.
16. Ernst E. The safety of massage therapy. *Rheumatology.* 2003;42(9):1101–1106.
17. Eyles K. Cancer Council Australia. Massage and Cancer: A Guide for People with Cancer, Their Families and Friends. SOS Print + Media Group; 2014.

18. <https://www.cancercouncil.com.au/wp-content/uploads/2018/04/UC-pub_Complementary-Therapies_CAN1141_lo-res_April-2018.pdf>.
19. Corbin L. Safety and efficacy of massage therapy for patients with cancer. *Cancer Control*. 2005;12(3):158–164.
20. MacDonald G. *Medicine Hands: Massage Therapy for People with Cancer*. 1st ed. Words Dist Company; 1999:24.
21. <https://www.ktmassageboise.com/wp-content/uploads/2019/04/article_infosheet_massageandcancer.pdf> Accessed 24.12.19.
22. Gecsedi RA. Massage therapy for patients with cancer. *Clin J Oncol Nurs*. 2002;6:52–54.
23. Dryden T, Moyer TA, eds. *Massage Therapy: Integrating Research and Practice*. Human Kinetics; 2012.

Index

Note: Page numbers followed by "*f*" and "*t*" refer to figures and tables, respectively.

D

Printed and bound by CPI Group (UK) Ltd, Croydon, CR0 4YY
03/10/2024
01040373-0004